Practical Geriatric Medicine

Practical Geriatric Medicine

EDITED BY

A. Norman Exton-Smith

CBE, MA, MD (Camb), Hon. DM (Nottm), FRCP (Lond)

Barlow Professor of Geriatric Medicine,
School of Medicine,
University College, London.
Honorary Physician,
University College Hospital, London.

Marc E. Weksler

MD

Irving Sherwood Wright Professor of Medicine,
Director — Division of Geriatrics and Gerontology,
Cornell University Medical College,
New York.

CHURCHILL LIVINGSTONE
EDINBURGH LONDON MELBOURNE AND NEW YORK 1985

CHURCHILL LIVINGSTONE
Medical Division of Longman Group Limited

Distributed in the United States of America by Churchill
Livingstone Inc., 1560 Broadway, New York, N.Y. 10036 and
by associated companies, branches and representatives
throughout the world.

First published 1985

ISBN 0 443 02702 1

British Library Cataloguing in Publication Data
Practical geriatric medicine.
   1. Ages——Diseases
   I. Exton-Smith, A.N.   II. Weksler, Marc E.
   618.97   RC952

Library of Congress Cataloging in Publication Data
Main entry under title:
Practical geriatric medicine.
   Includes index.
   1. Geriatrics. I. Exton-Smith, A.N. (Arthur Norman)
II. Weksler, Marc E. (Marc Edward), 1937–
[DNLM: 1. Geriatrics. WT 100 P8945]
RC952.P62 1985   618.97   84-21439

Printed in Great Britain by
Butler & Tanner Ltd, Frome and London

Preface

Successful treatment of young persons with acute diseases has dramatically altered the pattern of medical practice in much of the world. Today, physicians in every medical specialty must treat increasing numbers of elderly patients suffering from both acute and long-term illnesses. The majority of persons born this year will live into their eighth decade. Thus, the already high percentage of elderly patients now seen by family practitioners and specialists will continue to increase in the twenty-first century.

Unfortunately, increased responsibility for the care of the elderly has not been matched by increased education in geriatric medicine at either undergraduate or postgraduate levels. Although much progress has been made in the last few years, medical students and house officers still have inadequate contact with clinicians practising in geriatric departments. Geriatricians have only recently joined clinical science faculties in university hospitals. This situation has resulted in a shortage of teachers of geriatric medicine in many parts of the world. Furthermore, it has been difficult to find time in the medical curriculum to add new courses on gerontology or geriatrics. Attention to geriatrics in postgraduate medical courses has only just begun.

There are important consequences of inadequate geriatric medical education. The most serious is that subtle complaints of the elderly patient are often dismissed as due to 'old age'. Indeed many patients accept this view with the result that diseases remain untreated and opportunities for improving the health of older people are lost. New textbooks devoted to the care of the elderly patient attempt to make up for the deficit in geriatric education. These textbooks fall into two classes: introductory student handbooks and comprehensive textbooks of geriatric medicine. Neither format provides a practical, problem-oriented text for the primary care physician, house officer and medical student who care directly for elderly patients with common geriatric problems.

Practical Geriatric Medicine was conceived to fill the gap between introductory and comprehensive textbooks of geriatric medicine for the primary care provider. The major portion of this text provides a systematic, problem-oriented approach to geriatric medicine. The most important and most common problems faced by the primary care physician in dealing with elderly patients are carefully discussed. Symptoms and signs of disease in the elderly are presented in detail. Pathways to diagnosis are offered and strategies for the management of geriatric illness are provided.

Some aspects of medical care of the elderly are considered in general terms. For example, the discussion of cancer does not include a site by site review. Rather, the diagnostic approach to the elderly patient with a suspected cancer, the appropriateness of cancer therapy in the elderly cancer patient and the need for supportive care of the elderly cancer patient are presented. Specific cancer therapy, not usually the responsibility of the primary care physician but of the consulting oncologist, is not included. Similarly, a general consideration of infectious disease among elderly patients is presented. Once differences in susceptibility, presentation and drug tolerance are understood, the diagnostic approach and treatment of infection in the elderly do not differ significantly from site to site or from other adult groups. General discussions of preventive medicine in old age, the clinical approach to the elderly patient and age-related changes in drug therapy are included in the first part of the text.

The final part of the text is devoted to societal dilemmas in the care of the elderly. It has been said that, aside from world war, the greatest problem faced by our society concerns social, economic and health policy for elderly citizens. In a democratic society the resources allocated to health care including those for the elderly, although implemented by physicians, are decided upon by political consensus.

New models of geriatric care – home care, day hospitals and hospices – are attractive and humane. They are also expensive. Whether society will choose to support these health programmes for the elderly has not been settled. Physicians must appreciate that plans to provide health care for elderly patients depend not only upon their geriatric expertise but also on the will of the populace in placing limited resources at their disposal.

1985

A. N. Exton-Smith
M. E. Weksler

Contributors

Itamar B, Abrass MD
Co-Director, Geriatric Research, Education & Clinical Center, VA Medical Center, Sepulveda, California. Associate Professor of Medicine, UCLA School of Medicine, Los Angeles, California

Michael H. Alderman MD
Professor of Public Health, Associate Professor of Medicine, Cornell University Medical College, New York

Tom Arie BM, FRCP, FRCPsych, FFCM
Professor of Health Care of the Elderly, University of Nottingham and Hon. Consultant Psychiatrist to the Nottingham Hospitals

K. G. Arnold BSc, MB, BS, MRCP
Consultant in Geriatric Medicine, Bloomsbury Health Authority. Honorary Senior Lecturer in Geriatric Medicine, Faculty of Clinical Sciences, University College, London

Robert Austrian AB, MD
John Herr Musser Professor and Chairman, Department of Research Medicine, The University of Pennsylvania School of Medicine, Philadelphia

Laurie Barclay MD
Assistant Professor and Assistant Attending Neurologist, New York Hospital — Cornell University Medical College, Department of Neurology, New York. Staff Neurologist and Research Associate, The Burke Rehabilitation Center, White Plains, New York

John P. Blass MD, PhD
Professor of Neurology and Medicine, New York Hospital — Cornell University Medical College, New York. Director, Dementia Research Services, The Burke Rehabilitation Center, White Plains, New York

Mary R. Bliss MBBS, MRCP
Consultant Geriatrician, City and Hackney Health District, London

J. C. Brocklehurst MD MSc, FRCP
Professor of Geriatric Medicine, University of Manchester

Francis I. Caird MA, DM, FRCP
David Cargill Professor of Geriatric Medicine, University of Glasgow

Donna Cohen PhD
Head, Division of Aging and Geriatric Psychiatry, Montefiore Medical Center and Albert Einstein College of Medicine, New York

Harvey Jay Cohen MD
Professor of Medicine and Director, Geriatric Research, Education and Clinical Center, Veterans Administration Medical Center and Center for the Study of Aging and Human Development, Duke University, Durham, North Carolina

K. J. Collins MB, BS, DPhil (Oxon)
Member of Medical Research Council Staff. Honorary Senior Lecturer in Geriatric Medicine at University College Hospital, London

Jeffrey Crawford MD
Assistant Professor of Medicine, Divisions of Hematology, Oncology and Geriatrics, Veterans Administration Medical Center and Duke University School of Medicine, Durham, North Carolina

John L. C. Dall MD, FRCP
Consultant Physician, Geriatric Medicine, Victoria Infirmary, Glasgow. Honorary Clinical Lecturer, University of Glasgow, Glasgow. Visiting Professor (Geriatric Medicine), University of Ottawa, Canada

William Davison TD, MA, ChB, FRCPE
Consultant Physician, Department of Geriatric Medicine, Addenbrooke's Hospital, Cambridge

N. G. Dent MB, MRCP
Senior Registrar Addenbrooke's and Papworth Hospitals, Cambridge

Sandra C. Durmaskin MA
Gerontology Coordinator, Cornell University Medical College, Division of Geriatrics and Gerontology, New York

Carl Eisdorfer PhD, MD
President, Montefiore Medical Center. Professor, Departments of Psychiatry and Neuroscience, Albert Einstein College of Medicine, New York

J. Grimley Evans MA, FRCP, FFCM
Professor of Medicine (Geriatrics), University of Newcastle upon Tyne. Consultant Physician in Geriatric & General Medicine, Newcastle Health Authority

A. Norman Exton-Smith CBE, MA, MD, Hon. DM, FRCP
Barlow Professor of Geriatric Medicine, School of Medicine, University College, London. Honorary Physician, University College Hospital, London

P. A. Gardiner MD
Consultant Emeritus in Ophthalmology, Guy's Hospital, London

Aram Glorig MD
Associate Director of Research, House Ear Institute, Los Angeles, California

Edward A. Graber MD
Professor of Clinical Obstetrics and Gynecology Cornell Medical College. Attending Obstetrician and Gynecologist, New York Hospital — Cornell Medical Center, New York

E. M. D. Grundy MA, MSc
Research Officer, Dept of Health Care of the Elderly, Nottingham University

Cyril I. Gryfe MD, FRCP
Medical Director, Baycrest Centre for Geriatric Care, Toronto. Associate Professor of Medicine, University of Toronto

R. C. Hamdy MBChB, MRCS, LRCP, DM, MRCP
Consultant Physician in Geriatric Medicine, St John's Hospital London, Queen Mary's Hospital, London. Honorary Senior Lecturer, St George's Hospital Medical School, London

S. Mitchell Harman MD, PhD
Senior Investigator, Gerontology Research Center — Endocrine Section, National Institutes on Aging — Clinical Physiology, Baltimore City Hospitals, Baltimore, Maryland

Anita Herdan MD, PhD
Assistant Professor of Medicine, Cornell University Medical College, Division of Geriatrics and Gerontology, New York

Marion Hildick-Smith MD, FRCP
Consultant Physician in Geriatric Medicine, Nunnery Fields Hospital, Canterbury

Bernard Isaacs MD, FRCP
Charles Hayward Professor of Geriatric Medicine, University of Birmingham

O. F. W. James MA, FRCP
Consultant Physician, Reader in Medicine (Geriatrics), University of Newcastle, Newcastle upon Tyne

Rob Jones MB, ChB, DPM, MRCPsych
Senior Lecturer (Psychiatry), Department of Health Care of the Elderly, University of Nottingham

Robert M. Kark FRCP, MACP
Distinguished Emeritus Professor of Medicine, Rush Medical College. Consultant, Section of Nephrology, Rush-Presbyterian-St Luke's Medical Center. Section-Chief, Geriatrics, Hines Veterans Administration Hospital, Hines, Illinois

Dennis L. Kodner MSP
General Director, Elderplan, Inc., Metropolitan Jewish Geriatric Center, Brooklyn, New York. Adjunct Assistant Professor of Health Policy in Medicine, Cornell University Medical College, New York

Edmund J. Lewis MD
Professor of Medicine, Rush Medical College. Director, Section of Nephrology, Rush-Presbyterian-St Luke's Medical Center, Chicago, Illinois

David A. Lipschitz MD, PhD
Professor of Medicine, Director, Geriatric Research Education and Clinical Center, Little Rock VA Medical Center. Chief, Hematology/Oncology Division, Little Rock VA Medical Center and University of Arkansas for Medical Sciences, Little Rock, Arkansas

Robert B. McGandy MD
Professor of Nutrition, Schools of Medicine and Nutrition, Tufts University and U.S. Department of Agriculture, Human Nutrition Research Center on Aging, Tufts University, Boston, Massachusetts

James Malome-Lee MB, BS, MRCP
Senior Clinical Lecturer, University College, London

John Marshall DSc, MD, FRCP, FRCP, DPM
Professor of Clinical Neurology, University of London

Michael F. R. Martin MA, MB, B.Chir, MRCP
Consultant Rheumatologist, St James's University Hospital, Leeds and Royal Bath Hospital, Harrogate

J. C. Meadows MD, FRCP
Honorary Consultant Neurologist, St George's Hospital, London

Frances Meagher MB, MRCPI
Research Fellow, Department of Clinical Pharmacology,
Royal College of Surgeons in Ireland, Dublin

P. H. Millard MB, FRCP
Eleanor Peel Professor of Geriatric Medicine. Director of
the Geriatric Teaching and Research Unit, St George's
Hospital Medical School, London

Howard R. Nankin MD
Professor of Medicine and Director, Division of
Endocrinology and Metabolism, Department of
Medicine, University of South Carolina School of
Medicine and Dorn Veterans' Hospital, Columbia, South
Carolina

B. E. C. Nordin MD, FRCP, FRACP, DSc
Senior Research Fellow, Royal Adelaide Hospital.
Clinical Professor, University of Adelaide

Kevin O'Malley MD, PhD, FRCPI, FRCP
Professor of Clinical Pharmacology, Royal College of
Surgeons in Ireland, Dublin. St Laurence's Hospital &
Charitable Infirmary, Dublin

Ralph Pascualy MD
Director, Sleep Disorders Center, Providence Hospital,
Department of Psychiatry and Behavioural Sciences,
University of Washington School of Medicine, Seattle,
Washington

G. M. Ritchie MDS, LDSRCS, Dip Ed, FBIM AM,
FICD, FRIPHH
Professor and Head of Department of Prosthetic
Dentistry, National University of Singapore. Emeritus
Reader in Prosthetic Dentistry, London University

Laurence Z. Rubenstein MD, MPH
Chief, Division of Geriatric Medicine and Clinical
Director, Geriatric Research, Education and Clinical
Center, Veterans Administration Medical Center,
Sepulveda, California. Assistant Professor of Medicine,
UCLA School of Medicine, Los Angeles, California

Harvey C. Shapiro MD, FACP
Medical Director, Metropolitan Jewish Geriatric Center.
Associate Clinical Professor of Medicine, Albert Einstein
College of Medicine, Bronx, New York

John A. Spittell Jr., MD, FACP, FACC
Mary Lowell Leary Professor of Medicine, Mayo
Medical School. Consultant, Cardiovascular Division and
Internal Medicine, Mayo Clinic, Rochester, Minnesota

Margaret E. Stanback MPH
Department of Public Health, Cornell University
Medical College, New York

J. E. Stark MD, FRCP
Consultant Physician, Addenbrooke's and Papworth
Hospitals, Cambridge

Robert W Stout MD, FRCP
Professor of Geriatric Medicine, The Queen's University
of Belfast, Belfast

Julian Verbov MD, FRCP, MIBiol
Consultant Dermatologist, Liverpool Health Authority
and Isle of Man Health Services Board. Clinical Lecturer
in Dermatology, University of Liverpool

S. Webster MD, MA, MRCP
Consultant Physician, General and Geriatric Medicine,
Addenbrooke's Hospital, Cambridge

Babette B. Weksler MD
Professor of Medicine, Cornell University Medical
College, New York

Marc E. Weksler MD
Irving Sherwood Wright Professor of Medicine and
Director, Division of Geriatrics and Gerontology, Cornell
University Medical College, New York

J. Williamson MD, ChB, FRCPE
Professor of Geriatric Medicine, University of Edinburgh

P. H. L. Worth MA, MBBChir, FRCS
Consultant Urological Surgeon, University College
Hospital and St Peter's Hospital, London

V. Wright MD, FRCP
Professor of Rheumatology, Leeds University

Contents

General aspects

1

Epidemiology of aging

J. G. Evans

Aging is characterised by a loss of adaptability of an individual organism over time. On average, homeostatic mechanisms become less sensitive, less accurate, slower and less well sustained with age. Additionally their effective ranges become restricted. Ultimately the individual is unable to respond adaptatively to some challenge from the external or internal environment and death ensues. A rise in mortality rates with age is therefore an indicator of senescence. Human mortality rates rise continuously and exponentially from just before puberty, and this pattern is found in populations with widely different overall mortality levels. As an instance, the lowest point on the age-specific mortality curve is the same in England and Wales today as it was at the end of the last century. Many animal species in the feral state fail to show aging in the form of rising mortality rates because the risk of death from accidents, disease and predation is so high that the effects of aging are swamped and few individuals live long enough to show aging effects. In more protected environments it is clear that aging is a universal biological property of multicellular organisms.

Mortality is a crude index of aging but its continuous and broadly exponential increase is matched in some other indices of loss of adaptive capacity of the individual. Residence in institutions as revealed by Census data, the prevalence of disabling disease (Office of Population Censuses and Surveys (OPCS, 1975), and general practitioner consultation rates for non-gynaecological conditions (OPCS, 1974) also increase continuously and broadly exponentially over adult ages. These indices, like mortality rates, all reflect loss of adaptability of the organism as a whole. It does not follow that the pattern of change in a particular body organ or system will necessarily be similar. There are wide differences between systems in the rate and nature of age-associated functional change, with the greatest losses occurring in those functions requiring the co-ordinated activity of several different organs (Shock, 1981).

Although there is, therefore, no biological basis for distinguishing a group of the 'elderly' from other adults, human concern with aging has been dominated by such common crises of old age as dementia, falls, fractures,

hypothermia and inability to cope. The fact that such failures of adaptation are the end products of long preceding periods of diminishing adaptability has received less than appropriate attention. Furthermore the causes of loss of adaptability require more study. Because aging is universal it is easy to assume that all age-associated decrements are biologically inevitable and genetic in origin. The epidemiological study of human aging shows that this is not so and suggests that environmental causes of age-associated changes are more important than has been generally recognised.

THE EPIDEMIOLOGICAL MODEL OF AGING

The conventional model of human aging is to contrast 'normal' aging with 'abnormal' aging or disease. There is, however, no a priori basis for defining what is to comprise 'normal' aging, and attempts to operationalise the concept have often confused at least three different meanings of the word 'normal'. There is no reason to expect that what is 'normal' (in the sense of healthy) should occur 'normally' (in the sense of most frequently) in a general population, and even less reason why it should be distributed 'normally' (in the sense of the Gaussian distribution) around the observed population mean. The concept of normality is a relic of deterministic thinking which is properly superseded by the biologically more appropriate probabilistic approach to medical science.

The epidemiological model of aging is summarised in Table 1.1 which lists the processes contributing to differences observed between young and old people. True aging refers to those changes which occur in an individual as he grows older and which can be categorised as due to

Table 1.1 The epidemiological model of aging

True aging	Intrinsic
	Extrinsic
False aging	Cohort effects
	Aggravated aging
Secondary aging	Species
	Individual

3

the interaction of extrinsic (environmental) causes with intrinsic (genetic and constitutional) processes and properties. False aging refers to those differences between young and old which are not due to changes which have taken place within the older individuals. Secondary aging comprises adaptations to aging.

SECONDARY AGING

One of the basic biological enigmas of aging is the paradox that although the body can repair many forms of injury it is generally unable to repair the ravages of age. Some compensatory adaptations do however occur. In the individual the most obvious forms of adaptation to aging lie in the psychological sphere. The use of aids to supplement failing memory is a trivial instance but other psychological and behavioural changes can be viewed as adaptations to counter an age-associated increase in random 'noise' within the nervous system (Gregory, 1974). A desire for increased room lighting levels will lead to improve signal/noise ratio in the visual system. Studying problems for longer will increase temporal summation and informational redundancy so reducing the probability of mistakes due to neural noise; this adaptation may contribute to the greater 'caution' shown by old people in coming to conclusions in problem-solving situations.

With regard to physiological adaptation, one of the more plausible examples of adaptation to aging lies in the age-associated increase in sensitivity of hypothalamic osmoreceptors. It is unusual to find a homeostatic mechanism which increases its sensitivity with age and the explanation may be that this is a secondary and adaptive response to a decline (due to loss of nephrons) in the capacity of the kidney to handle fluid and electrolyte loads. Increase in sensitivity of the osmoreceptors thereby improves the 'early warning' of changes in fluid and electrolyte balance, but at the price, probably, of rendering the aging body more susceptible to hyper- and hyponatraemic syndromes in conditions of severe stress (Helderman et al, 1978).

At the species level, the female menopause may be an evolved adaptation to age-associated decline in reproductive efficiency rather than a primary aging change. The menopause conceptualised as an abrupt cessation of reproductive capacity approximately half-way through the maximum lifespan of the species appears to be unique to the human. Some individuals of certain other primate species may show a senescent loss of reproductive capacity (Graham et al, 1978) but this occurs only in extreme old age and is not universal within the species; it is therefore not analogous to the human menopause. Although the menopause is associated with an increase in the rate of age-associated loss of bone tissue and possibly with increased susceptibility to vascular disease (although this is by no

means unequivocally established) it also appears to be associated with a beneficial effect on the incidence of some cancers, notably that of the breast (Doll, 1971). In biological terms the likely origin of the menopause lies in the relatively long lifespan of the human and the role of the family in social structure. There is abundant evidence that the efficiency of reproduction as measured by the capability to produce viable offspring declines with age in the female of most animal species. Although the evidence is less complete, the same phenomenon probably occurs in the human. If reproductive efficiency declines with age there will come a point at which in biological terms it would be more profitable for a woman to cease increasingly unsuccessful attempts at producing offspring of her own, containing 50% of her genes, and instead to contribute to the raising of her grandchildren which contain 25% of her genes. An evolutionary development of this kind would only be relevant to the female of a mammalian species characterised by a family structure, a prolonged infancy, and a cumulative culture in which grandparents can make a crucial contribution to the survival of children (Evans, 1981; Dawkins, 1976).

FALSE AGING

False aging refers to those differences between young and old which are not due to changes that have occurred in the individuals as they grew older. One prevalent source of false aging lies with cohort effects in a developing society. People now aged 70 were brought up in a very different world from those now aged 20. Riley & Bond (1981) point out that only 38% of old people in the USA completed high school education compared with 66% of the middle-aged and 84% of the young. Psychological comparison between young and old therefore will involve the difficulties well-known to complicate cross-cultural comparisons between African tribes and urban Britons, or even black and white Americans. Schaie & Strother (1968) have shown the possible magnitude of these effects by comparing cross-sectional estimates of age-associated changes in psychological function with actual changes within individuals as they grow old. In general, age-associated decline in psychological functioning occurs later in life and is of smaller degree when people are assessed against their own previous performance than one would deduce from comparisons between old people and other younger persons. This effect will obviously only be seen in cultures which are undergoing rapid change and it must not be assumed that the result will always be to exaggerate aging changes. In the data of Schaie & Strother, one test of verbal fluency suggested that age-associated changes had in the past been underestimated because of secular decline in the verbal abilities of successive generations. The importance of cohort effects is that much of the popular view of aging and of the aged is based on cross-sectional comparisons which may be profoundly misleading.

Although it is in psychological functioning that cohort effects have been most clearly shown to have important and pervasive effects, similar influences on physical variables must be anticipated. Current changes in lifestyle between generations, for example in smoking habits, diet and exercise patterns, may be expected to contribute to future age-associated variations in the incidence and prevalence of cardiovascular disease (Havlik & Feinleib, 1979).

A second form of false aging may be regarded as an aggravation of age-associated changes. The recognition of aging as loss of adaptability implies the application of the same challenge to people at different ages and assessment of the response. In many ways society presents old people with more severe challenges than face younger adults. The relative poverty of elderly people is one example and inadequate housing another. Studies by Fox et al, (1973) in Britain have established that the incidence of hypothermia in the British elderly is high not only because of true age-associated decline in the efficiency of homeostatic mechanisms maintaining body temperature (Collins et al, 1982), but also because housing policy places old people on average in colder environments than younger adults have to endure. Survey data have shown that households headed by old people are more likely to have outside toilets and to lack central heating than households headed by younger adults (Wroe, 1973). The poorer quality of hospital care provided to elderly patients with age-associated mental impairments (Evans et al, 1980) and the shorter time spent by doctors in consultations with elderly patients (Keeler et al, 1982) are further examples of mechanisms which presumably aggravate the effects of aging. Sociological studies have also identified more subtle ways in which age-associated changes may be aggravated by unhelpful societal attitudes. Low expectations of elderly people and under-estimation of their functional abilities diminish the opportunities available to them to carry out activities unquestioned as among the rights of the young. The right to earn a living is a gross enough example but sexual activity is more directly revealing of social attitudes.

INTRINSIC AGING

Although improvements in public health over the last century in advanced countries have greatly extended the average lifespan there has been no change in maximum lifespan. Observation and breeding experiments show that every species of animal has a characteristic maximum lifespan, sometimes referred to as specific lifespan, which is inherited by natural populations largely as a polygenic characteristic. In some species a disproportionate maternal influence and even an effect of maternal age at conception on the longevity of offspring (the Lansing phenomenon)

raise the possibility that inherited cytoplasmic or mitochondrial factors may be active (Comfort, 1979). The processes determined by these genetic and other inherited factors which place an upper limit on the lifespan of an individual comprise intrinsic aging. Man, with a specific lifespan of approximately 110 years is the longest lived mammal and one of the longest lived of all animal species. There is no evidence which stands up to scientific scrutiny of groups of people living consistently beyond 110 years. At one time there was a fashionable view that aging and maximum lifespan were specifically evolved auto-destruct mechanisms preventing older organisms from competing with younger individuals of the same species. The reasoning behind this hypothesis was based on the view that selection pressure proceeds according to its beneficial effects on the species; modern theory regards the individual genes as the basic units of selection which would imply that other things being equal, selection would be towards prolongation or reproductive life of the individual. This appears to have been so among the higher animal groups. Death from intrinsic aging should therefore be regarded as due to ultimate failure of genetically determined survival systems rather than any kind of auto-destruction. Prolongation of maximum lifespan may have been achieved to some degree by selection pressure postponing the effects of deleterious genes later in the life of individuals as Medawar (1952), Hamilton (1966) and others have pointed out. This does not mean, as some commentators seem to have assumed, that all age-associated changes in later life are genetically caused. Indeed it is difficult to identify direct gene effects in human aging.

Most of the evidence on genetic effects on longevity in man is derived from comparison of young and old people with inevitable problems of smallness of samples and doubts about the validity of the comparison. Suggestions that longevity was associated with a high degree of heterozygosity at the human leucocyte antigen (HLA) loci or with particular lipoprotein patterns have been called in question by subsequent reports. Studies of long-lived families are also complicated by the fact that children inherit more than genes from their parents (Abbott et al, 1974). The social class of the father and the dietary practices of the mother probably have a more profound effect on lifespan than genetic differences from other families in the same racial group.

Cutler (1975) has provided evidence that there was a rapid increase in the specific lifespan of the early hominids which, if mutation rates at that time were similar to present levels, must have occurred through changes at a relatively small number of genetic loci. Two other lines of evidence also support the idea that a small number of genes may have an important effect upon determining maximum lifespan. King & Wilson (1975) have demonstrated that the genetic distance between the chimpanzee (maximum lifespan 30 years) and man is small, chimpanzee polypeptides being on average more than 99% identical with the corresponding polypeptide in the human. The implication is that a relatively small number of changes in systems controlling expressions of genes coding for structured proteins may explain the difference in lifespan between man and the lower primates. Martin (1978) has reviewed genetic determinants of segmental progeroid syndromes, that is to say, diseases which provide a partial imitation of accelerated aging. He points out that no single gene is an exact mimic of accelerated aging, but that a relatively small number of genes could be combined to produce a picture mimicking acceleration of intrinsic aging processes.

The suggestion that a relatively small number of genes may be important in prolonging life, raises the practical possibility that by biochemical or even genetic engineering means it may become possible in the near future to extend the maximum lifespan of man. There would seem little point in doing this if extrinsically determined diseases and disabilities continued to accumulate during the added years. Identification and prevention of extrinsic influences upon health and function in old age therefore seems to carry greater priority in human gerontological research at present.

EXTRINSIC AGING

The model of human aging outlined above and the epidemiological approach identifies two main methods for detecting the influence of extrinsic factors in the aging process. These may be called the comparative and the interventive.

Comparative methods

Comparison of the nature and rate of age-associated changes in populations living under different environmental circumstances is a potent method for detecting the effects of extrinsic factors. Clearly, there will be problems arising from possible cohort effects as described earlier if there is no longitudinal (follow-up) component in the study design. Also the validity of this method depends on collateral evidence that the differences observed are due to the environments and not to associated genetic differences. This can often be reasonably assumed where the people compared are living in the same country and are members of the same social strata of a racially homogeneous nation. Otherwise the hypotheses generated by observational methods must be tested by deliberate intervention or by studying the spontaneously occurring pseudo-experiments of migration or environmental development.

We may be able to obtain a better estimate of intrinsic aging from looking at the best that individuals of different ages can achieve, rather than age-associated changes in average performance. Data on marathon running times against age provide an example (Fries, 1980). This approach is a special instance of the comparative epidemiological method.

An early achievement of the comparative method was to demonstrate that the rise of blood pressure with age seen in Western populations is largely, if not entirely, environmentally determined. An epidemiological study of this type has recently shown how the traditional model of 'normal' aging versus disease may mislead. In Western populations mean electrocardiographic axis shifts towards the left even if individuals with hypertension or manifest coronary heart disease are excluded from the sample. On this basis it was assumed that leftward shift in the electrocardiogram (ECG) must therefore be a 'normal' or intrinsic aging process. However a population with no rise of blood pressure with age and at generally low risk status for coronary heart disease shows no significant leftward shift in electrocardiographic axis with age (Evans et al, 1982).

Disease states which are closely age-associated may also be demonstrated to be of extrinsic origin by the epidemiological approach. Most adult cancers follow a power-law relationship with age, that is to say age-specific incidence rises in proportion to age raised to a power (Doll, 1971). This type of function is compatible with a multi-stage process of accumulating random events. Such a process could be entirely intrinsic but variation in the incidence rates of most cancers around the world indicate that the majority, possibly 70%, of cancers are caused by environmental factors (Doll & Peto, 1981). The animal experiment of Peto and colleagues (1975) showed that the power-law rise in incidence with age was explicable in terms of cumulative exposure to carcinogens and older animals are no more susceptible to new carcinogens than are younger.

Cerebrovascular disease incidence also follows a power-law relationship to age, although its mortality rates show an exponential relationship to age. This latter fact taken with an apparent similarity of incidence rates in different countries led Kurtzke (1969) to postulate that cerebrovascular stroke was a more or less direct consequence of intrinsic aging processes. Since that time variation in stroke incidence with time (Matsumoto et al, 1979) and with region (Hansen & Marquardsen, 1977) have been more clearly established, indicating that some of the determinants of stroke must be extrinsic.

Extrinsic factors must be conceptualised as interacting with intrinsic. In the hypertensive rat for example, a high sodium low potassium diet produces hypertension only in genetically susceptible individuals (Meneely & Battarbee, 1976) and this may prove to be a model applicable to the human. Age-associated loss of bone density appears to be a universal process in the human (Garn et al, 1967) but Matkovic and colleagues (1977) have shown by comparison of populations in different parts of Yugoslavia that the overall pattern may be modulated by dietary intake of calcium. It seems likely that the effects of loss of bone density in terms of bone weakness and fractures may also be modulated by extrinsic factors. Solomon (1979) has presented evidence that although the South African Bantu have apparently less dense bones than the European, the latter have a greater incidence of proximal femoral fractures in old age. The solution to the paradox may lie with differences in physical activity as suggested by Chalmers & Ho (1970) who identified lower rates of proximal femoral fracture in Chinese than in European women.

There is the intriguing speculation that some extrinsic causes of aging may be so universally present throughout the world that they will not be detectable by epidemiological methods. In the presence of universal exposure to an environmental factor, differences between affected and unaffected individuals will appear to be entirely intrinsic. Thus if senile dementia of Alzheimer's type were due to aluminium toxicity, aluminium is so universally present throughout the human environment that the comparative method might be non-contributory.

Interventive studies

Changes in the functional status of an individual following modification of the environment may provide useful clues to the extrinsic component in aging. Bassey (1978) has reviewed the evidence for an important proportion of the decline in cardiorespiratory fitness seen 'normally' in Western populations to be due to culturally determined changes in activity pattern. Aniansson & Gustafsson (1981) have shown that physical retraining programmes in late middle age may produce not only improvements in cardiovascular and muscular fitness but may also bring about histological changes towards younger patterns in muscle biopsy.

Findings such as these raise some fundamental questions about the design of health and social services for the elderly. Much of what is provided for the elderly, particularly in domiciliary services is of prosthetic type; that is to say we provide people to do tasks that the old person no longer feels able to do for herself. By reducing the level of daily demands on the old person however this approach will inevitably lead to further deterioration in fitness. In a rational world no old person would be offered institutionalisation, a home help or other prosthetic intervention until medical assessment and attempted rehabilitation had demonstrated that she could not be made fit enough to continue fending for herself. Again the elderly can be seen to be the victims of inappropriate societal attitudes, particularly as applied in the context of the social work model of aging.

Interventive studies of this kind may underestimate the contribution of extrinsic factors since they will only detect the reversible effects of the environment. We may anticipate that most important environmental defects on the individual will be permanent and cumulative. In some instances extrinsically induced changes may be self-accelerating. Miall & Chinn (1973) postulated that once a rise of blood pressure had been triggered by environmental factors, pressure might continue to rise at a rate proportional to the achieved level. This suggestion was highly controversial at the time but data compatible with the hypothesis continue to emerge (Wu et al, 1980). The mechanism may lie in changes in the vessel wall and baroreceptors.

Problems in recognition of extrinsic factors

There are several factors which can lead to underestimation of the contribution of extrinsic factors to aging.

1. Most diseases and disabilities in old age are multifactorial in the sense that they are the final common pathway of a variety of possible antecedent causal chains. The relative significance of any single causative factor will therefore depend on the contributions from alternative causes of the same final pathway. The effects of different alternative environmental causes are likely to accumulate with age and as outlined above the theories of Medawar (1952) and Hamilton (1966) would also predict the accumulation of different genetic effects in old age.

2. Human aging is associated with increases in both between-individual and within-individual variation in physiological measurements. The latter reflects the decline in homeostatic mechanisms while the former also reflects variation in rates of intrinsic and extrinsic aging. Both will also be affected by changes in error variance. One would expect most homeostatic mechanisms to work on a logarithmic basis in that the feedback would be concerned with proportional rather than absolute changes in the controlled variable. An age-associated increase in the variance of variables measured in arithmetical rather than proportional scales (such as blood pressure or blood glucose), and whose mean values increase with age, must therefore be expected and is in one sense an artefact of measurement. True increases in variance will be partly due to true minute-to-minute variation within the individual owing to age-associated decline in the precision of homeostatic control. This has been demonstrated at a physiological level in the variability of blood pressure (Floras & Sleight, 1982) and at a behavioural level in the control of environmental temperature (Collins et al, 1981). It is also possible that error variance of some variables increases with age. It is for example more difficult to standardise the posture of elderly patients when blood pressure is being recorded. There are also problems of communication in interview data which may increase error. Both these effects mean that in order to categorise an elderly person accurately with regard to some risk factor or physiological variable, measurements have to be taken more often than they would in a younger person.

3. In epidemiological studies the risk variables that we measure may not be the responsible factors themselves but correlates of them. The relationship between the two may change with age. The relative contributions of low density lipoprotein (LDL) and high density lipoprotein (HDL) cholesterol to total serum cholesterol changes with age, and this may contribute to the poorer predictive power of total serum cholesterol for coronary heart disease at later ages.

4. Differential mortality may remove from a population those individuals susceptible to specific extrinsic causes of disease so that without a longitudinal study the cumulative effect of the environmental factor may be underestimated. There does not appear to have been a quantitative demonstration of this effect.

5. Cohort effects which as noted above can produce important differences between young and old people could theoretically modulate the effect of environmental factors particularly by varying the levels of interacting variables. Current changes in the USA in cigarette smoking, serum cholesterol, physical activity and in the treatment of blood pressure may interact in complex ways to change the age pattern of susceptibility to cardiovascular disease.

6. Probably the most important reason for underestimating the effects of environmental factors on aging lies with the use of current rather than past or cumulative measures of exposure to environmental factors. Feinleib et al, (1979) found that coronary artery insufficiency and left ventricular thickness at necropsy were more consistently correlated with serum cholesterol levels 9 years before death than with levels 1 year before death. The latter may reflect pre-terminal trends or changes due to symptomatic disease while the former were more representative of average lifetime values. In a prospective study of stroke incidence in a population sample of people aged 65 and over, it was found that current weight adjusted for height was not a predictor of stroke, but a history of relatively high weight for height at the age of 25 was (Evans, 1982). The same study produced some less clear-cut evidence that past hypertension might also be a better predictor of stroke than current blood pressure levels. These findings could imply that it is the cumulative lifetime dose of some environmental factor which is important and this may not be accurately reflected in a single estimate made in old age. The situation may be compounded by a 'ceiling' phenomenon whereby a maximal effect may have been arrived at by a particular age and by a variety of dose/time pathways. There is also the possibility that some risk factors are only baneful during vulnerable periods of susceptibility particularly in early

life. If these speculations have a factual basis they have important implications in the approach to and the scope of prevention in old age. First, an association between an environmental or physiological variable and morbidity that is causal in early adult life may be non-causal in later life. (By 'causal' we need imply no more than a reduction in risk of morbidity produced by change in the variable under study.) This would follow if the variable had already produced irreversible pathology or if changes in the variable in later life had only a negligible effect on life time cumulative exposure. Second it might be more profitable to seek prediction and prevention of morbidity in old age in 'mechanisms' rather than 'causes'. In the case of cerebrovascular stroke there may be less profit in old age in modifying the causes of vascular mechanisms in the form of hypertension or obesity than in interrupting the mechanisms whereby vascular disease is translated into thrombotic or embolic episodes. Among younger adults who will be less far down the natural history of disease, modification of primary causes would be the more appropriate strategy. It must also be recognised that loss of adaptability with aging would increase the probability of an undesirable outcome to the challenge of intervention. A fall with age in the magnitude of expected benefits from an interventive procedure may therefore result in the intervention doing, on average, more harm than good.

CONCLUSIONS: THE NEED FOR A MODEL OF AGING

Members of the general public have an implicit model of aging which colours their attitude and determines their actions towards old age and old people. As many studies have shown these models are in general negative and disparaging. Many professionals concerned with the elderly also have implicit models which may be inappropriate. The social work model which sees aging purely as a social process and relies heavily on prosthetic interventions, is as incomplete as the much lampooned medical model aimed at identifying those parts of the aging process which can be conceptualised as disease and dealt with by therapeutic intervention. The epidemiological model, arising from an ecological approach to the human species, offers an opportunity to transcend these profession-based models. As with all scientific models it is provisional and exists only to generate its successors. It does, however, offer a programme of hypotheses to be examined both in the care of the elderly and in the systematic study of the aging process.

REFERENCES

Abbott M H, Murphy E A, Bolling D R, Abbey H 1974 The familial component in longevity. A Study of offspring of nonagenarians. II. Preliminary analysis of the completed study. Hopkins Medical Journal 134: 1–16

Aniansson A, Gustafsson E 1981 Physical training in elderly men with special reference to quadriceps muscle strength and morphology. Clinical Physiology 1: 87–98

Bassey E J 1978 Age, inactivity and some physiological responses to exercise. Gerontology 24: 66–77

Chalmers J, Ho K C 1970 Geographical variations in senile osteoporosis. The association with physical activity. Journal of Bone and Joint Surgery 52B: 667–675

Collins K J, Easton J C, Exton-Smith A N 1982 The aging nervous system: impairment of thermoregulation. In: Sarner M (ed) Advanced Medicine 18 London, Pitman p 250–257

Collins K J, Exton-Smith A N, Dore C 1981 Urban hypothermia; preferred temperature and thermal perception in old age. British Medical Journal 282: 175–177

Comfort A 1979 The Biology of Senescence. Churchill Livingstone, Edinburgh

Cutler R G 1972 A working hypothesis of senescence. In: Strehler B L (ed) Advances in gerontological research. Academic Press, New York, vol 4, p 220–321

Cutler R G 1975 Evolution of human longevity and the genetic complexity governing aging rate. Proceedings of the National Academy of Sciences, USA 72: 4664–4668

Dawkins R 1976 The Selfish Gene. University Press, Oxford

Doll R 1971 The age distribution of cancer: implications for models of carcinogenesis. Journal of the Royal Statistical Society (Series A) 134: 133–155

Doll R, Peto R 1981 The causes of cancer. Oxford University Press

Evans J Grimley 1981 The biology of human aging. In: Dawson A M, Compston N, Besser G M (eds) Recent Advances in Medicine 18. Churchill Livingstone, Edinburgh p 17–38

Evans J Grimley 1982 'Stroke' predictors. In: Sarner M (ed) Advanced Medicine 18. Pitman, London, p 288–301

Evans J Grimley, Caird F I 1982 The epidemiology of neurological disorders in old age. In. Caird F I (ed) Neurological Disorders in the Elderly. Wright, Bristol, p 1–16

Evans J Grimley, Prudham D, Wandless I 1980 A prospective study of fractured proximal femur: hospital differences. Public Health (Lond) 94: 149–154

Evans J Grimley, Prior I A M. Tunbridge W M G 1982 Age-associated change in QRS axis: intrinsic or extrinsic aging? Gerontology 28: 132–137

Feinleib M, Kannel W B, Tedeschi C G, Landau T K, Garrison R J 1979 The relation of antemortem characteristics to cardiovascular findings at necropsy. Atherosclerosis 34: 145–157

Floras J S, Sleight P 1982 The lability of blood pressure. In. Amery A (ed) Hypertensive cardiovascular disability: pathophysiology and treatment. Martinus Nijkoff, Hague

Fox R H, Woodward P M, Exton-Smith A N, Green M F, Donnison D V, Wilks M H 1973 Body temperatures in the elderly: a national study of physiological, social and environmental conditions. British Medical Journal 1: 200–206

Fries J F 1980 Aging, natural death and the compression of mortality. New England Journal of Medicine 303: 130–135

Garn S M, Rohmann C G, Wagner B 1967 Bone loss as a general phenomenon in man. Federation Proceedings 26: 1729–1736

Graham C E, Kling O R, Steiner R A 1979 Reproductive senescence in female non-human primates. In: Bowden D M (ed) Aging in non-human primates. VanNostrand Reinhold, New York, p 183–202

Gregory R L 1974 Concepts and Mechanisms of Perception Duckworth, London p 167–227

Hamilton W D 1966 The moulding of senescence by natural selection. Journal of Theoretical Biology 12: 12–45

Hansen B S, Marquardsen J 1977 Incidence of stroke in Frederiksberg, Denmark. Stroke 8: 333–335

Havlik R J, Feinleib M (eds) 1979 Proceedings of the Conference on the Decline in Coronary Heart Disease. NIH Publication 79–1610, US Department of Health Education and Welfare, Washington DC

Helderman J H, Vestal R E, Rowe J W, Tobin J D, Andres R, Robertson G L 1978 The response of arginine vasopressin to intravenous ethanol and hypertonic saline in man: the impact of aging. Journal of Gerontology 33: 39–47

Keeler E B, Solomon D H, Beck J C, Mendehall R C, Kane R L 1982 Effect of patient age on duration of medical encounters with physicians. Medical Care 20: 1101–1108

King M C, Wilson A C 1975 Evolution at two levels in humans and chimpanzees. Science 188: 107–116

Kurtzke J F 1969 Epidemiology of cerebrovascular disease. Springer Verlag, Berlin

Martin G M 1978 Genetic syndromes in man with potential relevance to the pathobiology of aging. In: Bergsma D, Harrison D E, Paul N W (eds) Genetic Effects on Aging. Liss, New York, p 5–39

Matkovic V, Kostial K, Simonovic I, Brodarec A, Buzina R 1977 Influence of calcium intake age and sex on bone. Calcific Tissue Research Supplement 22: 393–396

Meneely G R, Battarbee H D 1976 High sodium — low potassium environment and hypertension. American Journal of Cardiology 38: 768–785

Matsumoto N, Whisnant J P, Furlan A J et al 1979 The declining incidence of stroke. New England Journal of Medicine 300: 449–452

Miall W E, Chinn S 1973 Blood pressure and ageing; results of a 15–17 years follow-up study in South Wales. Clinical Science and Molecular Medicine (Supplement) 45: 23–33

Medawar P 1952 An unsolved problem in biology. Lewis, London

Office of Population Censuses and Surveys 1974 Morbidity Statistics from General Practice: Second National Study 1970–71. HMSO, London

Office of Population Censuses and Surveys 1975 The General Household Survey 1972. HMSO, London

Peto R, Roe F L J, Lee P N, Levy L, Clack J 1975 Cancer and ageing in mice and men. British Journal of Cancer 32: 411–426

Riley M W, Bond K 1981 Beyond agism: postponing the onset of disability. In: Hess B B, Bond K (eds) Leading Edges: Recent Research on Psychosocial Aging. NIH Publication No 81–2390, Washington D C

Schaie K W, Strother C R 1967 A cross-sequential study of age changes in cognitive behaviour. Psychological Bulletin 70: 671–680

Shock N W 1981 Indices of functional age. In: Danon D, Shock N W, Marois M (eds) Aging: A Challenge to Science and Society Volume 1, Biology. University Press, Oxford, p 270–286

Solomon L 1979 Bone density in ageing Caucasian and African populations. Lancet 2: 1326–1330

Wroe D C L 1973 The Elderly. Social Trends 4: 23–34

Wu M, Ware J H, Feinleib M 1980 On the relation between blood pressure change and initial value. Journal of Chronic Diseases 33: 637–644

2

The elderly patient — special characteristics of disease in old age

A. N. Exton-Smith

Medical teaching based mainly on the experience of illness in younger people stresses the importance of unifying into a single diagnosis all the findings from the history, clinical examination and laboratory investigations. Such an approach is seldom appropriate in clinical practice in the elderly, the majority of whom suffer from multiple disorders. This is perhaps the most obvious way in which the older patient differs from the younger one; but there are other important differences which must be taken into account in the successful management of the elderly patient. The physician must have knowledge of the ways in which many physiological performances decline with age ultimately leading to impairment of homeostasis, an awareness that the manifestations of disease processes are modified, and the understanding of the aims of treatment and of the need to distinguish between disease and disability. Many of these special features are consequences of the structural and functional alterations which occur in the body in senescence.

SENESCENCE

With advancing years the maintenance and repair of body tissue gradually become less effective with the result that cells die and organ function declines. Bodily systems age differentially and this leads to individual variations in the rate of decline in function in these systems. There are two important consequences of this process: a lack of uniformity in the biological age of different organs and an increasing divergence between one individual and another.

Physiological performance

Shock and his colleagues (1972) have carried out measurements of physiological performances on the basis of cross-sectional studies comparing individuals within the age range of 30–80 years. The effects of age vary in different bodily systems and the average decrements during the 50 year period are as follows: nerve conduction velocity 15%, resting cardiac output 30%, vital capacity 50%, renal blood flow 50%, maximum breathing capacity 60%, maximum work rate 70% and maximum oxygen uptake 70%. It has been emphasised that the greatest age

decrements occur in tests carried out when stress is imposed on the organism, particularly in those functions requiring a co-ordinated activity of a number of bodily systems during exercise. There is considerable variation in the rate of decline between individuals but it is likely that deterioration in function is a universal phenomenon. That this is so has been shown from a few longitudinal studies; for example, Rowe and his colleagues (1976) have investigated renal function by repeated measurements in each individual and they have shown a decline in function which closely parallels that revealed by cross-sectional studies. This deterioration in renal glomerular excretion rate has a direct relevance to drug therapy in old age (see below) since the plasma levels of drugs for which the main route of elimination from the body is through renal excretion are likely to be elevated when the drug is given in doses appropriate for the younger adult.

Aging and disease

There have been many attempts to define the differences between 'normal' and 'abnormal' aging or between 'normal aging' and 'disease'. Evans (1981) regards this approach as unhelpful since apart from possible confusion between the implications of at least three entirely different meanings of the word normal there is no rational basis at present for defining normality (see chapter 1). These problems are particularly encountered when considering the diagnosis of such conditions as hypertension, hypothermia, diabetes, anaemia and osteoporosis. In the case of hypertension, for example, the diagnosis has often to be made from an 'operational' viewpoint, a level of blood pressure above which at a certain age an increased risk of morbidity and mortality would be associated. In this instance is is clearly important to make a distinction and no one would deny that every effort should be made to recognise hypertension and to treat it before the patient develops a cerebral haemorrhage. In other instances, however, the recognition of the distinction between the decline in function associated with normal aging from that due to a pathological condition may be largely academic. A few examples of these difficulties which face the clinician and influence overall management of the patient may be mentioned.

During the fourth and fifth decades the ability to change the focal length of the lens of the eye becomes impaired as the result of changes in the muscles of accommodation and of a loss of elasticity of the lens. Whereas in a younger person the focal length can be changed by 14 or more diopters, in persons over the age of 50 the maximum change may be only 1 diopter. In practice it matters little whether this impairment of accommodation leading to presbyopia be regarded as physiological or pathological since the lengthening of the focus of the lens can be corrected by appropriate spectacles. It is however interesting that measurement of the change in power of accommodation in the lens can be used as an index of the rate of aging, and it could be included in an aging test-battery of the type suggested by Comfort (1969). In addition there is some evidence that those individuals who show an accelerated development of presbyopia also show a more rapid rate of aging in other organs particularly in the vascular system (Bernstein & Bernstein, 1945).

The loss of bone tissue from the skeleton which occurs with increasing age has been determined in both cross-sectional and longitudinal studies. After the age of 35 this loss of bone tissue in both sexes leads to a diminution in radiographic density and to thinning of the cortex of the long bones. This process becomes accelerated in women after the menopause with the result that by the time old age is reached women have lost more bone than men and a clinical diagnosis of osteoporosis can be made in about half the women over the age of 75 years. When the duration of operative factors is prolonged over many years, as seems likely in most cases, before the clinical syndrome of osteoporosis develops it is inevitable that the disorder becomes more frequent with advancing age. In consequence the process will appear as a manifestation of aging and the problem is to determine whether the age-related changes are a universal phenomenon or whether they can be influenced by nutritional, hormonal or other means. Skeletal rarefaction is in itself of little consequence to the individual unless as a result of a fall he or she sustains a fracture of the femoral neck, or in the case of the spine minor trauma leads to a crush fracture of a vertebral body. When there is a better understanding of the pathogenesis of osteoporosis and when effective treatment becomes available it will clearly be important to make a distinction between physiological aging in the bone and pathological osteoporosis at a stage before fracture occurs.

There have been many studies which show that intellectual function declines with increasing age; these investigations have been based largely on the results of cross-sectional studies. Using Raven's progressive matrices for the measurement of intellectual performance in different ages, the results can be expressed in the form of percentile ranking curves. The maximum performance is at the age of 30; thereafter there is a steady decline and the mean performance at 65 years is about 25% less than at the age of 30. Moreover the curves show a divergence with increasing age and the decline in the lower percentiles occurs at a more rapid rate than in the higher percentiles. The interpretation of these findings is difficult, mainly because of the problems resulting from the intrusion of cohort effects. People aged 20 and people aged 70 are from very different cultural backgrounds and these cultural effects have considerable influence on the performance in the psychometric tests used. The fact that the downward trend in mental performance with age is greater in the lower percentiles than in the upper has been taken to mean decline is more rapid in those with poorer intellectual performance earlier in life and this may be related to the lack of use of mental faculties. Some support for this hypothesis is to be found in the work of Herron & Chown (1967) who have studied intellectual function in healthy subjects at different ages in various socio-economic groups in the population. Their findings indicate that there is a differential fall-off with age in non-verbal intelligence with those of the higher occupations showing a slower rate of decline. This matter merits futher investigation since it is clearly important to determine whether continued use of mental skills during working life will prevent or slow deterioration.

There is a further fact to which hitherto little attention has been paid and that is the effects of physical disease on mental performance. Studies of Birren and his colleagues (1976) have shown that the performance on a variety of psychometric tests may be affected by the physical health of the individual; thus subjects who are optimally healthy had higher scores than those suffering from impairment of health due largely to vascular disorders but asymptomatic in nature. It is possible that some of the divergence seen in the percentile ranking curves may be the results of the effects of unrecognised physical disease on mental performance especially in very old subjects. It remains to be seen whether treatment of these physical disorders will have any benefit in terms of improved mental function.

The few longitudinal studies which have been undertaken indicate that decline in intellectual function is very much less pronounced that that revealed by cross-sectional studies. Thus Schaie & Strother (1968) compared age-associated changes in mental abilities found by cross-sectional methods with the results derived from a longitudinal study based on follow-up of the same subjects. For most aspects of mental function the longitudinal study indicated smaller and later decrements with age than those suggested by cross-sectional data. It is clear that an important part of what appears to be the effect of aging in cross-sectional studies is due to differences in cultural backgrounds of successive generations and the influence of such variables as educational standards, length of time at school, standards of housing, nutrition and public health and in the case of the very old, to the effects of decline in physical health. At present we have no precise means of separating that fraction of decrease in physiological performance which is due to intrinsic processes from that which is due to environmental influences earlier in life. This is because few of the older people who are examined in cross-sectional studies have escaped the effects of exposure to disease and accidents. Longitudinal studies will provide the best means of making this distinction and will help to identify those environmental influences which have a particularly deleterious effect on the aging of the individual.

IMPAIRED HOMEOSTASIS

Homeostasis can be defined as the body's need to maintain a constant internal environment despite external changes. The more efficient the individual's control of homeostasis the better is his state of health. Under resting conditions the normal old person can maintain a constant internal environment within physiological limits which are similar to those found in a young person. Under basal conditions, blood glucose levels, plasma pH, plasma volume and osmotic pressure, for example, are variables which show little change with advancing age. Nevertheless, homeostasis is impaired as shown by diminished ability to react to stress.

In the case of blood glucose where the glucose load is imposed in both the oral and intravenous glucose tolerance tests, the rise in blood glucose levels is greater and the return to resting levels is slower in older people compared with the young. These features have been attributed to a decreased sensitivity of the pancreatic β-cells to hyperglycaemia and consequent sluggish insulin release (Andres, 1973) and to diminished insulin sensitivity (Soerjodibroto et al, 1979) resulting from decreased glucoreceptor response to insulin action on the cell membrane. These findings have important implications in clinical practice, namely in the diagnosis of diabetes mellitus in old age; when criteria used for the diagnosis of diabetes of glucose tolerance tests in younger adults are applied to the elderly a high proportion of the old age population have 'chemical' diabetes.

Impairment of blood pressure control in old age is believed to be due mainly to decline in function in the autonomic nervous sytem. A fall in systolic pressure of 20 mmHg or more on standing has been demonstrated in 14% of the elderly population (Exton-Smith, 1977). By contrast postural hypotension is rare in young people except when there is impairment of autonomic function due to such conditions as diabetic neuropathy. Additional factors account for the increasing frequency of the condition in old age are varicose veins, the use of certain drugs, anaemia, bacteriuria and hyponatraemia (Caird et al, 1973). Moreover in old age there exists a complex relationship between factors due to deterioration in other systems and this accounts for the serious consequences of postural hypotension. Whereas in the younger person auto-regulation within the cerebral circulation will maintain cerebral blood flow even when the systemic blood pressure decreases by as much as 60 mmHg, in the older person autoregulation in the cerebral vasculature is less precise, especially when following the precipitous fall of blood pressure in severe cases of postural hypotension or following a fall in cardiac output associated with myocardial infarction. The resultant brain cell ischaemia can lead to mental confusion, cerebral infarction with focal neurological signs, or when the border zones between the main arterial territories are affected, a condition of 'instant dementia' may result.

ATYPICAL FEATURES OF DISEASE

Problems in diagnosis of disease arise from differences in clinical manifestations of disease in the elderly. Thus certain diseases are more acute and others more benign when they appear in old age. Appendicitis may be mentioned as an example of the former; very often the onset is fulminating with the early development of gangrene and peritonitis. This atypical clinical picture probably results from atrophy of lymphoid tissue which predisposes to the rapid spread of infection and from the presence of arteriosclerotic vessels which become occluded by thrombosis. Thus in old age appendicitis is often a vascular event with the frequent and early occurrence of massive necrosis.

More often, however, the disease appears to be more benign in old age. Thus in carcinoma of the breast the neoplastic process can progress so slowly that marked general deterioration may not occur until many years have elapsed and indeed the patient may ultimately succumb to some unrelated disorder. In many other instances the insidious onset and the silent existence of the disease make its 'benign' nature more apparent than real. Thus cardiac infarction may have few of the dramatic features including severe pain and shock, seen in middle-aged individuals; in old age it may present with a confusional state, a slight increase in breathlessness or general weakness. A benign giant gastric ulcer measuring as much as 7–8 cm in diameter on the lesser curve may cause only mild discomfort in the left hypochondrium, and the first indication of its presence may be a complication such as perforation or haemorrhage. The patient with pulmonary fibroid tuberculosis may mention only the non-specific complaint of general weakness and the diagnosis may be missed until the disease has reached an advanced stage.

Bronchopneumonia in the elderly progresses insidiously and a diagnosis is often made only when extensive consolidation has occurred. McFadden and his colleagues (1982) have drawn attention to the importance of observing a raised respiratory rate. They have defined the normal respiratory rate in elderly patients as 16–25 breaths per minute. Most elderly patients with an acute lower respiratory tract infection develop a respiratory rate above the upper limit of this range and the tachypnoea is often present 24–48 hours before clinical diagnosis is made. Other acute illnesses, such as urinary tract infections, are not associated with a rise in respiratory rate. These authors conclude that an accurately measured respiratory rate above 25 breaths a minute in an old person should strongly suggest the possibility of a lower respiratory tract infection even before other clinical signs are manifest.

MULTIPLE AETIOLOGICAL FACTORS

Multiple pathology is a well recognised feature in old age (see below); it is less often emphasised that common clinical syndromes are usually the result of multiple aetiological factors. A good example is the clinical condition of hypothermia in which the deep body temperature falls below 35°C. Whereas in a young fit individual, hypothermia is due to a single cause namely exposure to severe cold on a mountainside or immersion in water, in the elderly accidental hypothermia is due to impairment of homeostatic mechanisms (see chapter 00) and the operation of several factors simultaneously. Thus hypothermia in older people can be attributed to:

1. An age-related impairment of function in the autonomic nervous system affecting thermoregulation within the vasomotor control zone. This impairment has been demonstrated in both cross-sectional and longitudinal studies (Collins et al, 1977).

2. Diminished shivering thermogenesis in response to cold (Collins et al, 1981).

3. Impaired thermal perception and decreased awareness of a cold environment (Collins et al, 1982); in consequence there is greater danger of the older individual overstressing a failing thermoregulatory system.

4. The lower room temperatures in the houses of old people in the winter months compared with those of the young, thus increasing the likelihood of their exposure to greater degrees of cold stress (Fox et al 1973; Wicks, 1978).

5. The presence of diseases in other bodily systems and the use of drugs which increase the likelihood of cold exposure and impair the thermoregulatory capacity (Exton-Smith, 1981).

In the majority of cases of accidental hypothermia it is possible to identify three or more of these groups of factors. It is important so far as is possible to identify each factor and to assess its relative contribution. Some are amenable to treatment or correction, whereas for those individuals with severe degrees of underlying physiological impairments the best that can be achieved is to protect them from undue cold exposure. It must also be recognised that survivors of hypothermia are prone to repeated episodes on further cold exposure (MacMillan et al, 1967).

In a younger person, congestive cardiac failure may well be ascribed to the effects of a single pathological process, namely rheumatic carditis. By contrast, the predisposing causes of cardiac failure in an individual of 75 years of age may be coronary insufficiency, aortic stenosis, hypertension and chronic anaemia; the precipitating factors may be pulmonary infection leading to increased myocardial anoxaemia, pulmonary infarction due to embolism or acute anaemia resulting from haemorrhage. If some of these underlying conditions can be treated the prognosis is better than in the individual who has a single untreatable cause.

MULTIPLE DISEASE

The main factors which favour the development of multiple diseases in the elderly may be summarised as follows:

1. Systemic interaction and the stress of disease in one bodily system leading to disorder in another in which there is already impairment of homeostatic control due to deterioration in functional capacity: e.g. congestive cardiac failure may be precipitated by a respiratory infection, cerebral ischaemia is a frequent consequence of cardiac infarction and paroxysmal disorders of heart rhythm, and acute confusional states may occur in a variety of physical illnesses.

2. The long periods of latency in development of many disorders (e.g. vascular disease in the brain, heart and limbs), during the course of which an acute process may be superimposed at any time.

3. An age-related increase in the incidence of common disorders and the effects of accumulation of injuries paticularly hypertension, arteriosclerosis, diabetes, neoplasia, spondylosis and osteo-arthritis. It is inevitable that several of these conditions will appear by chance in the same individual. In some cases two or more distinct diseases affect the same organ or bodily system e.g. the concurrence of Alzheimer type dementia and multi-infarct dementia.

4. Impairment of immune function and the greater likelihood of the occurrence of cancer, myxoedema and pernicious anaemia in the immuno-compromised host. Nutritional deficiencies may also lead to a further decrement in immune function.

5. Secondary consequences of immobility associated with a variety of neurological and locomotor disorders. In the elderly the risks of developing contractures, pressure sores, osteoporosis, urinary incontinence and infections, thrombo-embolism and bronchopneumonia are greater than in younger patients.

6. The high frequency of iatrogenic disease in older patients. This can be attributed to alterations in the pharmacokinetics leading to elevated blood levels of drugs, increased target organ sensitivity and use of multiple drug regimens.

IMPLICATIONS FOR TREATMENT

A thorough investigation of the elderly patient reveals that much disability which might otherwise be attributed to 'senility' is due to specific disease processes and these may be capable of amelioration by appropriate treatment. Often there will be found conditions which in themselves are not directly lethal but they can lead if neglected to progressive disablement. Effective management depends on the recognition of the distinction between disability and diseases which cause it and the assessment of the disabilities both physical and mental on a functional basis.

When a full clinical assessment of all the underlying pathological processes has been made by medical examination supported by appropriate investigations, treatment should be aimed first at the more serious conditions affecting the health of the patient. The therapeutic regimen should consist of the minimum number of the most effective drugs and a choice should be made of those drugs which are least likely to cause adverse effects. The possibility of interaction between drugs must be borne in mind; this is a relatively uncommon problem in the younger patient suffering from a single disease but in the elderly patient with multiple pathological processes, simultaneous treatment with more than one drug is an important factor in the production of adverse drug reactions. These problems are discussed in chapters 7 and 54.

Williamson and his colleagues (1964) emphasise the importance of the early ascertainment of disease, because preventive medicine is at least as important in old age as it is in earlier life and there are few conditions to which medical and social measures applied soon enough will not help. Early diagnosis and adequate treatment are required to prevent or to delay the progress of a disorder, to reduce the chance of development of 'vicious circles of regressive change' in which a lesion in one bodily system leads to disorder in another, and most important to institute appropriate rehabilitation measures to prevent or minimise dependency.

REFERENCES

Andres R 1973 Ageing and carbohydrate metabolism. In: Carlson L A (ed) Nutrition and Old Age, Alquist and Wiksell, Stockholm, p 24–29

Bernstein F, Bernstein M 1945 Law of physiologic ageing as derived from long range data, Refraction of the human eye. Archives of Ophthalmology 34: 378

Birren J E, Botwinick J, Weiss A D, Morrison D F 1971 Inter-relations of mental and perceptual tests given to healthy elderly men. In: Birren J E, Butler R N, Greenhouse S W, Sokoloff L, Yarrow M (eds) Human Aging I: A Biological and Behavioural Study. US Department of Health Education and Welfare, Rockville, National Instutute of Mental Health, p 143–156

Caird F I, Andrews G R, Kennedy R D 1973 Effect of posture on blood pressure in the elderly. British Heart Journal 35: 527–530

Collins K J, Doré C, Exton-Smith A N, Fox R H, McDonald I C, Woodward P M 1977 Accidental hypothermia and impaired temperature homeostasis in the elderly. British Medical Journal 1: 353–356

Collins K J, Exton-Smith A N, Doré C 1981a Urban Hypothermia: Preferred temperature and thermal perception in old age. British Medical Journal 282: 175–177

Collins K J, Easton J C, Exton-Smith A N 1982 impairment of thermo-regulation. In: Sarner M (ed) Advanced Medicine 18, Royal College of Physicians, Pitman, London, p 250–257

Comfort A 1969 A test battery to measure ageing in man. Lancet 2: 1411–1415

Evans J Grimley 1981 The biology of human ageing. In: Dawson A M, Compston N, Besser G M (eds) Recent Advances in Medicine 18, Churchill Livingstone, Edinburgh, p 17–37

Exton-Smith A N 1977 Functional consequences of ageing: Clinical manifestations. In: Exton-Smith A N, Grimley Evans J (eds) Care of the Elderly: Meeting the Challenge of Dependency, Academic Press London, p 41–52

Exton-Smith A N 1981 The elderly in a cold environment. In: Arie T (ed) Health Care of the Elderly, Croom Helm, London, p42–56

Fox R H, Woodward P M, Exton-Smith A N, Green M F, Donnison D V, Wicks M H 1973 Body temperatures in the elderly: A national study of physiological, social and environmental conditions. British Medical Journal 1: 200–206

Herron A, Chown S 1967 Age and Function. Churchill, London

McFadden J P, Price R C, Eastwood H D, Briggs R S 1982 Raised respiratory rate in elderly patients; a valuable physical sign. British Medical Journal 284: 626–627

MacMillan A L, Corbett J L, Johnson R H, Smith A C, Spalding J M K, Wollner L 1967 Temperature regulation in the survivors of accidental hypothermia in the elderly. Lancet ii: 165–169

Rowe J W, Andres R, Tobin J D, Norris A H, Shock N W 1976 The effect of aging on creatinine clearance in men; a cross-sectional and longitudinal study. Journal of Gerontology 31: 155–163

Schaie K W, Strother C R 1968 A cross sequential study of age changes in cognitive behaviour. Psychology Bulletin 70: 671–680

Shock N W 1972 Energy metabolism, caloric intake and physical activity of the ageing. In: Carlson A (ed) Nutrition in Old Age, Alquist and Wiksell, Stockholm p 12–20

Soerjodibroto W S, Hearn C R, Exton-Smith A N 1979 Glucose tolerance, plasma insulin level and insulin sensitivity in elderly patients. Age and Ageing 8: 65–74

Wicks M W 1978 Old and Cold: Hypothermia and Social Policy. Heinemann, London

Williamson J, Stokoe I H, Gray S, Fisher M, Smith A, McGhee A, Stephenson E 1964 Old people at home — their unreported needs. Lancet 1: 1117–1120

3

Geriatric assessment

L. Z. Rubenstein & I. B. Abrass

INTRODUCTION

Comprehensive assessment has become one of the corner-stones of geriatric medicine. By comprehensive assessment is meant the quantification of all relevant medical, functional and psychosocial attributes and deficits in order to achieve a rational plan for therapy and resource planning. Proper assessment relies on a thorough familiarity with principles of medical diagnosis, functional status determination, and psychosocial quantification. Because of its multifactorial nature, it is usually performed collaboratively with individuals from several disciplines, often forming a multidisciplinary team, and usually employs standardised assessment instruments to aid in quantification and reliability.

This chapter will provide a perspective on geriatric assessment by describing the purposes of assessment, and its different structural and functional components, surveying the different kinds of existing assessment programmes, and giving an overview of some of the most clinically useful of the different assessment instruments.

Purposes of assessment

Geriatric assessment has several major purposes, listed below.

Screening for treatable disease
Accurate diagnosis
Rational therapeutic planning
Ensuring appropriate use of services
Determining optimal placement
Documenting change over time

These include diagnosis (either screening or definitive), planning for therapy and for most appropriate use of services, determining optimal placement, and establishing baseline for documenting change over time. By accurate diagnosis is meant not only medical diagnosis but diagnosis of functional, psychological and social problems as well. This is especially important in light of the accumulating evidence which indicates that elderly individuals are often incompletely and inaccurately diagnosed when cared for in

the usual medical setting in the absence of a specialised and interdisciplinary geriatric approach (Williamson, 1964; Williams, 1972; Butler, 1975; Rubenstein, 1981). Several studies have shown that careful systematic assessment can lead to the discovery of important, previously-unrecognised, treatable problems (Brocklehurst, 1978; Cheah, 1980: Rubenstein, 1981). This improvement in diagnostic accuracy through assessment, stems from an orientation which pays special attention to functional deficits and psychosocial disabilities, and emphasises the value of searching systematically for unstated treatable problems, instead of simply responding to specific complaints.

Improvement in diagnostic accuracy relates directly to improvement in treatment. High rates of inappropriate drug regimens and iatrogenic illness have been documented among the elderly (Steel, 1981; Rubenstein, 1981; Ouslander, 1981; Jahnigen, 1982), and at least preliminary data suggest that careful assessment can help to ameliorate this problem.

Avoiding inappropriate use of service, especially those in institutional settings has been a major objective of most geriatric assessment programs on grounds of both compassion and cost. The US General Accounting Office (GAO) Report (1979) concluded that at least 10–20% of patients in skilled nursing facilities (SNF) and 20–40% of patients in intermediate level care facilities (ICF) receive unnecessarily high levels of care. Such inappropriate use is undesirable on several counts: it is wasteful of scarce resources, it can create further disability by leading to premature labelling of a patient as irremediably ill, and institutional environments are themselves hazardous to the aged (Steel, 1981). There is substantial and growing evidence that assessment can lead to improved appropriateness of placement (Williams, 1973; Brocklehurst, 1978; Rubenstein, 1981; Schuman, 1978; Sloan, 1980; Reed, 1979; Kleh, 1977). Finally, most assessment programmes are concerned about obtaining accurate data for documentation of patient improvement over time as well as for programme evaluation. Assessment, using any of a number of quantitative and validated instruments, can serve both purposes.

GERIATRIC ASSESSMENT PROGRAMMES

Types of programmes

The growing awareness of the vast health and psychosocial problems faced by elderly individuals, stemming from cumulative and interacting effects of age and disease, together with realisation that conventional care programmes deal inadequately with the elderly, has led a multitude of health care planners and providers to establish special programmes to assess and treat elderly patients. These programmes have a wide variety of structural and functional components, geared to differing types of populations and problems addressed, but they share some common characteristics. Virtually all programmes include the use of multidimensional assessment, utilising one or more sets of measurement instruments to quantify functional, psychologic, and social parameters. Most of them use interdisciplinary teams to pool expertise and enthusiasm in working toward common goals. Most attempt to couple their assessments with an intervention programme, such as rehabilitation, counseling or placement.

Some of the major characteristics which vary among programmes are listed below.

Intended function
  Assessment
  Rehabilitation
  Acute or chronic treatment
  Placement
  Education
  Research

Location/setting
  Acute hospital
  Chronic hospital
  Long-term care facility
  Out-patient clinic or office
  Freestanding unit
  Patient homes

Patient source
  Community (direct application or referral)
  Acute hospital
  Long-term care facility

Inclusion criteria for patients
  Minimum age (e.g. over 65, over 75)
  Type of problem (e.g. psychiatric, placement)
  Degree of disability (e.g. inability to function
    independently)

Exclusion criteria for patients
  Poor prognosis
  Unstable condition

Organisation
  Team composition
  Participating support service
  Size of unit
  Patient to staff ratio
  Payment source
  Follow up capacity
  Time allowed for assessment

Approach to assessment
  Dimensions included
  Testing of actual performance v presumed capability
  Use of test batteries v clinical judgments
  Types of record keeping formats

A variety of overall functions can be performed by geriatric assessment programmes. While assessment is common to all, many also include treatment and rehabilitation. Some include acute care while most include the determination of optimal placement. Research and education are important aspects of some programmes, and generally have profound impacts on programmatic structure.

Programme location largely determines the types of patients assessed and the functions performed. Assessment programmes in acute hospitals generally admit patients from acute inpatient services, though many also admit directly from the community if inpatient care is required. Hospital programmes usually combine treatment and rehabilitation with assessment and placement. Outpatient clinics or free standing units generally assess patients not requiring hospitalisation and usually do not perform substantial treatment or rehabilitation. Programmes performing assessment in patient homes can obtain unique insights into how patients live and function at home, but the cost and logistical problems associated with home visits limit the size and scope of home assessment programmes. Programmes in long-term care facilities or chronic hospitals assess patients on admission to determine care needs and appropriateness of placement, and some perform periodic reassessments for the same purposes as well as to document change over time.

The referral sources for patients, as well as the inclusionary and exclusionary admission criteria, also depend on the programme setting and intended functions. Although age criteria are admittedly arbitrary, programmes usually will insist that patients be at least 65, and some have a higher minimum age, to ensure that the programmes retain their 'geriatric' missions and do not become programmes caring for individuals with chronic disorders of all ages. The types of patients referred can vary widely between programmes. Some programmes have a geropsychiatric orientation and accept primarily patients with problems such as dementia and depression. Others, situated on acute medical services, accept patients with acute medical problems. Most, however, accept primarily patients with subacute and chronic problems not requiring acute medical or surgical hospitalisation yet who are at great risk for requiring long-term institutional care.

Programmes providing substantial inpatient treatment or rehabilitation can increase their impact by including only patients with reasonable 'rehabilitation potential'. However, prognostication is at best an inexact art, and every geriatrician knows many instances when patients not expected to do well have made remarkable recoveries. Some risks of failure must be taken, since accepting only patients expected to recover or rejecting patients on the basis of poor prognosis can become self-fulfilling.

Organisation of assessment programmes varies considerably, but most include a core team of a physician (or physician extender), nurse and social worker. To this core is added a variety of other specialists who either participate in the basic assessment or are called in on a consultation basis (e.g. psychologist or psychiatrist, occupational therapist, physical therapist, audiologist, dentist, optometrist or ophthalmologist, dietician, public health nurse et al). The size of the team is influenced by several factors, including programme goals, setting, patient load and funding or reimbursement levels. Most funding sources and insurance companies have restrictive limitations as to what services will be paid for, which profoundly affects what services can be offered. However, as evidence accumulates that these programmes can be cost-effective, not only in improving quality of life, but in reducing overall health care costs for the elderly, funding sources will probably expand.

Approaches to assessment vary among programmes depending upon programmatic goals and settings. Most include a multidimensional assessment in which most or all of the areas of medical problems, functional disabilities, psychologic status, as well as social network and needs are covered. Some programmes use a comprehensive test battery or multidimensional assessment to achieve this (e.g. CARE, PACE, OARS) (Kane, 1981), while others select from among the existing onedimensional instruments best suited to their particular programmes. In some programmes, individual team members complete separate assessment instruments pertaining to their own separate areas of expertise, while in other programmes a single individual, such as a nurse practitioner or a researcher, completes the entire assessment instrument(s). Some programmes make special efforts to ensure reliability and validity of their instruments in their own settings, while others simply use instruments validated in other places, and assume that the instruments are adequately reliable and valid. Some programmes use instruments from which data are easily computerised, while others are not concerned with data tabulation.

EVIDENCE FOR EFFECTIVENESS OF PROGRAMMES

Most geriatricians are firmly convinced of the effectiveness of geriatric assessment programmes for improving both the process and outcome of geriatric care, even though well-designed studies clearly leading to this conclusion are only beginning to appear. The many published reports on geriatric assessment units (GAU) show clear associations between the programmes and major improvements in care outcomes, though these reports are primarily based on simple descriptive or quasi-experimental studies. The reported improvements from GAUs, are summarised below.

Improved diagnostic accuracy
More appropriate placement
Less dependency on skilled nursing facilities
Improved functional status
More appropriate use of medications
Better co-ordinated use of available community support
    services
Improved emotional status and sense of well-being

The first reports on GAUs were published in Great Britain where the units originated. Dr Marjory Warren, generally considered one of the founders of modern geriatrics, initiated the concept of specialised geriatric assessment units during the late 1930s while in charge of a London workhouse infirmary. The infirmary was filled primarily with bedridden and largely neglected elderly patients who had not received proper medical diagnosis or rehabilitation. The high quality nursing kept the patients alive, while the lack of diagnostic assessment and rehabilitation kept them disabled. She systematically evaluated these patients and began policies of mobilisation and selective rehabilitation. She was able to get most of the long-term bedridden patients out of bed, often walking, and in some cases, even discharged home. As a result of her experiences, Dr Warren advocated comprehensive assessment and an attempt at rehabilitating all elderly patients before admitting them to long-term care hospitals, which has remained a basic principle of British geriatric policy. The present British system of 'progressive geriatric care' which is centered around geriatric assessment, is based largely on Dr Warren's reports, along with those of other pioneering geriatricians such as Lionel Z Cosin and W Ferguson Anderson.

The first report in North America describing the success of an American programme was T Franklin Williams's outpatient assessment programme in Monroe County, New York. Dr Williams's pioneering programme assessed all patients referred for nursing home placement in the county in an attempt to ensure the appropriateness of these placements and to decrease unnecessary use of long-term care facilities. They found that only 38% of patients referred for nursing home placement actually needed such long-term skilled nursing care, while 23% of patients were able to return to their homes and 39% to board and care facilities following careful assessment and recommendation of specific therapy. Expert judgments made by an independent team of observers as to appropriateness of placement locations before and after the initiation of the Monroe County programme indicated that major improvement in placement decisions were being made — from 50–60% appropriate before the 84% appropriate afterward. Several others have reported similar improvements in placement locations associated with assessments on GAUs (Bayne, 1977; Schuman, 1978; Reed 1979; Sloane, 1980; Rubenstein, 1982).

Several reports have examined patient functional status before and after treatment on those GAUs which include rehabilitation along with the assessment. These reports usually have used a validated measure of functional status, such as the Katz index of activities of daily living (ADL) to document change over time. They uniformly show that many if not most patients improve during their stays on the GAUs. However, the lack of control groups in most of the reports prevent a sceptical reader from concluding that the improvement came from the GAU, rather than from the effect of time alone.

Another major area of GAU impact is the improvement in diagnostic accuracy, usually indicated by the diagnosis of new, treatable problems. All studies reporting on this parameter have found many previously-undiagnosed problems resulting from careful GAU assessment. Depending on each study's criteria for considering newly documented problems as new diagnoses (some only counted major new treatable problems), new diagnoses were found in frequencies varying from 0.76 per patient to almost 4 per patient. Most of these new diagnoses seemed to stem from an awareness of the need to more thoroughly evaluate elderly patients and to search specifically for treatable problems, although they might also reflect a lack of diagnostic thoroughness in the referring services.

Improvement in quality of treatment is difficult to quantify. One measurable parameter, use of prescription drugs, was examined in several programmes. In those programmes, drug prescribing was generally made more appropriate and usually decreased in quantity despite a concurrent increase in the number of diagnoses identified.

Two recent controlled studies have begun to confirm these descriptive reports. They also show that the control group patients who survive the initial hospitalisation also tend to improve in functional status over time, indicating that not all the functional improvement can be attributed to the GAU itself. Nonetheless, the benefits from GAUs, at least to certain subgroups of elderly patients, are becoming more and more evident.

Dr Frengley's group in Cleveland recently reported data from a retrospective case-control study on their inpatient GAU at a rehabilitation hospital (Lefton et al, 1983). In their study, 50 consecutive patients aged 70 and over discharged from their GAU were compared retrospectively with 50 control patients discharged from other medical wards in the same hospital, matched for age, sex, and primary diagnosis. Mean length of stay for patients in the two groups were comparable and fairly long (68.0 and 70.7 days respectively), but reflected the extensive rehabilitation being performed along with the assessment. Discharge location was significantly better for the GAU group than the controls (80% v 62% were discharged to home settings and 20% v 38% to nursing homes respectively). Patients in the GAU were more likely than control patients to improve their functional status (Katz ADLs, independent ambulation, and continence status) during their hospitalisations. At follow-up evaluations, performed several months after discharge, the living locations had not substantially changed, and significantly more GAU than control patients were still at home. However, functional status of control patients had improved at follow up so as to approach the levels of the GAU patients, though only self-reported Katz ADL scores were assessed.

Our group at the Sepulveda VA Medical Center GAU has been conducting a prospective randomised controlled study, comparing inpatient candidates randomly assigned to enter the GAU or to continue receiving care on their acute hospital wards. Though the study is still in progress, preliminary data indicate significant reduction in one-year mortality and reduced overall use of institutional services by GAU patients as compared to control patients. In fact the savings in direct medical care costs for the GAU group appear to be substantial and more than enough to pay for the programme.

It is important to identify which subgroups of patients can be expected to benefit particularly from geriatric assessment programmes. While it might be argued that the majority of the elderly could benefit from careful assessment, the bulk of old people are generally healthy and the relative yield of assessment tends to be lower for healthy than for frail or ill elderly. In general, those individuals most likely to benefit from assessment are those who are on the verge of needing institutionalisation, who are in the lower socio-economic groups, who have had inadequate primary medical care and who have poor social support networks. These at-risk elderly seem to derive especially great benefit from assessment and associated therapeutic interventions.

GERIATRIC ASSESSMENT INSTRUMENTS

A geriatric assessment does not absolutely require the use of specific instruments and scales, especially if the individual providing the assessing is also the primary person providing therapy. However, the use of easy-to-administer, well-validated assessment instruments encompassing the major domains of geriatric assessment, makes the process of assessment considerably easier to perform and teach, and more reliable. In addition, these instruments facilitate transmission of understandable clinical information between health providers, permitting smooth teamwork to occur, meaningful and valid data to be tabulated, and therapeutic progress to be measured over time. In fact, it is doubtful that geriatric assessment programmes could have become as useful and as widely accepted as they are without the use of specific assessment instruments to facilitate documentation and communication, much less diagnosis. In our experience, the instruments most useful in supplementing the standard medical history and physical examination are those in the psychological and functional areas.

A recent book by the Kane Doctors provided an excellent analysis of the existing geriatric assessment instruments and described in detail which are best for which particular setting and patient population (Kane & Kane, 1981). The Kanes also discuss the theoretical and practical considerations involved in selecting assessment instruments from among the multitude available. Some of these important considerations are listed below.

Dimensions to be measured
Multidimensional *v* undimensional instruments
Source of information (e.g. patient, chart, proxy)
Reliability
Validity
Discrimination capacity in actual patient population
Practicality
Personnel and time needed to administer
Usefulness in repeated measurement

In this section, the basic domains of geriatric assessment (listed below) will be outlined, and our selection of one or two appropriate instruments for measuring each in the setting of a GAU will be suggested and described.

Physical health
   Diagnoses/conditions present
   Physiological Severity Indicators
   Quantification of medical services used
   Self ratings of health or disability
Functional ability
   Activities of Daily Living (ADL) scales
   Instrumental ADL scales
Psychological health
   Cognitive function (mental status)
   Affective function
Social parameters
   Social interaction network
   Social support needs and resources

Physical health

The quantification of physical health is probably the most difficult part of the assessment process. Most assessment programmes do not even make a true attempt at quantification, other than to simply list medical diagnoses and medications. Few instruments exist for actually quantifying physical health because it is so multifaceted and complex. Each organ system has its own set of parameters which could be quantified (e.g. cardiac output or ejection fraction for the heart, creatinine clearance for the kidneys, etc.). In addition, each medical diagnosis has a wide spectrum of severity, not conveyed by merely stating the diagnosis. Moreover, two individuals with the same diagnoses are often physiologically more disparate than two individuals with different diagnoses. A few diagnostic entities have been reasonably well scaled (e.g. the New York Heart Association classification for heart disease), but most have not. (A potentially useful concept which needs to be developed is an AQ or 'age quotient', analogous to the IQ test, in which physiologic age would be determined for each major organ system, contrasted with actual age, and weighted according to the relative importance of each organ system in determining life expectancy.) Existing instruments for measuring physical health tend to suffer from being either too disease or organ system specific (and thus not providing a common denominator score for comparing patients with different diagnoses) or else too non-specific and dependent on judgment.

We are thus left with either disease-specific scales, such as pulmonary function test scores or the New York Heart Association Classification for coronary heart disease, or scales based on general functional level, such as exercise tolerance level. In each scale, only a part of physical health is being described, either narrowly disease-specific (ignoring other organ systems) or else based on broad functional capacity (ones emphasising certain measurable aspects of function while ignoring potentially serious elements not yet affecting function).

Other parameters which could be measured and which bear a quantitative but not precise relationship to actual physical health include: use of medical services (e.g. hospital days, physician visits), restricted activity days, the presence of and number of specific diagnostic entities, the presence of specific symptoms or physical signs, and self-ratings of pain, discomfort and general health level.

Although all of these parameters could serve as proxy measures of physical health, and certainly bear some relation to it, most are limited by either subjectivity (in the self-ratings) or by difficulty in quantification (in the case of diagnostic entitites, symptoms or signs). Use of services is an objective phenomenon and is quantifiable; yet it, too, only imperfectly reflects true health, since many very ill individuals use few services and many high users of services may not be proportionately 'ill'.

Thus, no reasonably good scale of global physical health

exists, as opposed to the areas of functional status and psychological health, as will be seen. Nonetheless, certain aspects of health are measurable and are useful in certain circumstances (e.g. physiological measures of specific organ systems, exercise tolerance, use of medical services, identification of specific diagnostic entities). Though categorical or organ specific data may be difficult to quantify between patients, it is essential to gather for purposes of diagnosis and care planning in individual patients, as well as for monitoring change over time.

Functional ability

Measurement of functional ability — the ability to perform functions necessary for independent living — is one of the most useful parts of geriatric assessment. Not only is functional ability possible to quantitate in a way that general physical health is not, but it is an area which is very amenable to intervention so that improvement can clearly be documented. As well, functional status is probably the largest determinant of the living situation in which an individual can reside following treatment and of how much assistance will be required.

Measures of functional ability can be usually grouped into two levels: scales quantifying such as basic activities of daily living (ADL) that an individual needs to perform in order to live independently without very frequent assistance, and scales describing more complex 'instrumental' ADLs (IADL) that an individual needs to perform in order to be able to live completely independently in a community without any assistance. The basic ADL scales usually include such functions as feeding, continence, bathing, dressing, transferring and getting to the toilet. Instrumental ADL scales include such functions as using the telephone, handling finances, using out-of-home transportation, preparing meals, shopping and handling medications.

Perhaps the best-studied and most well-known and valid of the measures of basic ADLs in the Katz Index of ADL (Katz, 1970). It includes the six functions of bathing, dressing, getting to the toilet, transferring, remaining continent and feeding. Each function is scored by a knowledgeable rater in a dichotomous fashion, depending on the subject's ability to perform the function without human assistance. Among this scale's particular attributes are its simplicity and that fact that for most individuals the six functions are lost and regained in a natural progression, as described in their order listed above, forming what is known as a Guttman scale. Thus, a score of C indicates that two functions are lost and that they are most likely those of bathing and dressing.

Two other well-studied basic ADL scales are worth mentioning: the Barthel Index (which lacks the Guttman scalability, but includes the additional functions in its score for grooming, walking and using stairs) (Mahoney, 1965); and the Philadelphia Geriatric Center Physical Self-

Maintenance Scale (PSMS) (which is similar in content and scalability to the Katz but has been validated as a self-report measure, not requiring the input of a knowlegeable caregiver). Thus, the Barthel index might be more useful in a rehabilitation setting, where more precision and breadth is required; and the PSMS might be more useful in a setting where a caregiver is unavailable for reporting. There may be a problem, however, in relying purely on a self report, as subjects have been shown in some settings to over-state their functional abilities relative to reports from caregivers; so caution must be excercised in using self-report data (Rubenstein, 1982b).

Among the most useful of the IADL scales is the one developed by Lawton at the Philadelphia Geriatric Center (Lawton, 1969). It includes the functions of shopping, telephoning, housekeeping, taking medications, handling finances, doing laundry and using public transportation. This scale is especially useful because of its simplicity, ease of administration, and Guttman scalability.

In choosing instruments to assist in assessing physical function, several considerations help to determine the choice. First is the paticular purpose for which the assessment is being performed: to determine care needs, to decide upon placement, to document functional status progress over time, to determine eligibility for services, to screen for disabilities, etc. Second is the location and patient population which is being assessed: nursing home, acute hospital, community clinic, patient home, etc. Third is the source of data: patient interview, patient questionnaire, family member, professional caregiver, etc. Each available instrument was developed for a particular purpose, with a particular population, and using a particular data source. Some have also been subsequently used and validated with different purposes, populations, and data sources. It is important to use the most well-matched instrument to ensure maximum reliability and validity.

Mental functioning

Caregivers frequently need to assess the mental status of the elderly. Extensive psychological testing of each individual would be costly and impractical. The geriatric caregiver does, however, need to have some screening measures for initial assessment to aid in decisions for further intervention. This section, therefore, addresses assessment instruments which might best be used to meet this goal. More detailed psychometrics should be performed in conjunction with psychologists. Differential diagnoses and evaluation for etiology are discussed in specific chapters of this book.

Mental status assessment involves measurement of both cognitive and affective functioning. Impairment of intellectual ability and depressive states are both prevalent among the elderly. Objective instruments are available to assess both these components of mental functioning. Such instruments are useful not only for screening and identifying individuals at risk but also for assessing change. Such tools can provide reliable information about the progress of persons under care and are useful in documenting the effects of care.

The interrelationship between physical and mental impairments is particularly acute in the elderly. In this age group, mental status changes are often associated with acute and chronic illnesses. Sensory deprivation may also produce symptoms of mental impairment. Many over-the-counter and prescribed drugs can affect mental function; iatrogenic problems are easily overlooked.

Although cognitive and affective disorders occur separately, they may coexist in the same individual. Distinguishing them may be difficult, even though determining the primary problem is often important.

Just as in the interrelationship of physical and mental functioning, social functioning affects mental parameters. Suspicion and loneliness may be based on reality. On the other hand, social interaction is often used as an indicator of mental health.

Mental functioning can be assessed in a variety of ways including unstructured 'mental-status examinations,' structured and semi-structured interviews that permit scoring, self-completed questionnaires, observer ratings, and formal psychological tests (Kane & Kane, 1981).

Structured interviews for assessing mental functioning maximise reliability and validity ensuring that each judgment is based on very similar content. Some structured interviews are also designed to collect information about possible physical or social problems that could bias the results. Less structured interviews, though less formal to administer, have several disadvantages. They depend on a more cooperative subject, tend to be lengthier, and rely more on judgment in rating than structured interviews.

Self-administered scales are available for assessment of affective functioning. They have the advantage that the subject does not need to reveal sensitive topics directly to the interviewer and the interviewer does not influence the test results. The disadvantage is that answers may be based on misunderstanding of the items. In the elderly, visual and motor deficits may interfere with completion of self-administered tests. The validity of orally presenting such tests is unclear until separate validation procedures are performed.

Observer ratings are useful in supplementing information obtained from the subject and have been used in institutional settings. Such ratings have problems of rater subjectivity with bias to both under- and overstatement. Such scales may also have the problems of the time-frame for the observation where immediate rating may have a sampling error for overall behaviour and extended rating may be biased by selective recall.

Psychological tests are in the realm of the psychologist.

Many of these tests need more study before they can be used diagnostically in the elderly. Some have been developed particularly for elderly subjects, but problems in administration still remain.

Cognitive functioning

Cognitive functioning includes a variety of subcategories ranging from simple orientation to time, place and person, to abstract thinking and problem solving. An assessment need not include all the dimensions. With severe disorientation and memory loss, higher reasoning abilities may be assumed to be absent. Conversely, lower abilities can be assumed to be present in individuals who can perform complex tasks. The direction and depth of the assessment can often be addressed during the gathering of identifying information (name, age, birthdate).

The following paragraphs describe what, in the authors' opinion, are some of the most useful screening tests for cognitive function in the elderly. The Mental Status Questionnaire (MSQ) is a brief, 10 item test which has been used extensively in geriatric research and practice (Kahn et al, 1960 a,b). The test is administered by interview with scoring done by counting errors yielding three levels of disability determined on the basis of cut-off scores. Test-retest reliability is high. Two items which occur on this test and several other mental-status examinations, that is, the present and immediate past president, which tap awareness of current events and memory for more distant events, have come under some criticism. Such items may become increasingly irrelevant to the elderly, especially those residing in institutions.

The Short Portable MSQ (SPMSQ) is another 10 item test which has several items similar to the MSQ but also taps other spheres (Duke University, 1978). The item on 'mother's maiden name' is a test for remote memory, but unlike the question on past president is likely to have once been learned. The question on telephone number (or street address) is a practical question about self-care skills in the community. One drawback of these two questions is that they require knowledge of the correct answers by the test administrator. The serial subtraction from 20 by 3s is an indication of mathematical ability. A marked advantage of the SPMSQ is that norms have been developed. Both the MSQ and SPMSQ are only screening tests since they have a true positive rate of only about 55% and a true negative rate of 96%. Few with cognitive deficits will be missed. However, those with positive tests require further evaluation for correct diagnosis.

The Face-Hand Test is based on the ability of the individual to recognise simultaneous tactile stimulation on cheek and palm (Fink et al, 1952). Although this test probably adds little additional information to the mental-status examination it is useful for distinguishing psychotic patients from those with brain damage since psychotic patients can identify the locus of the stimuli.

The Set Test is an easily used test that identifies the presence and level of senile dementia (Isaacs & Kennie, 1973). The subject is asked to name as many examples of animals, fruits, colours and towns as possible. One point is awarded for each, up to 10 in each category. A score under 15 closely approximates the diagnosis of senile dementia. Although used in the United Kingdom, its use has not been reported in the United States.

Affective functioning

Measuring affective functioning is one of the great challenges in geriatric care. Little consensus has emerged on how to measure depression in the elderly. Depression is loosely used in common language to depict a gloomy mood and has thus led to ambiguity in its use. The third edition of the Diagnostic and Statistical Manual (DSM III) has provided operational diagnostic criteria for depression (American Psychiatric Association, 1978). The application of these criteria to the elderly have not been well defined, particularly as to dysphoric symptoms that are related to medical disorders and other problems. There is also little information as to the incidence and prevalence of depression in community-based elderly and thus a lack of norms for development of scales.

Depression scales rely heavily on the presence of somatic indicators of depressed mood state. Such symptoms may relate to poor physical health rather than to depression. Depression scales often contain items regarding preoccupation with own health and death. Such thoughts may have much less negative significance for the elderly. Many depression scales are complex instruments and thus may present difficulty in administration for the elderly, particularly those with some physical deficit.

Despite these difficulties several measures are available to assess depression in the elderly. The Zung Self-Rating Depression Scale (Zung SDS), which is clinically derived, has been used widely in geriatric research (Salzman & Shader, 1979). The scale choices range from 'a little of the time' to 'most of the time' and thus may antagonise the elderly person by forcing him or her to concede having a symptom. Some advocate using a 'none or a little of the time' choice instead. Many items have a substantial psychophysiological component prompting some gerontologists to suggest dropping some items, particularly those related to libido. Further analysis of the somatic items is indicated before such scales are applied generally to the elderly population. Scores on the Zung scale do, however, improve after therapy of depression.

Items on the Beck Depression Inventory are also clinially derived (Beck et al, 1961). The statements are read to the subject who selects the most personally pertinent. Extensive work has been done on the reliability and validity of the inventory. It is reliable in rating the depth of depression and registers changes in intensity of depression over time. In the elderly, it has been shown that this scale measures improvement after psychotherapy. Elderly subjects may become fatigued by the full instrument. A shortened version has however, been shown to be reliable (Sherwood et al, 1977).

The 13 depression items on the Hopkins Symptom Checklist are easily administered to aged subjects. It is a promising instrument for measuring the existance of a dysphoric mood apart from psychophysiological symptoms (Gallagher et al, 1980).

Social functioning

Geriatric caregivers have the responsibility to assess social functioning to the same extent as physical and psychological factors. Objective indicators of social well-being need to replace subjective judgments. However, developing an efficient and accurate way of assessing social well-being of elderly patients is a challenge. Despite the difficulties discussed below, assessment of social functioning is critical in the care of the elderly since social functioning correlates with physical and mental functioning, social well-being enhances the ability to cope with health problems and functional limitations, and adequate social functioning is an important outcome in itself.

Several problems exist in assessing social functioning among the elderly. Concepts in social health are exceedingly general. Universal agreement on the components has not been achieved. Norms are not available for many of the measures. Rating of components is difficult due to the subjective nature of many of the parameters. Aspects such as 'quality of life' have differing subjective qualities both from the subject's and rater's perspective. It is difficult to assign a score to relationships (numbers, intensity, proximity). What is perceived as adequate by one subject may not be by another. Monitoring for a change in social functioning may, however, be more helpful. Evidence for determination may indicate the individual at risk for dysfunction.

The geriatric provider must decide which aspects of social functioning are important components of the geriatric data base, how to gather trustworthy information, the degree of detail that should be sought, and the way that social information should be interpreted and used. In consideration of such factors, one of the authors in conjunction with his colleagues has developed a social assessment form to be used as part of the data base in the care of geriatric patients (Kane et al, 1984). This form includes parameters the authors have found useful in their experience with elderly patients.

A discussion of the long arrays of instruments that measure some aspect of social functioning is beyond the scope of this chapter.

REFERENCES

American Psychiatric Association 1978 Diagnostic and statistical manual of mental disorders. 3rd edn. Task Force on Nomenclature and Statistics, Washington, DC

Applegate W D, Akins D, Vanderzwaag R, Thoni K, Baker M G 1983 A geriatric rehabilitation and assessment unit in a community hospital. Journal of the American Geriatrics Society 31: 206–210

Beck A T, Ward C H, Mendelson M, Mock J, Erbaugh J 1961 An inventory for measuring depression. Archives of General Psychiatry 4: 53–63

Brocklehurst J C, Carty M H, Leeming J T, Robinson J H 1978 Medical screening of old people accepted for residential care. Lancet 141: p. 141–2

Cheah K C, Beard O W 1980 Psychiatric findings in the population of a geriatric evaluation unit: Implications. Journal of the American Geriatrics Society 28: 153–156

Duke University Center for the Study of Aging and Human Development 1978 Multidimensional functional assessment: The OARS methodology. Duke University, Durham, NC

Fink M, Green M, Bender M B 1952 The face-hand test as a diagnostic sign of organic mental syndrome. Neurology 2: 46–59

Gallagher D, Thompson L W, Levy S M 1981 Clinical psychological assessment of older adults. In: Poon L (ed) Aging in the 1980's: Selected contemporary issues in psychology of aging. American Psychological Association, Washington, DC

Isaacs B, Kennie AT 1973 The set test as an aid to the detection of dementia in old people. British Journal of Psychiatry 132: 467–470

Jahnigen D, Hannon C, Laxson L, LaForce F M 1982 Iatrogenic disease in hospitalized elderly veterans. Journal of the American Geriatrics Society 30: 387–380

Kahn R L, Goldfarb A I, Pollack M, Gerber I E 1960a Relationship of mental and physical status in institutionalized aged persons. American Journal of Psychiatry 117: 120–124

Kahn R L, Goldfarb A I, Pollack M, Peck A 1960b Brief objective measures for the determination of mental status in the aged. American Journal of Psychiatry 117: 326–328

Kane R L, Kane R A 1981 Assessing the elderly: A practical guide to management. Lexington Books, Lexington, MA

Kane R L, Ouslander J G, Abrass I B 1984 Practical care of the geriatric patient. McGraw-Hill, New York

Katz S, Downs T, Cash H R, Grotz R C 1970 Progress in the development of the index of activities of daily living. Gerontologist 10: 20–30

Kleh J 1977 When to institutionalize the elderly. Hospital Practice 12: 121–134

Lawton M P, Brody E M 1969 Assessment of older people; Self maintaining and instrumental activities of daily living. Gerontologist 9: 179–186

Lefton E, Bonstelle S, Frengley J D 1983 Success with an inpatient geriatric Unit: A controlled study. Journal of the American Geriatrics Society 31: 149–155

Mahoney F I, Barthel D W 1965 Functional evaluation: The Barthel index. Rehabilitation 14: 61–65

Ouslander J G 1981 Drug therapy in the elderly. Annals of Internal Medicine 95: 711–722

Reed J W, Gessner J E 1979 Rehabilitation in the extended care facility. Journal of the American Geriatrics Society 27: 325–329

Rubenstein L Z, Abrass I B, Kane R L 1981 Improved care for patients on a new geriatric unit. Journal of the American Geriatrics Society 29: 531–536

Rubenstein L Z, Rhee L, Kane R L 1982a The role of geriatric assessment units in caring for the elderly: An analytic review Journal of Gerontology 37(5): 513–521

Rubenstein L Z, Schairer C 1982b Systematic biases in functional status assessment. Gerontologist 22(5): 142

Salzman C, Shader R I 1979 Clinical evaluation of depression in the elderly. In: Roskin A, Jarvik L (eds) Psychiatric symptoms and cognitive loss in the elderly: evaluation and assessment techniques. Hemisphere Publishing, Washington, DC

Schuman J, Beattie E J, Steed D A, Gibson J E, Merry G M, Campbell W D, Krauss A S 1978 The impact of a new geriatric program in a hospital for the chronically ill. Canadian Medical Association Journal 118: 639–645

Sherwood S J, Morris J, Mor V, Gutkin C 1977 Compendium of measures for describing and assessing long term care populations. Hebrew Rehabilitation Center for the Aged, Boston

Sloane P 1980 Nursing home candidates: Hospital inpatient trial to identify those appropriately assignable to less intensive care. Journal of the American Geriatrics Society 28: 511–514

Steel K S, Gertman P M, Crescenzi B S, Anderson J 1980 Iatrogenic illness on a general medical service at a university hospital. New England Journal of Medicine 304: 638–641

United States General Accounting Office Report 1979 Cost implications for Medicaid and the elderly. United States General Accounting Office, Washington, DC

Williams T F, Hill J G, Fairbank M E, Knox K G 1973 Appropriate placement of the chronically ill and aged: A successful approach by evaluation. Journal of the American Medical Association 226: 1332–1335

Williamson J, Stokel H, Gray S et al 1964 Old people at home, their unreported needs. Lancet I: 1117–1123

4

The evaluation of the elderly patient for surgery

M. E. Weksler

INTRODUCTION

The special concern for elderly candidates for surgery reflects not only their vulnerability but also the striking changes in our population with respect to age. The vulnerability of elderly surgical patients is documented by the fact that three-quarters of post-operative deaths are drawn from the 30% of surgical patients who are over 60 years of age. The number of persons over 65 years of age is increasing rapidly. In 1955, 14 million Americans were over the age of 65. Now, more than 25 million Americans are over 65 years of age. Today, a disproportionately large percentage of health care is devoted to elderly persons who spend, on the average, four times more per capita on health care than persons less than 65 years of age. Although the elderly represent only 11–12% of the United States population, they fill more than half of the doctor's ambulatory practice, and occupy almost 50% of hospital beds.

Despite this demographic imperative, medicine has been slow to respond to the changing needs of today's patients. Much of medical care remains cast in the mould established for acute, episodic diseases of the young patient. Furthermore the data base of geriatrics is limited. Specifically, the natural history of many diseases in the elderly is not known in sufficient detail in many cases to permit a rational decision between the risks of medical and surgical therapy. Nevertheless, medical experience has defined at least some of the special considerations required in evaluating the elderly for surgery.

EVALUATING THE ELDERLY PATIENT FOR SURGERY

This chapter will describe the role of the geriatric consultant in evaluating the elderly patient for surgery. The consultation has several goals. The first goal is to review the need for surgery. The indications for surgery in the elderly are not always clear and at times a second surgical opinion may be helpful. Surgical second opinion programmes have revealed that certain operations are more frequently associated with conflicting recommendations (Finkel et al, 1982). Prostatectomy and cataract extraction, operations frequently recommended to elderly patients, are not recommended by the second surgeon in 20–40% of cases.

The second goal of the consultation is to identify risk factors which increase the morbidity and mortality of surgery. Many risk factors can be ameliorated and the patient's chance for uncomplicated surgery increased. The third goal is to provide the patient and family with a description of what can be expected before, during, and following surgery.

Homeostatic reserves are progressively narrowed with age. This age-associated process I have termed 'homeostenosis'. The limitation in physiological reserve described by this term suggests that 'fine tuning' of the physiological systems prior to surgery will maximise the capacity of the elderly patient to sustain the stress of surgery. The goal is to bring into balance the decompensated physiological systems that would otherwise complicate surgery. This can best be achieved if a geriatric evaluation is arranged four to six weeks prior to elective surgery. Obviously this is not possible when emergency surgery is necessary. Nonetheless, the pre-operative evaluation of the elderly patient who requires emergency surgery should consider the same risk factors within the time available.

Many authorities believe that morbidity and mortality following surgery increases (Fig. 4.1) with age (Polk, 1978). Some believe that surgical risk increases only in patients over the age of 70 (Goldman et al, 1977). Others believe age is not an independent risk factor but reflects the physiological limitations and diseases that accompany aging. (Djokovic & Headley-Whyle, 1979). This may be a semantic point for it is usually difficult to distinguish clearly aging from the pathological processes that accompany aging.

The reported surgical morbidity and mortality varies with operative procedure, the ratio of elective to emergency surgery and the population of patients. It is generally acknowledged that older patients are particularly

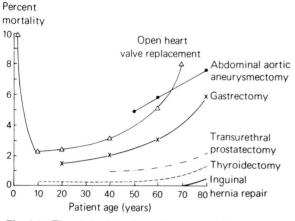

Fig. 4.1 The relationship of mortality to age with respect to several major surgical operations. (Polk, 1978.)

vulnerable to emergency surgery. The varied conclusions drawn from studies in which the distribution of these factors differ is to be expected. Recently the results of surgery in 500 patients over the age of 80 were reported (Djokovic & Headley-Whyle, 1979). Mortality approached 20% of exploratory laporatomies, usually performed on an emergency basis, whereas it was 12% for colectomy, 5% for open reduction and fixation of hip fracture and less than 2% for transurethral prostatectomy.

DISCUSSING THE OPERATION WITH PATIENT AND FAMILY

Acute decline in physical and intellectual function frequently follows surgery in the elderly. The family frequently believes the patient is worse off after surgery than before. A surgical success may be viewed by the patient or, more frequently, by the patient's family as a therapeutic failure, at least in the post-operative period. The patient who may have been leaving his bed at home only with difficulty may become bedridden, or worse yet incontinent, following surgery. For this reason the examination of the elderly patient prior to surgery should include an assessment of mental and physical function. A formal 'mini-mental' status should be administered to document the level of intellectual function. Similarly, if possible, the ability of the patient to get out of bed and walk should be tested. Intellectual and physical activity are critical determinants of independence and must be known in order to plan for convalescent care.

In part, the acute deterioration that occurs after surgery in the elderly represents the stresses of hospitalisation and surgery which fall disproportionately upon the elderly. In part however, these changes may be only apparent and reflect 'denial' by the patient and family of intellectual and physical impairment the patient has prior to surgery. Disorientation and 'sundowning' may become obvious for the first time following admission to hospital when the patient is in an unfamiliar environment. Confusion and delirium during the post-operative period are more frequent than commonly realised in all age groups. This is particularly true with older patients. Acute psychiatric disturbances are particularly common in intensive care units and when contact with the environment is compromised, as for example when visual or auditory function is lost. In careful studies, approximately 25% of post-operative patients have been found to suffer mental aberrations following surgery (Heller et al, 1970). It is helpful to warn the elderly patient that visual and/or auditory aberrations may occur after surgery. This information allays the anxiety that these psychological disturbances may otherwise provoke. Reorientation by the health care team is very helpful in the days following surgery and is far better than sedatives in quieting the agitated post-operative patient.

Fortunately the mental and physical deterioration that follows surgery is usually reversed with time although this may take as long as six to eight weeks. The use of a convalescent or intermediate care facility is of great benefit to the elderly patient following surgery. If the possible temporary deterioration of an elderly patient following surgery is anticipated and if this possibility is discussed with the patient and family prior to surgery, premature and inappropriate institutionalisation of the elderly patient can be avoided (Levilan & Kornfeld, 1981).

THE MEDICAL HISTORY

Most of the relevant information concerning the elderly patient's risk from surgery will be derived from the history. The patient's history should be reviewed with special emphasis on chronic diseases and impairments, current medications and past hospitalisations and operations, including in particular complications and unexpected problems that have developed in the past and might occur again. For example, post-operative deep vein thrombosis, wound infection or heamorrhage frequently recur. In medical history as in political history the past is often a prelude to the future.

A most important part of the history relates to medication. A knowledge of the drugs and anaesthetics taken in the past and those being taken prior to surgery is crucial to the pre-operative evaluation. For example, re-exposure to halothane may produce chills and fever and less frequently hepatic damage 7–14 days after surgery. Medications which have caused allergic or other untoward effects should be identified in order to prevent their use. Patients who have received corticosteroids for 10–14 days during the year prior to surgery should receive parenteral hydrocortisone pre-operatively and for 5–7 days after surgery to prevent acute adrenal insufficiency.

Some drugs e.g. levodopa and oral hypoglycemic agents, cannot be give parenterally. It must be decided whether these drugs can be discontinued during surgery and the immediate post-operative period or if alternative preparations which can be given parenterally, be substituted. Some patients with Parkinson's disease controlled with levodopa, may deteriorate if the drugs is withdrawn. To prevent this, drugs such as Cogentin which can be administered parenterally, may be used. Finally, some drugs should be discontinued prior to surgery. Aspirin which inhibits the haemostatic function of platelets should be discontinued at least one week prior to surgery. Clonidine and monamine oxidase inhibitors which potentiate the response to pressor agents should also be discontinued at least one week prior to surgery. Beta adrenergic blockers need not be discontinued. These drugs frequently used to treat angina, may protect cardiac patients from arrhythmias or reinfarction. Elderly patients with head trauma, infection and shock are at great risk from stress ulcers and may benefit from prophylactic antacids or cimetidine.

NUTRITION AND SURGERY

A dietary history including the use of alcohol is important. Signs and symptoms of alcohol withdrawal — tremor, confusion, delirium and convulsions — may occur in the post-operative period and if not recognised, can present a complex diagnostic problem.

Over- and under-nutrition are recognised to be risk factors for surgery. Obese patients are at greater risk of deep venous thrombosis, pulmonary emboli, atelectasis and pneumonia. Unfortunately, it is rare that significant weight reduction can be achieved prior to surgery. Weight loss may reflect a catabolic state or malnutrition. Malnutrition associated with serum albumin concentrations of less than 3.4 mg/ml, lymphopenia less than 1500 cells/mm^3 and anergy compromise wound healing and increase susceptibility to infection. Very thin elderly patients had significantly higher morbidity following hip fracture than did well nourished patients who were otherwise well matched (Bastow et al, 1983). There is increasing evidence that enteral or parenteral nutrition with vitamin and mineral supplements can replate nutritional deficits and decrease the complications following surgery. Thus patients given a short course of parenteral nutrition prior to surgery for gastro-intestinal carcinoma had decreased post-operative morbidity and mortality (Muller et al, 1982).

Many elderly patients without cancer who deny weight loss may be malnourished. Many elderly exist on a 'tea and toast' diet. A well-balanced diet is expensive, and its ingredients are heavy to carry home from the store. Furthermore, cooking is an effort especially if the socialisation that normally occurs at meal time is lacking. Not surprisingly vitamin and mineral deficiencies are common in these patients. As wound healing depends to a considerable extent upon adequate nutritional reserves of protein, vitamins, particularly vitamin C, and minerals, particularly zinc, it is reasonable to provide supplemental protein, vitamins and minerals when the nutritional state of a patient prior to surgery might be compromised.

RESPIRATORY DISEASE AND SURGERY

Pulmonary function shows the most rapid age-associated decline of any organ system. Lung volumes and flow rates at 65 years of age are only 60% of their values at 20 years of age. These changes increase the susceptibility of elderly patients to post-operative pulmonary complications. A history of obesity, obstructive pulmonary disease, cardiac disease, deep venous thrombosis, pulmonary emboli and smoking all increase the risk of post-operative pulmonary disease. Spirometry should be performed if there is significant exercise intolerance or a significant medical history.

Arterial blood gases should be obtained in patients with significantly impaired forced expiratory volume (FEV$_1$) prior to surgery. A raised $P\mathrm{CO_2}$ is associated with increased post-operative pulmonary complications. Similarly a $P\mathrm{O_2}$ below 55 mm Hg on room air places the patient at high risk. With significantly impaired pulmonary function, local or spinal anesthesia should be considered to avoid the 30–50% fall in tidal volumes which routinely occur following general anesthesia.

While many of the functional abnormalities are fixed in pulmonary disease, there is considerable evidence that discontinuing smoking, for as little as one to four weeks, significantly improves pulmonary function, decreases bronchial secretions and improves bronchial ciliary function. All patients should be urged to discontinue cigarette smoking before surgery. The benefit of prophylactic bronchodilators or antibiotics is debated.

An increased respiratory rate may be a clue to lung disease. Elderly patients who are obese or cigarette smokers must be suspected of having obstructive pulmonary disease. The physical examination of the lungs and pulmonary function tests should be used to measure respiratory function in the elderly patient. If severely compromised the stress of the operative procedure must be weighed against the degree of pulmonary insufficiency. Patients which chronic obstructive pulmonary disease should have pre-operative postural drainage with chest percussion. This has been shown to decrease pulmonary complications following surgery (Harman & Lillington, 1979).

THROMBO-EMBOLIC DISEASE AFTER SURGERY

Thrombo-embolic complications of surgery are very common. Patients with a history of deep venous thrombosis or pulmonary emboli are at very high risk of thrombo-embolic disease following surgery. The elderly patient is at particular risk as post-operative thrombo-embolic disease increases with age (Morrell et al, 1963). The chance of deep venous thrombosis and pulmonary emboli is increased following surgery not only because bedrest increases venous stasis, but also because the operative procedure may obstruct blood flow or traumatise vessels. Furthermore the fibrinolytic activity of the blood is reduced following surgery. Certain operations, for example hip surgery and prostatectomy, frequently performed on elderly patients, are associated with a particularly high rate of deep venous thrombosis and pulmonary emboli. Radio-isotope scanning or venography document deep venous thrombosis in 70% of elderly patients operated on for hip fractures, in 50% of elderly patients after prostatectomy and in 35% of all surgical patients over the age of 40 (Mitchell, 1979).

It appears therefore that all elderly patients, especially those for whom hip or prostate surgery is planned, should have prophylaxis for deep venous thrombosis and pulmonary emboli. What type of prophylaxis should be chosen? Early ambulation, physical therapy and pneumatic boots which compress calf muscles carry little risk and should be employed. Drugs used in the prophylaxis of deep venous thrombosis and pulmonary emboli include low-dose heparin, aspirin and dextran. Patients to be considered for such therapy must have normal coagulation studies and not be taking oral anticoagulants or aspirin.

Low dose heparin therapy (5000 U two hours prior to surgery and 5000 U two or three times per day for one week) prevents the activation of the clotting cascade and has been shown to decrease deep venous thrombosis and pulmonary emboli in patients undergoing major elective surgery (Medical Letter, 1977). Such therapy is not effective in decreasing deep venous thrombosis and pulmonary emboli after prostatectomy or hip surgery. Low dose heparin is inadequate for patients with an active thrombotic process. Heparin therapy should not be used prior to neurological or ophthalmic surgery. Aspirin (300 mg bid) has been shown to reduce deep venous thrombosis in men but not women following hip surgery, while Dextran has been reported to decrease both deep venous thrombosis and pulmonary emboli (Mitchell, 1979). When compared to low dose heparin, dextran produced a similar reduction in thrombo-embolic disease (Gruber et al, 1980). Although blood loss at surgery was not significantly different and transfusion requirements were the same, heparin therapy was associated with more wound haematomas.

CARDIAC DISEASE AND SURGERY

A history of cardiac disease is important in assessing the risks of surgery for the elderly patient. A history of angina or a previous myocardial infarction increases the risk of reinfarction in the post-operative period. The degree of risk is related to the interval between the myocardial infarction and surgery. Thus 37% of patients who had a myocardial infarction within the six weeks prior to surgery and 16% of patients who had a myocardial infarction between six weeks and six months prior to surgery, had a post-operative myocardial infarction (Tarhan et al, 1972). Most investigators believe that delaying surgery more than six months after myocardial infarction does not reduce the risk of postoperative reinfarction further. Post-operative myocardial infarction which occurs most frequently four to seven days after surgery, has a high (50%) mortality rate (Goldman et al, 1978). For this reason surgery should if at all possible, be delayed at least six weeks and preferably six months after myocardial infarction. One half of post-operative myocardial infarctions in the elderly patients are not associated with chest pain. These 'silent' myocardial infarctions may be manifested only by increasing congestive heart failure, by a fall in blood pressure or less frequently by a cardiac arrhythmia. Confusion or other mental aberrations, sometimes the result of reduced cerebral circulation, may be the only clue to a silent myocardial infarction.

Cardiac complications are a leading cause of post-operative morbidity and mortality in elderly patients (Djokovic & Headley-Whyte, 1979). A multifactorial analysis of cardiac risks in over 1000 patients who had non-cardiac surgery found that one third of post-operative death rate (the total death rate was 6%) was attributed to cardiac disease and 4% of patients who survived had life threatening, but non-fatal cardiac complications, following surgery (Goldman et al, 1977). A point system was devised to quantitate significant risk factors for post-operative cardiac complications (Table 4.1). Risks are detected by history, physical and laboratory examinations of the surgical candidate. Two historical risk factors – age over 70 and a history of myocardial infarction less than six months prior to surgery – are highly significant risk factors. Other risk factors are detected by physical examination or laboratory examination.

The point system of cardiac risk provides a means to divide patients into four groups according to the degree of risk with respect to mortality and life-threatening but non-fatal complications (Table 4.2). The authors recommended that 'only truly life-saving procedures be performed on patients with risk index scores of 26 or more points'.

Table 4.1 Cardiac risk in non-cardiac surgery (Modified from Goldman et al, 1977).

Criteria	Points
History	
Age over 70 years	5
Myocardial infarction previous six months*	10
Physical examination	
S₃ gallop/jugular venous distention*	11
Significant aortic valvular stenosis	3
Laboratory examination	
EKG	
Premature artrial contractions or rhythm other than sinus	7
More than 5 premature ventricular contraction/minute	7
*General status**	3
Abnormal blood gases	
Electrolyte abnormalities	
Abnormal renal function	
Liver disease/bedridden	
Operation	
Emergency*	4
Intraperitoneal/intrathoracic/aortic	3
Total possible	53
*potentially reversible	28

Table 4.2 Correlation of cardiac risk points and post-operative cardiac problems. (Modified from Goldman et al, 1977)

Point total	Life threatening Complications (%)	Cardiac Deaths (%)
0–5	0.7	0.2
6–12	5.0	2.0
13–25	11.0	2.0
>26	22.0	56.0

Fortunately 28 of the 53 points are reversible to some degree and the geriatric evaluations should offer a therapeutic plan to lower these risks.

The pulse, taken for at least 30 seconds, may offer a clue to cardiac arrhythmias. All abnormal rhythms increase the risk of surgery. Premature atrial contractions add less to the risk to surgery than do premature ventricular contractions. Multifocal premature ventricular contracts, more than 5 premature ventricular contractions per minute and premature ventricular contracts exhibiting the 'R on T' phenomenon are of particular concern. If abnormal rhythms are suggested by history, physical or laboratory examination, a 24 hour Holter monitor recording should be obtained. Patients with serious arrhythmias may benefit from the insertion of a temporary pacemaker.

Many elderly patients have implanted cardiac pacemakers. Some operate only 'on demand'. As electrical interference from equipment in the operating room can disturb the operation of a demand pacemaker, fixed mode pacing should be instituted during surgery to prevent any malfunction during the course of the operation.

As many as 50% of elderly patients have blood pressures above 160/90. Although hypertension in the elderly is a significant risk factor for cardiovascular disease, it is not a risk factor with regard to cardiovascular morbidity and mortality following surgery (Goldman et al, 1977). If the diastolic blood pressure is less than 110, bed rest alone usually lowers the blood pressure so that antihypertensive therapy is not necessary prior to surgery. If hypertension contributes to congestive heart failure, anti-hypertensive therapy should be instituted as a means to improve cardiac function.

Auscultation of the carotid vessels is another important aspect of the pre-operative evaluation. If a bruit is discovered, symptoms of transient neurological deficits should be sought. If a history of a transient ischaemic attack is obtained, Doppler studies and angiography should be used to evaluate carotid blood flow. As the risk of cerebrovascular accidents during or following surgery is very high in patients with symptomatic carotid artery disease, vascular repair should be carried out before all except emergency surgery is performed. On the other hand if no symptoms of neurological disease are elicited, the course of action is less clear. As 15% of patients over 65 have bruits, it is not reasonble to subject all patients to angiographic studies. Perhaps candidates for coronary bypass surgery who are at particular risk of cerebrovascular accidents should have Doppler studies. Patients with carotid bruits without any history or signs of neurological deficit appear to be at no greater risk of cerebrovascular accidents following surgery than are patients without carotid bruits. Thus in a study of 700 patients examined prior to surgery, the frequency of cerebrovascular accidents was comparable in patients with and without carotid bruits (Ropper et al, 1982).

Cardiac disease in general and congestive heart failure in particular contribute much to the morbidity and mortality following surgery. Therefore, careful assessment of cardiac function is a crucial part of the pre-operative assessment. Cardiomegaly, jugular venous distension and hepatomegaly are important signs of congestive heart failure. Peripheral edema in the elderly is a less useful sign of congestive heart failure. Venous disease is a common cause of swelling of the lower extremities. Patients in heart failure or patients who have been in heart failure in the past are at greater risk of developing post-operative pulmonary edema. Therapy with digitalis, diuretics and/or agents which reduce cardiac afterload, improve cardic compensation and reduces the risk of acute post-operative heart failure. Venous disease increases the risk of thrombo-embolic disease and may suggest the need for anticoagulant therapy. Finally cardiac auscultation may reveal abnormalities in cardiac rhythm or valvular heart disease.

Patients who have had valvular heart disease and/or a prosthetic valve implanted, require special care prior to surgery. Many of these patients are receiving oral anticoagulant therapy. It is therefore necessary to provide a period of haemostatic competence during the surgical procedure without exposing the patient to undue risk of thrombo-embolic disease. This can be achieved by stopping the coumarin drug 24 hours prior to surgery and giving 50 mg of Vitamin K_1 intravenously. Intravenous heparin (1000U/hour) is begun 12 hours after surgery if there is no postoperative bleeding, and is continued until the effect of oral anticoagulants begun usually on the third postoperative day, is established.

INFECTIONS AFTER SURGERY

Increasing data suggests that patients given antimicrobial prophylaxis prior to certain operations have a lower incidence of sepsis and wound infection (Table 4.3). Patients with valvular heart disease, prosthetic heart valves or prosthetic joints are at particular risk for infections. These patients are at risk not only from sepsis but also from bactereamia which can result in bacterial colonization of

Table 4.3 Antibiotic propylaxis for surgery (Modified from Medical Letter 23:77 1981)

Operations	Antibiotic
Clean	
Cardiovascular	
Prosthetic valve insertions	
Vascular reconstruction	Cefazolin
Coronary bypass	
Orthopedic	
Joint replacement	Penicillinase
Internal Fixation Fracture	resistant Penicillin
Clean-contaminated	
Entry Upper Respiratory Tract	Penicillin
Gastric Surgery	
(a) with obstruction	
(b) with hemorrhage	Cefoxitin
Biliary Surgery	
(a) with jaundice	
(b) with cholecystitis	Cefoxitin
(c) age 70 or more	
Hysterectomy	Cefoxitin
Urologic with infected urine	antibiotic appropriate to bacteria
Colo-rectal	Cefoxitin plus oral erythromycin and neomycin
Dirty	
Ruptured viscus	Clindamycin Gentamicin Penicillin
Traumatic fracture	Cefazolin
Amputation with ulcer or compromised blood flow	Cefazolin

the prosthesis. Prophylactic antibiotics are given to such patients to prevent sepsis, bactereamia and wound infection. Patients with prosthetic valves or prosthetic joints (Table 4.4) require prophylactic antibiotics for surgical procedures involving the upper respiratory tract, e.g. for bronchoscopy, with penicillin; for procedures involving the urinary tract, e.g. cystoscopy, with penicillin and streptomycin; and for procedures involving the lower gastro-intestinal tract e.g. proctoscopy and barium enema, with penicillin and streptomycin. Even foot care is a potential risk in patients with prosthetic implants as an infected callus may be silent. A single dose of 500 mg of an oral penicillinase resistant penicillin should be given prior to podiatric surgery. If an infected area is uncovered, the antibiotic therapy should be continued for two days.

Table 4.4 Antibiotic prophylaxis for surgery

Antibiotic prophylaxis for patients with prosthetic valves or prosthetic joints in addition to that described in Table 4.3

I. Upper respiratory tract	
1) intubation	
2) bronchoscopy	Penicillin
II. Urinary tract Gastro-intestinal tract	
1) Barium enema	
2) Colonoscopy	
3) Cystoscopy	
4) Enema	Penicillin and Gentamicin
III. Podiatry — callus	
	Penicillinase-Resistant Penicillin

For most patients the advantages of antibiotic therapy prior to surgery outweigh the risk of untoward reactions (in the absence of known allergy) to these drugs. A concern in the use of prophylactic antibiotics is infection with drug-resistant micro-organisms. For this reason, antibiotics with a narrow spectrum which cover the most likely organisms should be chosen. Prophylactic antibiotics should be given for surgery in which foreign bodies such as prosthetic valves or joints are implanted. Drugs are given by the parenteral route immediately prior to surgery and continued for 24 hours after surgery, the period when bacteria are most likely to enter the blood stream. Surgical entry into the gastroduodenal tract or biliary system require prophylactic antibiotics only under special circumstances (Table 4.3). On the other hand, surgical procedures involving the upper respiratory tract, colon or an infected wound are always an indication for antibiotics. Cefazolin is frequently the drug of choice as it has a longer half life than other cephalosporins and injection is less painful. Cefoxitin is chosen when infections with anaerobic bacteria are likely. Urologic surgery in the absence of urinary tract infection does not require prophylactic antibiotics. If the urine is infected, appropriate antibiotics should be chosen based on the urine culture and sensitivity results. Gram negative sepsis may follow instrumentation of the urinary tract if the urine is infected.

HEMATOLOGIC DISEASE AND SURGERY

Polycythemia vera, multiple myeloma and chronic lymphocytic leukaemia occur most frequently in the elderly. These diseases may be associated with impaired hemostasis. Patients with polycythemia vera are at risk both from hemorrhage due to platelet dysfunction, and from thrombosis due to increased blood viscosity. Increased blood viscosity is due mainly to the increased erythrocyte count. These complications are minimised if the red blood cell and platelet count are in the normal range. Phlebotomy is the safest method to reduce the red cell mass but may stimulate thrombocytosis. Patients with platelet counts above 800,000/mm^3 should be treated with cytostatic drugs.

Patients with multiple myeloma may have impaired platelet function, due either to thrombocytopenia or the effect of myeloma proteins on the platelets or fibrin clot formation. Patients with multiple myeloma should have platelet function as well as platelet number tested. Patients with chronic lymphocyte leukaemia are at increased risk of pyogenic infection because of hypogammaglobulineamia. Parenteral gamma globulin should be given to enhance the opsonisation of bacteria.

ENDOCRINE DISEASE AND SURGERY

Diabetes mellitus is a very common disease among the elderly. Many patients with diabetes mellitus are treated with oral hypoglycemia agents. These agents cannot be used during the period when oral feeding is denied surgical patients. A decision must be made whether therapy for diabetes can be discontinued for a short time or whether insulin therapy is required to prevent hyperglycaemia. Careful attention to blood glucose homeostasis is particularly important as the elderly patient is particularly sensitive to the effects of both hypoglycaemia and hyperglycaemia. Most elderly patients have impaired renal function. Such patients are at particular risk for hyperglycaemia which in the face of peripheral resistance to insulin and a decreased capacity to clear glucose from the blood into the urine may develop to hyperosmolar, non-ketotic coma. It is usually reasonable to manage glucose metabolism during surgery and the immediate post-operative period with intravenous glucose and insulin. The dosage is established by frequent blood glucose determinations.

Thyroid disease is frequently difficult to recognise in the elderly. The signs and symptoms of hypothyroidism may be attributed to 'slowing down' with age. The signs of hyperthyroidism may be masked. Eye signs, tremors,

sweating and heat insensitivity frequently observed in the young, are usually not seen in the elderly hyperthyroid patient. One-third of elderly hyperthyroid patients do not have an enlarged thyroid. Atrial fibrillation may be the only clue to hyperthyroidism in the elderly. The danger of thyroid storm following surgery however is not any less in masked hyperthyroidism in the elderly patient. Despite greater awareness of apathetic hyperthyroidism, 10–30% of thyroid storm is still precipitated by surgery.

THERMOREGULATION AND SURGERY

Temperature regulation is known to be impaired in the elderly. Exposure of many elderly patients to cool temperatures fails to elicit the normal physiological responses to conserve heat, such as vasoconstriction or generation of body heat by shivering. Body temperature may therefore fall. Rectal temperature should be obtained on all elderly patients. Rectal temperature below 37°C may be of minor concern in the young patient but may be a clue to impaired thermoregulation in the elderly. Patients with low body temperatures have a higher risk of morbid and fatal events following surgery (Bastow et al, 1983). Surgery stresses the thermoregulatory capacity of the patient; the operating room is cool, intravenous fluids are at room temperature, peritoneal surfaces are exposed to ambient temperature and drapes conserve little body heat. Warming blankets used during surgery may be used to compensate for heat loss but nothing is more important than measuring body temperature during and after surgery. Hypothermia depressed cardiac and respiratory function and may lead to hypotension, impaired ventilation and cardiac arrhythmias. Such complications, frequently noted in the recovery room, may be due to hypothermia.

UROLOGICAL ABNORMALITIES AND SURGERY

Rectal examination should be performed on all elderly patients not only to obtain a stool specimen to be tested for occult blood, but also to detect rectal masses and an enlarged prostate. Rectal masses or prostatic hypertrophy may be the cause of a newly discovered hernia. Furthermore, an enlarged prostate presents a risk factor for urinary retention following surgery. In older men with prostatic hypertrophy, over-hydrations during or following surgery, anti-cholinergic drugs and bed rest may precipitate acute urinary retention. If the patient has prostatic hypertrophy, a history of urinary infection or will be subjected to a urological procedure, a urine culture should also be obtained to rule out bacteriuria. Appropriate treatment for bacteriuria should be given prior to surgery. Renal function may be estimated by blood urea nitrogen (BUN) and creatinine concentration. 'Normal values' in the elderly do not assure normal renal function. A loss of 50% of renal function is possible before either BUN or creatinine rises from the normal range. Furthermore in elderly patients with low protein intake and/or low muscle mass, even more renal function can be lost before BUN or creatinine levels become abnormal. If renal function may be compromised by infection, prostate enlargement, hypertension or prior renal disease, creatining clearance should be performed. The glomerular filtration rate not only documents the level of renal impairment, but also serves as a guide to the dose of many drugs excreted by the kidney. Impaired renal function does not become a significant risk to surgery until renal perfusion falls below 45–50 ml/min. Below this level of kidney function wound healing is compromised.

LABORATORY TESTS PRIOR TO SURGERY

A number of routine laboratory tests should be obtained prior to surgery (Table 4.5). Elderly patients should have a urinalysis, complete blood count, serum chemistries, a chest x-ray and an electrocardiogram prior to surgery. The integrity of the coagulation system should be tested by platelet count, prothrombin time and partial

Table 4.5 Routine tests obtained before surgery

Urinalysis
Complete blood count
Coagulation profile
  platelet count
  prothrombin time
  partial thromboplastin time
Serum chemistries
  BUN, Creatinine
  Alkaline phosphatase, SGOT, SGPT
  Electrolytes
Chest X-ray
Electrocardiogram

thromboplastin time. If there is any suggestion of a hemorrhagic diathesis or ingestion of drugs which inhibit platelet function a bleeding time should be performed. Finally, blood for typing and cross-matching should be obtained.

ACKNOWLEDGEMENT

The author wishes to thank Dr Kenneth P. Scileppi and Dr Anita Herdan for reviewing the original manuscript.

REFERENCES

Bastow M D, Rawlings J, Allison S P 1983 Undernutrition, hypothermia and injury in elderly women with fractured femur. An injury response to altered metabolism. Lancet I: 143–146
Djokovic J L, Headley-Whyle J 1979 Prediction of outcome of surgery and anesthesia in patients over 80. Journal of the American Medical Association 242: 2301–2306
Finkel M L, McCarthy E G, Ruchlin H S 1982 The current status of surgical second opinion programs. Surgical Clinics of North America 62: 705–719
Goldman L, Caldera D L, Nussbaum S R, Southwick F S, Krogstad D, Murray B et al 1977 Multifactorial index of cardiac risk in non-cardiac surgical procedures. New England Journal of Medicine 297: 845–850
Goldman L, Caldera D L, Southwick F S, Nussbaum S R, Murray B, O'Malley T A et al 1978 Cardiac risk factors and complications in non-cardiac surgery. Medicine 57: 357–370
Gruber U F, Saldean T, Brokop T, Eklof B, Eriksson I, Goldie I et al 1980 Incidence of fetal post operative pulmonary embolism after prophylaxis with Dextran 70 and low-dose heparin: An internal and multicare study. British Medical Journal 280: 69–72
Harman E, Lillington G 1979 Pulmonary risk factors in surgery. Medical Clinics of North America 63: 1289–1298

Heller S S, Frank K A, Malm J R, Bowman F O, Harris P D, Charlton M H, Kornfeld D S 1970 Psychiatric complication of open-heart surgery. New England Journal of Medicine 283: 1015–1020
Levilan S J, Kornfeld D S 1981 Clinical and cost benefits of liaison psychiatry. American Journal of Psychology 138: 790–793
Medical Letter 1977 Low-dose heparin prophylaxis and pulmonary embolism. 19: 71–72
Mitchell R A 1979 Can we really prevent post-operative pulmonary emboli? British Medical Journal I: 1523–1524
Morrell M T, Truelove S C, Barr A 1963 Pulmonary embolism. British Medical Journal II;. 830–835
Muller J M, Brenner U, Dienst C, Pilchmaier H 1982 Preoperative parenteral feeding in patients with gastrointestinal carcinoma. Lancet I: 68–71
Polk H C 1978 The mathematics of clinical judgement. In: Gardner B, Polk H C, Stone H H, Sugg W L (eds) Basic Surgery. Century-Crofts, New York, p 5–17
Ropper A H, Wechsler L R, Wilson L S 1982 Carotid bruits and the risk of stroke in elective surgery. New England Journal of Medicine 307: 1388–1390
Tarhan S, Moffitt E A, Taylor W F, Ginliani E R 1972 Myocardial infarction after general anesthesia. Journal of the American Medical Association 220: 1451–1454

5

Preventive medicine

J. Williamson

Of a land where even the old are fair

W B Yeats

'Prevention and Health: Everybody's Business' was the inspiring and optimistic title of a report from the Health Departments in Great Britain (Department of Health and Social Security, 1976). In this document the history of preventive medicine was outlined and the remarkable successes of the control and eradication of the great epidemic infectious diseases were described.

Unfortunately, the importance of prevention declined rapidly as the control of communicable disease progressed and in recent decades most Medical Schools have paid little or no attention to this fundamentally important field of medicine.

The report alluded to is interesting in one other respect — out of its 96 pages, a mere one and a half are devoted to 'Health problems of the aged' (p 36–37) and even in this short section, while the daunting scale of the problem is outlined, almost nothing is offered by way of 'practical prevention'.

Thus it is that we in geriatric medicine, find ourselves doubly disadvantaged in this context:

1. Prevention in general is an unfashionable field having been eclipsed to a large extent by the remarkable advances of 'curative' medicine; by pharmaceutical advances and, above all, by the spectacular achievements of medical technology.

2. The concept of prevention in old age is especially difficult to promote since it flies in the face of current negative stereotypes of old age which suggest that little can be done to influence the deterioration and dependency of old age let alone attempt their prevention.

Unfortunately, this misleadingly damaging nihilism has tended to be particularly prevalent among members of the medical professions presumably because they have, until very recently, received their training exclusively within hospital settings thus acquiring a most biased view of old age. In addition in recent years, the medical profession has often seemed to be almost bemused by increasingly complex technology with corresponding neglect of what are the fundamentally more important issues of prevention.

The pioneers of geriatric medicine in the United Kingdom were originally hospital orientated (Warren, 1943) but it was not long before they realised that since the vast majority of old people were within the community, attention should be paid to their needs therein. The next phase of development in geriatric care was the era of prevention and it is likely that this, along with the educational advances were the greatest contributions to medicine from British geriatric medicine.

What is certain is that only by constantly thinking in terms of prevention can we ever hope to cope with the ever increasing demands from the aging of populations (Williamson, 1979).

Having made this insistent plea for prevention, it must be admitted that the problems in old age are even more complex and puzzling than in younger age groups and those who venture into the field will inevitably encounter more questions than answers.

Firstly, many of the important diseases and disabling conditions which afflict the elderly are undoubtedly capable of partial or complete prevention but the prevention would have to be applied at much younger ages, e.g. in relation to the respiratory consequences of cigarette smoking, the target cell damage of hypertension or the ill effects of poor diet, obesity and sedentary life styles upon the arterial system. Nevertheless, even in old age, it is essential to think in terms of prevention especially with regard to earlier detection of disease or disability and in the slowing or reversal of progressive disability through effective rehabilitation. It must be emphasised also that in old age prevention does not concentrate solely upon the patient and disease but must also involve the health and welfare of family and other supporters in order that they may be able to continue their supportive roles for as long as possible. We may here take a useful lesson from the paediatricians who have taught for decades the importance of ensuring a healthy mother (and family) as a means towards achieving healthy children.

CLASSIFICATION OF PREVENTION

It is customary to divide prevention into primary, secondary and tertiary forms (Morris, 1975). Although the distinctions are more blurred in old age (especially as between secondary and tertiary phases), the classification has some merit for physicians with their inbred bias towards taxonomic niceties.

Primary prevention

This represents 'true prevention' whereby eradication or control of diseases may be achieved by measures aimed at whole populations or at specially vulnerable groups. Under this heading are also included the detection and control of states which have been shown to be precursors of disease (the process known as 'screening').

Ideally primary prevention results in the eradication of diseases as in the case of smallpox where strict segregation of cases plus aggressive world-wide vaccination programmes led to its final conquest. Diseases associated with poverty may be countered by economic and fiscal policies and malnutrition may be prevented by ensuring adequate food supplies at prices which ordinary people can afford and combining this with education on healthy eating.

Health education in old age

Since much of present day morbidity and mortality is related to unhealthy behaviour, health education must be seen as an important part of modern medicine. Its acceptance as such, however, has been slow and grudging largely due to the great difficulties encountered in proving its effectiveness and measuring its value. Great stress is now placed upon the importance of good diet, healthy exercise and the avoidance of unhealthy habits such as tobacco and alcohol abuse. Until quite recently however, a majority of doctors remained generally sceptical about the value of trying to persuade individuals to change their cherished habits and deny themselves immediate bodily and mental satisfactions in order to achieve somewhat nebulous benefits in the remote future. However recent trends in America and Australia have shown startling reductions in mortality from ischaemic heart disease and stroke, and while some of these benefits in relation to ischaemic heart disease may be due to better treatment (e.g. in coronary care units) and some of the reduction in mortality from stroke may be ascribable to more effective control of hypertension, the general concensus is that the main reasons for improvement are in reducton in smoking, reduced fat consumption and the realisation of the importance of exercise in securing better health (Walker, 1977; Stern, 1979).

For many years it seemed that these benefits were being denied to British people but recent publications have at last shown downward trends in mortality from ischaemic heart disease presumably for similar reasons (Heller et al, 1983).

While it has been shown to be possible to persuade young and middle-aged persons to embark upon healthier living there remains a reluctance to accept that similar efforts in old age are worthwhile. This is understandable since it is not easy to believe that healthy behaviour starting in old age can have any beneficial effects when it follows a life time of unhealthy activity. The picture is however not nearly so clear as this pessimistic view might suggest. For one thing, there will be relatively few aged persons who have pursued a genuinely unhealthy life since most of them will have succumbed earlier to related disease. Research results from deliberate attempts at improvement of fitness in old age are also much more encouraging than is widely believed.

Recent work from Sweden has shown that, in random samples of 70 year-old persons, the institution of simple regimes of physical training led to considerable improvement in general fitness as compared to 'untrained' controls. Thus the test groups showed a 26% increase in maximal oxygen consumption, lower heart rates after submaximal exercise and a marked increase in muscle strength. A most interesting observation was that type II muscle fibres in thigh muscle biopsy specimens showed significant increase after training regimes in test subjects (Anianson et al, 1980).

While changes in physical function associated with training are fairly easy to measure and their implications are readily understood, it is much more difficult to assess the effects of 'training' programmes upon social and mental function. Despite these difficulties, however, improvements in mental function and alertness have been demonstrated following deliberate attempts at training in 'figural relations' (Plemons et al, 1978).

Improvement in memory scores were also achieved by deliberate mental arousal in elderly subjects (Langer & Rodin, 1976). The same authors demonstrated the benefits to be expected in elderly persons in institutions when they were offered more choice and greater control over their daily lives (Langer et al, 1978).

It seems therefore that despite the general truth of the rule of linear decline in function due to age (Shock, 1977), a part of the observed loss of function in older subjects is often due to disuse and this may be wholly or partially recoverable. This, if widely confirmed, could be of momentous importance since it suggests that a substantial proportion of old people may be capable of significant improvement in fitness and independence through modification of behaviour and institution of schemes of retraining and reactivation. The time is therefore ripe for introduction of experimental schemes of health education aimed at counteracting the prevalent stereotype of old age that all is loss and more loss.

Some important aspects of primary prevention in old age

The general well-being and stability of any society have profound effects upon the health and happiness of all its members and since the aged are highly vulnerable to stress, this applies with greatest force to them. The aim must therefore be a society where old people retain dignity and self esteem both as members of their family groups and as elders in their communities. This may easily be lost sight of in modern urban and industrialised society with its insistence upon retirement at a fixed age, often with the consequence of abrupt decline in purchasing power due to relatively low pensions. This problem has been aggravated by current high unemployment in many countries which has increased the pressure upon older workers to retire earlier. They may be bribed to do so by apparently generous redundancy payments in order to make way for younger workers. The whole vexed question of reduced opportunity for work and increased leisure time requires radical rethinking. It seems fairly clear that the right to continuous employment for all is now under serious threat and in addition to considering ways of increasing employment, thought should be given to the provision of better opportunities for continuing education, hobbies, sport and other recreational and culturally satisfying activities. In this struggle for readjustment of roles, status and attitudes the elderly are especially vulnerable.

The importance of the physical environment

The elderly are less able to cope with environmental stress because of the reduced efficiency of homeostasis in old age. Some stresses may be easy to identify and measure and their effects accurately assessed, for example the increased risk of hypothermia in old age (Salvosa et al, 1971). Prevention of hypothermia in old age involves consideration of many aspects — adequate nutrition, adequate heating and insulation (at a price which the elderly can afford), education on suitable clothing and avoidance of accidents which may lead to an old person falling and being unable to rise. The medical profession has a special obligation to avoid drugs which may predispose to hypothermia either directly (through reducing metabolic activity as with major tranquillisers) or indirectly through increasing liability to falls (as with hypotensives or antidepressants which increase the risk of postural hypotension). In more extreme climatic conditions, reduced thermoregulatory efficency renders the elderly more liable to heat stress (Ellis et al, 1974).

Protection of the elderly who have reduced capacity for thermoregulation is thus a matter for old people themselves, for their families and the communities in which they live as well as the authorities responsible for housing, heating and ventilation.

Housing as a preventive service

Most old people wish to live on in the areas in which they have settled. They often have brought up their families there and have put down deep social and psychological roots. Even in middle age it may be quite traumatic to move to new areas and in old age this stress may be intolerable.

Due attention to this should be paid by planners and others who frequently may determine housing patterns of individuals or even of whole communities. When the time comes to move every effort must be made to prepare the old person and to alert family members to the need for extra support. Wherever possible, they should be able to remain in the same district and thus retain local links and support. In the United Kingdom there has been a romantic but mistaken idea that people should migrate to the country or the seaside when retired with the generally rosy notion that this would ensure a perpetual holiday atmosphere. The sad fact is that, while this second honeymoon may last for a few years, there usually comes a time when the wife finds herself a widow amongst strangers. Those who practice geriatric medicine in the south coast of England or other favourite retirement areas are well aware of the loneliness and distress that commonly ensues.

In urban communities in the nineteenth and early twentieth centuries it was common to find members of extended families living close together in downtown areas. The elderly were then easily able to keep in close touch with their siblings and their own offspring and thus retain active family roles and eventually to receive extended family support. With the decay of inner city areas and the frightful depredations of the town planners of recent decades, family members have often tended to be scattered within anonymous outlying housing estates and the elderly left in relative isolation. Under these circumstances families have often to go to great extremes and sacrifices in order to keep in touch with their elders.

All is however not uniformly depressing, and some hopeful developments have taken place. Most important has been the growth of grouped or sheltered housing for the elderly. This involves the provision of small enclaves of specially designed flats for single old people or elderly couples. These are situated within 'normal' housing areas surrounded by younger folk and their families and by different socio-economic classes. They are also close to shops and other amenities and are designed to cope with residents who vary from 'fit elderly' to those who may be frail and moderately dependent. An essential ingredient is the Warden (Supervisor) who acts as a guardian and ensures day by day that each resident is coping adequately. Where this is not the case the Warden's responsibility is to alert the appropriate service or individual whether that be a relative, the family doctor or district social worker. A useful provision is a two-way communication system whereby the resident may contact the Warden in an emergency or the Warden may reassure herself that all is well.

The scope for the use of alarm systems has been widened recently by the provision of small radio alarm systems which may be offered to 'at risk' old people living in ordinary housing. There are clear indications for the installation of such devices, for example the old lady who is liable to falls and who cannot be relied upon to get off the floor. At the same time there is a risk that some local authorities may see this as a cheap, easily provided universal panacea for coping with many old people living alone and this may be to the neglect of more appropriate support in some cases. These is already evidence that this may have occurred, for example in reports that an alarm was not activated even when a definite crisis had occurred (Butler & Oldman, 1981). More research in this field is urgently required.

It will be apparent that this list of general primary preventive measures could be almost indefinitely extended and we would end up describing a Utopia where everyone loved his neighbour, where poverty and avarice did not exist and everyone retained satisfying roles throughout life. In addition no one would be afraid to go out at night and it would not be necessary to lock doors and windows. Some would have us believe that at present we experience unprecedented violence, robbery and dishonesty and that not so long ago there was a golden age as described in the preceding sentences. When I hear such talk I always ask myself why it is that all the ground floor windows in my comfortable Edinbourgh house have stout iron bars — the house was built in 1820!

The detection of risk factors for disease in old age
It has already been pointed out that primary prevention encompasses the planned detection and amelioration of precursors of disease. This process is known as screening and has been defined (Department of Health and Social Security, 1976) as 'Screening differs from ordinary clinical practice in that it involves seeking out people with no overt symptoms of disease and asking them to undergo examination and tests to see whether the condition to be identified is present'. Commonly sought risk factors are asymptomatic hypertension, hypercholesterolaemia, increased intra-occular tension and metaplasia of the cervix uteri. This appears such a rational and sensible procedure that even to question it has often been regarded as almost heretical. It has certainly proved to be a popular medical activity by encouraging the use of new technology for preventive purposes, and which appealed to the informed layman (fed by the media of mass communication with the wonders of medical science). The result was a rapid growth of what came to be known as multiphasic screening centres to which were attracted apparently healthy individuals who were then subjected to batteries of tests and procedures designed to detect deviations from 'normal' in a number of measurements. Blood pressure measurements, electro-cardiography, blood and urine assays of numerous constituents and respiratory function tests were carried out. Chest X-rays, cervical smears, mammograms and sometimes sigmoidoscopy were performed. Personality 'inventories' and assessments of mood, anxiety and cognitive function were also offered and the data were then analysed by computer and a profile sent to the individual's

nominated primary physician who then had to decide what should be done. It was confidently asserted that this form of screening would lead to effective therapeutic intervention and reduction in morbidity and mortality. It was also hoped that there would be an ensuing reduction in demand for health and social services.

It will be obvious that the evaluation of such a complex process would be difficult and likewise an assessment of its cost effectiveness. Only well planned controlled trials could answer these questions and such trials have been very few. Even the most enthusiastic protagonists of multiphasic screening have been hard pressed to demonstrate convincing benefits and one of the most elaborate and comprehensive centres failed to show reduction in mortality or morbidity among screened subjects (Cutler et al, 1973).

A London study was promoted with the specific purpose of determining whether multiphasic screening was an activity which should be fostered by the National Health Service. This study failed to show any significant differences in morbidity, mortality or use of services between subjects randomly allocated to screened and control groups (South East London Screening Study Group, 1977). Predictably these findings were criticised, mainly on the grounds that the failure was not one of screening but in the failure of the primary care physician to take proper action after being informed of the detection of an existent risk factor. This argument is difficult to sustain since, whatever the deficiencies of general practice may be within the National Health Service, the practitioners who collaborated in the London Study were all highly motivated and enthusiastic individuals who wished to contribute to the success of the project. It is inconceivable that screening activities dependent upon less highly motivated general practitioners would be more successful. This Study involved individuals aged 45 to 64 and it seems certain that similar activities involving older subjects would be no more successful.

Screening for hypertension in old age
The problem of screening for hypertension and its management in old age is so complex and disputed that it warrants special consideration. This is a field in which doctors tend to hold very strong views despite the dearth of valid research on the significance of raised blood pressure and the effects of lowering it in this age group. The dangers of over-enthusiasm in the use of drugs to reduce blood pressure have recently been spelled out clearly by Oliver (1982). He indicated that only a minority of individuals with a given risk factor will actually develop the disease yet if all such individuals are treated with drugs to counteract the risk then they are all exposed to the risks of adverse drug reactions and so the net result may be increased morbidity (or even increased mortality). Oliver also states that 'aggressiveness in the use of these drugs should be

inversely proportional to age' and this would be supported by most open-minded geriatricians.

The Framingham Study appears to show that the harmful effects of raised systolic and diastolic pressures persist into the age group 65–74. The corollary that it must therefore be beneficial to lower raised pressures at this (or an older) age group cannot be accepted on existing evidence. If the aim of reducing raised pressure is to prevent or minimise resultant target tissue damage then many might argue that it is rather late to be attempting this in someone aged 74 (or even more so in someone aged 85!). This is, of course, especially so where target damage is already manifest as in the stroke patient or the individual with multi-infarct dementia.

It is necessary to ask the question as to whether a raised systolic pressure in an 80 year-old with a rigid, inelastic arterial tree has the same significance as a similar pressure in a 40 year-old who retains normal elastic artery recoil. The answer is almost certainly negative and it may be argued that in order to deliver a given quantity of blood to a distant organ through a rigid artery, the pressure wave will necessarily have to be higher than in the case of normally elastic arteries. To lower the pressure by drug therapy in such circumstances may have the potentially dangerous effect of reducing tissue perfusion. If we relate this to the perfusion of the most important organ, the brain, then we find that in young and healthy subjects any fall in blood pressure is immediately compensated for by cerebral vasodilation as a result of which cerebral perfusion is maintained, although perfusion of other less vital tissues may be reduced. This vital process of cerebral autoregulation is liable to be lost or impaired in certain elderly subjects (Wollner et al, 1979). In subjects who have impaired cerebral autoregulation, reduction in blood pressure may thus result in a corresponding reduction in cerebral perfusion. This would help to explain the relatively common occurrence of stroke soon after the start of hypotensive therapy in some elderly subjects.

Nor is the available literature at all clear upon the relationship of raised blood pressure to stroke or ischaemic heart disease in the elderly. Two recent UK prospective studies of random population samples of old people have failed to show significant correlations between initial blood pressures and incidence of stroke (Evans, 1980; Milne, 1981). Both these studies confirmed the phenomenon of 'regression towards the mean', i.e. those who started with high pressures tended to drift down while those with low pressures showed increase with the passage of time.

The lesson therefore is plain — we do not yet possess evidence to suggest that lowering blood pressure in old subjects who do not have left ventricular strain or angina, is beneficial and we are not entitled to extrapolate from studies on younger individuals. the policy must therefore be *extreme caution*.

The place of immunisation in primary prevention in old age

The raising of immunity by immunisation and vaccination has been one of the great success stories of medicine. It has already been pointed out in this volume (page 000) that immune competence declines with age and hence it may be expected that aged subjects will be more liable to acquire infection, the ensuing illness will be more severe and prolonged and the chance of complications will be greater. The practical implications of this are fairly obvious, i.e. that old people should be protected from infection and this may involve treatment at home as opposed to hospital (where particularly virulent and antibiotic resistant organisms abound).

In the United Kingdom each year the Health Departments issue advice to physicians that high-risk individuals should be offered immunisation against influenza. Among the designated high-risk groups are the 'institutionalised elderly'. The final decision on this action is, however, left to the discretion of the individual physician. How is he to make up his mind in this contentious sphere? The early influenza vaccines were often of low potency and also relatively impure so that immunity was dubious and adverse reactions common (Ruben, 1982). In these earlier times it was also not certain that similar degrees of protection by immunisation would be afforded to the old as to the young, although it had been established that influenza vaccines would elicit a satisfactory increase in antibody titres (Douglas et al, 1977). An increase in antibody titres may not necessarily lead to enhanced immunity so it is significant that Barker & Mullooly (1980) were able to demonstrate that influenza vaccination led to a 70% reduction in hospitalisation and almost a 90% reduction in mortality from influenza and pneumonia among vaccinated elderly subjects. These authors conclude that the benefits of influenza vaccination are as great in the elderly as in younger age groups.

The question therefore is — what advice do we offer the physician as regards influenza vaccination for his elderly patients? It may be stated that for the fit elderly living in their own homes, the policy must be the same as for other ages, i.e. if an epidemic threatens due to a strain for which there is an available vaccine then protection should be offered; the elderly in these circumstances are indeed a priority group. The problem of the protection of the elderly in institutions is less clear cut however, and there is certainly no justification for annual vaccination in the hope that the vaccine used will be effective against the strain of the virus which may eventually pose a threat. In long stay hospitals and nursing homes there will always be a proportion of patients for whom death would be a merciful release and a short sharp influenzal illness may in these circumstances be seen as acceptable a terminal illness as any other. It may usefully be emphasised here that, in this context, it is perhaps more important to protect caring staff against a threatened influenzal epidemic. All who have worked with the elderly are acutely aware of the adverse consequences of reduced staffing levels in institutions upon elderly patients with increased incidence of pressure sores, incontinence and other results of reduction in levels of nursing care.

There have been suggestions in recent years that since pneumonia is such an important cause of death and invalidism in old age, it would be prudent to offer vaccination with polyvalent pneumococcal vaccines. The recommendation of the Food and Drug Administration of the United States (1978) is that persons over 50, especially those in institutions, should be given pneumococcal vaccine. Bently et al (1981) cast serious doubts upon the validity of this recommendation however. At the time of writing it seems therefore that there is no valid reason to advocate the use of available pneumococcal vaccines in older subjects.

Secondary prevention

This involves the earlier detection of disease, generally at a stage at which the pathology can be reversed. The diseases detected in this way are usually at a subclinical stage of evolution and are accompanied by minor symptoms which may become apparent only after specific challenge. The benefits of detection of disease at this stage are obvious — indeed the notion of early diagnosis has remained the cornerstone of medicine from its earliest history. By earlier diagnosis of disease we may hope to reduce its severity, its speed of progression and frequency of sequelae. In old age (especially in extreme old age) early diagnosis is absolutely essential because the reduction of reserves of function render the aged subject liable to multisystem failure if early diagnosis and effective treatment cannot be offered.

Special problems exist in old age in that the onset of disease may be masked or disguised and its existence only become apparent as a form of crisis presentation. The non-specific presentation of disease in the elderly creates problems for the doctor who may not fully appreciate the fact that almost any disease may signal its occurrence by vague failure of health, the development of mental confusion or the onset of falls and postural instability. For secondary prevention the most urgent requirement is that Medical Schools should resolutely set about the task of producing graduates who are knowledgeable about the complexities of the clinical medicine of late life (Svanborg & Williamson, 1980).

Tertiary prevention

This phase of prevention implies the detection of disabling conditions and provision for their optimum management. Generally there are irreversible changes due to chronic disease, many of the patients will be under some degree of medical supervision and in the elderly many of the sufferers face some degree of loss of independence in basic activities of daily living. It might be thought that there is remarkably little scope for preventive activity in such circumstances and this generally pessimistic view has certainly coloured the thinking of many members of the medical and paramedical professions. However the main thrust of geriatric medicine in recent years has been towards counteracting this nihilistic view, since treatment, rehabilitation and proper general management may frequently ensure that deterioration is slowed or reversed, relapse is made less likely, complications and sequelae are reduced and the individual is maintained at a higher level of independence for much longer. In addition, if we include family members and other carers, tertiary prevention has an important role in ensuring that they are protected from excessive stress and thus enabled to continue their supportive roles for much longer periods of time.

Tertiary prevention in old age is thus quite distinct from screening as already defined under primary prevention, since it involves the detection of chronic disabling conditions which are already causing distress and dependency and if unchecked will be sure to produce more hardship and increased demands upon medical and social services. The earlier these disabling conditions are detected, the greater is the chance that effective treatment and rehabilitation will reduce dependency and that supporting relatives will be able to continue their caring roles.

It will be apparent from what has been said that while the eventual goal must remain the primary prevention of disease and disability, any pragmatic approach must be based upon the acceptance that at present tertiary prevention offers the most important form of prevention with the most tangible dividends in return for invested resources. As already emphasised, the demarcation line between secondary and tertiary prevention in this age group is frequently blurred and indistinct.

One of the greatest triumphs of modern geriatric medicine has been the demonstration that in very old subjects, some degree of rehabilitation is generally possible even in such unfavourable conditions as stroke, osteoarthritis and dementia. By meticulous care in diagnosis, by treatment of concomitant disease and by restoration of confidence and morale in patient and carers, it is almost always possible to improve independence and to enable old people to remain in the community for longer periods. In the era preceding the introduction of the principles of geriatric medicine, it was almost universally accepted that care of the elderly was a simple matter of custody. If anyone wishes to obtain an insight into the thinking of doctors and others in this era they ought to read the decription by Thomson (1949) of the care of elderly patients in so-called 'chronic wards' prior to the advent of modern geriatric care. It should be noted that the conditions described in this paper refer to a situation which existed in the United Kingdom less than 40 years ago.

These old fashioned, paternalistic and prohibitively expensive practices persist to this day in many countries of the world where geriatric medicine has failed to flourish.

In an effort to secure earlier detection of disabling conditions and reduced social competence among the elderly Anderson & Cowan (1955) proposed that preventive centres should be widely established so that old people with significant problems could be helped by medical and social intervention. This initiative led to further research in which it was established that self-reporting of disability by elderly sufferers was often inadequate and incomplete. A sample of old people in Edinburgh was investigated and their medical and social needs determined. These needs were then compared to the information held by their general practitioners and it was found that many important, disabling and unpleasant conditions had not been reported by the elderly (or their families) to their general practitioner (Williamson et al, 1964).

Similar studies in different parts of the world have confirmed this iceberg phenomenon of unreported and unmet need among the elderly. Its true explanation is uncertain but is probably multifactorial. The old tend to have a fatalistic attitude towards disability — 'it's only my age' is a commonly heard remark among elderly subjects suffering from a wide range of disabilities. For younger subjects there are powerful incentives to seek medical help when disability threatens; for men there is the threat of becoming unemployable and for women (in addition to the threat to employment) there are obvious threats to her efficiency as mother, wife and household manager. The

incentives to seek medical help are reduced or absent in old age and many old people also harbour certain fears which act as disincentives, e.g. the fear of being put into an institution, the fear of losing control over their own affairs and consequent loss of independence. These fears may often be based upon a real appreciation of the dangers of being old in a materialistic society in which doctors and other health professionals frequently possess little genuine understanding of the needs of the elderly and tend often to think in negative terms of 'disposal' rather than the fundamental needs of the individual. The Edinburgh Study (Williamson et al, 1964) tended to suggest that old people were somewhat selective in how they reported their disabilities. Disabling conditions associated with the respiratory system, the cardiovascular system and the central nervous system tended to be well reported and known to general practitioners. Thus the patient who had cough, breathlessness and wheeze and produced sputum was likely to seek medical help. It might be added that doctors are generally programmed to welcome such patients since they clearly fit into the general pattern of medical interest. However, there is another spectrum of disabling states about which elderly patients and their doctors are much more ambivalent. These are depicted in Figure 5.1 which shows the relative proportion of certain conditions known and not known to general practitioners.

Figure 5.1 indicates that disabilities arising from the locomotor system, the urinary bladder and mental disturbances are very liable to be unreported and unknown. These, of course, are the conditions which many doctors

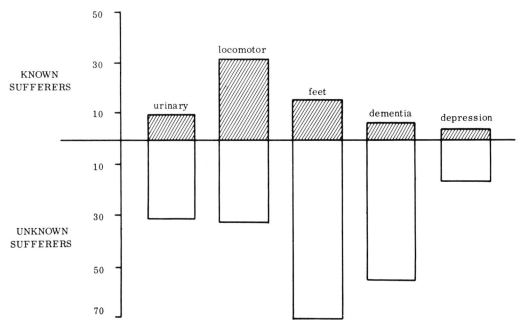

Fig. 5.1 Unknown disabilities in older persons. In disabilities where most of the iceberg is submerged, the practitioner's awareness is low. (Arie, 1981: With the permission of the editor and Croom Helm Publishers)

tend to shy away from since they are traditionally seen as unrewarding to diagnose and treat. The sufferers are not among the 'popular patients'! However, they are extremely important in several respects:

1. Anything which limits mobility is liable to lead to secondary consequencs of reduced social life and eventually to reduced ability to cope with the essentials of daily living.

2. Conditions associated with bladder disturbance are particularly irksome and the old lady who suffers from stress incontinence or the old man with prostatism are not only inconvenienced by their condition but are liable to be aware that their clothes may become malodorous and their social acceptance and confidence are eroded.

3. Any mental disturbance whether it be dementia or depression will have obvious dangers and treatment and appropriate support may be urgently necessary if rapid deterioration is to be avoided.

THE PROCESS OF CASE FINDING IN OLD AGE

The planned attempt to uncover some of the submerged iceberg or poorly reported disabling states is known as case finding which is now accepted as an important contribution of primary medical care towards the health and well-being of the elderly.

There has been a persistence of confusion over the roles of screening (as described previously) and case finding, and the development of case finding has perhaps been retarded because of the criticisms that have been levelled at some aspects of multiphasic screening. Attempts to validate case finding have also proved extremely difficult mainly because the search tended to be centred upon the identification of pathology and, in old age, the results of pathological changes may be extremely variable, for example one old person with a measured degree of hearing loss (on pure tone audiometry) may have better effective hearing than another with the same audiogram but who also has a significant degree of dementia. It is common knowledge that a degree of osteoarthrosis of knees which renders one individual severely dependent, may in another lead only to minor incapacity. Chamberlain (1973) tried to investigate the accuracy and reproducibility of case finding in the elderly but, because the search was for pathology, found the results very discouraging.

It is therefore logical in case finding to concentrate upon the detection of functional loss as opposed to the identification of pathological processes. The process embraces the detection of loss of physical function, mental function and social (including family) function. Clearly such a broad-based enquiry involving not only the patient but her family and other supporters must be the responsibility of the primary medical care team. It would seem fairly obvious that the team member most appropriate for this form of case finding is the Health Visitor (or Public Health Nurse) who possesses extra training in preventive

medicine. However it is probable that interest and natural aptitude are at least as important as formal training in this field, and it has been shown that a nurse (with general training only) may rapidly acquire proficiency in the assessment of medical and psychiatric problems in the elderly (Milne et al, 1972).

The case finding procedure

There remains uncertainty as to the actual scope of case finding and where it should be carried out. If the search is for pathology or for the detection of precursors of disease then the process is most appropriately conducted at the doctor's office or at a 'screening centre' since the technical requirements may be concentrated there. Pike (1976) carried out a screening exercise in which elderly subjects were encouraged to come to his office and be interviewed by team members. This process was shown to be of some benefit to elderly subjects but relatively poor acceptance rates were achieved.

The author is convinced that, for case finding aimed at the detection of loss of function as outlined above, the correct place to do it is in the patient's home. It is after all her ability to live comfortably and safely in that environment which is the principal concern of the enquiry and this can only be determined by seeing the patient there. A home visit paid by an experienced observer will yield a huge amount of vital information not only upon the patient's general health and function but also about the dangers from the environment, the suitability of equipment and furniture, the adequacy of cooking and heating equipment etc. The general state of the household may tell at a glance just how capable the old person is of safe living in her home.

Inspection of medication in the household is also an important part of any such enquiry (Arcand & Williamson, 1981). The general atmosphere within the house particularly the state of mind and morale of family members (or other carers) may likewise be of the greatest importance and this also can best be assessed at a home visit.

I have suggested that the case finding nurse might follow a simple check list of items for enquiry and these I have divided into two levels– 1. observations which the nurse makes and acts upon herself (Table 5.1) and 2. observations which she makes and which lead to referral to the general practitioner (Table 5.2).

In addition to what is described in Table 5.1 the nurse observer should enquire as to the existence of more specifically medical problems and if present, patients should be referred to the general practitioner.

Tables 5.1 & 5.2 therefore list the most important categories of functional loss which should be included in any case finding scheme. The next problem is to decide to whom this process should be offered. Some have suggested

Table 5.1 Suggested check list for case finding in the home: Level 1 – Detect and act

Observation	Action
Evidence of loneliness social isolation and withdrawal	Counselling patient and family. Invoking voluntary agencies, day centre attendance
Effects of relocation (rehousing, admission to institution etc)	Counselling. Introduction to local agencies and facilities. Stimulation of family activity
Family neglect or inadequacy	Find out the background cause. Counsel family, contact voluntary agencies. Help towards installation of telephone
Family under stress – expressions of resentment, anger culminating in 'rejection'	Counsel family. Arrange help, e.g. day centre attendance, respite admission. Offer of future continuing help
Apprehension and mis-giving in patient's mind (fear of falls, vandalism, violence)	Reassurance. Installation of radio alarm system. Make environment safer. Alert family or other protectors
Dangers of hypothermia – cold damp rooms, inadequate heating or insulation	Advice on clothing, heating insulation, draught suppression. Financial help with heating costs etc
Diet — assessment of food intake, dentition, cooking arrangements adequacy of food stores	Dietary advice. Weight reduction. Adequate fibre in diet
Medication – inspect drugs in the home, check if patient understands the purpose and regime	Patient should be aware of drug use and the recommended dosage. Simplify regime or invoke help from a family member or other carer

Table 5.2 Suggested check list for case finding in the home: Level 2 – Detect and refer

Nature of problems for enquiry and referral to a GP	
Cardiorespiratory	Cough, dyspnoea, orthopnoea, wheeze, sputum production Presence of cyanosis, cardiac dysrhythmia or oedema
Locomotor disability	Difficulty in walking due to pain or joint stiffness. Examine gait and footwear, look at joints
Bladder disturbance	Existence of frequency, nocturia, dysuria. Any form of incontinence or prostatism
Bowel disturbance	Constipation or diarrhoea. Recent change in bowel habit. Painful defaecation, blood in stool. Laxative abuse
Postural disturbance	History of falls, syncope or unsteady gait. Evidence of postural hypotension, hazards in the home environment
Vision	Simple assessment of ability to read newsprint, recognise individuals across the street. Examination of existing spectacles
Hearing	Is conversation strained or difficult? Is it necessary to raise the voice or make repetitions?

that case finding of some sort should be offered to all old people 'on demand'. This would certainly be a gross waste of scarce resources and its main result would be to reduce the help available to the most needy. Some form of selection is therefore necessary and the following suggestions are advanced:

1. The aged, i.e. those aged 85 years or more. Akhtar et al (1973) showed that four-fifths of this age group needed help to cope with the ordinary demands of day-to-day living. This is therefore a group which warrants surveillance since those who are not receiving necessary help may be headed for trouble and deterioration in health.

2. The lonely or isolated who have suffered loss of social contacts and are suffering as a result. This is a difficult group to identify since some although apparently lonely are in their own eyes entirely self-sufficient and require no help at all.

3. The bereaved, the most common sufferer being a widow who originally married a man older than herself and whose life expectancy is, in any case, greater than his in virtue of her female sex.

4. Those who have recently been in hospital. It must be emphasised that for those who manifested any evidence of self neglect at the time of admission, some special form of surveillance is essential after discharge because of the virtual certainty of future deterioration and trouble.

5. Those who have been relocated for any cause whether it be rehousing or admission to any form of institutional care.

6. Those already labelled as having special difficulties, e.g. in receipt of supplementary benefits, home help or community nursing services.

In addition to the above suggestions each district should take steps to identify individual high risk groups of elderly, for example those living in large housing estates where vandalism may be rife or those in deprived inner city areas where petty crime and violence may bear especially hard upon the elderly.

Barber et al (1980) attempted to identify old people in special need by sending them a simple questionnaire of nine items to which a simple Yes/No response was requested. This achieved an 81% response rate and could be used as a means of deciding which individuals warranted further case finding activity.

How valuable is case finding?

As in so many medical activities which seem to be logical and generally 'a good idea', thorough evaluation of case finding has not yet been carried out. An Edinburgh study reported the outcome of a case finding programme among 300 consecutive patients at 18–30 months after initial involvement (Lowther et al, 1970). This case finding was rather a mixture of screening as defined earlier and case finding and at follow-up 29% of the total were judged to be still benefiting from their involvement. Williams (1974) found that 27% of subjects were classed as benefiting at a yearly follow-up and Pike (1976) claimed that screening as practised by him and his team-mates led to lower consultation rates (compared to those reported in the National Morbidity Study). Tulloch and Moore (1979) described a randomised controlled trial of case finding among persons aged 70 and over. This study centred upon one practice and numbers were hence rather small. The only significant difference between test and control subjects over a two year period was that the former group had shorter hospital inpatient stay.

The present position is that there is an urgent need for clarification upon the exact screening process, how and where it ought to be carried out and by whom. Once these requirements have been met it will be necessary to conduct careful research to determine benefits in terms of enhanced life satisfaction, degree of independence, use of services and family satisfaction with results.

SUMMARY

Prevention, having been in the doldrums for some decades is now re-establishing its value. Primary prevention must always remain the ideal to be sought after but its application must generally be among the younger members of society. Screening for precursor states in old age has little present value and there are dangers of diverting scarce resources into this field with little or no ensuing benefits.

Secondary prevention means 'early diagnosis' and is therefore even more relevant in old age than in younger groups.

Tertiary prevention in the form of case finding is the most directly relevant aspect of prevention in old age. There is a need to define more accurately the groups who justify special surveillance, to describe in more detail the actual case finding process and to evaluate its effects upon individual old people, their families and health and social services.

REFERENCES

Akhtar A J, Bore G A, Crombie A , McLean W M R, Andrews G R, Caird F I 1973 Disability and dependency in the elderly at home. Age and aging 2: 102–111
Anderson W F, Cowan N 1955 A consultative health centre for older people: The Rutherglen Experiment. Lancet 2: 239
Anianson A, Grinby G, Rundgren A, Svanborg A, Orlander J 1980 Physical training in old men. Age and Ageing 9: 186–187
Arcand M, Williamson J 1981 An evaluation of home visiting of patients by physicians in geriatric medicine. British Medical Journal 283: 718–720
Arie T (ed) 1981 Essays in Health Care of the Elderly, Croom Helm, London
Barber J H, Wallis J B McKeating E 1980 Postal screening questionnaire in preventive geriatric care. Journal of Royal College of General Practitioners 30: 49–51
Barker W H, Mullooly J P 1980 Influenza vaccination of elderly persons. Reduction in pneumonia and influenza hospitalizations and deaths. Journal of the American Medical Association 244: 2547–2549
Bently D W, Ha K, Mamot K, Moon D, Moore L, Poletto P, Springett A 1981 Pneumococcal vaccine in the institutionalised elderly: Design of a nonrandomised trial and preliminary results. Review of Infectious Diseases 3 (supplement): 71–81
Butler A, Oldman C 1981 Alarm Systems for the Elderly: Report of a workshop held at the Univeristy of Leeds. Sept 1980. Department of Social Policy and Administration, University of Leeds
Chamberlain J O P 1973 Screening elderly people. Proceedings of the Royal Society of Medicine 66: 38–39

Cutler J, Ramcharan S, Feldman R, Siegelaub A B, Campbell C, Friedman G D, Dales L G, Collen M F 1973 Multiphasic check-up evaluation study, 1–3. Preventive Medicine 2: 197
Department of Health and Social Security 1976 Prevention and health: Everybody's business. HMSO, London
Douglas R G, Bently D W, Brandriss M W 1977 Responses of elderly and chronically ill subjects to bivalent influenza A/New Jersey/8/76 (HSW INT) – A/Victoria 3/75 (H3N2) Vaccine. Journal of Infectious Diseases 136 (supplement): 526–533
Ellis F P, Nelson F, Pincus L 1974 Mortality during heat waves in New York City July 1972 and August-September 1973. Environmental Research 10: 1–13
Evans J G, Prudham D, Wandless I 1980 Risk factors for stroke in the elderly. In: Barbagallo-Sangiorgi G, Exton-Smith A N (eds) The Ageing Brain. Plenum Press London p113–126
FDA Drug Bulletin 1978 Pneumococcal vaccine, polyvalent licensed. Jan-Feb 8: 4–5
Heller R F, Hayward D, Hobbs M S T 1983 Decline in rate in death from ischaemic heart disease in the United Kingdom. British Medical Journal 286: 260–262
Langer E J, Rodin J 1976 The effects of choice and enhanced personal responsibility: A field experiment in an institutional setting. Journal of Personality and Social Psychology 34: 191–198
Langer E J, Rodin J, Beck P, Weinman C, Spitzer L 1978 Environmental determinants of memory improvement in late adulthood. Journal of Personality and Social Psychology 37: 2003–2013
Lowther C P, McLeod R D M, Williamson J 1970 Evaluation of early diagnostic services for the elderly. British Medical Journal 3: 275–277

Milne J S 1981 A Longitudinal study of blood pressure and stroke in older people. Journal of Clinical and Experimental Gerontology 3: 135–159

Milne J S, Maule M M, Cormack S, Williamson J 1972 The design and testing of a questionnaire to assess physical and mental health in older people using a staff nurse as observer. Journal of Chronic Diseases 25: 385–405

Morris J N 1975 The Use of Epidemiology. Churchill Livingstone, Edinburgh

Oliver M F 1982 Risks of correcting the risk of coronary disease and stroke with drugs. New England Journal of Medicine 306: 297–298

Pike L A 1976 Screening the elderly in general practice. Journal of the Royal College of General Practitioners 26: 698–703

Plemons J K Willis S L, Bates P B 1978 Modifiability of fluid intelligence in aging: A short-term longitudinal training approach. Journal of Gerontology 33: 224–231

Ruben F L 1982 Prevention of influenza in the elderly. Journal of the American Geriatrics Society 30, 9: 577–580

Salvosa Carmencita B, Payne P R, Wheeler E F 1971 Environmental conditions and body temperatures of elderly women living alone or in local authority homes. British Medical Journal, ii: 656–659

Shock N 1977 Systems Integration. In: Hayflick L, Fiuch C E (Eds) Handbook of the Biology of Aging. Van Norstrand Rheinhold p 639–665

South-East London Screening Study Group 1977. International Journal of Epidemiology 6: 357

Stern M P 1979 The recent decline in ischaemic heart disease mortality. Annals of Internal Medicine 91: 630–640

Svanborg A, Williamson J 1980 Health Care of the elderly: Implications for education and training of physicians and other health care professionals. World Health Organisation Discussion Paper EUR/HCE/80/1

Thomson A P 1949 Problems of ageing and chronic sickness. British Medical Journal 2: 244–250 & 300–305

Tulloch A J, Moore V 1979 A randomised controlled trial of geriatric screening and surveillance in general practice. Journal of the Royal College of General Practitioners 29: 733–742

Walker W J 1977 Changing United States life-style and declining vascular mortality: Cause or coincidence? New England Journal of Medicine 297: 163–165

Warren M W 1943 Care of chronic sick. A case for treating chronic sick in blocks in a general hospital. British Medical Journal ii: 822–823

Williams I 1974 A follow-up of geriatric patients after sociomedical assessment. Journal of the Royal College of General Practitioners 24: 341–346

Williamson J 1979 Notes on the historical development of geriatric medicine as a medical specialty. Age and Ageing 8: 144–148

Williamson J, Stokoe I H, Gray S, Fisher M, Smith A, McGhee A, Stephenson E 1964 Old people at home: Their unreported needs. Lancet i: 1119–1120

Wollner L, McCarthy S T, Soper N W, Macy D J 1979 Failure of cerebral autoregulation as a cause of brain dysfunction in the elderly. British Medical Journal 1: 1117–1118

6

Nutrition

R. B. McGandy

INTRODUCTION

Improvements in nutrition and environmental quality, along with gains in health care, have lead to an increased average life expectancy at birth from 47 years in 1900 to 73 years in 1980. A greater proportion of our population survives to older age. Those over age 65 now constitute about 11% of the US population (about 13% in Europe), and this proportion is projected to rise to 17% by the year 2030. Thus medical practitioners will be devoting an increasing proportion of their time and efforts to the care of the elderly, a group which in the US today already accounts for over half of all federal health expenditures. Chronic, disabling conditions, as well as acute medical illnesses, occur more frequently and persist longer with increasing age. In the US in 1980, the elderly averaged 6.4 physician visits per year, a quarter required a period of hospitalisation, and 45% had a condition limiting their activity (Metropolitan Life Foundation, 1982). In the UK (Exton-Smith, 1982) men over age 65 have an average of 3.26 and women 3.42 diseases. Leading causes of restricted activity, either job or home (Metropolitan Life Foundation, 1982) are arthritis and rheumatism (12%), heart conditions (11%), hypertension (5.6%), visual impairments (2.9%) and diabetes (2.9%). Data such as these have raised interest in the possible role of nutrition in improving the quality of life among the elderly, in retarding some of the chronic diseases associated with aging, and even perhaps in mitigating some of the underlying age changes themselves.

But the possibilities of further gains in disease prevention and extension of longevity — by dietary modifications, control of deleterious personal health habits or sophisticated direct medical care — must be considered in the light of age-specific, secular trends in longevity. As provocatively presented by Fries (1980), there appears to be an upper limit on maximum life span. Since 1900, the increase in average life expectancy is almost completely attributable to decreased mortality in the first 3–4 decades of life. At age 45, average life expectancy has increased by only 9 years since 1900 and a part of this gain is due to the substantial decline in cardiovascular diseases within the past 15 years (Levy, 1981). For individuals at age 75 years,

life expectancy has improved by less than one year in this century. From these secular trends, Fries then predicts that the attainable average life expectancy in Western societies will be 85 years (slightly less for males and more for females) with a standard deviation of 4 years. Thus 95% of all deaths will occur in persons between 77 and 93 years of age. With this compression of mortality, owing to the prevention of 'premature' deaths in the 6th, 7th and 8th decades of life, further improvements in preventive practices and medical care will serve only to compress further the age range of terminal morbidity. Superimposed upon the increasing metabolic fragility of the aged and the concurrent presence of multiple chronic diseases, the average duration of terminal morbidity will be shortened.

Nutritional problems associated with aging throughout adult life and with the elderly have come to the forefront for several reasons. The first is that nutritional status surveys of the elderly have revealed a low to moderate prevalence of possible deficiencies in both institutionalised and non-institutionalised population groups. These judgements are based upon assessments of energy and nutrient intake, measurements of biochemical levels relevant to various specific nutrients, and on observations of clinical signs thought to be specifically associated with nutrient deficiencies. Uncertainty about standards of comparison presents a continuing problem in the interpretation of these sorts of data. Dietary and biochemical standards applicable to growth and development in early life and to pregnancy and lactation are more securely established than are standards applicable to adults. For many nutrients, adult standards have been derived from populations showing significant frequencies of deficiency disease or from studies in which deficiencies have been experimentally induced. For the elderly, present recommended dietary allowances are based upon extrapolations of our best estimates of nutrient requirements in healthy, young adults. In the US, there is some unease in the Food and Nutrition Board's (1980) catagorising individuals in a group of '51 years and above'. In light of present knowledge regarding the increased biological variability of the elderly — variability associated with the presence of one or more chronic diseases and with their increasingly restricted social circumstances — it seems unlikely that such a generalisation will ultimately be found appropriate. Developing ways of determining nutrient requirements in the elderly is a high priority of current nutrition research.

Secondly, nutrition has been linked to many of the chronic diseases which afflict older adults and the elderly. We are not yet certain of the potential of their retardation through dietary means. Salt, obesity and hypertension, fats and atherosclerotic cardiovascular disease, diet and cancer, diet and osteoporosis — each of these is a condition of multifactoral cause, each is an area of current investigation and even current controversy.

Thirdly, there is the question of whether nutritional status may modify the rates of decline in a wide variety of organ system functions. Most of our present knowledge of this facet of aging derives from laboratory animal studies and is still of uncertain relevance to human aging.

NUTRITION, THE AGING PROCESS, AND AGE ASSOCIATED CHRONIC DISEASES

The quest for dietary elixers to retard, prevent, or restore age-related decrements in cosmetic, physical and psychological functions is as old as recorded history. Even today the basis for much of the faddism and mystique of special foods and the use of dietary supplements, is their presumed role in maintaining youthful health and vigour. Aside from whatever imagined benefits these may confer, there is no acceptable evidence from laboratory animal studies — much less from human observations — that progressive, involutional changes can be retarded by supplements (Barrows & Roeder, 1977; Shock, 1982).

Present knowledge of age changes over adult life derives almost entirely from average rates of decrement in function inferred from a very limited number of cross-sectional population studies. Virtually all organ systems investigated in age decade groups averaging from 30 to 80 years show linear decreases in function, and particularly in complex, integrative functions examined by stressing the organ system to assess reserve capacity. This age-related loss of reserve capacity is mainly the result of cell loss with aging, the attrition of functional redundancy of young adulthood. To an unknown but probably lesser degree, it represents altered metabolism of remaining cells. As shown by the Baltimore Aging Study (Shock, 1977) from age 30 to 80 years, the rates of loss show a wide range. Nerve conduction time slows by 15%, resting cardiac index by 30%, vital capacity and renal blood flow by 50%, and maximal oxygen uptake by 70%. Similarly, there is an increasing delay in the time of return of blood sugar concentration to fasting level after an oral glucose tolerance test (Shock, 1977). Cross-sectional studies show no increase in fasting blood glucose with age, an example of a stress test

being needed to unmask age changes in a complex regulatory system. Other functional changes with age have been described for erythrocyte sedimentation rate (Sparrow et al, 1981), pulmonary capacities (Bosse et al, 1980) and immune response (Makinodan, 1978). Declines in the latter system may well have some relationships to nutritional status (Beisel et al, 1981) as may the linear increment in age pigment within human myocardial fibres reported by Strehler et al (1959).

With each of these age changes, however, there is almost as much variability between individuals within an age group as between age decade groups (Norris & Shock, 1966). This means that there are some 60 or 70 year old individuals with functional tests equivalent to the average 30 or 40 year old and, conversely, there are some younger individuals with reserve capacities equivalent to the average elder.

As cautioned by Exton-Smith (1982), there must be many reservations in conclusions based upon cross-sectional studies. The different age groups represent cohorts of individuals with quite different past dietary, environmental, and disease exposure. The older cohorts increasingly represent privileged survivors. There is the underlying problem of separating 'true' age changes from organ system alterations owing to the presence of a specific disease process. Causality can not be inferred from cross-sectional studies. Clearly we need longitudinal studies designed to uncover determinants of functional changes in the same individuals over time. Such studies are logistically complicated, expensive, and need to be of long duration.

What this means is that we cannot presently assign a net estimate of biological age (a functional index) to an individual. This makes it very difficult indeed to design satisfactory studies of factors, such as nutritional status, which may influence the rates of these involutional changes. The basis for at least some potential regulatory power of nutrition to shape these changes are the observations (Barrows & Roeder, 1977) the calorically undernourished laboratory animals, restricted from early life, have a considerable increase in average life expectancy and in maximal life span. These animals show a retardation in the rate of loss of many of the same functions which mark human aging (Everitt, 1982); they also show a delay in the chronological time of onset of the spectrum of specific types of degenerative diseases and neoplasia found in these species (Berg & Simms, 1960). There is the question, of course, as to what relevance these studies have to practical dietary habits and human aging.

There are inevitable age changes in body composition. It is presumed that a complex interplay of nutrition and other life style factors — exercise being an important one — can influence the rate of these compositional changes. Additionally, body composition changes may have implications for energy and nutrient requirements. Cross-sectional studies show an **age-related** loss in lean body mass

(Forbes & Reina, 1970; Cohn et al, 1982) and bone (Garn, 1978; Cohn et al, 1982). The former is accompanied by a compensatory gain in adipose tissue (Rossman, 1977). The major contributor to the loss in lean body mass is skeletal muscle which may decline as much as 45% over adult life (Cohn et al, 1982). Cellular loss in liver, kidneys, heart and lung (Rossman, 1977) leads to a decline in the weights of these organs and contributes to the overall loss in lean body mass. Loss of bone mass occurs in both sexes, though among women there is a marked acceleration after menopause. This, along with the initially smaller bone mass in young women, accounts for the greater frequency of osteoporosis-related fracture in older women than men. Many nutrients influence bone integrity. In particular, calcium and vitamin D may be closely related to adult loss in bone mass. As will be discussed presently, there is already some suggestion that the allowances for these nutrients should be increased.

As has been already mentioned, separating inevitable age-related organ system changes from changes related to specific chronic diseases has been a problem confounding aging studies. This is particularly true of diseases of the cardiovascular system because of the almost universal presence of atherosclerosis among adults and the elderly in industrialised societies. The subclinical presence of ischaemic disease, along with other degenerative diseases, must temper the many investigations reporting on 'healthy' or 'normal' elderly populations. Nonetheless, diet appears to play some role in several degenerative processes and thus offers the potential for some degree of retardation in the major contributors to morbidity and mortality.

Atherosclerotic vascular disease
In many countries, but not in the UK (Anonymous, 1982), there has been a 25–35% decline in mortality rates from atherosclerotic coronary heart disease over the past decade or so (Levy, 1981). As shown by Stern (1979), this decline is also shared by the elderly, even those over age 85. Changes in diet, smoking and exercise habits may be responsible. But the independent roles of the several possible contributing factors, including effective pharmacological management of hypertension, is now known. Attempts to demonstrate that modifications in the amount and type of dietary fats can lead to a reduced risk of ischaemic heart disease, have been inconsistent (Turpeinen et al, 1979; Multiple Risk Factor Intervention Trial Research Group, 1982) and controversial (Oliver, 1981). It appears that the predictive value of blood lipids (Bierman, 1978) and physical activity (Paffenbarger et al, 1970) diminish rapidly past age 50. And since the histopathology of atherosclerotic lesions in the fourth and fifth decades of life shows extensive fibrosis and calcification — surely less amenable to reversibility than the predominantly lipid lesions of younger adults — it may reasonably be argued that preventive efforts should begin in young adulthood.

Hypertension
While there is convincing evidence that drug therapy of hypertension can reduce mortality (Hypertension Detection and Follow-up Program Cooperative Group, 1979), the potential for prevention of the age-related rise in blood pressure and of hypertension through reduction of dietary sodium (Liu et al, 1979) or control of obesity (Reisin et al, 1978) is still uncertain (Tobian, 1979).

Cancer
The differences in site-specific cancer mortality rates between countries, between vegetarians and omnivores in the US, along with secular trends in some particular cancers have presented a new area for nutritional epidemiology. Gori (1979), Peto et al (1981) and Kolonel et al (1981) have reviewed this topic. The dietary components suggested by epidemiological or experimental animal studies are quite broad: high fat diets may be related to breast and colon cancer; insufficient vitamin A or its plant precursor, beta carotene, and vitamin C may enhance the carcinogenesis process. Certain non-nutrient components of food will also prove to be important. Among these are fibre, mixed-function oxidase inducers, and protease inhibitors. While vitamin E is popularly assumed to protect against cancer, experimental animal work does not support its effectiveness (Wattenberg, 1978).

Belloc & Breslow (1972) have shown that physical health status among elderly individuals is significantly related to nutritional health habits. Regularity of eating breakfast, infrequent snacking between meals, maintenance of weight within −5 to +20% of desirable weight, were independently and additively (along with sleeping, activity, smoking and alcohol habits) associated with better health. A subsequent report (Belloc, 1973) showed these health practices also to be good predictors of mortality after 5 years of follow-up.

Thus, the potential role of nutrition in human aging and chronic disease experience encompasses some elements of hope, some areas of controversy, and considerable investigative challenge.

EFFECTS OF AGE ON ESTIMATED ENERGY AND NUTRIENT REQUIREMENTS

Observations of daily food intake of populations show that from about the third decade of life, energy intake progressively decreases. On the whole this trend is paralleled by decreases in protein, minerals, and vitamins, although trends in specific micronutrients depend upon food choices. While the US Food and Nutrition Board (1980) provides for downward adjustments in energy allowances, neither protein nor micronutrients are so adjusted. The latter are maintained at middle-aged adult levels, the assumption being that consumption of mixed, varied diets will continue to meet the protein and micronutrient requirements of 95% of healthy persons. Is this so? Although we are far from certain about precise nutrient allowances for the elderly, there is accumulating evidence of potential problems which must be addressed in future deliberations of allowances for the elderly. The evidence derives from nutritonal status surveys of elderly population groups.

Data on food intake in large surveys is subject to errors. In particular, the variance between individuals is overestimated when one, two or even three day observation periods are used (Beaton et al, 1979). While it is assumed that average values of daily energy and nutrient intake are fairly comparable among surveys, the proportions at the low (and high) end of the distributions are exaggerated in studies utilising the relatively short observation periods. Nonetheless, it appears uniformly true that very low levels of average energy intake have been reported in studies of mainly urban elderly in the US, Canada, and Europe. Groups over age 70 years commonly appear to consume less than 1800 kcal per day in males and as low as 1300 kcal per day in females. And as is well known to dieticians, at energy intakes below 1800–2000 kcal, it demands increasingly judicious food selection to meet the allowances for many nutrients. In addition to this there are many problems faced by the elderly: poor food choices owing to living alone, poverty or mental depression; restricted ability to shop or to prepare foods owing to physical or mental disabilities; conditions affecting appetite; dentition problems; alcoholism; and less commonly, malabsorption or the use of drugs which influence nutrient metabolism. It is perhaps no surprise then that a significant proportion of the elderly fall below current dietary standards. The problems, however, are that the proportion not meeting one or another nutrient standard is exaggerated in surveys based upon short observation periods and that a low dietary intake does not, by itself, prove deficiency.

Nutritional surveillance and assessment should also include measurements of nutrient levels in body tissues, most commonly blood. Modern laboratory technology has allowed us, by these techniques, to get closer to estimates of biochemical adequacy in studies both of individuals and of populations. But here too there remain questions of the standards by which the nutrient values are interpreted. Levels labeled 'deficient', 'borderline' or 'low' may occur with significant prevalence in surveys of the elderly and yet, without clinical evidence of frank deficiency. It is very difficult to relate these to a quantifiable, functional impairment. Thus a central problem in evaluating nutrient requirements in older persons is the lack of appropriate criteria of adequacy.

Energy

The adult energy allowances of the US Food and Nutrition Board (1980) are proposed as average needs adequate to maintain a desirable body weight. These are expressed as a range ± 400 kcal which is the approximate size of one standard deviation of energy intakes observed in population studies. Thus about 70% of a specific age and sex group's energy needs would be expected to lie within this range. For males and females aged 51 to 75 years, adult allowances are reduced by 200 kcal per day, and by 500 kcal per day in individuals over the age of 76. For females in the older age group the allowance is 1600 kcal (1200–2000 range) and for males 2050 kcal (1650–2450 range).

These decreased allowances beyond the age of 50 are partly based upon the approximate 2% per decade decline in basal metabolic requirements (owing to the decline in lean body mass). But the more important contributor is ascribed to the diminished levels of discretionary energy expenditure associated with contemporary, urban, Western societies. For example, in a cross-sectional survey of middle-class males in Baltimore, McGandy et al (1966) observed a decline in average energy intake of 2700 kcal at the age of 30 to 2100 kcal per day at the age of 90. Of the 600 kcal per day decline, 200 kcal were accounted for by decreased basal needs and 400 kcal by decreased physical activity. Low intakes of energy in individuals over the age of 65 years have been observed in many other studies as well. In the US nutrition survey (Abraham et al, 1979a), intakes in this age group were 1800 kcal in males and 1300 kcal in females. Among nursing home patients observed by Stiedemann et al (1978), male and female energy intakes averaged 1720 kcal and 1333 kcal respectively. Thus the observed intakes are below the recommended allowances, particularly among females. The impact of a more active lifestyle on total food intake has been demonstrated by the careful dietary studies by Debry et al (1977) of urban and rural elderly women in the Lorraine region of France. Among women over the age of 74, the daily energy intake of the urban group was 1592 kcal and of the rural group, 2155 kcal — a difference of over 500 kcal per day! This in itself, of course, has important implications for dietary quality in terms of protein, vitamins and minerals. The allowances for the latter assume overall food intakes often considerably exceeding the observed levels, especially among females.

A corollary question is whether or not desirable weights (at low levels of energy expenditure) are actually being achieved. In the US (Abraham et al, 1979b; Bowman & Rosenberg, 1982) the prevalence of obesity as assessed by relative weight for height is high: 12% of males and 30% of females aged 65–74 years were 20% or more over ideal weights. Furthermore, in the decade between 1960 and 1970 the trends were toward increasing obesity, particularly among males (Bowman & Rosenberg, 1982). While the reputed mortality disadvantages of obesity at levels of up to 20% above desirable weight have been questioned (Andres, 1980; Keys, 1980), the contribution of physical inactivity both to obesity and to morbidity and well-being of the elderly should be further examined. Improvements in cardiovascular and pulmonary functions, lessening of stress on weight bearing osteoarthritic joints, perhaps even retarding the rate of bone loss would seem reasonable goals in programmes aimed at modest increases in physical activity and prevention of gross obesity among the elderly. Even small increases in food intake would improve dietary quality.

Protein
The protein allowance is 0.8 g/kg body weight; for the 'average' 55 kg female this is 44 g per day and for a 70 kg male, 56 g per day. Considering that the average daily protein intake in the US (Abraham et al, 1979a) is below the recommended level, and that the elderly may have increased variability in their individual requirements owing to the more frequent stress of illness (Munro, 1981), there may be a significant proportion of this age group at an increased risk of deficiency. The recent report of Gersovitz et al (1982) has shown that not all of their elderly study subjects remained in nitrogen balance at 0.8 g/kg.

On the other hand, among younger adults the intake of protein in the US (Abraham et al, 1979) is well above the recommended allowance. Brenner et al (1982) have expressed the concern that relatively high protein diets may be a major cause of the progressive loss of reserve renal function with aging.

Fat
As discussed earlier in this chapter, there is not yet complete certainty that diets lower in total fat, saturated fat and cholesterol can retard the risks of atherosclerotic vascular disease, certainly not among the elderly. On the other hand, such diets would seem to be prudent advice for the elderly, particularly if the fat 'deficit' were compensated for by an increased consumption of whole cereal grains, vegetables, and fruits — all sources of fibre and many micronutrients.

Carbohydrate
Both dental and peridontal disease in the elderly have been associated with refined dietary carbohydrates, sucrose being the major example (Bierman, 1979). Deemphasis on refined sugars and the substitution of complex carbohydrates from grains and vegetables would also enhance micronutrient intake. It would also lead to an increased intake of dietary fibre. The potential health benefits of perhaps doubling the current 'typical' fibre intake of 15–20 g per day have been reviewed by Mendeloff (1977). Several epidemiological studies have suggested significant health benefits either from dietary fibre itself (Kromhout et al, 1982) or from the lower dietary fat intake which inevitably accompanies the high fibre diets consumed by Seventh-Day Adventist populations in the US (Marsh et al, 1980; Gorbach et al, 1982). This vegetarian religious group has lower mortality rates from cancer and atherosclerotic vascular disease; post-menopausal women have less osteoporosis than omnivorous, comparison females. The situation is, however, not completely clear since Adventists also do not smoke or use alcohol; additionally, they may differ in other life style factors — physical activity, for example — which could also influence disease risk.

Micronutrients
For the US dietary intakes presented below, the percentage of the population consuming less than two thirds of the recommended allowance of the specified nutrient is cited. This is a common way of expressing the proportion 'at risk' of an inadequate intake. These data are derived from the publication of Bowman & Rosenberg (1982) and are based on the health and nutrition examination survey (HANES) results concerning persons aged 65–74 (Abraham et al, 1979a). Comparison intake data from Belfast, similarly expressed, are cited from the publication of Vir & Love (1979); these are based upon a very careful investigation of 196 subjects over the age of 65.

Calcium
In HANES, up to 60% of the males and 66% of the females had a low intake of this mineral. Heaney et al (1982) have extensively reviewed the literature relating calcium intake and the loss of bone which accompanies aging. Calcium intake is low in most Western adult and elderly population groups. Dairy products are consumed with decreasing frequency and overall energy consumption is low. Furthermore, calcium absorption decreases with age. These authors have concluded that the allowance for this nutrient should be increased to 1200 or even 1500 mg per day.

Iron
Both HANES and Belfast elderly showed a substantial prevalence of low dietary iron: 25–50%. Although haemoglobin concentration tends to diminish with age, Lynch et al (1982) have concluded that the still limited data on iron stores in the elderly do not document an important iron deficiency problem in this age group.

Trace metals
Incomplete food table values and limited studies utilising newer chemical methods leave us with very little data on zinc, copper, chromium and selenium status of the elderly. Sandstead et al (1982) have concluded that zinc deficiency, owing to low dietary intake, is a potential problem and one that requires further research because of the relationship of zinc nutriture to wound healing and immune function.

Vitamin A
Based upon dietary intake and vitamin A serum levels, neither HANES nor Belfast have suggested a basis for

concern regarding this micronutrient. On the other hand, liver vitamin A levels measured in an autopsy survey in Canada (Hoppner et al, 1969) showed a high frequency of very low values among adults. This raises the question as to the appropriateness of a blood level to the assessment of nutrient status. This is yet another area of research needed to provide the basis for determining nutrient requirements.

Vitamin D
Serum 25, hydroxyvitamin D levels were measured in a subsample in the Belfast study and in a group of elderly in the US (Omdahl et al, 1982). In both populations there was a substantial prevalence of low values, particularly among females. This study also showed a seasonal trend in the serum levels; values were highest at the end of the summer season. Parfitt et al (1982) have reviewed the data relating vitamin D to bone loss in the elderly. They have concluded that age-related decrease in vitamin D intake, the decreased intestinal absorption and the decreased skin synthesis of this vitamin, all contribute to the low serum values observed. They recommend that the daily allowance be increased to 15 to 20 μg (600 to 800 IU).

Thiamin
Both HANES and the Belfast studies showed that 20–40% of the population had an inadequate intake of this vitamin. Enzymatic functional assessment (red blood cell transketolase) of thiamin status in Belfast showed low or deficient values in 15% of the group. There is current uncertainty as to whether some common peripheral and central nervous system changes in the elderly (loss of reflexes, disturbances of gait, loss of memory, dizziness) are related to a deficiency of this vitamin. In a recent review of thiamin and aging (Iber et al, 1982), the authors have concluded that there is yet no proof of an association other than in elderly alcoholics with frank thiamin deficiency.

Riboflavin, niacin, vitamin B-6
For each of these water-soluble vitamins there is some evidence of a significant prevalence of low intakes and of low biochemical indices. But it remains to be determined whether or how these nutrients are related to the health of the elderly.

Vitamin C
In the United States, the prevalence of low serum ascorbic acid levels has been very small. This is in contrast to the Belfast study in which up to one half of some subgroups had low serum levels. Serum distributions of this nutrient are lower in elderly males than in females (even though dietary intakes are higher among males); levels are also lower in smokers than non-smokers. In an elderly population in New Mexico, Garry et al (1982b) have examined the relationship between dietary intakes and serum levels of vitamin C. They concluded that, in order to

maximise the body ascorbic acid pool, the daily dietary allowances would need to be 150 mg and 75 mg for males and females respectively. Here too, there remains the key issue as to whether measurable health benefits would be achieved. This issue was addressed, but not resolved, in the supplemental vitamin C study reported by Schorah et al (1979). These authors noted equivocal improvements in the clinical status of elderly hospital patients given large daily supplements (1000 mg) of this nutrient.

Folacin
Rosenberg et al (1982) have reviewed the issue of the status of this nutrient to the relative anaemia of the aged. In the US, up to 20% of elderly groups have low serum folacin levels; in Belfast the prevalence of low values was as high as 60% in some subgroups. Rosenberg et al have concluded, however, that folacin deficiency is not an important cause of the anaemia of the elderly and have pointed out that alcohol intake, which can depress folate absorption, may be partly responsible for low serum values.

Vitamin B-12
There is little evidence from US surveys (Bowman & Rosenberg, 1982) or from the Belfast survey (Vir & Love, 1979) that a deficiency of this vitamin is a significant haematologial or health problem in the elderly.

Use of vitamin-mineral supplements in elderly populations
In several recent studies within the US, the use of nutritional supplements among elderly groups has been assessed. In ambulatory, non-institutionalised populations in Florida (Hale et al, 1982) and New Mexico (Garry et al, 1982a), regular use of single or multiple vitamin-mineral supplements was observed in up to 60% of the population. As has been shown by Vir & Love (1979), these supplements do indeed improve the biochemical indices and do reduce the prevalence of low serum values. While the health risks of doses within the ranges of recommended allowances are negligible, the health benefits are unknown and the economic costs to many elderly are substantial.

CONCLUSION

Since age changes in body function and composition progress throughout adult life, nutritional and other health practices aimed at slowing involutional changes in the elderly must become life-long habits. Beyond this, there is no current evidence that use of dietary supplements will provide a simple solution to the assurance of a healthy and vigorous old age. Frank nutrient deficiencies seen in the elderly are usually associated with serious illness, prolonged hospitalisation, alcoholism, malabsorptive states or social isolation. As with younger adults, these must be recognised and treated. Present criteria for determining nutritional adequacy still leave uncertainty as to the health consequences of the marginal nutritional status found in some elderly population groups. Nutrient intakes of many elderly could be significantly improved by increasing food intake; with even modest increases in physical activity, this can be done without leading to weight gain. Moreover, increased activity may well lead to improved

cardiovascular-pulmonary function and to a sense of well-being.

The most likely contribution of diet to better health of the elderly will be through its role in reducing or delaying several major chronic diseases: atherosclerotic vascular disease, hypertension, osteoporosis and neoplasia. Each has evidence for nutritional involvement in its pathogenesis; each awaits proof from clinical trials that practical dietary modifications are in fact effective.

REFERENCES

Abraham S, Carroll M D, Johnson C L, Dresser C M V 1979a Caloric and selected nutrient values for persons 1–74 years of age: United States, 1971–1974. US Department of Health, Education and Welfare Publication No (PHS) 79–1657, Hyattsville, Maryland

Abraham S, Johnson C L, Najjar M F 1979b Weight by height and age for adults 18–74 years: United States, 1971–74. US Department of Health, Education and Welfare Publication No (PHS) 79–1656, Hyattsville, Maryland

Andres R 1980 Effect of obesity on total mortality. International Journal of Obesity 4: 381–386

Anonymous 1982 Mortality from coronary heart disease. Lancet ii: 507

Barrows C H, Roeder L M 1977 Nutrition. In: Finch C E, Hayflick L (eds) Handbook of the Biology of Aging, Van Nostrand Reinhold, New York, ch 23

Beaton G H, Milner J, Corey P, McGuire V, Cousins M, Stewart E et al 1979 Sources of variance in 24-hour dietary recall data: implications of nutrition study design and interpretation. American Journal of Clinical Nutrition 32: 2456–2559

Beisel W R, Edelman R, Nauss K, Suskind R M 1981 Single nutrient effects on immunological functions. Journal of the American Medical Association 245: 53–58

Belloc N B 1973 Relationship of health practices and mortality. Preventive Medicine 2: 67–81

Belloc N B, Breslow L 1972 Relationship of physical health status and health practices. Preventive Medicine 1: 409–421

Berg B N, Simms H S 1960 Nutrition and longevity in the rat. Journal of Nutrition 71: 255–263

Bierman E L 1978 Atherosclerosis and aging. Federation Proceedings 37: 2832–2836

Bierman E L 1979 Carbohydrates, sucrose, and human disease. American Journal of Clinical Nutrition 32: 2712–2722

Bosse R, Sparrow D, Garvey A J, Costa P T, Weiss S T, Rowe J W 1980 Cigarette smoking, aging and decline in pulmonary function: a longitudinal study. Archives of Environmental Health 35: 247–252

Bowman B B, Rosenberg I H 1982 Assessment of the nutritional status of the elderly. American Journal of Clinical Nutrition 35: 1142–1151

Brenner B M, Meyer T W, Hostetter T H 1982 Dietary protein intake and the progressive nature of kidney disease. New England Journal of Medicine 307: 652–659

Cohn S H, Vaswani A N, Vartsky D, Yasumura S, Sawitsky A, Gartenhaus W et al 1982 In vivo quantification of body nitrogen for nutritional assessment. American Journal of Clinical Nutrition 35: 1186–1191

Debry G, Bleyer R, Martin J M 1977 Nutrition of the elderly. Journal of Human Nutrition 31: 195–203

Everitt A V 1982 Nutrition and the hypothalamic-pituitary influence on aging. In: Moment G B (ed) Nutritional Approaches to Aging Research, CRC Press, Boca Raton, ch 13

Exton-Smith A N 1982 Epidemiological studies in the elderly: methodological considerations. American Journal of Clinical Nutrition 35: 1273–1279

Food and Nutrition Board 1980 Recommended Dietary Allowances, 9th edn. National Academy of Sciences, Washington, DC

Forbes G B, Reina J C 1970 Adult lean body mass declines with age: some longitudinal observations. Metabolism 19: 653–663

Fries J F 1980 Aging, natural death, and the compression of morbidity. New England Journal of Medicine 303: 130–135

Garn S M 1978 Bone loss and aging. In: Farmer F A (ed) Nutrition of the Aged, University of Calgary, Alberta

Garry P J, Goodwin J S, Hunt W C, Hooper E M, Leonard A G 1982a Nutritional status in a healthy elderly population: dietary and supplement intakes. American Journal of Clinical Nutrition 36: 319–331

Garry P J, Goodwin J S, Hunt W C, Gilbert B A 1982b Nutritional status in a healthy elderly population: vitamin C. American Journal of Clinical Nutrition 36: 332–339

Gersovitz M, Motil K, Munro H N, Scrimshaw N S, Young V 1982 Human protein requirements: assessment of the adequacy of the current Recommended Dietary Allowance for dietary protein in elderly men and women. American Journal of Clinical Nutrition 35: 6–14

Goldin B R, Adlercreutz H, Gorbach S L, Warram J H, Dwyer J T, Swenson L S et al 1982 Estrogen excretion patterns and plasma levels in vegetarian and omniverous women. New England Journal of Medicine 307: 1542–1547

Gori G B 1979 Dietary and nutritional implications in the multifactoral etiology of certain prevalent human cancers. Cancer 43: 2151–2161

Hale W E, Stewart R B, Cerda J J, Marks R G, May F E 1982 Use of nutritional supplements in an ambulatory elderly population. Journal of the American Geriatrics Society 30: 401–403

Heaney R P, Gallagher J C, Johnston C C, Neer R, Parfitt A M, Whedon G D 1982 Calcium nutrition and bone health in the elderly. American Journal of Clinical Nutrition 36: 986–1013

Hoppner K, Phillips W E J, Erody P, Murray T K, Perrin D E 1969 Vitamin A reserves of Canadians. Canadian Medical Association Journal 101: 736–738

Hypertension Detection and Follow-up Program Cooperative Group 1979 Five-year findings of the hypertension detection and follow-up program. Journal of American Medical Assocation 242: 2562–2571

Iber F L, Blass J P, Brin M, Leevy C M 1982 Thiamin in the elderly — relation to alcoholism and to neurological degenerative disease. American Journal of Clinical Nutrition 36: 1067–1082

Keys A 1980 Overweight, obesity, coronary heart disease, and mortality. Nutrition Reviews 38: 297–307

Kolonel L N, Nomura A M Y, Hirohata T, Hankin J H, Hinds M W 1981 Association of diet and place of birth with stomach cancer incidence in Hawaii Japanese and Caucasians. American Journal of Clinical Nutrition 34: 2478–2485

Kromhout D, Bosschieter E B, Coulander C L 1982 Dietary fibre and 10-year mortality from coronary heart disease, cancer and all causes. Lancet ii: 518–522

Levy R I 1981 The decline in cardioavascular disease mortality. Annual Review of Public Health 2: 49–70

Liu K, Cooper R, McKeever J, McKeever P, Byington R, Soltero I et al 1979 Assessment of the association between habitual salt intake and high blood pressure: methodological problems. American Journal of Epidemiology 110: 219–226

Lynch S R, Finch C A, Monsen E R, Cook J D 1982 Iron status of elderly Americans. American Journal of Clinical Nutrition 36: 1032–1045

Makinodan T 1978 Mechanism of senescence of immune response. Federation Proceedings 37: 1239–1240

Marsh A G, Sanchez T V, Mickelsen O, Keiser J, Mayor G 1980 Cortical bone density of adult lacto-ovo-vegetarian and omniverous women. Journal of The American Dietetic Association 76: 148–151

McGandy R B, Barrows C H, Spanias A, Meredith A, Stone J L, Norris A H 1966 Nutrient intakes and energy expenditure in men of different ages. Journal of Gerontology 21: 581–587

Mendeloff A I 1977 Dietary fibre and human health. New England Journal of Medicine 297: 811–814

Metropolitan Life Foundation 1982 Health of the elderly. Statistical Bulletin 63: 3–5

Multiple Risk Factor Intervention Trial Research Group 1982 Multiple risk factor intervention trial. Journal of American Medical Association 248: 1465–1477

Munro H N 1981 Nutrition and aging. British Medical Bulletin 37: 83–88

Norris A H, Shock N W 1966 Aging and variability. Annals New York Academy of Sciences 134: 591–601

Oliver M F 1981 Serum cholesterol — the knave of hearts and the joker. Lancet ii: 1090–1095

Omdahl J L, Garry P J, Hunseker L A, Hunt M A, Goodwin J S 1982 Nutritional status in a healthy elderly population: vitamin D. American Journal of Clinical Nutrition 36: 1225–1233

Paffenbarger R S, Laughlin M E, Gima A S, Black R A 1970 Work activity of longshoremen as related to death from coronary heart disease and stroke. New England Journal of Medicine 282: 1109–1114

Parfitt A M, Gallagher J C, Heaney R P, Johnston C C, Neer R, Whedon G D 1982 Vitamin D and bone health in the elderly. American Journal of Clinical Nutrition 36: 1014–1031

Peto R, Doll R, Buckley J D, Sporn M B 1981 Can dietary beta-carotene materially reduce human cancer rates? Nature 290: 201–208

Reisin E, Abel R, Modan M, Silverberg D S, Eliahou H E, Modan B 1978 Effect of weight loss without salt restriction on the reduction of blood pressure in overweight hypertensive patients. New England Journal of Medicine 298: 1–6

Rosenberg I H, Bowman B B, Cooper B A, Halsted C H, Lindenbaum J 1982 Folate nutrition in the elderly. American Journal of Clinical Nutrition 36: 1060–1066

Rossman I 1977 Anatomic and body composition changes with aging. In: Finch C E, Hayflick L (eds) Handbook of the Biology of Aging. Van Nostrand Reinhold, New York, ch 8

Sandstead H H, Henriksen L K, Greger J L, Prasad A S, Good R A 1982 Zinc nutriture in the elderly in relation to taste acuity, immune response, and wound healing. American Journal of Clinical Nutrition 36: 1046–1059

Schorah C J, Newill A, Scott D L, Morgan D B 1979 Clinical effects of vitamin C in elderly inpatients with low blood vitamin C levels. Lancet i: 403–405

Shock N W 1977 Systems integration. In: Finch C E, Hayflik L (eds) Handbook of the Biology of Aging, Van Nostrand Reinhold, New York ch 25

Shock N W 1982 The role of nutrition in aging. Journal of the American College of Nutrition 1: 3–9

Sparrow D, Rowe J W, Silbert J E 1981 Cross-sectional and longitudinal changes in erythrocyte sedimentation rate in men. Journal of Gerontology 36: 180–184

Stern M P 1979 The recent decline in ischemic heart mortality. Annals of Internal Medicine 91: 630–640

Stiedemann M, Jansen C, Herill I 1978 Nutritional status of elderly men and women. Journal of The American Dietetic Association 73: 132–139

Strehler B L, Mark D D, Mildvan A S, Gee M V 1959 Rate and magnitude of age pigment accumulation in the human myocardium. Journal of Gerontology 14: 430–439

Tobian L 1979 The relationship of salt to hypertension. American Journal of Clinical Nutrition 32: 2739–2748

Turpeinen O, Karvonen M J, Pekkarinen M, Miettinen M, Elosuo R, Paavilainen E 1979 Dietary prevention of coronary heart disease: the Finnish mental hospital study. International Journal of Epidemiology 8: 99–118

Vir S C, Love A H G 1979 Nutritional status of institutionalised and noninstitutionalised aged in Belfast, Northern Ireland. American Journal of Clinical Nutrition 32: 1934–1937

Wattenburg L W 1978 Inhibitors of chemical carcinogenesis. Advances in Cancer Research 26: 197–226

7

Pharmacological aspects of therapeutics

K. O'Malley & F. Meagher

INTRODUCTION

Pharmacology can be taken to mean virtually all matters to do with drugs so that it may lean heavily on sociology, psychology and epidemiology in addition to a consideration of the physical interaction of man (or animal) with drugs. In the present chapter some of the broader implications will be dealt with because often in the elderly these may dominate in determining how the patient responds (or fails to respond) to the drug prescription written by his doctor (Table 7.1). However, most emphasis will be placed on the physiological, biochemical and pathological changes attendant on aging that may affect the pattern of response observed.

Table 7.1 From prescription to drug effect

Prescription
Administration
Pharmacokinetics
  Absorption
  Distribution
  Metabolism
  Excretion

Drug Concentration at site of action
Pharmacodynamics
  Receptors
    number
    affinity
  Post receptor events
    biochemical
    physical
    electrical

Aging is a process which involves deterioration of structure and function and as drug effects represent perturbation of pathological and physiological systems, altered response both qualitative and quantitative can be expected. Similarly, the social circumstances of the aging population gradually change such that the interaction of the elderly with the health care system must also change. One of the most important aspects of this change is that there is an increased dependence on the facilities available. In the present context this entails an increase in prescription rate. Related problems include compliance (see also Chapter 54) and adverse drug reactions.

COMPLIANCE

Compliance has been defined as 'the extent to which the patients' behaviour coincides with the clinical prescription' (Sackett, 1976). The prescription may involve, in addition to drug therapy, a modification of life style e.g. smoking habits etc. The bulk of the literature however, concentrates on various aspects of patients' compliance with drug therapy.

An accurate assessment of the magnitude of the problem of non-compliance is not possible because of the difficulty in the qualitative and quantitative interpretations of the above definition. The non-compliant patient has variously and arbitrarily been defined as one who takes less than 30%, 50% or 90% of his treatment. Further confusion arises from the failure to distinguish between the deliberate and unintentional non-complier.

It is not surprising therefore that the estimated incidence of non-compliance shows marked variability. Most studies have shown that at least one third of patients fail in some way to comply with prescriptions but in some cases the incidence of non-compliance has been found to be as high as 93%. In spite of the potentially significant effect of age on compliance, there is a remarkable paucity of data in the literature on compliance in the elderly compared with the young. The suspicion that the non-compliance rate among elderly patients is higher than that for young patients may be a correct one. Because of the occurrence of multiple diseases they are prescribed more medications than young people. This polypharmacy increases the likelihood of errors. The problem is further compounded by poor vision, mental impairment and reduced manual dexterity. Three drugs is the maximum number that the average alert elderly patient can manage. Those patients who err are likely to make multiple mistakes. Schwartz and colleagues (1962) found that the average number of errors per error-making patient was 2.6. The most frequent error was of omission, followed by errors in drug dose, timing and sequence. On the other hand, it may well be that relatively healthy elderly patients take their medication as reliably as younger patients. They are more likely to have a regular routine on which they superimpose their medicine taking.

The consequences of non-compliance among elderly patients are serious. Omission of therapy, deliberate or accidental, results in lack of the anticipated therapeutic effect. It has been shown that non-compliance is a factor relating to hospital admission. Unnecessary hospitalisation is clearly undesirable in any patient irrespective of age but more so in elderly patients for whom change of environment and daily routine is deleterious. Unnecessary diagnostic procedures and/or prescribing of more powerful, potentially toxic drugs are further consequences of non-compliance.

Adverse drug reactions

The last few years has seen a growth in concern about the problem of drug induced disease. As shown in the study of Hurwitz (1969) adverse drug reactions are more common in the elderly (Table 7.2). Iatrogenic disease reflects partly the increased number and potency of available drugs, but also

Table 7.2 Age and drug reactions (Hurwitz, 1969)

Age of Patients (years)	No of given drugs	No with reactions	Rate %
60	667	42	6.3
60+	493	76	15.4

the high level of drug consumption. The elderly are particularly susceptible to adverse drug reactions as they are prescribed more drugs than are young patients. In a general practice survey (Law & Chalmers, 1976) 87% of those over 75 years of age received regular drug treatment, 34% taking 3 or 4 different drugs each day. Altered drug handling by the elderly may contribute to their increased susceptibility to adverse drug effects. The overall rate of adverse reactions is increased in patients with decreased renal function, a common finding among the elderly. Patients' sex has also been shown to be a predisposing factor in adverse drug reactions — women being more susceptible. The high rate of adverse drug effects in the elderly is arguably due to the high ratio of women to men in the geriatric population, although the greater number of drugs taken by women is most likely a contributing factor. In a multicentre study of 1998 geriatric patients 81% of patients were receiving drugs and 15% of these had an adverse reaction (Williamson, 1979). The rate of adverse reactions in patients receiving a single drug was 10% but in those receiving six drugs it was 27%. Approximately 10% of all admissions were judged to be the direct consequence of adverse drug effects. Some studies have found that the duration of hospital stay is significantly prolonged in patients who have an adverse drug reaction. Unfortunately, none of these studies relates the prolongation of hospital stay to age but it is tempting to suggest that this is more marked in the elderly.

As can be seen in Table 7.3 cardiovascular and central nervous system drugs dominate when listing drugs that are most likely to be associated with adverse drug reactions in the elderly. The underlying mechanism may be pharmacokinetic as with digoxin, or pharmacodynamic as is the case with the adrenergic neuron blockings drugs (debrisoquin, guanethidine and bethanidine).

Table 7.3 Some drugs with higher incidence of adverse drug reactions (ADR) in the elderly

Drug	Comment
Digoxin	Digoxin toxicity
Heparin	Bleeding
Isoniazid	Hepatotoxicity
Propranolol	Higher ADRs
Phenylbutazone	Bone marrow depression
Benzodiazepines	CNS depression
Disopyramide	Urinary retention
Phenothiazines	Postural hypotension
Diuretics	Dehydration, low potassium
Adrenergic neurone blocking drugs	Postural hypotension
Aminoglycosides	Ototoxicity

Regular review and reassessment of elderly patients' drug therapy is important in attempting to optimise pharmacotherapeutic geriatric care. Without a clear idea of the therapeutic end-point, the doctor may find himself prescribing drugs on a 'repeat' basis when they are no longer necessary or beneficial to the patient. They may in fact be detrimental to well being. Psychotropic drugs serve to illustrate this point. Walker (1971) found that in a sample of his patients over 70 and over 80 years of age approximately 45% and 60% respectively were on repeat prescriptions many of these being for psychotropic drugs. Patients may have been taking these drugs for many years with inadequate supervision. In a survey of psychotropic prescribing in general practice, Dennis (1979) found that repeat prescriptions were often given without the patients seeing the doctor. His analysis showed that the longer the drug had been prescribed, the older the patient was likely to be and the less closely they were monitored by the general practitioner. Reliance on self-referral by the elderly is unsafe and this makes this area all the more problematic.

Coping with adverse drug reactions and poor compliance

The problem of poor compliance and adverse drug reactions are closely related and the methods of dealing with both are therefore similar. If drug therapy is considered necessary by the physician he must ensure that the minimum number of drugs is prescribed. If more than one drug is given he must give appropriate consideration to their possible interaction as this may result both in adverse effects and consequent reduced compliance. If possible the doctor should pre-determine the therapeutic end-point of each drug thus ensuring that the patient takes the drug for the minimum period necessary. This will, depending on the toxicity of the drug, minimise, to a variable extent, the likelihood of adverse effects. It has also been shown that adherence to drug therapy diminishes with time. Once commenced on treatment, elderly patients must be regularly supervised. The physician must have a high index of suspicion of non-compliance and take the appropriate corrective steps. He must also actively seek adverse drug effects. Elderly patients are more often tolerant of symptoms, attributing them to 'old age' or to a new development in their underlying illness. They may not even consider the new treatment to be the culprit and consequently they fail to report symptoms of drug toxicity. Adverse effects and non-compliance are more likely to occur in elderly patients on long term unsupervised medication. The practice of issuing such 'repeat' prescriptions is to be deplored. Impaired comprehension and retention of information, poor vision and hearing are additional factors that militate against compliance in the elderly. They also predispose the old to adverse drug reactions. Clear concise simple written instructions supplemented with written material help to mimise these problems (Wandless & Davies, 1977). The labelling of medicines should be legible and easily understood. Instructions 'to be taken as directed' are clearly inappropriate. It has been suggested that occupational therapists could successfully incorporate the active teaching of geriatric patients into their activities of daily living programme. An additional factor worthy of consideration is that of drug packaging. Drugs should be supplied to the elderly in containers that allow the tablets to be clearly visualised and that open without undue difficulty.

PHARMACOKINETIC CONSIDERATIONS

Pharmacokinetics refers to four simultaneous processes whereby drugs are handled in the body — absorption, distribution, metabolism and excretion. A number of extensive reviews of pharmacokinetics in relation to aging have been published in recent years (Triggs & Nation, 1975; Crooks et al, 1976; Richie & Bender, 1977; Greenblatt et al, 1982). The more important changes in drug handling in the elderly are summarised in Table 7.4.

Absorption

Despite the often repeated litany of age related changes in gastrointestinal structure and function associated with aging which might be expected to cause changes to the pattern of drug absorption (Bender, 1968) there are few data to indicate significant alterations in drug absorption in

Table 7.4 Major pharmacokinetic changes with aging

Absorption
No significant change
Distribution
Volume of distribution
↑ for lipid soluble
↓ for water soluble
Protein binding
↓ for acidic drugs
↑ for basic drugs
Metabolism
Variable
some ↓ but environmental factors important
↓ first pass metabolism
Renal excretion
↓ in proportion to renal function

the elderly. Absorption of the following drugs has been studied and has been shown to be unchanged in the elderly — aspirin, paracetamol, atenolol, cimetidine, oxazepam, antipyrine, dextropropoxyphene, sotolol and theophylline. Some delay in absorption has been described for digoxin, lorazepam and chlordiazepoxide. However, relatively minor changes in the rate of absorption are not important. Evidence has been presented for a decrease in the extent of absorption of prazosin but this is indirect. In summary, we can dismiss changed drug absorption as an important contributing factor to altered drug response in the elderly.

Distribution

Body composition changes with aging — lean body mass decreases, fat making up the deficit initially. As the distribution of drugs depends among other things on partitioning to fat and water it comes as no surprise that drug distribution changes in the elderly. In fact, the volume of distribution of water-soluble drugs such as antipyrine, sotolol and paracetamol decreased while that of more fat-soluble drugs such as diazepam, lignocaine, salicyclates and methyldiazepam is increased. These changes have two related consequences. Firstly, for a given dose of water-soluble drugs the plasma level will be higher in old people. Secondly, the magnitude of effect may be greater. The converse applies to the lipid-soluble drugs.

Protein binding of drugs is a major determinant of drug distribution and as many drugs are bound to either plasma albumin which decreases with age or alpha$_1$-acid glycoprotein which increases with age this mechanism must be taken into account. In general, acidic drugs bind to albumin whereas basic drugs are associated with alpha$_1$-acid glycoprotein. Thus, the binding of phenytoin is increased whereas that of lignocaine is decreased.

The significance of protein binding resides in the fact that the unbound (free) drug is the pharmacologically active moiety. Thus, the extent of protein binding is inversely related to the intensity of effect. In the short term, protein binding is important as for example when phenylbutazone displaces warfarin from binding sites on albumin. However, in long-term use such changes are of relatively little significance because the excess free drug is available not only to exert a more pronounced pharmacological action but also it is available to be more rapidly eliminated.

While knowledge of the degree of protein binding and of the volume of distribution give us a general idea of how a drug is distributed in the body it tells us nothing of regional differences; most importantly it tells us nothing of access of drugs to its site of action — usually the receptor. As aging is associated with alterations in membrane structure and function, it is not beyond the bounds of possibility that penetration of drugs to their site of action is altered.

Metabolism

Most drugs that are metabolised undergo transformation in the liver often under the influence of microsomal enzymes. From animal studies there is good evidence for a decrease in drug metabolising capacity with aging. In man the evidence is indirect. For some drugs handling in the liver is dependent on liver blood flow and such drugs have a high extraction ratio so that the rate limiting step is the rate at which they are presented to the liver for metabolism (Wilkinson & Shand, 1975). Example include lignocaine and propranolol. On the other hand, some drugs have a very low extraction ratio and in such cases the rate of elimination depends on the activity of drug metabolising enzymes in the liver. Examples include phenylbutazone, diazepam and the test drug antipyrine.

Liver blood flow decreases with age and there is also a decrease in liver mass with aging. However, there is no change in the standard clinical indices of liver function. There is evidence for a decrease in the clearance of low extraction drugs including various benzodiazepines and antipyrine (Greenblatt et al, 1983). However, it has been suggested that some of the apparent age related decrease in elimination may be the result of environmental (Wood et al, 1979; Vestal et al, 1975) differences between old and young rather than an effect of aging itself.

There are a number of low extraction drugs, the rate of elimination of which is not significantly reduced in the elderly. These drugs are conjugated in the liver rather than metabolised by oxidation, and they include various benzodiazepines and possibly paracetamol, though there is some debate about the latter. Alcohol is metabolised by the non-microsomal enzyme alcohol-dehydrogenese and its rate of elimination is not altered in the elderly (Vestal et al, 1977). Isoniazid is also metabolised by non-microsomal enzymes and the proportion of slow and fast acetylators has been found not to change with age.

First pass metabolism

A considerable number of drugs when absorbed after oral administration are avidly taken up by the liver prior to reaching the systemic circulation — presystemic elimination. Drugs so treated include propranolol, labetalol, chlormethiazole and lignocaine, and in each case the fraction of drug reaching the circulation has been shown to be increased in the elderly. Bioavailability can be more than doubled from young adulthood to old age so that for drugs with lower therapeutic index, dosage adjustment is appropriate (O'Malley & Kelly, 1982).

Enzyme induction

A mater of theoretical if not practical interest is the question of whether enzyme induction occurs and if so does it occur to the same extent in the elderly as in young people? The evidence is that induction does occur in response to cigarette smoking and various inducing drugs in the elderly but probably to a lesser extent than in the young. The only clinical significance is that the potential for drug interactions by this mechanism is thereby reduced in the elderly population.

Excretion

The classical studies of Shock and his colleagues (1952) in the 1950s have amply demonstrated that many facets of the renal circulation and of kidney function deteriorate with aging in the apparent absence of renal disease. Thus, renal blood flow and glomerular filtration rate both decline from the third decade onwards so that by the eighth or ninth decade they may be reduced by as much as 50% of the value pertaining in young adulthood. There is also a decrease in renal tubular function so that for example the maximum reabsorptive capacity for glucose falls. Similarly, urine concentrating ability falls with aging. It is important for the clinician to realise that the serum creatinine does not usually rise in these circumstances because firstly, in the young creatinine clearance must fall by about 70% before the serum creatinine rises. Furthermore, in the elderly creatinine production falls so that an even greater decrease in glomerular filtration rate must take place before it is reflected in an increase in serum creatinine.

Drugs are handled in the kidney by three processes — glomerular filtration, renal tubular secretion and non-ionic diffusion. It can reasonably be anticipated that the elimination of renally handled drugs irrespective of the particular process will be diminished in old age. Many drugs have been studied — digozin, penicillin, dihydrostreptomycin, gentamicin, kanamycin, phenobarbitone, quinidine, and tetracycline — and in each case the rate of elimination has been shown to be diminished (for reviews see Kampmann & Molholm-Hansen, 1979). This is important particularly for those drugs with a low therapeutic ratio such as digoxin and the aminoglycosides but less so for relatively safe drugs like penicillin and tetracycline.

PHARMACODYNAMICS

Pharmacodynamics refer to that which the drug does to the organism. Direct drug effects are brought about either by a specific interaction with receptors be they on the cell surface or inside the cell, or by generalised membrane effects. Drugs may exert their effects indirectly as for example acting on a bacterium.

Aging may effect responsiveness to drugs in various ways (O'Malley & Kelly, 1980) at different levels of organisation from the receptor-drug interaction itself through to the final biochemical, mechanical or electrical event. Homeostatic mechanisms operate less effectively in the elderly. Membrane composition is altered and superimposed on the aging process are various pathological changes, many of which occur commonly and in combination in this age group. As drugs act by perturbing physiological systems we confidently expect to see differences in responsiveness in the elderly. We suspect, however, only a small fraction of altered responsiveness has so far been characterised.

Receptors

Relatively few studies have been carried out in the elderly to ascertain the state of receptor function. The most convenient systems to examine are those present on formed elements of the blood as these can be removed and examined without putting the patient at risk. Such studies however, suffer from the major disadvantage of being indirect and therefore the findings are not necessarily applicable. Nevertheless, in the case of the beta adrenoceptor they provide us with interesting insights. Contrary to initial expectation, beta adrenoceptor mediated responses are decreased in the elderly — this applies both to agonists such as isoprenaline and terbutaline as well as to antagonists such as propranolol. Thus, the heart rate response to these drugs is diminished with advancing age. The receptors are apparently unaltered but there is a diminished ability to convert the receptor drug interaction into a response. The pharmacokinetic changes with aging tend to increase plasma levels of beta adrenoceptor blocking drugs. Renal elimination of nadolol, sotalol and atenolol is diminished and first pass metabolism of propranolol and labetalol is decreased. Thus there are opposing pharmacodynamic and pharmacokinetic influences and it may well be that the state of health or otherwise of the drug recipient may be the final arbiter of whether or not the patient responds appropriately. Thus disturbance of sino-atrial node function is more common in the elderly and it may well be that adverse drug reactions are more common not because of changes in responsiveness or kinetics but because of the high prevalence of relevant disease.

Alpha adrenoceptor mediated responses do not change significantly with age in man even though animal data suggest that there is a decrease in response. Interestingly,

alpha$_2$ receptors on platelets have been described as falling with age but the physiological importance of this is not known.

Drugs acting on the central nervous system

As indicated in Table 7.3 the central nervous system active drugs are a major source of unwanted effects in the elderly. While barbiturates should only be of historical interest in this context, the benzodiazepines by virtue of their being extensively prescribed are of key importance (Thompson et al, 1983). It has been amply demonstrated that the adverse drug reactions are more common in the elderly and this usually involves either increased intensity or duration of central nervous system depression. Greenblatt et al, (1977) studied flurazepam and showed convincingly that not only was the frequency of adverse drug reactions related to age but also to dose. In fact, the age related increase in frequency was not apparent at doses below 15 mg per day but became obvious at doses between 15 and 30 and was striking at daily doses of 30 mg and above.

With some of the benzodiazepines such as diazepam and chlordiaxepoxide there is marked lengthening of half life in the elderly. The practical significane of this is that it takes longer to achieve steady state concentrations and the duration of action is longer. Thus the potential for prolonged hang-over effect is very considerable in the elderly. By contrast the pharmacokinetics of three benzodiazepines — oxazepam, lorazepam and nitrazepam — are not significantly altered. Nevertheless the duration and intensity of the effect of nitrazepam for example, is markedly increased in the elderly and this raises the possibility of increased sensitivity in the elderly. Possible mechanisms for this include altered susceptibility of sleep pattern in the elderly, a change in the benzodiazepine receptor with aging or changes in access of drug to the site of action in the brain. As with younger patients, if benzodiazepines must be used as hypnotics, the shorter acting members of the group such as oxazepam, lorazepam, alprazolam or triazolam should be used.

Many drugs have unwanted central nervous effects including the beta adrenoceptor blocking drugs, methyldopa, clonidine and ketotofen, and while specific data are lacking with many drugs, clinical experience suggests that such effects are more common in the elderly. As a general principle it is best to avoid those drugs which produce unwanted affects on the central nervous system as these usually take the form of depression including psychological depression, daytime drowsiness, sleep disturbances, lack of energy and lethargy.

Homeostatic mechanisms

One of the hallmarks of aging is a deterioration in the ability of homeostatic mechanisms to maintain the status-quo (see chapter 10). This is well illustrated in the case of the baroreflex; the elderly have a diminished ability to counter alterations in blood pressure. Thus they are paticularly at risk with drugs known to cause postural hypotension, the best example being the adrenergic neuron blocking drugs. By this reasoning the elderly would be at increased risk with many vasodilator drugs and drugs such as the phenothiazines which are potent alpha adrenoceptor blocking drugs. The increased incidence of bleeding associated with heparin in the elderly represents another form of altered homeostasis. In this case it may well be that pathological as well as age-related change in blood vessels and/or the clotting system are at fault.

CONCLUDING REMARKS

In attempting to explain the altered responses observed in the elderly we must examine each determinant of drug effect. The altered social circumstances, or the presence of various infirmities, may be of importance. Alternatively changes in pharmacokinetics as for example with renally excreted drugs, or change in pharmacodynamics as with adrenergic neuron blocking drugs, may be responsible. In no case in medical therapeutics is it more important to individualise drug therapy than in the elderly. This entails taking into account not alone the indication for drug treatment but also the way other changes associated with aging can influence the patient's response to the prescription. Geriatric pharmacotherapy provides the physician with a challenge which if taken up can significantly improve the quality of life of our elderly population.

REFERENCES

Bender A D 1968 Effect of age on intestinal absorption: Implications for drug absorption in the elderly. Journal of American Geriatrics Society 16: 1331–1339

Crooks J, O'Malley K, Stevenson I H 1976 Pharmacokinetics in the elderly. Clinical Pharmacokinetics 1: 280–296

Dennis P J 1979 Monitoring of psychotrope prescribing in general practice. British Medical Journal 2: 1115–1116

Greenblatt D J, Allen M D, Shader R I 1977 Toxicity of high dose flurazepam in the elderly. Clinical Pharmacology & Therapeutics 21: 355

Greenblatt D J, Divoll M, Abernethy D R, Harmatz J S, Shader R I 1982 Antipyrine kinetics in the elderly: Prediction of age-related changes in benzodiazepine oxidizing capacity. Journal of Pharmacology and Experimental Therapeutics 220: 120–126

Greenblatt D, Sellers E, Shader R 1982 Drug disposition in old age. New England Journal of Medicine 306: 1081–1088

Hurwitz N 1969 Predisposing factors in adverse reactions to drugs. British Medical Journal 1: 536–539

Kampmann J P, Molholm-Hansen J 1979 Renal excretion of drugs. In: Crooks J, Stevenson I H (eds) Drugs and the Elderly, Macmillan, London, p 77–88

Law R, Chalmers C 1976 Medicines and elderly people: a general practice survey. British Medical Journal 1: 565–568

O'Malley K, Kelly J G 1980 Drug response at extremes of age. In: Turner P (ed) Clinical Pharmacology & Therapeutics, Macmillan, London, p 124–131

Richey D P, Bender A D 1977 Pharmacokinetic consequences of aging. Annual Review of Pharmacology & Toxicology 17: 49–65

Sackett D L 1976 Introduction. In: Sackett D L, Haynes R B (eds) Compliance with therapeutic regimens. The Johns Hopkins University Press, Baltimore and London

Schwartz D, Wang M, Zeitz L, Goss M E W 1962 Medication errors made by elderly chronically ill patients. American Journal of Public Health 52: 2018–2019

Shock N W 1952 Age changes in renal function. In: Lansing A I (ed) Cowdreys problems of ageing. Williams and Wilkins, Baltimore p 614–630

Thompson T L, Moran M, Nies A S 1983 Psychotropic drug use in the elderly. New England Journal of Medicine 308: 134–137

Triggs E J, Nation R L 1975 Pharmacokinetics in the aged: A review. Journal of Pharmacokinetics and Biopharmaceutics 3: 387–418

Vestal R E et al 1975 Antipyrine metabolism in man: Influence of age, alcohol, caffeine and smoking. Clinical Pharmacology & Therapeutics 18: 425–432

Vestal R E. McGuire E A, Tobin J D, Andres R, Norris A H, Mesey E 1977 Aging and ethanol metabolism. Clinical Pharmacology & Therapeutics 21: 343–354

Walker K 1971 Repeat prescription recording in general practice. Journal Royal College General Practitioners 21: 748–751

Wandless I, Davie J W 1977 Can drug compliance in the elderly be improved? British Medical Journal 1: 359–361

Wilkinson G R and Shand D G 1975 A physiological approach to hepatic drug clearance. Clinical Pharmacology & Therapeutics 18: 277–390

Williamson J 1979 Adverse reactions to prescribed drugs in the elderly. In: Crooks J, Stevenson I H (eds) Drugs and the Elderly. Macmillan Press, London p 243

Wood A J J, Vestal R E, Wilkinson G R, Branch R A, Shand D G 1979 Effect of aging and cigarette smoking on antipyrine and indocyanine green elimination. Clinical Pharmacology & Therapeutics 26: 16–19

8

Cancer

H. J. Cohen & J. Crawford

EPIDEMIOLOGY

The relationship between cancer and aging may be best expressed by an epidemiologic approach. In the United States over one-half of all cancer occurs in the 11% of the population over the age of 65 (Butler, 1979). At age 25 the probability of developing cancer within five years is 1 in 700, while at age 65 it is 1 in 14 (Lancet, 1976). Despite the prevalence of cancer in the aged, many misleading statements exist (Crawford & Cohen, 1984). Because many textbooks quote the 'peak' incidence and mortality of cancer to be in the 60–75 age-range, the misleading

impression is that cancer becomes less common in the elderly. In fact, cancer incidence and mortality continue to rise with age if one looks at age-specific rates which allow for the decreasing population size with progressive age (Fig. 8.1).

Because of the co-existence of other diseases or the 'compression of morbidity' in the elderly (Fries, 1980), and the less aggressive clinical course of some cancers in the elderly, another misleading clinical impression is that the elderly tend to die with cancer rather than of cancer. Although deaths attributable to cancer decrease from 30% at age 50 to 10% or less at age 85 (King, 1982), this

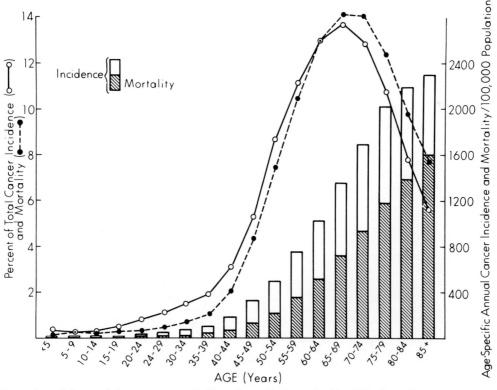

Fig. 8.1 Comparison of the age of the percent cancer incidence (o——o) and morality (●—●) for the total population versus the age-specific annual cancer incidence and mortality (bar graph). This data was tabulated from the National Cancer Institute Surveillance Epidemiology and End Results (SEER) Study, 1973-1977 (Young et al, 1981).

observation is largely due to the rapidly increasing denominator of deaths due to other causes with advancing age rather than to a decrease in cancer deaths. Despite the marked increase in cardiovascular related deaths with age, cancer remains the second leading cause of death in those over 65 (Libow, 1981). Furthermore, (See Fig. 8.1), the age-specific mortality of cancer rises with age at a rate that is actually greater than the rate of increase in incidence. This suggests that cancer may be even more lethal in the elderly than the young.

Figure 8.2 demonstrates that the age-related increase in cancer incidence occurs for all major types of cancer with males at greater risk than females. Only four cancers of adulthood have a median age of onset less than 50–Hodgkin's disease, acute lymphocytic leukaemia, bone and joint cancer and testicular cancer. Even these tumours have a second rise in incidence with advance aging. As shown in Figure 8.2, the rate of increase of breast and female genital tract cancer occurs earlier in life and the rate of rise is more gradual with age compared to the other major forms of cancer. If one looks at all these cancers collectively there is a logarithmic rise in incidence from the age of 30 to 80 (Dix, 1980). Current research evaluating common links between cancer and aging may well lead to better understanding of both related processes.

SCREENING

Cancer screening strategies such as the American Cancer society (ACS) recommendations, have concentrated on the earliest age at which screening should begin. Few adjustments in the specific recommendations have been made for the elderly despite the potential increased yield of accurate screening tests in this group with a high prevalence of cancer. Other modifications might also be appropriate in the debilitated elderly, but have not been addressed. Criticism of the ACS guidelines has been produced (Eddy, 1981); the factors involved in recommending a specific screening test are complex (Love, 1981) and the entire concept of a periodical health examination has come under closer scrutiny (Scherr, 1981). Thus, the American College of Physicians has recommended that each physician individualise his plans for patient examination. Unfortunately, screening for cancer in the elderly may not be performed at all, particularly because of the tendency to group the healthy along with the debilitated elderly.

A case in point is the pelvic examination in the elderly patient, which is often 'deferred' by the physician. The ACS recommends continuation of the annual pelvic examination, but discontinuation of pap smears at the age

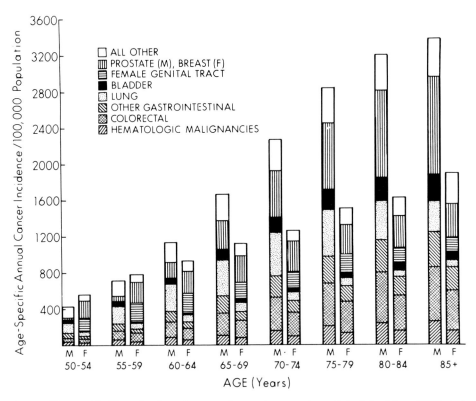

Fig. 8.2 Age-specific annual incidence for the major types of cancer by age and sex. Data derived from SEER study, 1973-1977 (Young et al, 1981).

of 65 *in those who have been previously screened.* The age-specific incidence and mortality of cervical cancer rise progressively to age 85 (Young, 1981) presumably due to patients who escape screening at a younger age. Thus pap smears may still be of value in this subgroup. Endometrial and ovarian cancer incidence and mortality are highest in patients over 70. Additionally vulvar carcinoma is uniquely a cancer of extreme age. Thus multiple reasons exist to continue the annual pelvic examination in the elderly, as recommended by the ACS. However, a current failure to effectively screen the elderly with pelvic examinations is suggested by the positive correlation of age and advanced stage of ovarian, endometrial and cervical carcinoma at diagnosis (Holmes, 1981).

From Figure 8.2 the potential value of cancer screening in the elderly should be clear. Age alone should not dissuade the physician from a vigorous health maintenance approach to the elderly. A regular screening programme should be instituted unless the patient's co-existing medical problems would preclude further diagnostic and therapeutic intervention if the screening tests were positive. Certainly an annual check-up including breast, pelvic and rectal examinations and a stool quaiac test are reasonable. The advanced stage of presentation of breast masses in the elderly (Holmes, 1981) suggest that breast self-examination and mammography are not being utilised to the same extent as they are in younger patients. Furthermore, the dramatic rise in colorectal carcinoma with age should warrant consideration of the periodic use of sigmoidoscopy in the elderly. Future health policy strategies must specifically address the questions of benefit versus risk for all these screening procedures in the elderly. Until that time, the elderly should be given the same attention with regard to screening examinations and health maintenance that are applied to younger populations.

THE DIAGNOSIS OF CANCER IN THE ELDERLY

In addition to inadequate cancer screening in the elderly, delays in diagnosis may result from the patient ignoring the warning signals of cancer. This may be partially explained by the pervasive attitude that 'feeling bad' is a normal part of aging and by the elderly patient's fear of cancer and its treatment.

Furthermore, delays in the recognition of neoplasia by both the patient and the physician may exist in the elderly patient with multiple disease processes (Hodkinson, 1978). Changes in bowel habits may be attributed to decreased motility rather than the possibility of colon cancer. Anemia is more common in the elderly (Cohen & Crawford, 1984) and may not alert the physician to other processes. General symptoms of anorexia, weight loss or decrease in performance status may be secondary to failing social competence, depression or early dementia, but may also be the first clue of malignancy. The age-related incidence of cancer emphasises the need to maintain a high index of suspicion for neoplasia in elderly patients despite complicating medical problems. Furthermore, the frequency of multiple primary cancers increases with age (Howell, 1980).

This index of suspicion must be balanced against the physicians judgment concerning the risk/benefit of a 'cancer workup' in an individual patient. As a group, the elderly receive more medical care, frequently resulting in abnormal lab tests that may lead to fruitless but expensive and often hazardous investigations. A study of the diagnosis of bronchogenic carcinoma at a major university hospital emphasises this dilemma for the physician (Cechner, 1980). In this autopsy study, men over 70 were the most likely group to have had clinically undetected lung cancer and also the most likely group to have had a mistaken clinical diagnosis of lung cancer.

CLINICAL COURSE OF CANCER IN THE AGED

Our understanding of neoplasia and aging is growing rapidly at the cellular level. Carcinogenesis has been divided into the stages of initiation (the initial genetic damage to cellular DNA), promotion (transformation from an initiated lesion into a neoplastic growth) and progression (local and/or metastatic spread of the cancer) (Farber, 1981). Human cell culture experiments have begun to explore the metabolic activation and inactivation of a variety of carcinogens and have shown a striking individual variation by as much as 50 to 100 fold in their metabolism (Harris, 1980). While a decline in drug metabolism has been described in elderly cancer patients (Highuchi, 1980), it is not yet clear what modifying effects age has on the ratio of activation to inactivation of carcinogens (Anisimov, 1981).

Conceptually is seems logical that the steps of promotion and progression in neoplasia might be altered in the setting of age-related decline in physiologic functions. Certainly the risk of neoplasia can be altered experimentally by hormone manipulation (Riley, 1981) and by nutritional influences (Fernandez, 1979). Widely implicated also has been the association of age-related decline in immune function, or immune senescence (Weksler, 1981). Of interest in this regard is the prevention of spontaneous tumours in aged mice by immunopharmacologic manipulation (Bruley-Rosset, 1981). The interrelationship of these and other systems in the genesis and promotion of cancer is reviewed in detail elsewhere (Holland, 1982; DeVita, 1982).

Moving from the cellular level to the patient, the devastating influence of neoplasia on the aged is clear to anyone who has cared for elderly cancer patients. Progressive decline in physiological function with age accompanied by co-morbid diseases and a loss of social and financial support systems often makes cancer even more ominous in the elderly than in the young. The diagnosis and therapy of cancer often overwhelm the adaptive ability of the elderly patient in the absence of support from the family and/or community.

The influence of aging on the clinical course of neoplasia is less clear, with some believing cancer is more indolent in the elderly where others believe it is more aggressive (Peterson, 1979). The time-honoured marker of success, the five year survival rate, may not be an accurate means of comparing young and old patients, particularly at the extremes of age or in the presence of co-morbid diseases. Unfortunately, more accurate measurements of clinical doubling-time (Shackney, 1978) or in vitro kinetic studies of tumours (Hansen, 1981) have not been systematically evaluated with respect to patient age. Clinical observations are often biased by marked variations in lead time; e.g. the shortened survival of the patient diagnosed to have late stage cancer for the reasons cited above, versus the apparent longer survival of patients with the same cancer detected fortuitously at an earlier stage because of medical attention for other problems.

Despite these uncertainties, some variations in biological aggressiveness with age have been suggested for several cancers. Malignant melanoma has a relatively constant five year survival for women until aged 60, after which a sharp decline occurs (Shaw, 1978). Increasing age has been correlated with increasing depth of skin penetration by melanoma at the time of diagnosis, a major prognostic factor (Levine, 1981). Whether this is a failure of early detection of the melanoma in the aged or a biologically more-aggressive cancer in the elderly cannot be answered at this point. In thyroid cancer, however, age greater than 60 is a risk factor for death that is independent of histological type, extent of tumour or type of treatment (Cady, 1979). Additionally, differences in histologic subtypes exist. Anaplastic carcinoma of the thyroid, the more malignant counterpart of the better differentiated forms, occurs predominantly in the elderly. Thus changes in the biology of cancer with age may in some situations relate to changes in grade or subtype of cancer rather than to effect of age per se. Another example of this change in subtype occurs in breast cancer where a clinical impression exists that this disease has a more benign course in the elderly. This is supported by the increased frequency of oestrogen receptor positive breast cancer in post-menopausal women (Lemon, 1982). The presence of the oestrogen receptor protein is associated with better prognosis, longer disease free survival and a more slowly growing tumour. Thus, each type of cancer, and its potential confounding variables, must be studied in detail before drawing conclusions about the influence of age per se on neoplasia.

CLINICAL DECISION MAKING

Estimates of the benefits versus risks of diagnostic and therapeutic interventions in the elderly are often difficult. To predict accurately the benefit/risk ratio for an intervention, the physician needs to know the 'functional reserve' of the patient. While known disease processes can be considered in some semi-objective fashion, chronologic age alone cannot. Unfortunately, there is no simple practical way to measure physiologic age at a tissue level that would tell us the 'margin of safety' that exists in aging cardiovascular, pulmonary, or renal systems (Kark, 1980). In some situations pre-operative monitoring by invasive means may be warranted to make an accurate assessment (Del Guercio, 1980). Too often because the risk of procedures is not clear to the physician, the elderly patient may be inappropriately excluded from good medical care. A case in point is fibroptic bronchoscopy which contrary to popular opinion has recently been shown to be safe, useful and acceptable in patients older than 70 even with severe pulmonary impairment (MacFarlane, 1981). Until more studies such as this are available, the physician must apply his clinical judgment to assess how aggressive an approach to pursue in the individual patient.

The first consideration must be whether making a diagnosis and undertaking treatment will in some way alter the patients quality or quantity of life. In some situations a combination of advanced age and co-morbid disease may make an evaluation difficult and the rewards for diagnosis nil if the patient were unable to withstand appropriate therapy. Too often, however, chronologic age alone has been used to exclude patients from standard diagnostic and therapeutic approaches without understanding the normal survival of the elderly. In fact, the average life expectancy for a 70 year-old man is 11 years and for a 70 year-old woman it is 15 years (Kovar, 1977). At age 85, men have a life expectancy of 5.3 years and women of approximately 7 years. In oncologic terminology, the median 5 year survival for a 70 year-old is 93% and for an 80 year-old is 63%. Without intervention any cancer that is not indolent should be expected to alter survival.

What is more difficult to assess than quantity of life, but generally more important to the aged patient, is quality of life. In addition to the impact of diagnostic and therapeutic interventions on health status and functional level, the physician must consider the impact of the financial and social status of the patient.

THERAPY

Supportive care

The goal of therapy in any patient with cancer must be clearly understood first, i.e. is it a curative attempt or one aimed at improving the quantity and/or quality of life?

Extreme age and co-morbid disease may limit the physicians attempts at curative therapy. Palliative therapy, a mainstay of cancer treatment at most ages, achieves increased significance in the elderly where maintenance of function is more difficult. Thus the second question must be what are the patients expectations of therapy and what support systems exist for achieving such expectations? Is there a spouse in good health? What is the proximity and willingness to help of family and friends? The team concept has been well developed in dealing with elderly patients (Hogue, 1978) and in cancer patients (Dugan, 1984). Care of such patients requires the skills of a physician, nurse oncologist, social worker, psychologist and chaplain with assistance from the dietician, dentist and physical therapist working together with the patient, family and friends. Such teams can vary in members and services as well as formal versus informal organisation, but the presence of a support group of health professionals provides the best basis for cancer management in the elderly. Such a group can provide patient counselling (Linn, 1981) as well as a better overall asessment of the cancer patients needs (Lucas & Brown, 1982). Similarly, the unique needs of the dying patient and the needs of the professionals involved with the dying patient (Lucas & Siegler, 1982) can be best met within the framework of a team approach to the patient. Further discussion of the roles of hospice and other supportive services is found elsewhere in this book.

The primary goal of treatment is relief of suffering. Guidelines for the medical treatment of cancer pain have recently been reviewed (Medical Letter, 1982). Oral morphine on a regular basis titrated to a dose that achieves freedom from pain is a treatment of choice for severe cancer pain in the younger patients. Differences in pain perception (Kaiko, 1980) and response to analgesics (Harkins, 1980) need to be further characterised in the elderly before general conclusions can be made about the best pain regimen. With regard to narcotics, it is wise for the practitioner to begin with reduced doses because of the prolonged half-life of these drugs in the elderly. Critical to the management of the pain patient is the recognition and treatment of associated depression, as well as the use of adjunctive procedures such as radiation therapy for local painful bony metastases and neurosurgical procedures such as percutaneous cordotomy for intractable pain.

Treatment induced nausea and vomiting has received more attention in recent years (Siegel & Longo, 1981). In addition to phenothiazines, newer anti-emetic agents have been developed including intravenous metoclopromide (Gralla, 1981) and natural and synthetic cannabinoids (Laszlo, 1981). All of these agents have central nervous system side effects which may be exacerbated in the elderly. For example dysphoria from cannabinoids is more common in the aged. Until formal anti-emetic trials are completed in the elderly patient, these drugs will have to be titrated in each individual, beginning with reduced doses.

Surgery

The topic of surgery in the elderly has been well reviewed (Johnson, 1982). Numerous studies document that chronologic age per se is not a contra-indication to surgical intervention although large surgical series do show an overall increase in mortality in patients over 70 (Turnbul, 1977; Schein, 1979) with even greater increases in mortality in patients over 80 (Santos, 1975). Deaths are most commonly due to cardiac events, pulmonary emboli, pneumonia and other infections.

Thus part of the increased surgical mortality in patients over 70 may relate to our inability to assess adequately cardiopulmonary reserve (Goldman, 1977). By invasive pre-operative monitoring of the elderly, 23% of the group of patients who had been 'cleared' for surgery were found to have unacceptable risks for major surgery under general anaesthesia (Del Guercia, 1980). Thus, careful pre-operative assessment is critical in the elderly patient (Feigal, 1979) and some situations may warrent invasive monitoring.

In one surgical series of 500 patients over 80 years of age, the hospital mortality was 6.2% within one month of surgery (Djokovic, 1979). This low mortality was attributed to improvements in pulmonary care and management of infectious complications, along with the use of low-dose heparin therapy and early mobilisation. However, the ability to predict post-operative myocardial infarction was poor.

Risk for complications varies with the procedure. Surgery for gynaecologic malignancy in patients over 75 resulted in a higher incidence of wound complications but otherwise resulted in no differences in complications than for younger patients (Pierson, 1975). Operative mortality was 6% and 4% in two series of patients over 65 undergoing craniotomy for brain tumours (Stewart, 1975; Tomita, 1981).

In another study, a thorough evaluation of operative risk factors for colon resection in the elderly revealed a mortality rate of 5% for the age-group 70–80 and 17% for those patients over 80, with a relatively constant morbidity rate of between 30–35% for all patients over age 50 (Boyd, 1980). Mortality rate correlated best with the number of pre-existing medical conditions. Patients over 70 with two or more complicating medical conditions had an operative mortality of 16% whereas no patient without a pre-existing medical condition died regardless of age. These data are quite encouraging for the elderly healthy patient and further supports the need to consider aggressive screening for colorectal cancer in this group.

Thoracotomy in elderly patients is frequently complicated by direct compromise of the cardiopulmonary system, which undergoes a significant age-related decline apart from any specific disease process (Libow, 1980). Thus functional reserve has even greater importance here. In 150 patients with lung cancer who had 'lung sparing' procedures, the hospital mortality was 4% compared to a 17% mortality in other reported series (Breyer, 1981). Moreover, the five year survival for this group was 27% which is comparable to other series which involve more aggressive surgical resection.

In the past, undertreatment was a common problem for the elderly woman with breast cancer. Recent studies showing similar survival rates for women over and under 70 who have undergone surgery, suggests that denying standard surgical procedures such as mastectomy and axillary lymph node dissection on the basis of age alone is inappropriate (Herbsman, 1981). Similarly for small breast masses, quadrantectomy and axillary dissection with post-operative radiotherapy may provide a comparable alternative to mastectomy (Veronesi, 1981).

Thus, chronologic age does not preclude surgery. But it does increase the probability of co-existent decline in functional reserve and complicating disease which must be carefully evaluated. Moreover one must consider not only immediate post-operative problems, but more long-term problems of recuperation, difficulty in returning to pre-operative functional status and the potential for further complications during that prolonged recuperative phase (Schein, 1979). Clinically, this is a well recognised problem for the elderly, but little data exists to assess objectively these parameters. Clinical experience and common sense would suggest that the narrower the functional reserve of the patient pre-operatively, the more difficult it will be for rehabilitation. However, despite the uncertainties involved in intra- and post-operative recovery, the marginally compensated elderly patient may often be able to tolerate the acute stress of surgery better than the chronic stress of radiation treatment or chemotherapy.

Radiation therapy

No clinical evidence exists that a given cancer varies in its radiosensitivity as a function of patient age. However the radiation effect on normal tissue is said to be enhanced by 10–15% in the elderly (Gunn, 1980). Those organs with most marked physiological decline such as the lungs would be in most jeopardy. Also side effects may be more hazardous as in radiation therapy delivered to the oropharyx or oral cavity, because of the resultant loss of taste, dryness of the mucous membranes and involution of the salivary glands. Combined with the precarious nutritional intake in the elderly, this can be lethal unless careful attention is given to nutritional support (Ching, 1979). Additionally, the usual treatment schedules often must be altered for the elderly due to their inability to tolerate daily treatment secondary to nausea, weakness etc. Treatment may be compromised by decreased daily dose rate, unscheduled absences from treatment or decreases in planned total dose. Anticipation of these problems may be handled by an altered regimen, such as a split-dose schedule. With these adjustments potentially curative radiation therapy can even be given. In other situations, palliative radiation as a means of pain control or to treat local obstructive symptoms can be used very effectively in elderly patients.

Chemotherapy

Because of the marked heterogeneity of the elderly as a population with respect to both variations in physiological aging and comorbid diseases, the clinical dictum has been for individualisation of therapy. While this is an important concept in many elderly patients, it has been often inappropriately applied so that older patients frequently have been excluded from systematic treatment protocol studies, the standard source from which oncologists gain information on response to the toxicity of therapy (Begg, 1980).

Although knowledge is beginning to accumulate in regard to drug metabolism in the elderly (Ouslander, 1981), little data exists in regard to altered handling of specific chemotherapeutic agents in this group. Because of the variability in the biology of tumours in the elderly, no conclusions can be reached about chemotherapeutic responsiveness of specific tumours as a function of age per se. However more information is available concerning the toxicity of these agents in aged patients. The major limiting factor for most drugs is bone marrow toxicity. In aged patients with anaemia, a decrease exists in granulocyte reserve as measured by CFU-C or bone marrow precursor cells (Lipschitz, 1980). Furthermore, long-term cultures of mouse bone marrow cells indicate a reduced proliferative capacity of normal stem cells in aged mice (Reincke, 1982; Manch, 1982). In a retrospective review of elderly patients entered on the Eastern Cooperative Oncology Group (ECOG) protocols, only two drugs, methyl CCNU and methotrexate were associated with excessive toxicity compared to that in younger patients (Carbone, 1982). It was postulated that the methotrexate toxicity may have been related to failure to appropriately reduce the dose for an age-related decline in renal function. Methyl CCNU is a nitrosourea which may more severely suppress the normal bone marrow stem cell. However another recent study using another nitrosourea, Bischloroethyl nitrosourea (BCNU) in combination with cyclophosphamide and prednisone in patients with myeloma showed no increased toxicity in elderly patients (Cohen, 1983). Clearly, further studies are warranted to determine drug dosage in elderly patients and the risk factors predisposing to excessive bone marrow toxicity.

Regarding other drug toxicity, patients over 70 do appear at increased risk for pulmonary toxicity from bleomycin (Ginsberg, 1982). The cardiotoxicity of adriamycin in the elderly is more controversial. In one series, age was a risk factor (Bristow, 1978), but in a larger series, pre-existing cardiac disease rather than age was the major predisposing factor (Praga, 1979). In other situations it is not clear if age per se is a predisposing risk factor, but because of age-related increase in the frequency of co-existing diseases, toxicity may be more common and the result of toxicity more dramatic. A case in point is the neuropathy associated with vincristine. Peripheral neuropathy is much more frequent in the elderly but may be subclinical until a neurotoxic agent is administered. Furthermore a younger patient may be able to compensate for paraesthesias or even some degree of motor weakness, whereas the complications may be disastrous in an elderly patient who already has compromised strength and balance. Other general toxicities of chemotherapy have been well reviewed (Perry, 1982).

It is not surprising given this range of known and unknown toxicities that there has been a bias against aggressive chemotherapy in the elderly. However, in retrospective reviews of elderly patients entered on protocols, the aged have equivalent responses in terms of chemotherapy (Begg, 1980; Cohen, 1983). Another series of small cell lung cancer with patients over 70 also showed a beneficial effect for the use of combination chemotherapy (Clamon, 1982). All these studies are retrospective and may be inherently biased in terms of selection of the elderly patient. However, they should lessen the tendency to withhold chemotherapy based on chronologic age alone. Prospective studies should be done to further evaluate specific benefits and toxicities for chemotherapy in the elderly as has been done for younger patients.

One area where this is currently being studied is adjuvant chemotherapy in breast cancer (Bonnadona, 1981). From the early trials of adjuvant chemotherapy in breast cancer, dose reductions were commonly made in women over the age of 60. The conclusion of the studies was that post-menopausal women did not receive the same benefit from chemotherapy that pre-menopausal women did. However when the data were reviewed retrospectively, it was clear that the subgroup of post-menopausal women who had received full dose chemotherapy similar to the pre-menopausal women, received the same benefit of treatment.

In attempts at curative treatment with chemotherapy, dose appears to be a critical factor (Frei, 1981). Even if the elderly are able to receive full dose chemotherapy, there may still be a difference in the biology of the tumour that may alter responses compared to younger patients. An example of this may be Hodgkin's disease where patients greater than 60 years of age with advanced disease were treated with combination chemotherapy. Even when the analysis was restricted to patients who received greater than 90% of their projected drug dosages, the complete remission rate and the median time of recurrence and duration of survival were all much shorter than in younger patients (Peterson et al, 1982).

In most situations currently, cancer chemotherapy is used as a palliative treatment. The haematologic malignancies in general show a striking age-related increase

in incidence. Experience with nodular lymphomas, chronic lymphocytic leukaemia, and multiple myeloma in the elderly.

In other situations such as acute leukaemia, both the disease and the treatment are more desperate. Controversy continues as to the best management of the elderly patient with acute leukaemia (Peterson, 1982). The patient may have increased infections and bleeding complications during bone marrow aplasia from aggressive chemotherapy, but with the current supportive care available at major leukaemia centers, identical remission rates can be achieved for patients under and over 60 (Foon, 1981). However, elderly patients are more likely to have antecedent haematological disorders, or 'pre-leukaemia' which adversely influence prognosis (Keating, 1981). Treatment decisions in these situations must be made with the assistance and expertise of a skilled haematologist with therapy designed to meet the goals of an informed patient and family.

Hormonal therapy
Hormonally responsive cancers offer an additional therapeutic option in the elderly with breast or prostate cancer. The likelihood of response to hormonal therapy is 50–60% in the estrogen receptor positive patient and 5% in the estrogen receptor negative patient (Holland, 1982). If the estrogen receptor status is not known or not obtainable, in the setting of indolent metastasis, a therapeutic hormonal trial is reasonable. Tamoxifen is generally favoured over diethylstilbestrol as initial therapy because of the lowered cardiovascular morbidity, although it is more expensive. Relapse of a hormonally responsive tumour can often be successfully treated with subsequent hormonal manipulation such as hormone withdrawal, aminoglutethimide, steroids, androgens or progesterones. A skilled breast oncologist can often manage an elderly patient with metastatic breast cancer for many years with hormonal manipulation.

Systemic treatment of prostate cancer should await symptomatic or progressive metastatic disease. Orchiectomy produces fewer cardiovascular side effects than diethylstilbestrol, with equivalent response (Garnick, 1982). Any elderly man with a diagnosis of metastatic adenocarcinoma of unknown primary should have a careful examination for prostate carcinoma including an acid phosphatase, a skeletal survey looking for osteoblastic lesions and a prostate biopsy if the prostatic examination is abnormal.

CONCLUSION

Screening, diagnosis and treatment of cancer in the aged provide many challenges to the practitioner. Appropriate application of research to improve our understanding of cancer in the aged will lead to easier management decisions in the future. The primary care provider should play an important role by working together with the oncologist and patient care team to optimise benefit and minimise risk in the treatment plans. The elderly patient, to an even greater extent than the younger patient, can benefit from such an approach.

REFERENCES

Anisimov V N, Turusov V S 1981 Modifying effect of aging on chemical carcinogenesis, a review. Mechanisms of Ageing and Development 15: 399–414

Begg C B, Cohen J L, Ellerton J 1980 Are the elderly predisposed to toxicity from cancer chemotherapy? Cancer Clinical Trials 3: 369–379

Begg C, Carbone P P, Elson P J, Zelen H 1982 Participation of community hospitals in clinical trials: Analysis of Five Years of Experience in the Eastern Cooperative Oncology Group. New England Journal of Medicine 306: 1076–1080

Bonnadonna G, Valgussa P 1980 Dose-response effect of adjuvant chemotherapy in breast cancer. New England Journal of Medicine 304: 10–15

Boyd J B, Bradford B, Watne A L 1980 Operative risk factors of colon resection in the elderly. Annals of Surgery 192: 743–746

Bristow M R, Mason J W, Billingham M E, Daniels J R 1978 Doxorubicin cardiomyopathy: Evaluation by phonocardiography, endomyocardial biopsy, and cardiac catheterization. Annals of Internal Medicine 88: 168–175

Breyer R H, Zippe C, Pharr W F, Jensik R J, Kittle F, Faber L P 1981 Thoractomy in patients over age seventy years. Journal of Thoracic and Cardiovascular Surgery 81: 187–193

Bruley-Rosset M, Hercend T, Martinez J, Rappaport H, Mathé G 1981 Prevention of spontaenous tumors of aged mice by immunopharmacologic manipulation: Study of immune antitumor mechanisms. Journal of the National Cancer Institute 66: 1113–1119

Butler R N, Gastel B 1979 Aging and cancer management part III: research perspectives. Ca 29: 333–340

Cady B 1979 Risk factor analysis in differentiated thyroid cancer. Cancer 43: 810–820

Cechner R L, Chamberlain W, Carter J R, Milojkovic-Mirceta L, Nash N P 1980 Misdiagnosis of bronchogenic carcinoma. Cancer 46: 190–199

Ching N, Grossi C, Zurawinsky H, Jham G, Angers J, Mills C 1979 Nutritonal deficiencies and nutritional support therapy in geriatric cancer patients. Journal of the American Geriatrics Society 27: 491–494

Clamon G H, Audeh M W, Pinnick S 1982 Small cell lung carcinoma in the elderly. Journal of the American Geriatrics Society 30: 299–302

Cohen H J, Bartolucci A 1983 Influence of age on response to treatment and survival in multiple myeloma. Journal of the American Geriatrics Society 31: 272–277

Cohen H J, Crawford J 1982 Haematologic problems in the elderly. The Practice of Geriatric Medicine. W. B. Sanders, Philadelphia. (in press)

Crawford J, Cohen H J 1982 An approach to monoclonal gammopathies in the elderly. Geriatrics 37: 97–112

Crawford J, Cohen H J 1983 Aging and neoplasia. Annual Review of Gerontology and Geriatrics 4, in press

Del Guercio L R M, Cohn J 1980 Monitoring operative risk in the elderly. Journal of the American Medical Association 243: 1350–1355

DeVita V T, Hellman S, Rosenberg S A, (eds) 1982 Principles of Surgical oncology. J B Lippincott, Philadelphia

Dix D, Cohen P 1980 On the role of aging in cancer incidence, Journal of Theoretical Biology 83: 163–173

Djokovic J, Hedley-Whyte J 1979 Prediction of outcome of surgery and anesthesia in patients over 80. Journal of the American Medical Association 242: 2301–2306

Dugan S O, Scallion L M 1984 The elder with cancer: a developmental perspective. In: McIntire S, Ciotpa A (eds) Cancer Nursing: A Developmental Approach, John Wiley & Son Inc, New York

Eddy D 1981 ACS Guidelines: One year later. The Internist May: 9–11

Farber E 1981 Chemical carcinogenesis, New England Journal of Medicine 305: 1379–1389

Feigal D W, Blaisdell F W 1979 The estimation of surgical risk. Medical Clinics of North America 63: 1131–1143

Fernandes G, West A, Good R A 1979 Nutrition, immunity and cancer-a review. Part III. Effects of diet on the diseases of aging. Clinical Bulletin 9: 91–106

Foon K A, Zighelboim J, Yale C, Gate R D 1981 Intensive chemotherapy is the treatment of choice for the elderly patients with acute myelogenous leukemia. Blood 58: 467–470

Frei E, Canellos G P 1981 Dose: a critical factor in cancer chemotherapy. American Journal of Medicine 69: 585–594

Fries J F 1980 Aging, natural death, and the compression of morbidity, New England Journal of Medicine 303: 130–135

Garnick M B, Prout G R, Canellos G P 1982 Cancer of the prostate. In: Holland J F, Frei E (eds) Cancer Medicine. Lea & Febiger, Philadelphia

Ginsberg S J, Comis R L 1982 The pulmonary toxicity of anti-neoplastic agents. Seminars in Oncology 9: 34–51

Goldman L, Caldera D L, Nussbaum S R, Southwick F S, Krogstad D, Murray B 1977 Multifactorial index of cardiac risk in noncardiac surgical procedures. New England Journal of Medicine 297: 845–850

Gralla R J, Itri M, Pisko S E, Squillante A E, Kelsen D P, Braun D W 1981 Antimetic efficacy of high-dose metoclopramide: randomised trials with placebo and prochlorperazine in patient with chemotherapy-induced nausea and vomiting. New England Journal of Medicine 305: 905–909

Gunn W G 1980 Radiation therapy for the aging patient. Cancer 30: 337–347

Hansen H, Koziner B, Clarkson B 1981 Marker and kinetic studies in the non-Hodgkin's lymphomas. American Journal of Medicine 71: 107–123

Harkins S W, Warner M H 1980 Age and pain. Annual Review of Gerontology & Geriatrics 1: 121–131

Harris C C, Mulyhill J J, Thorgeirsson S S, Minna J D 1980 Individual differences in cancer susceptibility. Annals of Internal Medicine 92: 809–825

Herbsman H, Feldman J, Seldera J, Gardner B, Aflonso A E 1981 Survival following breast cancer surgery in the elderly. Cancer 47: 2358–2363

Higuchi T, Nakamura T, Uchino H 1980 Effect of age on atipyrine metabolism in patients with gastric cancer. Journal of the National Cancer Institute 65: 897–900

Hodkinson H M 1978 Cancer in the aged. In: Brocklehurst J C (ed) Textbook of Geriatric Medicine and Gerontology, Churchill Livingstone, Edinburgh

Hogue C C 1978 Professional teamwork: implementation of a good idea. In: Assessment and Evaluating Strategies in Aging: People, Populations and Programs, Duke University Center for the Study of Aging, Durham, North Carolina

Holland J F, Frei E (eds) 1982 Cancer Medicine. Lea & Febiger, Philadelphia

Holmes F F, Hearne III E 1981 Cancer stage-to-stage relationship: implications for cancer screening in the elderly. Journal of the American Geriatrics Society 29: 55–57

Howell T H 1980 Multiple primary neoplasms in the elderly. Journal of the American Geriatrics Society 28: 65–67

Johnson J 1982 Surgery in the elderly. In: Brown F, Goldman D, Levy W, Slapp G, Sussman E (ed) Medical Care of the Surgical Patient, J B Lippincott, Philadelphia

Kaiko R F 1980 Age and morphine analgesia in cancer patients with post-operative pain. Clinical Pharmacology and Therapeutics 28: 823–826

Kark A E, Wardle D F G 1980 Management of malignant disease in old age. In: Denham M J (ed) The Treatment of Medical Problems in the Elderly, University Park Press, Baltimore

Keating M J, McCredie K B, Benjamin R S, Bodey G P, Zander A, Smith T L 1981 Treatment of patients over 50 years of age with acute myelognous leukemia with a combination of rubidazone and cytosine arabinoside, vincristine, and prednisone (ROAP). Blood 58: 584–591

King D W, Pushparaj N, O'Toole K 1982 Morbidity and mortality in the aged. Hospital Practice 17(2): 97–109

Kovar M G 1977 Elderly people: the population 65 years and over, Health United States. In: National Center for Health Statistics 1976–1977, National Center for Health Statistics, United States Department of Health, Education and Welfare

Lancet Ed. 1976 Aging and Cancer. Lancet 1: 131–132

Laszlo J, Lucas V S, Pharm B S 1971 Emesis as a critical problem in chemotherapy. New England Journal of Medicine 305: 948–949

Lemon H M 1982 Estrogens. In: Holland J F, Frei E (eds) Cancer Medicine, Lea & Febiger, Philadelphia

Levine J, Kopf A W, Rigerl D S, Bart R S, Hennessey P, Friedman R J 1981 Correlation of thicknesses of superficial spreading malignant melanomas and ages of patients. Journal of Dermatological Surgery and Oncology 7: 311–316

Libow L S, Sherman F T (eds) 1981 The Core of Geriatric Medicine. C. V. Mosby Co., St. Louis

Linn B S, Linn M W 1981 Late stage cancer patients: age differences in their psycho-physical status and response to counseling. Journal of Gerontology 36: 689–692

Lipschitz D A, Thompson C 1980 Leukocyte reserve in anemic elderly. Clinical Research 28: 318A

Love R R, Camilli A E 1971 The value of screening, Cancer 48: 489–494

Lucas R, Brown C 1982 Assessment of cancer patients. In: Keefe F J, Blumenthal J A (eds) Assessment Strategies in Behavioural Medicine. Grune & Stratton, New York, 351–369

Lucas R A, Siegler I C 1983 The dying patient. In: Blazer D G, Siegler I C (eds) A family Approach to Health Care of the Elderly. Addison-Wesley, Menlo Park

MacFarlane J T, Storr A, Ward W J, Smith W H R 1981 Safety, usefulness and acceptability of fibreoptic bronchoscopy in the elderly. Age and Ageing 10: 127–131

Manch P, Botnik L E, Hannon E C, Obbagy J, Hellman S 1982 Decline in bone marrow proliferative capacity as a function of age. Blood 60: 245–252

The Medical Letter on Drugs and Therapeutics, Drug Treatment of Cancer pain 1982 The Medical Letter 24, October 29, 95–98

Ouslander J G 1981 Drug therapy in the elderly. Annals of Internal Medicine 95: 711–722

Perry M C 1982 Toxicity of chemotherapy, Seminars in Oncology 9: 1–4

Peterson B A 1982 Acute nonlymphocytic leukemia in the elderly. Biology and treatment. In: Bloomfield C P (ed) Acute Leukemia I, Martinus Nijhoff Publishers, The Hague, p 199–235

Peterson B A, Kennedy B J 1979 Aging and cancer management Part I: clinical observation, Cancer 29: 322–332

Peterson B A, Pajak T F, Cooper M R, Nissen N I, Glidewell O J, Holland J F 1982 Effect of age on therapeutic response and survival in advanced Hodgkin's Disease, Cancer Treatment Reports 66: 889–898

Pierson R L, Figge P K, Buchsbaum H J 1975 Surgery for gynecologic malignancy in the aged. Obstetrics and Gynecology 46: 523–527

Praga C, Beretta G, Vigo P L, Lemaz G R, Pollini C, Bonadonna G 1979 Adriamycin cardiotoxicity: A survey of 1273 patients. Cancer Treatment Reports 63: 827–834

Reincke U, Hannon E C, Rosenblatt M, Hellman S 1982 Proliferative capacity of murine hematopoietic stem cells in vitro. Science 215: 1619–1622

Riley V 1981 Psychoneuroendocrine influences on immunocompetence and neoplasia. Science 212: 1100–1109

Santos A L, Gelperin A 1975 Surgical mortality in the elderly. Journal of the American Geriatrics Society 23: 42–46

Scherr L 1981 Periodic health examination: a guide for designing individualized preventive health care in the asymptomatic patient. Annals of Internal Medicine 95: 729–732

Schein C J 1979 A selective approch to surgical problems in the aged. In: Rossman I (ed) Clinical Geriatrics. J B Lippincott Co, Philadephia

Seligman P A 1982 Hematologic and oncologic problems in the elderly. In: Schrier R W (ed) Clinical Internal Medicine in the Elderly. W B Sanders, Philadelphia, p 280–296

Shackney S E, McCormack G W, Cuchural G J 1979 Growth rate patterns of solid tumors and their relation to responsiveness to therapy. Annals of Internal Medicine 89: 107–121

Shaw H M, Milton G W, Farago G, McCarthy W H 1978 Endocrine influences on survival from malignant melanoma. Cancer 43: 669–677

Siegel L T, Longo D L 1981 The control of chemotherapy-induced emesis. Annals Internal Medicine 95: 352–359

Stewart I, Millac P, Shephard R H 1975 Neurosurgery in the old patient. Postgraduate Medicine Journal 51: 453–456

Tomita T, Raimondi A J 1981 Brain tumors in the elderly, Journal of the American Medical Association 246: 53–55

Turnbull A D, Gundy E, Howland W S, Beattie E J 1978 Surgical mortality among the elderly. An analysis of 4,050 operations (1970–1974). Clinical Bulletin 8: 139–142

Veronesi U, Saccozzi R, del Vecchio M, Banfi A, Clemente C, de Lena M 1981 Comparing radical mastectomy with quadrantectomy, axillary dissection, and radiotherapy in patients with small cancers of the breast. New England Journal of Medicine 305: 6–11

Weksler M E 1981 The sensescence of the immune system. Hospital Practice 16(10): 53–64

Young J L, Percy C L, Asire A J, Berg J W, Cusano M M, Gloeckler L A 1971 Surveillance, epidemiology, and end results: Cancer Incidence and Mortality in the US 1973-77. National Cancer Institute Monograph 57: 1–187

9

Infection

A. M. Herdan, S. C. Durmaskin & M. E. Weksler

The elderly are highly vulnerable to infectious diseases. This is documented by an age-related increase in the severity and frequency of these diseases. For example, the risk of death from pneumonia doubles every decade after the age of 20 (Besdine & Rose, 1982). The greater severity of infectious disease in the elderly results from a decline in defence mechanisms which prevent dissemination of local infection and from a loss of homeostatic forces which maintain normal physiological functions even during disease.

The increased susceptibility, with age, to infectious disease may appear at first sight paradoxical as immunity to many infections is acquired from prior exposure to microbial agents. Lifelong immunity, acquired during early and middle age, explains the relatively rare occurrence of viral infections such as measles or mycoplasma infections in old age (Foy et al, 1979). However two factors, immune senescence and anatomic defects which facilitate bacterial growth, make the elderly more susceptible to infection despite their immunological experience.

The immune system changes with age. The most dramatic changes involve the involution of the thymus at sexual maturity and the decline in the concentration of thymic hormone in the blood. There are also subtle alterations in the balance among regulatory T lymphocyte populations. Functional changes include a loss of cell mediated and humoral immune responses to foreign antigens and an increased response to autologous antigens. The increased frequency of auto-antibodies and circulating immune complexes in elderly people may cause tissue damage and contribute to the diseases of aging.

The importance of anatomic changes which accompany aging to infectious disease is obvious. For example, anatomic factors such as weakened perineal support and prostatic enlargement probably contribute to the increased incidence of urinary tract infection. Similarly a decreased cough reflex, weakened force of expiration and poor mucociliary clearance contribute to the occurrence of pulmonary infection. While the consequences of anatomic change are apparent, the precise contribution of impaired IgA antibody mediated immunity to urinary or bronchial infection has been more difficult to define.

The phrase 'immunocompromised host' refers to individuals who are highly susceptible to infection because of congenital or acquired immune deficiency. Young patients may have one of a heterogeneous group of rare congenital immunodeficiency diseases: DiGeorge's syndrome, X-linked agammaglobulinemia, or severe combined immunodeficiency. These diseases are usually fatal at early ages. Acquired immune deficiency in the young and middle-aged adult patient most commonly results from neoplastic disease or cytotoxic drug therapy although common variable immune deficiency and the acquired immune deficiency in homosexual men may represent primary diseases of the immune system itself. However, the most common immunodeficient state in middle-aged and older adults is that associated with normal aging.

Local defence barriers which normally limit the spread of infection include both the inflammatory and local immune responses. Bacteraemia which so frequently follows urinary tract infection and pneumonia in old age is a consequence of the failure to localise infection. The increased adherence of gram-negative bacteria to the epithelial surfaces of the oropharynx and lower respiratory tract also reflects altered local defence mechanism. It is clear that bacterial colonisation is inversely related to the general health of the patient. Thus, 20% of elderly people in the community, 40% in nursing homes and 60% in chronic disease hospitals have gram-negative bacterial colonisation of mucosal surfaces (Valenti et al, 1978). Gram-negative bacterial adherence to epithelial surfaces is increased in the elderly and seriously ill patients. Although prospective studies have not been reported, it is reasonable to believe that the colonised patients are the ones most likely to have gram-negative infections.

The symptoms and signs of infection in the elderly frequently are the same as those observed in young patients. However, the usual indications are absent in 10–20% of elderly patients with infection. Another problem is that symptoms and signs of infections when present, are sometimes erroneously attributed to non-infectious diseases common to the elderly. For example confusion, a sign of sepsis in the elderly may be attributed to cerebrovascular insufficiency. Fever may not be expressed by the elderly patient with localised or even disseminated infection. Afebrile bacteraemia was found three times more frequently in persons over 65 as compared to those under 65 years of age (Gleckman & Hilbert, 1982). In addition, one third of bacteraemic patients did not have a leukocytosis. Sometimes bacteraemic patients became afebrile and were thought to have responded to antibiotic therapy although antibiotic-resistant bacteraemia persisted. In treating the elderly patient the possibility of infection must always be considered even though the classic symptoms and signs may be lacking. A clue to infection in the afebrile patient is a shift to the left in the differential white cell count. This finding has been recorded in about 90% of elderly with afebrile bacteraemia (Gleckman & Hilbert, 1982). In addition, blood culture, which should be obtained if infection is a possibility, allows the identification and antibiotic sensitivity of the organism to be determined.

The usual symptoms or signs which help to identify the site of infection are less prominent in the elderly. There is a decreased sensitivity to pain, in part because of the loss of skin turgor. Chest pain or cough may be absent in pneumonia; dysuria may not be sensed in urinary tract infection; and pain may be absent with abscesses. The most common sources of sepsis in the elderly are the urinary tract, the gastro-intestinal and biliary tracts and the respiratory system (Esposito et al, 1980). A careful physical examination may be more productive than the elicitation of symptoms in finding the source of infection. The examiner should look for lesions such as a pressure sore, peri-rectal abscess or prostatic enlargement. In about one third of all cases, no source of infection can be identified. At other times symptoms or signs of infections in the elderly can be deceptive: bibasilar rales may reflect chronic bronchial disease or congestive heart failure and not acute pneumonia; bacteriuria, frequently present in women, may not indicate acute urinary tract infection.

When considering the possibility of infection in an elderly patient it is important to recognise that the symptoms may be non-specific. Fatigue, tiredness, somnolence or confusion may be the only clues to infection. The initial manifestation of endocarditis may be a neurological deficit, resulting from a septic embolus. This is sometimes misdiagnosed as a cerebrovascular accident, and the underlying endocarditis overlooked. In one study of X-ray diagnosed cases of pneumonia, more than half the patients failed to show signs of consolidation on physical examination (Osmer & Cole, 1966). Similarly, some patients with bacterial meningitis lack classical physical signs and present only with confusion and somnolence.

BACTERIAL DISEASES

There is a striking difference between the types of bacterial infection acquired in the community and those found in institutionalised patients (Garb et al, 1978). Pneumococcal pneumonia is predominant in community-acquired disease whereas patients in hospital more frequently develop gram-negative bacterial or staphylococcal pneumonia infections. Elderly patients are especially subject to 'nosocomial' infections. Altered host susceptibility and the increased exposure to infection from other patients and hospital staff, infected mechanical equipment and a reservoir of multiple antibiotic resistant and atypical bacteria all increase the incidence of unusual infections in hospitalised elderly patients. Approximately 5% of the population over 65 years in the USA are in long-term care institutions where the incidence of infection increases in proportion to the level of care provided (Garibaldi et al, 1981).

Pneumonia

While cough, rigors and fever can herald pneumonia in the elderly as in the young, it more often appears insidiously, presenting with non-specific symptoms such as malaise or confusion. If the history and physical examination suggest the possibility of bacterial pneumonia in an elderly patient, a complete blood count, sputum smear, blood culture and chest X-ray should be obtained. In severe pneumonias or in patients with chronic respiratory diseases, measurements of blood gases and serum electrolytes to detect hypoxia and electrolyte imbalance are also recommended.

It may be difficult to obtain sputum from an elderly patient whose cough reflex is depressed and who is too feeble to raise sputum. The yield of sputum is sometimes improved with the aid of gentle physiotherapy and postural drainage. It is important to Gram-stain a fresh sputum specimen. Specimens with polymorphonuclear cells showing intracellular bacteria are highly suggestive of an acute bacterial pneumonia. Such specimens are suitable for culture. If there are many squamous epithelial cells in a low power field, the specimen is probably from the upper respiratory tract and should be discarded. However it should be noted that the sputum is negative in more than 50% of pneumococcal pneumonias (Barrett-Connor, 1971). In hospital-acquired pneumonia it is important to establish whether the organisms (usually gram-negative bacteria or staphylococci) are pathogens of the lungs or only oropharyngeal commensals. Transtracheal aspiration can provide an uncontaminated lower respiratory tract aspirate. The white blood count might be normal in bacterial pneumonia but in such cases it is important to check for the presence of band forms on the blood smear. Bacteraemia occurs in over 30% of cases (Austrian & Gold, 1964) and a positive culture can identify the pathogen when the sputum specimen is inadequate. Chest X-rays can reveal pneumonia even when other signs are not present.

There are general therapeutic measures which can be applied to all elderly patients but the choice of a specific anti-microbial therapy will depend on the most probable pathogen, since therapy generally has to be started before laboratory identification. A broad spectrum antibiotic such as ampicillin or amoxicillin can be used with the addition of gentamycin if gram-negative infection is likely or the patient appears critically ill. Aminoglycosides because of their nephrotoxicity must be used with caution and frequently in reduced dosages. There is an age related decline in renal function with reduced capacity to excrete these drugs. Creatinine clearance is a better estimate of renal function than the serum creatinine level. Creatinine clearance can be estimated using the following equation (Cockcroft & Gault, 1976):

For men:

$$\frac{(140 - \text{Age in years}) \times \text{Weight in kg}}{72 \times \text{Serum Creatinine in mg/dl}}$$

For women: Multiply result by 0.85

The elderly are especially susceptible to the effects of lack of oxygen. Confusion or agitation in patients with pneumonia may be due to hypoxaemia and may respond to oxygen therapy. Sedation of the agitated elderly patient should be avoided, if possible, as it depresses respiration and increases the chance of aspiration. If sedation is essential, a short-acting benzodiazepine can be used. Fluid loss and electrolyte imbalance due to fever, poor oral intake or hyperventilation should be corrected. Fluid balance must be carefully monitored. Pneumonia can precipitate congestive cardiac failure and may necessitate the use of diuretics or rapid digitalisation. Physical therapy and postural drainage can be of great benefit in clearing lung secretions. Many patients are poorly nourished and can become hypo-albuminaemic with the stress of infection. Special attention to nutritional requirements is essential during convalescence. Abdominal distension, usually due to air swallowing, may cause considerable discomfort. This can be relieved by a naso-gastric tube.

Pneumococcal pneumonia
More than half of adult pneumonias are due to the pneumococcus. The overall mortality rate of pneumococcal pneumonia for all ages is about 10%. Bacteraemia following pneumonia is more common and more lethal in the elderly (Mufson et al, 1974). *Streptococcus pneumoniae*, a gram-positive bacteria, is a normal inhabitant of the upper respiratory tract. Many individuals harbor virulent pneumococci at times. Pneumococcal pneumonia is therefore a disease of carriers. Its occurrence reflects a breakdown in the host defence mechanisms of the elderly and debilitated. An upper respiratory tract viral infection which impairs these defence mechanisms is a frequent antecedent. Pneumococci penetrate into the alveoli and provoke an intense inflammatory response and profuse fibrinous edema.

The sputum usually contains numerous red blood cells and polymorphonuclear cells frequently with intracellular gram-positive cocci in pairs. Blood culture is positive in a third of cases (Austrian & Gold, 1964). The classic radiologic pattern shows alveolar infiltration with air bronchograms. The basal segments and posterior segments of the upper lobes are more frequently involved. Treatment with penicillin should be continued for at least seven days. If there is a history of penicillin allergy, erythromycin or an intravenous cephalosporin can be substituted. Bacteraemia is by far the most common extra-thoracic complication in pneumococcal pneumonia; meningitis, endocarditis and septic arthritis occur less frequently. Resolution is slow and it may take weeks to months before the lungs appear clear (Jay et al, 1975). Preventive therapy by vaccination, which hopefully will be more widely used, is fully discussed by Austrian elsewhere in this volume (chapter 28).

Staphylococcal pneumonia
Staphylococcal pneumonia is a common nosocomial infection. The bacteria are normal inhabitants of the nasopharynx, oropharynx and skin and the carrier rate can be as high as 70%. In a closed community such as a hospital ward, bacteria shed from desquamated epithelial cells, are found on clothing and bedding and can also be cultured from air samples. Only a few of the many phage types are pathogenic (Nahmias & Schulman, 1972). Mechanical ventilators have been a source of infection and a haematogenous spread of skin staphylocci has occurred following the use of intravenous or arterial catheters. Staphylococcal pneumonia may also be acquired in the community following a viral infection such as influenza.

If gram-positive organisms resembling staphylococci are identified in the sputum, treatment with a penicillinase resistant penicillin should be started immediately. To eradicate the staphylococcal infection and prevent a relapse or haematogenous spread, treatment should continue for a minimum of three to four weeks. The bacterial drug sensitivity will dictate the final choice of an appropriate antibiotic for prolonged therapy. Lung abscess and empyema are the most frequent complications.

Aspiration pneumonia
Aspiration pneumonia is a common problem in the frail elderly. A number of conditions contribute to this such as neurological damage and depressed consciousness. Important too is the decline with age of protective mechanisms which normally guard against aspiration such as cough, pharyngeal and laryngeal reflexes. In addition as previously described, increased colonisation of the oropharynx with gram-negative organisms occurs in the elderly.

The type and severity of the pulmonary reaction will depend on the inoculum. Aspiration of highly acidic gastric juice causes a chemical pneumonia and may cause the adult respiratory distress syndrome. When infection develops following aspiration of oropharyngeal secretions, the organisms are frequently mixed anaerobes, especially bacteroides and anaerobic streptococci. Symptoms can range from a typical pneumonia to a feeling of non-specific malaise. Chest X-ray shows focal or diffuse pulmonary infiltrates. If the inflammatory reaction progresses, lung abscess and empyema sometimes develop. Repeated aspiration can lead to fibrotic lung changes.

Elderly patients who tend to aspirate should not be given prophylactic antibiotics. However if they become infected, the culture report will determine the appropriate antibiotic therapy. Usually gentamycin and clindamycin can be given until the report is available. The risk of aspiration pneumonia is reduced by careful attention to oral hygiene and feeding of elderly patients in the sitting position.

Gram-negative pneumonia

The incidence of pneumonia due to gram-negative bacteria is increasing, particularly in hospitals and nursing homes. Although primarily associated with chronic aspiration, bacterial contamination of mechanical ventilating equipment may also be a source of infection. Pneumonia due to *Klebsiella, Proteus, Pseudomonas* and *Serratia* can all cause serious lung disease with a high fatality rate. *Klebsiella pneumonia* is responsible for less than 3% of primary bacterial pneumonia in the community. However one third of hospital acquired pneumonias are due to *Klebsiella* (Kreger et al, 1980). Alcoholics and those with chronic respiratory disease are the most susceptible.

All patients with suspected gram-negative pneumonia should be admitted to hospital. Early antibiotic therapy is imperative and should include a cephalosporin and aminoglycoside. Therapy can be modified once the bacteria are isolated and the antibiotic sensitivity determined. The severe and toxic nature of this pneumonia usually necessitates oxygen administration and frequent tracheal suction to remove tenacious secretions. The fatality rate is high in spite of therapy.

Haemophilus influenzae pneumonia

In recent years an increasing number of primary infections with pathogenic *Haemophilus influenzae* have been reported in the elderly (Berk et al, 1982). *Haemophilus influenzae* is a gram-negative pleomorphic rod which is found in the oropharynx of healthy individuals. This organism has been associated as a secondary pathogen following a viral infection, such as influenza. Since most individuals acquire antibodies to *Haemophilus* in childhood, patients with *Haemophilus* pneumonia usually have an acquired immune-deficiency associated with chronic lymphocytic leukaemia, lymphoma, or less commonly with immune senescence.

Blood cultures, in such patients, are frequently positive.

The radiological appearance is similar to that of pneumococcal pneumonia but there is often a more marked pleural reaction. Treatment is begun with intravenous ampicillin or amoxicillin. Since 10% of *Haemophilus influenzae* bacteria are resistant to ampicillin, the critically ill patient should be started on intravenous chloramphenicol until antibiotic sensitivity is determined.

Legionnaires' disease

The reported incidence of Legionnaires' disease has been increasing since the much publicised outbreak in 1976. The organism, *Legionella pneumophila*, does not appear to be related to other known micro-organisms. It is gram-negative, aerobic and motile. Although specific tests for the bacterium have become more readily available, the epidemiology of Legionnaires' disease is still uncertain. This pneumonia occurs more frequently in the elderly and in particular in men with a history of smoking. Asymptomatic disease occurs in the general population as evidenced by a rise in specific antibodies.

The most frequent symptoms are an acute, rapidly rising fever, a dry cough, pleuritic pain (often severe) and haemoptysis. Diarrhoea, vomiting and abdominal pain can also be prominent. However the predominant symptoms may be those associated with the central nervous system including lethargy, confusion or delirium and hypoxaemia. There may be a moderate leukocytosis and a shift to the left. Liver function tests may be abnormal and the serum glutamic-oxaloacetic transaminose (SGOT) level is elevated in 90% of cases. Proteinuria and occasional haematuria are also found. The cerebrospinal fluid is normal. The X-ray picture is that of a progressive broncho-pneumonia in the majority of cases but occasionally nodular infiltrates or pleural effusions may be present (Kirby et al, 1978). The mortality rate is about 15% and is higher in patients with serious underlying disease. Intravenous erythromycin is indicated as relapses have been reported with oral therapy.

It is often difficult to make a firm diagnosis at the onset of the disease but an atypical pneumonia in the presence of unexplained encephalopathy, abnormal liver function tests and haematuria suggest the possible diagnosis of Legionnaires' disease. The indirect fluorescent antibody test is the most commonly used diagnostic test. The diagnosis is confirmed by a fourfold rise in serum antibody titer. The culture of this bacterium is difficult and is possible only in specialised laboratories. Recently, a rapid diagnostic test has been developed which demonstrates the presence of bacterial antigens in the urine using an enzyme-linked immunoabsorbent assay (ELISA) (Tilton, 1979).

Pulmonary tuberculosis

Tuberculosis is now primarily found in the elderly population (Stead, 1981). This age group still has a reservoir of mycobacteria which can become active during the period of immune senescence. Since the elderly may not show the characteristic constellation of signs and symptoms of tuberculosis, it is always important to consider this diagnosis. Sometimes a patient will recall a long forgotten illness or period of prolonged therapy and this may suggest a past infection. Patients may be asymptomatic or may have vague, ill-defined complaints; they rarely present with fever, night sweats, loss of weight, productive cough and X-ray changes found in younger patients.

Skin testing with purified protein derivative (PPD) should be done. Hypersensitivity to *Mycobacterium Tuberculosis* develops two to six weeks after initial exposure, but usually declines after 60 years of age. False negative PPD tests occur in as many as 20% of elderly individuals tested at the standard dose of 5 Tuberculin Units. While induration of 10 mm or more at 48–72 hours is considered unequivocally positive, smaller indurations may be found in the elderly and require repeated testing for a clear result. Thus reactions measuring between 5 and 9 mm in diameter which are regarded as doubtful positive, can occur in patients with active tuberculosis. Anergy, which frequently occurs with severe malnutrition and in debilitating diseases can also give a false negative result. Therefore when skin testing with PPD, at least one other antigen which commonly gives a positive reaction in most persons, such as *Candida*, should be administered to test for anergy.

The definitive diagnosis for tuberculosis is made by culture. However, characteristic granuloma may be seen in bone marrow or liver biopsy. This evidence is sufficient to warrant treatment pending the culture result since these bacteria grow slowly and may take several weeks to produce a positive culture.

The treatment of tuberculosis requires two drugs, each with a different action on the mycobacteria. Isoniazid and rifampin or ethambutol are the first line drugs.

Urinary tract infection

The epidemiology of bacteriuria is well documented (Brocklehurst et al, 1968; Sourander, 1966). The prevalence rises sharply after age 65, especially among women. In the age group 70–80, urinary tract infection is found in more than 30% of women and about 20% of men. For those under 60, the rate is 6% for women and 3% for men (Brocklehurst, 1968). Because bacteriuria is such a frequent laboratory finding and is often without symptoms, efforts have been made to determine whether it has clinical significance. One study, conducted in a nursing home over a ten year period, showed an association between asymptomatic bacteriuria and a shortened life span (Dontas et al, 1981). Other studies concerned with hypertension (Marketos et al, 1970) and renal function (Kass et al, 1978), found no significant correlation with bacteriuria.

Certain age-related structural changes in the genito-urinary tract contribute to the high incidence of infection. In men, enlargement of the prostate gland and associated obstruction generally causes pooling of urine in the bladder, which is then a site for infection. In women, the prime causes of infection are atrophy of the urethral mucosa, cystocele and perineal soiling. Colonisation of the peri-urethral region by faecal bacteria often precedes the onset of infection (Gruneberg, 1969).

The majority of urinary tract infections are asymptomatic and are picked up on routine screening. However, when elderly patients present with such non-specific complaints as fever and lethargy, the possibility of a urinary infection should be included in the differential diagnosis. Many patients also present with the classical signs of urinary tract infection such as dysuria, frequency or transient incontinence.

It is not always possible to collect a clean-catch sample of urine from an incontinent patient. However, the use of a urinary catheter should be a last resort. The colony count of gram-negative enteric bacteria in the urine is a reliable diagnostic test for infection. A count of 100 000 colonies per ml is regarded as positive. If the count is less than 100 000 per ml, the test is inconclusive and should be repeated. *Escherichia Coli* is the pathogenic organism in the great majority of urinary tract infections. It is also the major pathogen in hospital acquired infection, but other enteric bacteria such as *Proteus mirabilus*, *Pseudomonas aeruginosa* and *Klebsiella pneumoniae* are also frequently encountered. Bacteria encountered in the hospital environment are frequently resistant to antibiotics.

Urinary tract infections in the elderly are generally chronic and recurrent because they result from structural changes of aging. Asymptomatic bacteriuria seems to be reasonably well tolerated and need not be treated. Symptomatic infection due to *Escherichia coli* usually responds to sulfonamides, ampicillin or amoxicillin. It may be difficult to eradicate the organisms and further therapy should be given only if symptoms recur. It is important to be alert to the consequences of bacteraemia with the development of septic shock, in any chronic urinary tract infection.

Septicaemia

Septicaemia is a serious and often fatal complication of bacterial infection. Urinary tract infection, pneumonia, malignancy and decubitus ulcers are some of the disorders frequent in the elderly which increase the risk of septicaemia. In some cases, no underlying disease is found (Esposito et al, 1980).

The majority of septicaemias are caused by a single organism, most frequently gram-negative bacteria such as *Escherichia coli*, *Kelbsiella*, *Proteus* or *Bacteroides*. *Staphylococcus aureus*, *Streptococcus pyogenes* or *Streptococcus pneumoniae* can also cause septicaemia. In about 5–10% of all cases more than one organism is involved. The physician should be alert to the possibility of an occult neoplasm in the gastro-intestinal tract or to a perforated diverticulum if such enteric organisms as group *D streptococci*, *Clostridia* or *Bacteroides* are reported on culture (Klein et al, 1977).

If sepsis is suspected, a minimum of three blood cultures should be taken immediately and antibiotic and supportive therapy started without waiting for microbial culture results. The complex of hypovolaemia, poor renal perfusion, adult respiratory distress syndrome and disseminated intravascular coagulation may occur in septicaemia and the patient should be treated in an intensive care unit where multi-system failure can be monitored. Much of the toxicity of gram-negative bacterial diseases is thought to be due to endotoxin derived from the cell wall. Antibodies to the core glycolipid of the cell wall of gram-negative bacteria have now been produced and used to treat gram-negative bacteraemia with promising results (Ziegler et al, 1982). In the future, immunisation with the core glycolipid may benefit elderly patients who are at high risk of gram-negative sepsis as for example would be patients with an indwelling urinary catheter.

Infectious endocarditis

Infectious endocarditis, which has a mortality rate of over 50% among patients of all ages, is particularly threatening to the elderly because the symptoms may be so vague that diagnosis and treatment are delayed. Transient bacteraemia can occur after such procedures as dental or urological surgery. If there is a pre-existing heart valve lesion such as calcification of a bicuspid or degenerative aortic valve, then infectious endocarditis may follow. A prosthetic heart valve is sometimes the site of endocardial infection. In some instances no underlying heart lesion is present. About one third of cases involve the aortic valve but the mitral valve or both valves may also be affected.

Fever, almost a universal symptom of infectious endocarditis in the young, is absent in one third of all elderly patients. This may be due to previous anti-microbial therapy or the blunted fever response of the elderly. Over 90% of elderly patients with infectious endocarditis develop heart murmurs and this may be the only clinical sign of infection. Splenomegaly occurs in about 50% of cases. Neurological complications may be the first presenting symptom or sign of infectious endocarditis. Emboli causing hemiplegia or coma are more frequent in the elderly.

Repeated blood cultures may be required to identify the infecting organism in infectious endocarditis. *Streptococcus viridans*, *Staphylococcus aureus*, *Staphylococcus epidermidis* and intestinal streptococci are the organisms most frequently found on culture. Echocardiography can be used to detect vegetations or other valvular damage.

Untreated patients with infectious endocarditis will die of heart failure. Prompt diagnosis remains critical to a decrease in mortality. Treatment with an appropriate antibiotic should be given in high doses intravenously for a period of 4–6 weeks. Antibiotic therapy can then be stopped but blood cultures should be taken at weekly intervals for an additional month. The majority of relapses occur during the first month after antibiotic treatment has been completed, but relapses can occur after many months.

Skin infections

In old age, the skin is a frequent site of local infection and occasionally the source of systemic bacteraemia. A decrease in the barrier function of the stratum corneum may make the epidermis more susceptible to bacterial penetration (Kligman, 1979). Inadequate skin hygiene increases the risk of infection.

The patient's response to infection may be minimal and it is important to inspect the skin routinely in all immobilised patients. Boils and carbuncles in the hair-bearing areas are sometimes not noticed on the back, buttocks and thighs. Treatment with systemic antibiotics and surgical incision of larger lesions is indicated.

Pressure sores are a major site of infection. They occur in 5–10% of hospital patients and 5–30% of nursing home patients. Special matresses of the water-filled or alternating pressure type can be very helpful in treatment and prevention of early lesions. Decubiti should be monitored by repeated bacterial culture and X-ray of the underlying bone. Timely treatment can prevent the development of septicaemia and osteomyelitis. In an established pressure sore, dead tissue must be removed regularly, either by topical enzyme application or excision. If this treatment fails then skin grafting may be necessary. Skilled nursing care including attention to hygiene and frequent turning to relieve pressure points can reduce morbidity. Attention to nutrition and correction of any anaemia encourage healing.

The elderly diabetic is prone to develop infection in foot ulcers and around the toe nails. Tissue hypoxia due to poor peripheral circulation and anaesthesia from neuropathy contribute to these infections. The lesions are frequently colonised by anaerobic bacteria and treatment with an appropriate antibiotic is essential. If left untreated, gangrene and osteomyelitis develop.

VIRAL DISEASES

The most common viral diseases of old age are influenza and herpes zoster. There are, however, increasing reports of other viral diseases occurring in nursing homes, particularly viral hepatitis B and viral gastroenteritis but it is still too early to assess their prevalence.

Influenza

In healthy young people, influenza is usually a self-limiting disease but among old people, pulmonary complications and death are frequent. Epidemics occur every few years with sporadic cases at other times. Resistance to influenza is in part associated with the level of residual antibody from a previous attack.

The symptoms of abrupt onset of fever, sore throat, dry cough, headache, and myalgia occur in both young and old, but among the old a secondary bacterial infection is common. The invading organisms are usually *Pneumococci, Staphylococci, Streptococci* or *Hemophilus influenzae.* During epidemics, physicians are alert to the typical signs and symptoms but at other times the diagnosis is more difficult and requires isolation of the virus or testing for a rise in serum antibody titre. The influenza patient should be carefully observed for complications but many bacterial and viral infections also produce flu-like symptoms and alternative diagnoses must always be considered.

No specific anti-viral agents are yet available, however amantidine has been shown to inhibit the replication of type A influenza virus and possibly type B at higher dose levels. As a preventive therapy in patients who have not been vaccinated, amantidine can be given throughout the epidemic for a period of 5–8 weeks. If treatment is started at the onset of symptoms there is some evidence that a 3–5 day course of amantidine can lessen the severity of the illness. The prophylactic dose is 100 mg twice daily and this same dose can be tried at the onset of a presumed type A influenza. This dosage appears to reduce the incidence of side effects, especially confusion, hallucination, depression, seizures and coma. Careful monitoring for central nervous system changes is recommended if amantidine is used.

The best treatment is prophylaxis. Since there is often a variation in antigenic strain from year to year, the current vaccine should be administered to all persons over 65 years of age in the autumn of each year. The value of immunoprophylaxis is discussed by Austrian (chapter 28).

Herpes zoster

Susceptibility to Herpes Zoster increases sharply with age. The *Varicella-Zoster* virus remains dormant in dorsal root ganglia after an attack of chicken pox and can be reactivated decades later. The triggering mechanisms of viral replication are not yet well understood but certainly diminished immune response appears to be an important factor. When the virus is reactivated, particles spread along axons to the regional dermatome.

Zoster may present with fever, chills and general malaise. Usually a prodrome of pain and paraesthesia lasting several days precedes a sudden eruption of the characteristic vesicles in a dorsal nerve root distribution, but this sequence of events may vary. The thoracic root segments are involved in 50–60% of cases and the trigeminal nerve in 10–15% (Fulginiti et al, 1979). Since the vesicles are infectious, contact in a non-immune individual can lead to chicken pox. A vesicle on the tip of the nose is a sign of involvement of the opthalmic division of the trigeminal nerve. Ophthalmic herpes can cause serious corneal damage and the eye should be carefully monitored. The incidence of post-herpatic neuralgia increases with age and by the seventh decade it is about 50%. The very serious complications of generalised zoster, pneumonia and encephalitis are quite rare.

A three week course of steroids, if begun within five days of onset of the rash may reduce post-herpetic neuralgia. Steroids should be given in ophthalmic zoster. Pain usually passes in a few weeks or months but sometimes persists permanently. At present, there is no satisfactory anti-viral agent for Varicella Zoster infection, however, systemic anti-viral drugs are being explored.

SUMMARY

The infections which occur with greatest frequency among the elderly have been reviewed. The most common sites are the lung and bladder where infections tend to be recurrent and chronic. Since the symptoms and signs of infection are often muted they are difficult to detect and thus effective therapy may be delayed. Nosocomial infections are common in elderly patients in acute as well as chronic care institutions. Antibiotic resistant bacteria, prevalent in these institutions, complicate therapy. Prophylactic vaccines for the pneumococcus and influenza virus are now available and should be considered in the routine care of the elderly population. Current research on immune senescence and mechanisms of host resistance hopefully will provide new approaches to limit or prevent infection. This should profoundly alter the future treatment of infectious disease.

REFERENCES

Austrian R, Gold J 1964 Pneumococcal bacteremia with especial reference to bacteremic pneumococcal pneumonia. Annals of Internal Medicine 60: 759–776

Barrett-Connor E 1971 The nonvalue of sputum culture in the diagnosis of pneumococcal pneumonia. American Review of Respiratory Diseases 103: 845–848

Berk S L, Holtsclaw M S, Wiener S L, Smith J K 1982 Nontypeable *haemophilus influenzae* in the elderly. Archives of Internal Medicine 142: 537–539

Besdine R W, Rose R M 1982 Aspects of infection in the elderly. In: Eisdorfer C, Besdine R W, Cristofalo V, Lawton M P, Maddox G L, Schaie K W, Starr B D (eds) Annual Review of Gerontology and Geriatrics, 3, Springer, New York

Brocklehurst J C, Dillane J B, Griffiths L, Fry J 1968 The prevalence and symptomology of urinary infection in an aged population. Gerontology Clinic 10: 242–253

Cockcroft D W, Gault M H 1976 Prediction of creatinine clearance from serum creatinine. Nephron 16: 31–41

Dontas A S, Kasviki-Charvati P, Chem L, Papanayiotou P C, Marketos S G 1981 Bacteriuria and survival in old age. New England Journal of Medicine 304: 939–943

Esposito A L, Gleckman R A, Cram S, Crowley M, McCabe F, Drapkin M S 1980 Community-acquired bacteremia in the elderly: Analysis of one hundred consecutive episodes. Journal of the American Geriatrics Society 28: 315–319

Foy H M, Kenny G E, Cooney M K, Allen I D 1979 Long-term epidemiology of infections with mycoplasma pneumoniae. Journal of Infectious Disease 139: 681–683

Fulginiti V A, John J T, Sieber O F 1979 Herpes zoster In: Dennis J D, Dobson R L, McGuire J (eds) Clinical Dermatology 3, Harper & Row, New York

Garb J L, Brown R B, Garb J R, Tuthill R W 1978 Differences in etiology of pneumonias in nursing home and community patients. Journal of the American Medical Association 240: 2169–2172

Garibaldi R A, Brodine S, Matsumiyas S 1981 Infections among patients in nursing homes, policies, prevalence, and problems. New England Journal of Medicine 305: 731–735

Gleckman R, Hilbert D 1982 Afebrile bacteremia; a phenomenon in geriatric patients. Journal of the American Medical Association 248: 1478–1481

Gruneberg R N 1969 Relationship of infecting urinary organism to the faecal flora in patients with symptomatic urinary infection. Lancet 2: 766–768

Jay S J, Johanson W G J, Pierce A K 1975 The radiographic resolution of Streptococcus Pneumoniae pneumonia. New England Journal of Medicine 293: 798–801

Kass E H, Miall W H, Stuart K L, Rosner B 1978 Epidemiologic aspects of infection of the urinary tract. In: Kass, E H and Brumfitt, W (eds) Infections of the Urinary Tract. University of Chicago Press, Chicago

Kirby B D, Snyder K M, Meyer R D, Finegold S M 1978 Legionnaires' disease: Clinical features of 24 cases. Annals of Internal Medicine 89: 297–309

Klein R S, Recco R A, Catalano M T, Edberg S C, Casey J, Steigbigel N H 1977 Association of streptococcus Bovis with carcinoma of the colon. New England Journal of Medicine 297: 800–802

Kligman A M 1979 Perspectives and problems in cutaneous gerontology. Journal of Investigative Dermatology 73: 39–46

Kreger B E, Craven D E, Carling P C, McCabe, W R 1980 Gram-Negative Bacteremia III. Reassessment of etiology, epidemiology and ecology in 612 patients. American Journal of Medicine 68: 332–343

Marketos S G, Dontas A S, Papanayiotou P, Econonou P 1970 Bacteriuria and arterial hypertension in old age. Geriatrics 25: 136–147

Mufson M A, Kruss D M, Wasil R E, Metzger W I 1974 Capsular types and outcome of bacteremic pneumococcal disease in the antibiotic era. Archives of Internal Medicine 134: 505–510

Nahmias A J, Schulman J A 1972 Staphylococal infections: Clinical aspects In: Cohen J O (ed) The Staphylococci, J. Wiley & Sons, New York

Osmer J C, Cole B K 1966 The stethoscope and roentgenogram in acute pneumonia. Southern Medical Journal 59: 75–77

Sourander L B 1966 Urinary tract infection in the aged: An epidemiological study. Annales Medicinal Internae Fenniae 55: Suppl 45 1–55

Stead W W 1981 Tuberculosis among elderly persons: An Outbreak in a nursing home. Annals of Internal Medicine 94: 606–610

Tilton R C 1979 Legionnaires' disease antigen detected by enzyme-linked immunosorbent assay. Annals of Internal Medicine 90: 697–698

Valenti W M, Trudell R G, Bentley D W 1978 Factors predisposing to oropharyngeal colonization with gram-negative bacilli in the aged. New England Journal of Medicine 298: 1108–1111

Ziegler E J, McCutchan J A, Fierer J, Glauser M P, Sadoff J C, Douglas H, Bravde A T 1982 Treatment of gram-negative bacteriuria and shock with human antiserum to a mutant Escherichia coli. New England Journal of Medicine 307: 1225–1230

10

Disorders of homeostasis

K. J. Collins

One of the fundamental characteristics of mammalian species is the ability to adapt to internal and external environmental changes through a series of physiological adjustments which restore equilibrium and maintain the constancy of the 'milieu interne'. Homeostasis reflects the sum of all physiological and biochemical regulations that maintain the steady-state condition. In adaptive processes, the nervous (particularly autonomic) and endocrine systems play a primary role, but clearly the maintenance of homeostasis involves to some extent the integrated function of all organs and systems.

It is well-recognised that aging is accompanied by a decline in adaptive ability, but nevertheless in resting conditions there is no marked difference in intracellular composition between young and old individuals (Timiras, 1972) and vital extracellular equilibrium levels such as blood sugar, pH and osmotic pressure are regulated closely and maintained even into advanced old age. Displacement of these levels evokes adjustments to restore equilibrium, but with aging, the steady-state level appears to be restored more slowly. Differences with age also become apparent in the ability to co-ordinate complex functions, manifested as an altered sensitivity and reduced flexibility of reflex responses. Functional changes in the motor and sensory components of the central nervous system (see chapters 2, 9 & 20) have been described and it has been postulated that it may not be a loss of neurones which contributes mainly to these changes but a decline in the quality of nerve cell functional processes (Bowen & Davison, 1978). Thus it is perhaps not the loss of any specific functional component which first leads to a decline in adaptive ability with age, but a progressive imbalance or desynchronisation of responses. The functional capacity rather than functional ability of an organ system may, however, diminish with age as a result of decreased cellular mass following involution (Bellamy, 1970). The decline in basal metabolic rate with age, for example, appears to be related to a reduction in the mass of functioning cells rather than to a decline in their metabolic activity. The functional capacity of many systems such as respiratory vital capacity, renal clearance and cardiac performance show a linear regression with age (Shock 1972) Figure 10.1.

In effect, should a functional decrement occur, compensatory processes intervene to help re-establish homeostasis and this ensures biological competence even in old age. There is considerable reserve to protect the performance of the organism, but accumulating pathological events with aging can seriously compromise performance. If repair of pathological changes fails to take place, especially when there are alterations occurring in immune reactions with age (see chapter 9), there then follows a progressive breakdown of adaptive mechanisms, of homeostasis and eventually complete failure of the organism. Disorders of homeostasis with age may therefore be considered to arise not by changes in equilibrium levels but in the efficiency with which they can be re-established once displacement has occurred. In old age, disturbances of adaptation are revealed as a decreased resistance to environmental stresses such as a reduced capacity to adapt to physico-chemical changes in the environment. This is sometimes expressed as an increased risk of death following stress in the elderly. With respect to traumatic injury it has been disputed that older individuals have less chance of survival (Collins, 1950). In controlled animal studies however using haemorrhage as a cause of mortality (Simms, 1942), it is shown that a relatively small linear change in homeostasis results in a large logarithmic increase in death-rate.

NEURO-ENDOCRINE RELATIONSHIPS

Almost all metabolic responses involve regulation by hormones and during development the actions of the endocrine system become indispensable to adaptive reactions. A loss in capacity to adapt to environmental changes is likely to involve changes in neuro-endocrine control. Central to these homeostatic regulations are the hypothalamo-pituitary-adrenal and thyroid axes.

The evidence for alterations in endocrine control with aging is mostly equivocal. A full appreciation is required of the dynamic equilibria which operate in both the resting condition and with stress displacement. Changes in blood hormone levels by themselves are not an adequate guide to

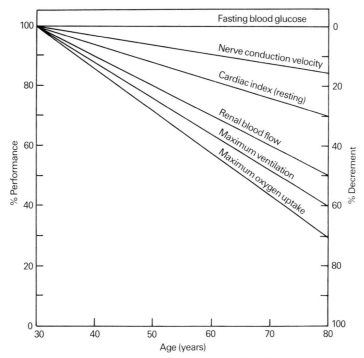

Fig. 10.1 Schematic linear projections to show age decrements in physiological functional capacity in males. Mean values for 20–35 year old subjects are taken as 100%. (Shock, 1972).

functional alterations, and particularly in non-steady stress states blood hormone levels depend on changes in secretion rates, metabolic and renal clearance, plasma protein carrying capacity and possible changes in target organ response (Collins & Few, 1979). It is difficult therefore to be sure of endocrine relationships without a comprehensive assessment of the physiological dynamics.

Though certain general features of senescence such as diminished motor responses, impaired muscle bulk, susceptibility to cold and hair thinning are suggestive of hypothyroidism, no profound differences have been shown in thyroid function between healthy young and old adults. Under resting conditions there are a number of reports of apparently normal levels of adrenal and thyroid hormones in healthy elderly individuals (Tyler et al, 1955; Gregerman & Solomon, 1967) but whether this represents the sum of changes in the turnover, secretion and metabolism of these hormones with age and whether the neuro-endocrine capacity to respond to stress is as efficient remains to be clearly established. Although there have been extensive studies, little consistent evidence has been obtained of an inability to cope with stress in old age due to deficiency in the function of the hypothalamo — pituitary — adrenal system. Hochstaedt et al (1961) have claimed that there is a significant diminution in the adreno-corticol response of old people to insulin hypoglycaemia. A later investigation by Cartlidge et al (1970) however failed to confirm any age differences. More detailed studies by

Romanoff et al (1961) suggest that there is negligible change in blood cortisol levels over the age range 10–90 years and that decreased removal of cortisol from the circulation in old age correlates with decreased muscle bulk.

An interesting generalisation advanced by Frolkis (1968a) suggests that homeostasis may fail during aging as the result of the diminishing influence of neural control on effector organs coupled with an increasing sensitivity to hormones. Evidence for the first observation appears to bear out the view that nervous co-ordination may indeed be compromised in old age. That for increased target-organ sensitivity to hormones is less well-founded. Increased sensitivity to exogenous thyroxine with age has often been shown (Belasco & Murlin, 1941) but data for other hormones suggests a decreased rather than increased sensitivity. Silverstone et al (1957) are of the opinion that for insulin, target-organ sensitivity is reduced, possibly in association with a fall in the rate of turnover of the hormone.

Another approach has been explored by Bellamy (1970) who contends that not only is homeostasis affected by a decreased capacity of hormone secretion but that there is a failure with age of the ability of hormones to elicit the correct 'pattern' of response in the target organ. There is however apparently no consistent direction in the changing pattern of effector responsiveness. The aging kidney appears in animal experiments to become less sensitive to anti-diuretic hormone (Dicker & Nunn, 1958) and other target organs are similarly shown to be less sensitive to insulin, growth hormone and adrenocorticotrophic hormone (ACTH). Some hormones on the contrary have been shown to be more effective in the elderly than in the young as mentioned above. Thyroid hormones in equivalent doses produce a greater increase in resting metabolism in old compared with young animals, an age difference in response not observed after thyroidectomy (Grad, 1969). Such differences in direction of changes in response with age are similar to the contrasting effects of different pharmacological agents on nervous structures. A reduced responsiveness of target tissues may be due to a decline in tissue sensitivity or to an impaired capacity to respond, while in tissues showing increased sensitivity compensatory mechanisms may counter-balance the reduced reactivity (Frolkis, 1968a). Whatever alterations occur in the secretion and action of endocrines some of the most consistently reported changes with age can be ascribed to the effects of neuro-transmission. Such changes can have a profound effect on endocrine feed-back mechanisms regulated in the brain and in neuro-endocrine control, and are therefore likely to be an important factor underlying alterations in adaptative capability. A loss of sensitivity of hypothalamic neurones to feedback signals, neural or endocrine, has been postulated (Dilman, 1971) as playing a key role in development, aging and disease.

THE AUTONOMIC NERVOUS SYSTEM

The autonomic nervous system plays an essential part in reflex regulations which help to maintain homeostasis. Abnormalities of sweating and vasomotor reflexes, orthostatic hypotension, gastrointestinal and bladder dysfunction, disorders of pupillary reflexes, impotence etc which occur more frequently in old age are all regarded as indications of autonomic impairment. Some of these disorders are associated with systemic degenerative disease but a component of age-related changes in autonomic function is often present (Exton-Smith, 1982). Methods of testing autonomic nervous system function in elderly patients have been described (Collins, 1982).

Essential differences can be discerned in the intensity of autonomic responses as well as the duration of reactions as for example in cold-induced sympathetic vasoconstrictor reflexes (Fig. 10.2). When autonomic reactions are repeatedly evoked there is a pronounced increase in the recovery time for function to return to initial levels after stimulation and the onset of fatigue is more pronounced in old age. In this respect both sympathetic and parasympathetic effects on organs and tissues can be shown to decline with aging. At an unsophisticated level of investigation it is observed that old animals require a much

stronger electrical current to stimulate autonomic nerves. Thus bradycardia is caused by a current of 0.35 V when the vagus nerve is stimulated in young adult rats but only with a stronger current of 0.53 V in old animals (Frolkis, 1968b). The functional capacity of autonomic ganglia appears to decline in old animals and the number of impulses the ganglion is able to transmit per second also falls. Peripheral autonomic nerves are reported to show equivalent age-related changes in structure to those in somatic nerves. These include an increasing incidence of random damage to Schwann cells which can be detected histologically as scattered segmental loss, thinning or abnormal shortness of the myelin sheath around axis cylinders and even some loss of nerve fibres with their replacement by finer axons (Ochoa & Mair, 1969). Physiologically these changes result in a slowing of conduction velocity and a diminution of reflex responses. Other evidence from animal experiments of failing autonomic function with aging suggests that there is reduced synthesis of acetylcholine in autonomic ganglia, an attenuation of baroreceptor reflexes and altered responses to hypothalamic stimulation (Timiras, 1972).

With the decline in parasympathetic and sympathetic nervous effects with age there is an apparent increase in the sensitivity of cells and tissues at postganglionic synapses and of autonomic ganglia to neuro-transmitters. In older animals smaller concentrations of transmitters will elicit a given change in heart rate and contractility, blood sugar level and endocrine function than in the young. There is a similarity in this respect to the exaggerated responses to noradrenaline infusion in patients with chronic autonomic failure (Bannister et al, 1979). Increased sensitivity to neuro-humoral transmitters in the autonomic nervous system could represent an important adaptive mechanism tending to maintain cellular neuro-humoral regulation in old age in spite of failing autonomic function. A decline in the density of functional sympatho-adrenal nerve terminals with aging has been postulated by Thulesius (1976) and this may go hand in hand with supersensitivity due to proliferation of receptors similar to that induced by denervation (Famborough & Hartzell, 1972). A rise in sensitivity to substances that stimulate is also accompanied by increased susceptibility to substances that block autonomic nervous transmission and this gives further credence to the view that neurones become more receptive but less competent with aging (Timiras, 1972). As noted earlier in discussing changes in sensitivity to hormones, there is not a complete concensus for the view that aging increases target-organ sensitivity. Reduced beta-adrenoceptor sensitivity has been demonstrated by Vestal et al (1979) who further suggested that there was a reduction in the number of receptors with increasing age. An age-associated loss of adrenergic nerve responsiveness has similarly been ascribed by Schocken & Roth (1977) to diminished beta-adrenoceptor concentration on the cell surface of lymphocyte cell fractions. The sum of the

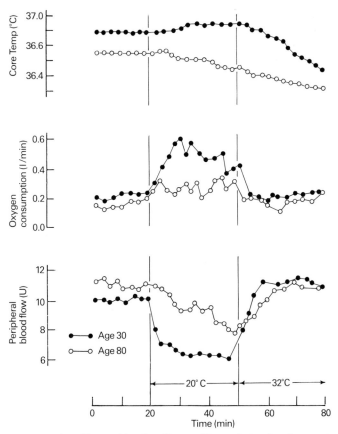

Fig. 10.2 Thermoregulatory responses in a 30 year-old and an 80 year-old man during forced convective cooling in air at 20°C followed by warming in air at 32°C.

evidence nevertheless argues for changes in one or other direction in the quality of autonomic neuro-humoral function with age. This may in turn reduce the adaptive capability of the organism by removing the 'fine' control but at the same time shielding cells and tissues from the effects of powerful disturbances in the central nervous system.

CONTROL AND IMPAIRMENT OF HOMEOSTASIS

Processes maintaining homeostasis in old age are influenced by alterations in the quality of central nervous, autonomic and neuro-endocrine control which leads to a loss of flexibility to adapt efficiently to environmental changes. Such changes in the internal or external environment may be expected to have a wide-ranging influence on the function of all bodily systems. Some of these systems have, however, been studied more intensively with respect to the effects of aging and may be singled out as examples of changes in physiological response which will ultimately determine the integrated performance of the whole organism. The specific systems which will now be

considered are those controlling thermoregulation, body fluid balance and blood sugar regulation, all of which involve multiple feed-back systems integrated in the hypothalamus. Age-related changes in hypothalamic-pituitary function for example, would potentially have a profound effect on all of these systems. According to some investigators (Finch, 1975), input signals to the hypothalamus from other parts of the brain conveyed by biogenic amines play an important part in regulating the aging process and changes in the function of hypothalamic cells may lead to declining control of homeostasis. Theories proposing that the hypothalamus performs a dominant role in the aging process owe much to investigations of the sensitivity threshold changes in neuro-endocrine response (Dilman et al, 1979), though at present the evidence for hypothalamic dysfunction remains inconclusive.

Thermeostasis in the elderly
Many integrated neuro-humoral control systems ensure that body temperature is kept constant over a wide range of environmental temperatures. Thermal lability in old age, i.e. an inability to maintain thermeostasis occurs for two main reasons. Firstly, thermal control of the body may be

inefficient because of changes in the intrinsic regulatory system or because of the presence of drugs which interfere with normal regulation. Secondly there are external factors such as a stressful climatic temperature which may be too severe for an impaired thermoregulatory system to cope with. A moderately cold or warm environment may be well-tolerated by a young person but it may be too severe for an elderly person if the responsiveness of the control mechanism is depressed. Two well-known examples of thermal lability in old people testify to this fact. During the coldest winter months in Great Britain there is usually an increase in the number of cases of hypothermia admitted to hospital, especially elderly patients (Maclean & Emslie-Smith, 1977; Collins et al, 1977). In central and southern States of the USA it is the summer epidemics of heatstroke in the hottest months which are of concern and this usually involves elderly city dwellers more than the younger population (Ellis, 1972).

Thermogenesis

Metabolic rate is lower in older people whether this is measured as heat produced per kilogram of body weight or per square metre of body surface. The reason why internal heat production is less in old people is a fundamental one. The proportion of body mass made up of functioning cells is usually smaller in the elderly and this results in an overall decrease in the total heat production of the body. When related to the total body water which also declines with age, basal oxygen consumption however is found to be constant (Shock et al, 1963). In addition the more sedentary life-style of the older age group results in a smaller contribution to overall heat production from muscular activity.

Most of the evidence for thermogenesis as the result of shivering when challenged with a cold environment suggests that the shivering process is reduced or less efficient in the elderly (Horvath et al, 1955). Recent investigations using convective cooling in air have shown that shivering ability is not lost with aging even in those over 80 years of age but changes occur in the character of the shivering response (Collins et al, 1981a) (Fig. 10.2).

High peaks of muscle contraction achieved by young people are usually not attained by the elderly and there is often a longer latent period required to initiate maximum shivering. Though many elderly people do not shiver during mild cold stress, some shiver quite well and in those that do there is often a marked loss of efficiency in the vasoconstrictor response to cold. Together with a reduced speed and intensity of the maximum response in the elderly a contributory factor may be a loss of motor power in the muscles themselves (Gutmann & Hanzlikova, 1976; Ermini, 1976). In the adult human, non-shivering thermogenesis does not seem to play a major role in thermoregulation. If there is any contribution to internal heat production from brown-fat in later years it is likely to be small, for though a few cells of brown-fat have been found in tissues of younger adults they disappear almost entirely by the eighth decade (Heaton, 1972).

Vasomotor responses

In the zone of vasomotor control i.e. in the intermediate zone of body temperature control between the points at which shivering or sweating occur, vasoconstriction or vasodilatation of the skin blood vessels form the first line of defence against temperature stress. A number of investigations have shown abnormal vasoconstrictor patterns in elderly people exposed to cold. Some elderly people, perhaps 20% of a normal healthy group, do not constrict significantly on cooling. Furthermore, in longitudinal studies the proportion showing non-constrictor responses to cooling increased during the course of a four-year period, and this was even more marked after eight years (Collins et al, 1982).

In most people it is possible to demonstrate transient bursts of vasoconstrictor activity, occuring a few times each minute. This rhythm is one which is generated by the central nervous control system because electrical recording from nerves supplying the blood vessels show a similar pattern of waxing and waning responses in a neutral temperature environment (Bini et al, 1980). With the additional stimulus of cold, the rhythmic activity increases in frequency until the vasoconstrictor response becomes continuous. In some elderly people this rhythmic activity is absent or difficult to detect (Collins et al, 1982) and it suggests altered sensitivity of the vasomotor control system.

Another aspect of blood flow control can be demonstrated during rewarming after cold exposure. One of the reasons for an 'after-drop' in body temperature when rewarming follows a mild cold exposure in air is a redistribution of cold blood from the skin as the blood vessels start to dilate. It might be expected that if blood vessels do not constrict very well in the cold, then on rewarming, the after-drop in body temperature would be reduced. This is found to be the case in elderly people who vasoconstrict poorly in the cold (see Fig. 10.2).

Temperature perception

As a general rule sensory systems in the body become blunted in old age and there are variable losses of vision, hearing and the senses of taste and smell. At least part of this decline in sensitivity appears to be due to changes in the nervous system itself, e.g. the degeneration of hair cells in the hearing organs and changes in the auditory nerves leading to losses in hearing acuity. Less is known about age-related changes in warmth and cold sensation and other modalities of skin sensation — pain, touch, pressure and vibration. It is known that cold receptors in the skin of primates such as the ape are highly dependent for optimum function on a good oxygen supply (Iggo & Paintal, 1977). In old age the vascular supply to skin tissues is reduced and the number and sensitivity of functioning nerve cells may alter. Both of these factors could influence the efficiency of thermal perception. An increase in threshold of cutaneous sensibility might also be due to changes with age in collagen and elastic tissues of the skin (Hall, 1976).

The results of tests of ability to discriminate between objects heated to different temperatures have shown that whereas nearly all young people can discriminate differences of about 1°C between two objects, old people were not usually able to match this, sometimes being unable to detect a temperature difference of 4°C or more (Collins & Exton-Smith, 1981). On the whole, the elderly perform much worse than young in tests of ability to perceive temperature differences. But an alternative explanation could be that older people were less confident in reporting different sensations of temperature rather than being less capable of detecting the differences. By the method of signal detection analysis, account can be taken of the ways such decisions are made by the individual. Such tests show that there were no differences in the criteria upon which decisions were taken by young and old groups in these particular experiments and this indicates that the differences in temperature perception were probably a true indication of an age effect. A lowered ability to sense the cold may put some old people at risk if they cannot detect a fall in environmental temperature. One study of elderly people aged between 74 and 86 years (Watts, 1972) showed that most responded to cold discomfort by an appropriate action to produce a warmer environment. Some however only experienced the feeling of cold at unusually low temperatures and did not regulate the indoor climate so promptly. Investigations of behavioural thermoregulation in controlled temperature conditions confirm that some elderly people lack the precision of environmental temperature control shown by younger people (Collins et al, 1981b).

Sudomotor responses
Impairment of the thermoregulatory system due to diminished or absent sweating is an important cause of heat exhaustion and heat stroke in hot conditions. In the elderly, sudomotor dysfunction will considerably increase the thermal strain and this is suggested by the increased mortality in persons aged 65 years or more in heat-waves of moderate severity in New York City in 1972 and 1973 and in London in 1968. Deaths in the elderly during heat waves when there is no air-conditioning can usually be ascribed to heart disease and cerebrovascular disease exacerbated by heat stress and only a small proportion directly to primary thermoregulatory failure (Ellis, 1972). Nevertheless, the sweating response to thermal and neurochemical stimulation in people aged 70 years or more has been found to be markedly reduced in most subjects compared to younger adults (Foster et al, 1976). Similarly there is a significantly higher core temperature threshold at which

sweating can be initiated (Collins et al, 1977) and a delayed development of vasodilatation (see Fig. 10.2) with heating. Deficient sweat and vasomotor responses may reflect deterioration in effector function as well as autonomic control. A further consideration is whether previous 'training' (acclimatisation) of the sweat glands in older people is less likely to have occurred in comparison with the young.

Central nervous control of thermeostasis
Body temperature varies with a well-marked circadian rhythm with deep-body temperature falling to a minimum during sleep at night and rising to a maximum during the day time. The body temperature rhythm appears to be synchronised with the sleep-wake cycle, but it has been found that there is an inherent difference in the way these two rhythmical changes are generated by 'pacemakers' in the brain. In some cases when a person is deprived of 'cues' which time these rhythms, the sleep-wake cycle operates free and with a different periodicity from the body temperature rhythm. When this happens, and it can be induced for example by constant illumination instead of a normal light-dark cycle, it has been observed that in a cold environment the body temperature decreases significantly (Moore-Ede & Sulzman, 1981). There is some evidence that desynchronisation of the circadian rhythms arises more frequently with increasing age (Wever, 1979) and if this is so it would increase the risk of hypothermia in elderly people.

The reduced efficiency of thermoregulatory processes in a proportion of elderly can be traced to structural and functional changes in the nervous system and to a reduced blood supply to central and peripheral effector systems. The hypothalamic threshold of sensitivity may be a primary cause of altered thermeostasis, both in 'setting' deep-body temperature (which is often low in older people, but there are few well-controlled studies to show that 'neutral' temperature is in fact lowered with age) and in functional responses to temperature stress. In responding to temperature change physiological responses in the elderly are more variable as body temperature is allowed to oscillate uncontrolled between wider limits of internal temperature.

Body fluid balance
The percentage of water in the body of an elderly person is smaller than that of a young adult and considerably smaller than an infant. Cross-sectional data suggest that there is an age-related decrease in total body water (Moore et al, 1963), with a more marked decrease in intracellular than extracellular volume (Fig. 10.3). Sodium, potassium, chloride, calcium and magnesium concentrations in serum are not significantly altered with age when measured under basal conditions (Korenchevsky, 1961).

The kidney obviously performs an important regulatory

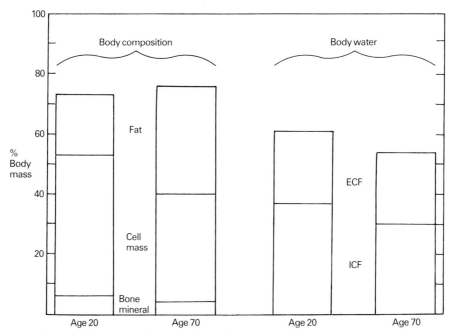

Fig. 10.3 Representation of the changes in body composition and body water during ageing in normal males.

role in maintaining body fluid balance as well as electrolyte and acid-base equilibria, and any alteration in renal efficiency is likely to have a profound effect on the ability to control homeostasis. Imbalance in body fluid regulation can arise, however, not from intrinsic renal changes with age but from extrarenal pathology, which in turn influences renal regulatory mechanisms. Several renal functions are reported to change with age, the most consistent being changes in glomerular filtration rate and renal blood flow (see chapter 43). Creatinine clearance rates fall from a mean of 81 ml min^{-1}/m^2 at 25–34 years of age to a mean of 56 ml min^{-1}/m^2 at 75–84 years, while serum creatinine concentrations do not change significantly (Lindeman, 1981). There is a proportional decrease in creatinine production in the body which reflects the decrease in cell mass with aging. Since normal kidney function depends on an adequate circulation, many aspects of renal pathology are related to circulatory disturbances. Shock (1960) concluded that though there are marked individual differences, the amount of blood flowing through the kidney reduces by about 6% per decade and between the age of 20 and 90 years renal blood flow is reduced by about half its original value. Glomerular filtration is decreased with aging and the capacity of the renal tubules to excrete and reabsorb is also impaired. Structural changes in the kidney bring about an involution with a reduced number of nephrons and degenerative changes in the remaining nephrons result in a decline in transport mechanisms, enzyme activity and membrane permeability of tubular and glomerular cells.

It remains undetermined whether the effects of changes in blood flow with aging affect renal function by local or systemic action. Local changes in the renal vascular tree i.e. the structure of renal arterioles or their degree of constriction, have been described, but the influence of changes in cardiac output or extensive atherosclerotic pathological changes in major vessels with age are also often implicated. An increased vasoconstriction of renal arterioles may divert blood normally directed to the kidney toward other tissues of the body. However when pyrogen is administered to young adult and elderly subjects to induce vasodilatation, there is a greater vasodilatation in the afferent arterioles of the older subjects which suggests a greater vasoconstriction exists in the resting state (McDonald et al, 1951). This appears to rule out the possibility of permanent structural defects in the renal arterioles which would render them incapable of dilatation. Hollenberg et al (1974) later found that renal blood flow varied with salt intake in young subjects but not in older subjects, and it was suggested that the renal vasculature in the elderly was in a relatively greater state of baseline vasodilatation or had a greater capacity to vasodilate. This finding is in contrast to the earlier data suggesting a relative state of resting vasoconstriction and the issue clearly has still to be resolved. Most of the evidence at present points to arteriolar vasoconstriction as a feature of the aging kidney, a feature which is aggravated by any general impairment of the circulatory system.

Homeostasis in body water balance depends partly on the response of tubular cells of the kidney to anti-diuretic hormone and, as noted earlier, tubular responsiveness to this hormone is markedly reduced in the aged. Contributing to this is a reduced activity of enzymes essential for renal transport mechanisms (Barrows et al, 1960), and a decreased functional capacity of the tubules (Adler et al, 1968). In the ability to produce ammonia, tubular capability was found to be unchanged and that reduced glomerular filtration was the primary factor in the observed decrease in ammonia excretion. Functional decline in the kidney does not therefore appear to be generalised but there are disproportionate decreases in separate excretory functions with aging. Despite such changes, the kidney remains capable under basal conditions of exerting a regulatory role to help maintain the constancy of body water balance, electrolytes, osmotic pressure and pH even in advanced old age.

If the equilibrium of body fluids is challenged, for example by an abnormal increase in acid or base, older individuals do however appear less capable of restoring acid-base balance to normal. The time required to return the pH value of arterial blood to normal after excess bicarbonate or ammonium chloride is measurably longer in the elderly. Another example of the slow response is illustrated in the ability to conserve sodium under conditions of dehydration. Epstein & Hollenberg (1976) have found that older subjects fail to conserve sodium as rapidly and efficiently as did younger subjects and that they are more likely to develop an exaggerated natriuresis after a water or saline load.

Glucose homeostasis

Changes in body composition with aging (see Fig. 10.3) partly reflect altered endocrine homeostasis and insulin-glucose relationships. The increase in adipose cell mass is associated with decreased insulin sensitivity which has been attributed to a reduction in effective insulin receptors (Archer et al, 1975). Thus aging man, even at a constant body weight, would be expected to show a decline in insulin sensitivity. In some individuals a relatively normal glucose homeostasis may be maintained at the cost of a higher rate of insulin secretion. Others may have an impaired insulin secretion and impaired glucose homeostasis. Defective insulin secretion with aging might occur according to Duckworth & Kitbachi (1972) because of a larger proportion of the less biologically active precursor, pro-insulin, appearing in the circulation. In addition there may also be a diminishing capacity of beta-cells to secrete insulin in response to a glucose load (Andres & Tobin, 1974).

Following intravenous or oral glucose loads, glucose tolerance is progressively impaired with aging (Fig. 10.4). There appears to be little change in the fasting unstressed blood glucose level and after a glucose load, blood glucose rises equally in all age groups for the first 40 minutes. After two hours, although there are large variances at all ages, the elderly show a significantly higher blood glucose level. In these studies (Andres & Tobin, 1974), the subjects were all considered to have no family history of diabetes, no diseases known to influence carbohydrate metabolism and no drug intake likely to influence glucose tolerance.

Under resting conditions blood sugar levels remain essentially unchanged throughout life. A balance is maintained by mechanisms that promote storage of glucose as glycogen in the liver and muscle when blood sugar levels

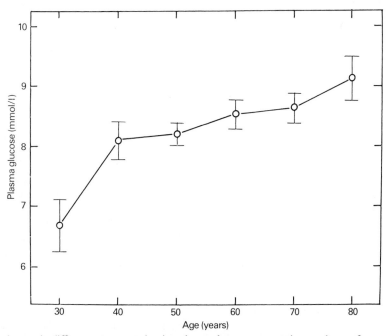

Fig. 10.4 Glucose tolerance in different age groups showing plasma glucose concentration two hours after an oral glucose load.

are high, those that release glucose from these stores for metabolic and functional needs, and those that induce overflow of glucose when blood levels are above the renal threshold. The regulation of blood sugar is multifactorial in nature and provides a good example of homeostasis which is maintained into old age by many possible compensatory adjustments which can be brought into play in the event of a decrement in any of the normal control mechanisms.

REFERENCES

Adler S, Lindeman R D, Yiengst M J, Beard E, Shock N W 1968 The effect of acute acid loading on the urinary excretion of acid by the ageing human kidney. Journal of Laboratory and Clinical Medicine 72: 278–289

Andres R, Tobin J D 1974 Aging and the disposition of glucose. In: Cristofalo V, Roberts T, Adelman R (eds) Advances in Experimental Medicine and Biology 61 Plenum, New York, p 239–249

Archer J A, Gordon P, Roth J 1975 Defect in insulin binding to receptors in obese man. Amelioration with calorie restriction. Journal of Clinical Investigation 55: 166–174

Bannister R, Davies B, Holly E, Rosenthal T, Sever P 1979 Defective cardiovascular reflexes and supersensitivity to sympathomimetic drugs in autonomic failure. Brain 102: 163–176

Barrows C H, Falzone J A, Shock N W 1960 Age differences in the succinoxidase activity of homogenates and mitochondria from the livers and kidneys of rats. Journal of Gerontology 15: 130–133

Belasco I J, Murlin J R 1941 The effect of thyroxin and thyrotropic hormone on the basal metabolism and thyroid tissue respiration of rats at various ages. Endocrinology 28: 145–152

Bellamy D 1970 Ageing and endocrine responses to environmental factors: with particular reference to mammals. In: Benson G K, Phillips J G (ed) Hormones and the Environment Cambridge University Press p 307

Bini G, Hagbarth K E, Hynninen P, Wallin B G 1980 Thermoregulatory and rhythm-generating mechanisms governing the sudomotor and vasoconstrictor outflow in human cutaneous nerves. Journal of Physiology 306: 537–552

Bowen D M, Davison A N 1978 Biochemical changes in the normal ageing brain and in dementia. In: Isaacs B (ed) Recent Advances in Geriatric Medicine 1. Churchill Livingstone, Edinburgh

Cartlidge N E, Black M M, Hall M R P, Hall R 1970 Pituitary function in the elderly. Gerontologia Clinica 12: 65–70

Collins D D 1950 Mortality in traumatic abdominal injuries in the elderly. Journal of Gerontology 5: 241–244

Collins K J 1982 Autonomic failure in the elderly. In: Bannister R (ed) Autonomic Failure Oxford University Press 489–507

Collins K J, Doré C, Exton-Smith A N, Fox R H, MacDonald I C, Woodward P M 1977 Accidental hypothermia and impaired temperature homeostasis in the elderly. British Medical Journal 1: 353–356

Collins K J, Easton J C, Exton-Smith A N 1981a Shivering thermogenesis and vasomotor responses with convective cooling in the elderly. Journal of Physiology 320: 76P

Collins K J, Easton J C, Exton-Smith A N 1982 The ageing nervous system: impairment of thermoregulation. In: Sarner M (ed) Advanced Medicine Pitman, Bath 250–257

Collins K J, Exton-Smith A N 1981 Urban hypothermia: thermoregulation, thermal perception and thermal comfort. In: Adam J M (ed) Hypothermia — ashore and afloat. Aberdeen University Press

Collins K J, Exton-Smith A N, Doré C 1981b Urban hypothermia: preferred temperature and thermal perception in old age. British Medical Journal 282: 175–177

Collins K J, Few J D 1979 Secretion and metabolism of cortisol and aldosterone during controlled hyperthermia. Journal of Physiology 292: 1–14

Dicker S E, Nunn J 1958 Antidiuresis in adult and old rats. Journal of Physiology 141: 332–336

Dilman V 1971 Age-associated elevation of hypothalamic threshold to feedback control, and the role in development, ageing and disease. Lancet 1: 1211

Dilman V M, Ostroumova M N, Tsyrlina E V 1979 Hypothalamic mechanisms of ageing and of specific age pathology. II. On the sensitivity threshold of hypothalamic-pituitary complex to homeostatic stimuli in adaptive homeostasis. Experimental Gerontology 14: 175–181

Duckworth W C, Kitbachi A E 1972 Direct measurement of plasma proinsulin in normal and diabetic subjects. American Journal of Medicine 53: 418–427

Ellis F P 1972 Mortality from heat illness and heat-aggravated illness in the United States. Environmental Research 5: 1–58

Epstein M, Hollenberg N K 1976 Age as a determinant of renal sodium conservation in normal man. Journal of Laboratory and Clinical Medicine 87: 411–417

Ermini M 1976 Ageing changes in mammalian skeletal muscle. Gerontology 22: 301–316

Exton-Smith A N 1982 Disorders of the autonomic nervous system. In: Caird F I (ed) Neurological Disorders in the Elderly. Wright P S E, Bristol p 182–201

Famborough S M, Hartzell H C 1972 Acetylcholine receptors: number and distribution of neuromusuclar junctions in rat diaphragm. Science 176: 189–191

Finch C E 1975 Aging and the regulation of hormones: a view in October 1972. In: Cristofalo V, Roberts T, Adelman R (eds) Advances in Experimental Medicine and Biology 61 Plenum, New York, p 229

Foster K G, Ellis F P, Doré C, Exton-Smith A N, Weiner J S 1976 Sweat responses in the aged. Age and Ageing 5: 91–101

Frolkis V V 1968a Regulatory process in the mechanism of ageing. Experimental Gerontology 3: 113–123

Frolkis V V 1968b The autonomic nervous system in the ageing organism. Triangle 8: 322–328

Grad B 1969 The metabolic responsiveness of young and old female rats to thyroxine. Journal of Gerontology 24: 5–11

Gregerman R I, Solomon N 1967 Acceleration of thyroxine and triiodothyroxine turnover during bacterial pulmonary infection and fever: implications for the functional state of the thyroid during stress and in senescence. Journal of Clinical Endocrinology and Metabolism 27: 93–105

Gutmann E, Hanzlikova V 1976 Fast and slow motor units in ageing. Gerontology 22: 280–300

Hall D A Ageing of Connective Tissue. Academic Press London

Heaton J M 1972 The distribution of brown adipose tissue in the human. Journal of Anatomy 112: 35–39

Hochstaedt B B, Scheenbaum M, Shadel M 1961 Adrenocorticol responsivity in old age. Gerontologia Clinica 3: 239–246

Hollenberg N K, Adams D F, Solomon H S 1974 Senescence and the renal vasculature in normal man. Circulation Research 34: 309–316

Horvath S M, Radcliffe C E, Hutt B K, Spurr G B 1955 Metabolic responses of old people to a cold environment. Journal of Applied Physiology 8: 145–148

Iggo A, Paintal A S 1977 The metabolic dependence of primate cutaneous cold receptors. Journal of Physiology 272: 40–41P

Korenchevsky V 1961 Physiological and pathological ageing. G H Bourne (ed) Karger: Basel, Switzerland p 129

Lindeman R D 1981 Age changes in the kidney. In: Danon D, Shock N W, Marois M (eds) Ageing and challenge to science and society. 1. Biology Oxford University Press, Oxford, p 227

Maclean D, Emslie-Smith D 1977 Accidental Hypothermia. Blackwell Scientific Publications, Oxford p 286–311

McDonald R K, Solomon D H, Shock N W 1951 Ageing as a factor in the renal hemodynamic changes induced by a standardized pyrogen. Journal of Clinical Investigation 30: 357–362

Moore F D, Olesen K H, McMurrey J D, Parker H V, Ball M R, Boyden C M 1963 In: The body cell mass and its supporting environment. Body Composition in Health & Disease. W B Saunders & Co, Philadelphia.

Moore-Ede M C, Sulzman F M 1981 Internal temporal order. In: Aschoff J (ed) Handbook of Behavioural Neurobiology. Plenum, New York, p 215–241

Ochoa J, Mair W C P 1969 The normal sural nerve in man. Part 2: Changes in the axons and Schwann cells due to ageing. Acta Neuropathologica 13: 217–239

Romanoff L P, Morris C W, Welch P, Rodriguez R M, Pincus G 1961 The metabolism of cortisol-4-C^{14} in young and elderly man. I. Secretion rate of cortisol and daily excretion of tetrahydrocortisol, allotetrahydrocortisol, tetrahydrocortisone and cortolone (20 and 20). Journal of Clinical Endocrinology and Metabolisn 21: 1413–1445

Schocken D D, Roth G S 1977 Reduced beta-adrenergic receptor concentrations in ageing man. Nature 267: 56–58

Shock N W 1960 Age changes in physiological functions in the total animal: role of tissue loss. In: Strehler B L, Ebert J D, Glass H B, Shock N W (eds) The Biology of Aging. American Institute of Biological Sciences, Washington p 258–264

Shock N W 1972 Energy metabolism, caloric intake and physical activity of the aging. In: Carlson L A (ed) Nutrition in old age. Almqvist & Wiksall, Uppsala, p 12

Shock N W, Watkin D M, Yienst M J, Norris A H, Gaffrey G W, Gregerman R I, Falzone J A 1963 Age differences in water content of the body as related to basal oxygen consumption in males. Journal of Gerontology 18: 1–10

Silverstone F A, Brandfoubrener M, Shock N W, Yiengst M J 1957 Age differences in the intravenous glucose tolerance tests and the response to insulin. Journal of Clinical Investigation 36: 504–514

Simms H S 1942 The use of a measurable cause of death, (haemorrhage) for the evaluation of ageing. Journal of General Physiology 26: 169–178

Thulesius O 1976 Pathophysiological classification and diagnosis of orthostatic hypotension. Cardiology 61 (Suppl 1): 180–190

Timiras P S 1972 Developmental Physiology and Ageing. Macmillan, London & New York

Tyler F H, Eik-Nes K, Sandberg A A, Florentin A A, Samuels L T 1955 Adrenocorticol capacity and metabolism of cortisol in elderly patients. Journal of the American Geriatrics Society 3: 79–84

Vestal R E, Wood A J, Shaud D G 1979 Reduced beta-adrenoreceptor sensitivity in the elderly. Clinical Pharmacology and Therapeutics 26: 181–186

Watts A J 1972 Hypothermia in the aged: a study of the role of cold sensitivity. Environmental Research 5: 118–126

Wever R A 1979 The circadian system of man. Results of experiments under temporal isolation. Springer-Verlag, New York

Illness in the elderly

11

Evaluation and treatment of the cognitively impaired patient

L. Barclay & J. P. Blass

INTRODUCTION

Cognitive impairment in the aging population is becoming a public health problem of epidemic proportions. Approximately 10% of the population over the age of 65 have clinically significant intellectual impairment, and by the early 21st century the number of elderly patients in nursing homes will probably increase to over three million (Beck et al, 1982). With the cost in America of nursing home care in 1979 at $22 billion, it is apparent that even a small decrease in the number of patients institutionalised could result in considerable savings of health care dollars, as well as in improvements in individual quality of life.

Diagnosing treatable forms of dementia therefore becomes of paramount importance to prevent unnecessary institutionalisation of salvageable patients. About 15% of patients referred for evaluation of dementia in several series proved to have treatable causes, and the proportion increased to 20% of patients under 65 years of age (Smith & Kiloh, 1981). Successful symptomatic management of untreatable forms of dementia can also forestall institutionalisation while improving the quality of life of the patient and his caretakers and family. As new developments in research promote better understanding of Alzheimer's disease and other currently untreatable dementias, there is always hope that these diseases may eventually be treatable, at least if detected in early stages.

Evaluation and treatment of the cognitively impaired patient is not only a problem for the neurologist, geriatrician or psychiatrist, but for the internist or family practitioner as well. Efficient and effective management requires knowledge of the wide differential diagnosis of diseases that can lead to cognitive impairment, a thorough evaluation to detect treatable conditions, and alleviation of symptoms when a treatable etiology cannot be found.

COMMON CAUSES OF COGNITIVE IMPAIRMENT

By far the most common cause of cognitive impairment in the elderly is Alzheimer's disease, accounting for 40%–50% of patients referred to most centres (Garcia et al, 1981). At autopsy, approximately half of the patients with dementia are found to have the argyrophilic plaques and neurofibrillary tangles characteristic of Alzheimer's disease (Terry & Davies, 1980). The clinical, pathological and research aspects of this disorder are well summarised in several recent reviews (Terry & Davies, 1980; Wilkins & Brady, 1969). Age of onset can be either presenile (less than 65) or senile (greater than 65), with insidious onset and steady progression. Whether or not distinctions based on age of onset have biological validity is still debated (Bondareff et al, 1982). Early features include forgetfulness, decreased problem solving ability and mild anomia, with disorders of language, orientation, praxis and spatial abilities following close behind. Eventually, patients are unable to care for themselves, and become mute, vegetative and bedridden. Neurological signs and symptoms are rarely seen. As of yet, there is no proven treatment for this disorder.

Many cognitively impaired patients are found at autopsy to have multi-infarct dementia, a condition in which multiple infarcts affecting large or small vascular territories lead to a state of chronic intellectual impairment. They often have a history or the physical findings of hypertension, cardiac or peripheral vascular disease, or small strokes. Characteristically, the onset of symptoms is abrupt, with stepwise deterioration, fluctuating course, emotional lability, nocturnal confusion and focal neurological signs and symptoms. These clinical features can be quantitated using the Hachinski ischaemic score (Hachinski et al, 1974), which has been modified by Rosen et al (1980) (Table 11.1). Although multi-infarct dementia

Table 11.1 Modified Hackinski Ischaemic Score. This score measures the likelihood that a patient has multi-infarct dementia, and has been pathologically verified by Rosen et al (1980).

Feature	Point value
Abrupt onset	2
Stepwise deterioration	1
Somatic complaints	1
Emotional lability	1
History of hypertension	1
History of strokes	2
Focal neurological symptoms	2
Focal neurological signs	2

is not reversible, good control of hypertension and appropriate anticoagulation is indicated in the hope of preventing further deterioration.

Depression can mimic dementia closely enough to fool even experienced diagnosticians. The combination of mild organic brain disease and severe depression is a particular trap. This error was made in 30% of a series of patients seen at the Maudsley Hospital (Ron et al, 1979). Others have made similar observations (Garcia et al, 1981). Depression can cause a subjective sensation of cognitive difficulty. Unlike patients with Alzheimer disease, these patients characteristically complain of their memory problems. They can score poorly on cognitive tasks because of poor effort, with many 'I don't know' responses (Wells, 1970). Past history or family history of depression should be a red flag alerting the clinician to the probability of depressive 'pseudodementia'. Patients often respond well to treatment with antidepressants, even if they have co-existent organic brain disease. Of course depression does not protect patients against the subsequent development of Alzheimer's disease, stroke or other disorders. Several centres have found similar incidences of these disorders (Table 11.2).

The classical clinical features of Alzheimer's, depressive pseudodementia and multi-infarct dementia are listed in Table 11.3. This table is not intended as an aid to diagnosis for the individual patient, as patients rarely have all the classical features of a given disease. Rather, it is intended as a description of the idealised presentation of these common causes of intellectual impairment.

DIAGNOSTIC APPROACH TO INTELLECTUAL DYSFUNCTION

The clinician's first objective in evaluating a patient whose chief complaint is intellectual impairment is to ascertain whether there is objective evidence of cognitive impairment. Among the brief psychometric tests which are helpful in making this distinction are the 'mental status' questionnaire (MSQ) of Kahn et al (1960) (Table 11.4) and the 'mini-mental status' examination (MMS) of Folstein et al (1975). The former is a set of 10 questions testing orientation and long-term memory for personal information, whereas the latter comprises 20 questions testing orientation, recent memory, attention, language and spatial constructions. Since the 'mini-mental status' examination involves reading, writing and copying, visual or motor impairment may lower the score. On the MSQ, clearly demented patients often score 7 or less, patients with milder cognitive impairment usually score 8 or 9 and cognitively intact patients usually score 9 or 10. The number of errors on the Kahn correlates with poor performance on verbal learning and recall tasks, even when only one or two errors are made (Zarit et al, 1978). Indeed orientation difficulties correlate with the number of plaques found at autopsy (Kurucz et al, 1981).

In patients without objective evidence of cognitive impairment, it is necessary to determine whether depression or other psychiatric illness and failure to pay attention to the task might be contributing to their subjective sense of intellectual dysfunction. When depressed patients score poorly on the MMS, their errors are often on the delayed three item recall task, unlike demented patients who score equally poorly on all items (LaRue, 1982).

Patients with mild cognitive impairment might have benign senescent forgetfulness (BSF), a relatively stable non-progressive condition associated with mild forgetfulness and anomia in the elderly. In comparison with demented patients, these patients tend to forget remote rather than recent events, and relatively unimportant parts of events rather than entire events. They are typically aware of their deficit and may have strategies for coping with it (Kral, 1978). Other patients with mild cognitive

Table 11.2 Frequency of diagnoses in patients referred to major centres for the evaluation of dementia.

Authors, location & number of patients	Smith & Kiloh, Sydney, Australia, 200	Marsden & Harrison, London, UK, 106	Malletta & Pirozzolo, 100	Garcia et al, White Plains, New York, 100
Demented:	*90.0%*	*79.2%*	*71.0%*	*63.0%*
AD	32.9%	45.3%	43.0%	39.0%
MID	13.6%	7.5%	10.0%	8.0%
MIX	—	—	—	—
Possibly Treatable	7.9%	13.2%	8.0%	—
Other	27.6%	13.2%	10.0%	9.0%
Not Demented	*10.0%*	*14.1%*	*28.0%*	*26.0%*
Depressed	5.0%	7.5%	24.0%	15.0%
Other	5.0%	6.7%	4.0%	11.0%
Dementia uncertain:	—	*6.6%*	*1.0%*	*11.0%*

AD – Alzheimer's disease; MID – multi-infarct dementia; MIX – mixed dementia

Table 11.3 Check points in the evaluation of the demented patient. Rows represent different points in the evaluation of the demented patient; columns represent expected findings in classical cases of Alzheimer's disease (AD), multi-infarct dementia (MID), depression and subcortical dementias. This table is intended merely as a descriptive guideline to the classical presentations of these disorders; it should not be used for taxonomic diagnosis.

	Alzheimer's	Multi-infarct	Depression	With subcortical signs
HISTORY				
Onset	Insidious	Abrupt	Variable, often after precipitating event	Variable
Progression	Steady decline, sometimes with plateaus	Stepwise decline	Uneven, fluctuating	Steady decline
Typical presenting symptoms	Memory or cognitive	Focal neuro Sx may occur	Personality change; concern over ↓ memory	Gait, speech, movement
Hx of strokes, ASCVD	Usually absent	Prominent	Usually absent	Usually absent
Risk factors for vascular disease	Usually absent	Prominent	Usually absent	Usually absent
Hachinski ischemic score	<4	>5	<4	Variable
Psychiatric history	Absent	Absent	Prominent to absent	Absent
Family history	Sometimes + for AD	Often + for ASCVD	Often + for depression	+ in Wilson's, Huntington's
Review of systems	Usually negative	+ for vascular Sx	+ for vegetative Sx	Myoclonus suggests CJ Seborrhea suggests Parkinson's
Sleep pattern	Often disturbed	Often disturbed	Early A.M. awakening	Hypersomnolence
Appetite	Eating apraxias common	Variable	Usually decreased	Often hyperphagic
PHYSICAL EXAM				
Appearance	Preserved initially	Self-care may be impaired	Sad; self-care often impaired	Disheveled
Alertness	Alert	Alert	Alert	Inattentive or lethargic
Affect	Cheerful, inappropriate	Labile	Depressed, anxious	Inappropriate
Attitude	Unconcerned, usually cooperative	May be hostile	Poor cooperation, apathetic or anxious	Often inappropriate
Awareness of deficit	Unaware	Unaware	Keenly aware	Unaware
Activity	Normal or increased	Variable	Bradykinetic	Bradykinetic
Gait	Normal or senile	May be hemiparetic	Normal	Festinating, ataxic
Station	Normal	May be hemiparetic	Normal	Stooped or dystonic
Movements	Normal	May be unilaterally impaired	Normal	Ataxic or tremulous
General physical exam	Usually normal	↑ BP, PVD, ASCVD (MID)	Usually normal	Usually normal
Neurological exam	Normal	Focal findings	Normal	Abnormal speech, tone, movements
Frontal lobe release signs	Present	Present	Absent	Present
PSYCHOMETRIC TESTING				
Language	Impaired (anomia, paraphasia) Vocabulary may be preserved	Impaired	Normal	Initially preserved
Praxis	Impaired	Impaired	Normal	Initially preserved
Memory	Short-term impaired more than long term	Impaired	Long-term impaired more than short term	Poor retrieval
Cognitive tasks	Wrong answers; coverups	Impaired	'I don't know' answers	Eventually impaired
Spatial constructions	Impaired	Impaired	Slow due to poor cooperation	Sloppy due to movement disorder

Table 11.3 (*contd*)

	Alzheimer's	Multi-infarct	Depression	With subcortical signs
Kahn MSQ / Folstein MMS	Usually < 7 / Decreased	Usually < 7 / Decreased	Usually > 7 / Usually normal with sufficient time & encouragement	Usually < 7 / May be decreased due to movement disorder
WAIS	Performance impaired relative to language	Variably decreased	Language = performance; timed tasks impaired	Variable
Behavioural rating scales	Behavioural impairment usually follows cognitive impairment	Impaired	Usually unimpaired	Behavioural impairment may precede cognitive impairment
LABORATORY TESTS				
Blood chemistries	Normal	May reveal end-organ damage (↑ BUN) or risk factors (↑ FBS; cholesterol)	Normal	Normal / Abnormal LFTs in Wilson's
CBC, ESR	Normal, may be anemic 2° to deficient diet	Normal, may be anemic 2° to deficient diet	Normal	Normal
B$_{12}$, folate	Normal, may be low 2° to deficient diet	Normal; may be low 2° to deficient diet	Normal; may be low 2° to deficient diet	Normal
Thyroid function tests	Normal	Normal	Normal	Normal
VDRL	Negative	Negative	Negative	+ in syphilis
CXR, urinalysis	Normal	May reveal cardiomegaly or renal disease	Normal	Normal
EKG	Normal	Abnormal	Normal	Normal
CTT	Mild atrophy, or normal	Infarcts; asymmetrical atrophy	Normal	Variable
EEG	Diffuse slowing	Asymmetrical or focal slowing	Normal	1 Hz repetitive spikes in C-J
Lumbar puncture	Normal	Normal	Normal	May reveal chronic meningitis
Cerebral blood flow	Diffusely & posteriorly decreased	Patchily decreased	Slightly decreased	Variable
Ceruloplasmin	Negative	Negative	Negative	+ in Wilson's
Red cell/plasma choline ratio	May be elevated	Normal	May be elevated	Normal
Dexamethasone suppression	Usually normal; may have false +	Variable	Usually abnormal	Abnormal in hypothalmic involvement
Long-latency event-related potential	May be abnormal	Variable	Normal	Variable
Brain & meningeal biopsy	Plaques & tangles; may be normal	Usually normal	Normal	May reveal chronic meningitis or C-J

C-J – Creutzfeldt-Jakob disease; Sx – symptoms; Hx – history; ASCVD – arteriosclerotic cardiovascular disease; PVDS – peripheral vascular disease; BUN – blood urea nitrogen; FBS – fasting blood sugar; LFT – liver function tests; CBC – complete blood count; ESR – erythrocyte sedimentation rate; VDRL – serological test for syphilis; CXR – chest X-ray; MSQ – mental status quotient; MMS – mini-mental status; WAIS – Wechsler adult intelligence scale; TPP – thiamine pyrophosphate.

Table 11.4 'Mental Status Questionnaire' of Kahn et al (1960) One point is scored for each correct answer.

Name of this hospital?
What city are you in now?
What year is it?
What month is it?
What is the date today?
What is the year of your birth?
When is your birthday?
How old are you?
Who is the present president?
Who was the previous president?

---

impairment eventually show the more malignant deterioration associated with Alzheimer's disease or other forms of dementia; careful follow-up should distinguish these conditions.

Moderate or severe cognitive impairment can be acute (duration less than six months) rather than chronic. Causes of acute cognitive impairment or delirium include hypertensive encephalopathy, drug toxicity, herpes encephalitis or other acute infections of the central nervous system, or metabolic encephalopathy. Delirium is generally associated with a fluctuating or decreased level of consciousness, making it relatively easy to distinguish from dementia, in which level of consciousness is generally preserved. Chronic cognitive impairment can either be present from childhood, in which case it is defined as mental retardation, or can occur de novo in adulthood, in which case it is defined as dementia. Patients can of course have an acute impairment of cognition superimposed on a chronic one.

The decision tree for analysing the chief complaint of intellectual dysfunction is summarised in the flow sheet of Figure 11.1.

DIAGNOSTIC APPROACH TO DEMENTIA

The diagnosis of dementia conventionally requires global (not just focal) cognitive impairment, lasting at least six months and in a clear sensorium. Focal lesions can lead to cognitive impairments which vary with the location of the lesion. If large enough, they can also lead to global impairments, i.e. to 'dementia', perhaps through pressure effects or oedema. However mass lesions giving rise to focal neurological deficits should not be confused with global intellectual impairment. For example, relatively circumscribed left hemisphere lesions can cause language impairment, and right hemisphere lesions can cause difficulties with spatial constructions. Common causes of mass lesions in the elderly include brain tumour and subdural hematoma; cerebrovascular accidents can also cause focal deficits with or without corresponding lesions on computerized transaxial tomogram (CTT) scan.

Multifocal lesions can cause multifocal cognitive deficits which may merge imperceptibly into 'global' dementias. The neurological examination, CTT scan and electroencephalogram (EEG) may reveal multiple areas of deficit, with impairment of several cognitive functions and multifocal lesions of motor, sensory or other neurological pathways. Most patients with multifocal dementia have multi-infarct dementia, although cerebral vasculitis, end-stage multiple sclerosis, carcinomatous meningitis, progressive multifocal leucoencephalopathy, and dementia pugilistica or other forms of dementia following head trauma are also in the differential diagnosis. Most of these conditions pose no diagnostic difficulty due to the clear historical or physical evidence of associated disorders.

Cerebral vasculitis, however, can occur in the absence of systemic vasculitis, and cerebral amyloid angiopathy can be particularly difficult to distinguish from multi-infarct dementia, as these patients often present with progressive dementia and episodes resembling transient ischemic attacks (Okazaki et al, 1979). This distinction can be important, as treatment of these patients with anticoagulants may predispose to lobar haemorrhage. Unfortunately, definitive diagnosis is only possible at brain biopsy. Certainly patients with past history of cerebral haemorrhage should not be given anticoagulants or antiplatelet agents in any event.

A number of disorders lead to both global cognitive dysfunction and evidence of subcortical damage. Since there are diffuse projections from the cerebral cortex to the diencephalon and other subcortical structures and vice versa, it is not surprising that disease processes affecting subcortical regions can also give rise to dementia. Similarly diffuse cortical dementias such as Alzheimer's disease are often associated with degenerative changes in the nucleus basalis, locus coeruleus, and other subcortical structures (Whitehouse et al, 1981). The distinction between diffuse cortical dementia and 'subcortical' dementia is artificial. However, neurological lesions in subcortical structures such as the basal ganglia and thalamus may be detectable early in the course of certain forms of dementia and may alert the clinician to the possibility of a set of differential diagnoses distinct from those associated with so-called 'cortical dementias'. Involvement of basal ganglia or extra-pyramidal pathways may be manifest as hypophonic or dysarthric speech, or as abnormalities of tone, posture, gait and movement. Involvement of thalamic or hypothalamic nuclei may cause hyperphagia, hypersomnolence or hyper-sexuality. Patients with 'subcortical' dementia may tend to have less cognitive impairment but more depression than Alzheimer patients with comparable functional impairment, although patterns of neuropsychological test performance are similar in the two groups (Mayeux et al, 1983).

Rapidly progressive dementia is seen in Creutzfeldt-

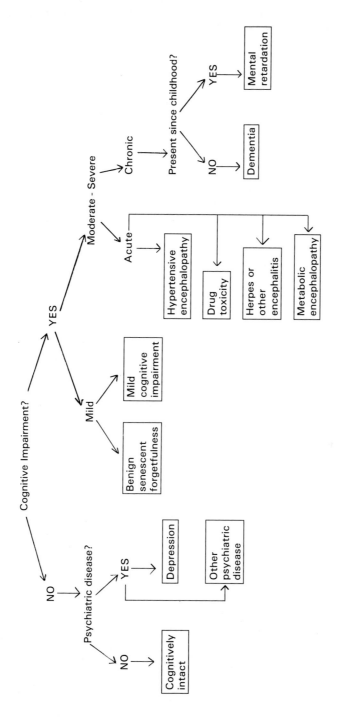

Fig. 11.1 Flow sheet for the differential diagnosis of intellectual dysfunction. Arrows represent decisions made in evaluating the patient with a chief complaint of intellectual dysfunction; boxes represent final diagnoses. See text for further explanation.

Jakob disease, a virally transmissable disease associated with myoclonus, periodic paroxysmal spike-and-wave discharges in EEG, and pyramidal, extrapyramidal and cerebellar signs (Roos et al, 1973). Progressive supranuclear palsy, characterised by supranuclear paralysis of vertical gaze, Parkinsonian signs, pseudobulbar symptoms and subcortical dementia, may be partially treatable with dopamine agonists such as bromocriptine and pergolide (Jackson et al, 1983). Although dementia is commonly seen in Parkinson's disease, a disorder affecting subcortical extrapyramidal pathways, recent autopsy evidence suggests that the associated dementia is usually Alzheimer's disease (Hakim & Mathieson 1979).

Hereditary causes of dementia associated with lesions of subcortical structures include Wilson's disease or hepatolenticular degeneration (Dobyns et al, 1979) and Huntington's chorea. Sporadic causes include chronic basilar meningitis such as syphilis or sarcoid which can be detected by lumbar puncture.

'Normal pressure' hydrocephalus, a condition with enlarged ventricles but normal or low cerebral spinal fluid pressure, can be detected by CTT scan and is often associated with the classic triad of dementia, gait disturbance and incontinence, due to early involvement of periventricular corticospinal fibres supplying the legs and perineal region. Cases with early and prominent gait disturbance or with a past history of known antecedent factors, such as head trauma, meningitis, or subarachnoid haemorrhage, generally respond best to shunting (Hakim & Adams, 1965). Patients who improve on psychological tests after lumbar puncture and removal of 40-50 ml of cerebrospinal fluid may be better candidates for shunt procedure than patients with no improvement after lumbar puncture (Wikkelso et al, 1982).

Most patients with dementia have diffuse cortical dysfunction, with global impairment of highest integrative functions and absence of localising findings on neurological examination. The largest category of diffuse cortical dementias is the degenerative category, including Alzheimer's and Pick's disease. The clinical distinction between these two disorders is not generally made in the United States as the prognosis and lack of specific treatment are the same in both. In some parts of Europe, early onset of personality change and 'frontal lobe behaviour' suggest the diagnosis of Pick's disease, with characteristic Pick bodies seen in frontal and temporal regions at autopsy.

The causes of diffuse cortical dysfunction are however multiple, and include systemic disorders which indirectly impair cognitive functions. Cardiopulmonary disorders including congestive heart failure and systemic infections including endocarditis can either present as dementia or can further impair cognitive functions in patients with other causes of dementia. Other such conditions are hepatic, uraemic, post-hypoxic and other forms of metabolic encephalopathy (Blass, 1980); endocrine causes including hypo- or hyperthyroidism, hypopituitarism and Cushing's disease; toxin exposure including alcoholic degeneration, heavy metal poisoning and substance abuse; and deficiency states including Korsakoff's psychosis and B_{12} or folate deficiency. All can impair cognitive function, and certainly can 'tip' patients with Alzheimer's disease or other dementing disorders into severe cognitive failure. Since these conditions are potentially treatable, early detection may help reverse cognitive impairment in patients with these disorders. Cancer not directly involving either the brain or meninges can cause diffuse cortical dysfunction through a poorly understood 'remote effect' (Brain & Adams, 1965).

Rarely metachromatic leucodystrophy can present in adult life as diffuse cortical dementia (Skomer et al, 1983). Another genetic cause of degenerative dementia is lipomembranous polycystic osteodysplasia, which is associated with progressive dementia resembling Alzheimer's except for increased frequency of seizures, calcification of basal ganglia and multiple bone cysts with pathologic fractures (Bird et al, 1983).

The decision tree for the differential diagnosis of dementia is summarised in the flow sheet of Figure 11.2.

EVALUATION OF THE PATIENT WITH COGNITIVE IMPAIRMENT

As indicated above, evaluation of a patient with a chief complaint of intellectual dysfunction requires ascertaining whether cognitive impairment or dementia exists, discerning the cause as exactly as possible, and determining whether there is a treatable component to the patient's complaints. History taking should focus on the presenting symptoms, onset, progression and duration, as these features help distinguish the major causes of cognitive impairment. History of drug or alcohol abuse, family history, cardiovascular history, review of systems and analysis of sleep and eating patterns may also give important clues to aetiology. The Hachinski ischaemic score measures the likelihood that a patient has multi-infarct dementia (Table 11.1).

The main function of the physical examination is to rate the general appearance, activity and affect of the patient and to determine whether systemic illness or vascular disease is present. The neurological examination should be geared to detecting extrapyramidal features or speech disturbances typically associated with pathology in subcortical structures, and corticospinal or other long tract signs seen in the multifocal dementias. Brief bedside testing of mental status, including the Kahn MSQ and the 'mini-mental status' of Folstein et al should help determine the presence and degree of cognitive impairment (Table 11.4).

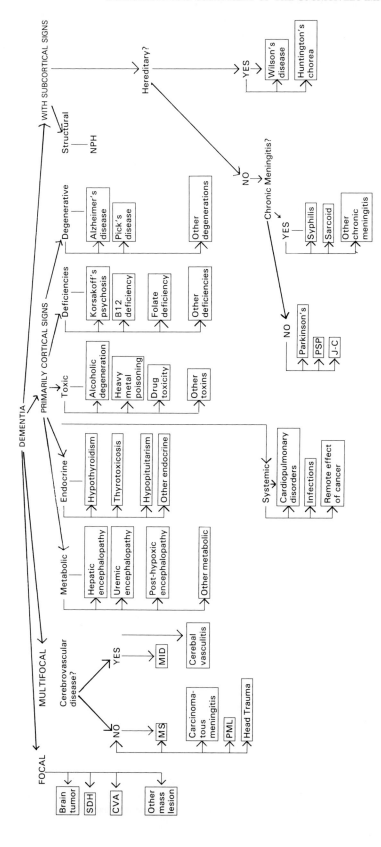

Fig. 11.2 Flow sheet for the differential diagnosis of dementia. See text and legend of Fig. 11.1 for further details. Focal lesions only give rise to global cognitive impairment, i.e. dementia, if large enough to cause significant edema or mass effect. Focal cognitive impairment should not be confused with dementia. SDH — subdural hematoma; CVA — cerebrovascular accident; MS — multiple sclerosis; PML — progressive multifocal leucoencephalopathy; MID — multi-infarct dementia; PSP — progressive supranuclear palsy; JC — Jakob-Creutzfeldt disease; NPH — normal pressure hydrocephalus.

Behavioural rating scales are useful in measuring the functional limitations of cognitively impaired patients and can be used to follow progression. Quantitative measures of behavioural impairment in Alzheimer's disease are correlated with number of plaques and tangles seen at autopsy (Blessed et al, 1968). Similarly a detailed social history can shed some light on the degree of social and behavioural impairment of the patient, and can help determine environmental or social factors which may be endangering the welfare of the patient or his family.

Laboratory evaluations should help rule out treatable causes of dementia and should include complete blood count, sedimentation rate, blood chemistries, a serologic test for syphilis, B_{12} and folate levels, thyroid function tests, chest x-ray and urinalysis. Electrocardiogram can help detect clinically silent cardiovascular disease. CTT scan with contrast is mainly useful to rule out mass lesions, infarcts or normal pressure hydrocephalus. Atrophy below the age of 60 suggests Alzheimer's disease or other organic cause of diffuse cortical dysfunction. Above the age of 60, overlap with non-demented controls is so extensive that 'atrophy' loses its diagnostic value. Indeed overinterpretation of CTT 'atrophy' has been an important source of overdiagnosis of dementia (Garcia et al, 1980). Low CTT numbers have been reported in Alzheimer's disease (Naeser et al, 1980). CTT density numbers are not routinely reported in most centres, but where available they may be a useful aid to diagnosis. All these tests should be done routinely in the evaluation of the cognitively impaired patient (Table 11.3).

Ancillary studies may be indicated to help rule out treatable factors compromising cognitive function. Audiologic evaluation may reveal treatable deafness leading to decreased ability to communicate (Herbst & Humphrey, 1980). Lumbar puncture, urine for heavy metals and aryl sulfatase assay should be done if there is reason to suspect chronic meningitis, heavy metal poisoning or adult-onset metachromatic leucodystrophy respectively. Despite its risks and expense, a brain biopsy may on occasion be justified to rule out cerebral vasculitis or other potentially treatable disorder.

Recently developed techniques may eventually prove to be useful in distinguishing the more common forms of dementia. Cerebral metabolic rate and blood flow typically fall in dementias, and several groups are trying to adapt their measurement as diagnostic aids (Zemcov et al, 1983). The dexamethasone suppression test is positive in 50% of depressed patients and only 4% of normals, but there is also a high rate of false positives in patients with Alzheimer's disease (Carrol et al, 1981). The P3 component of the novel event-related cortical potential, as measured by computer-averaged electro-encephalography, has been reported to be abnormally delayed in organic dementia but not depression (Goodin et al, 1978). Biochemical assays may eventually aid in the diagnosis of Alzheimer's disease (Barclay et al, 1982).

MANAGEMENT OF THE COGNITIVELY IMPAIRED PATIENT

A familiar and predictable environment can reduce the demented patient's disorientation and psychological discomfort. Regular and predictable routines, repeated explanations, constant reminders of time, place and person, and strategic placement of calendars and clocks can have a similar effect. Allowing the cognitively impaired patient to make simple but relatively restricted choices can allow him or her to feel in control without the frustration associated with choices that may be too difficult (Rabins, 1981). The essence of successful management is to present only as much new information as the patient can handle comfortably, and to present it over and over again.

Safety measures should include night-lights and brightly lit passages and stairs, locked doors or gates to prevent wandering, and keeping medications and poisons out of reach. Nutritional status can be better preserved if the patient is given well-balanced meals that are easy to eat, such as sandwiches, as eating apraxias are common in moderately advanced dementia. Daily exercise can promote a sense of physical well-being while decreasing restlessness, agitation and insomnia. Day Hospital programmes such as at the Burke Rehabilitation Centre, White Plains, New York, can be helpful in the behavioural mangement of these patients. This programme focuses on providing relief for the primary caretaker by caring for the patient three days per week, and on providing orientation, socialisation, dance therapy, recreational therapy and group therapy for the patient, with medical management as needed.

Social intervention can assist the family with obtaining home help, including homemakers, visiting nurses and Meals-on-Wheels programme. Transfer of financial and legal affairs should be expedited whenever necessary. Counselling and support groups for relatives can help them deal with their grief over gradually losing a loved one, their anger at the patient for deserting them or becoming a burden, and their guilt over their feelings of anger (Rabins et al, 1982).

Similarly, medical professionals working with demented patients need to be aware of their own problems in confronting this difficult task. Limitations of staff and physical resources often prevent adequate implementation of the behavioural measures described above; modern medical education is geared toward diagnosis and treatment of acute illness rather than management of chronic disease, and confronting a demented patient tends to induce psychological discomfort in physicians who may feel helpless when confronting untreatable conditions (Cassel & Jameton, 1981).

Finally, medical management should include diagnosis and treatment of congestive heart failure, systemic infections, drug toxicity or other reversible conditions exacerbating cognitive impairment. Medical management of depressive symptoms can be difficult, as the tricyclic antidepressants have an anticholinergic effect which may worsen cognitive function. Trazodone, a newer antidepressant with fewer anticholinergic effects, can be useful. A conventional starting dose is 25 mg at bedtime. This can be increased slowly in divided doses as tolerated. Neuroleptics commonly used in younger patients for treatment of delusions, hallucinations or marked agitation can markedly depress cognitive functions in elderly patients, and often cause tardive dyskinesia. Our preference is to use Oxazepam, a rapidly metabolized benzodiazepine, as a first drug of choice in 'sundowning', agitation or catastrophic reactions, resorting to butyrophenones or phenothiazines if minor tranquillizers and antidepressants fail. Our customary starting dose is 10 mg of Oxazepam at bedtime which is then increased to 10 mg thrice a day or more if needed. Altered pharmacokinetics in the elderly necessitates reduced dosage of most drugs (Ouslander, 1981).

EXPERIMENTAL THERAPY OF DEMENTIA

Experimental evidence suggests that central cholinergic systems are deficient in Alzheimer's disease. In postmortem specimens, choline acetyltransferase and acetylcholinesterase are decreased in the cortex, hippocampus, caudate and putamen in Alzheimer brains relative to controls. Furthermore the decrease of cortical choline acetyltransferase in Alzheimer patients is correlated with the number of plaques and with the degree of intellectual impairment (Perry et al, 1978). Similarly, acetylcholine synthesis is relatively decreased in biopsy samples from the temporal lobe of Alzheimer patients, and there is selective loss of cholinergic neurons in the nucleus basalis, which provides diffuse cholinergic input to the neocortex (White et al, 1981). Cholinergic manipulation in Alzheimer patients in vivo has included trials of the acetylcholine precursors choline or lecithin, which have been ineffective. However, the acetylcholinesterase inhibitor physostigmine, when used alone at the appropriate dose or in combination with precursors, led to statistically significant improvement on selected tasks in Alzheimer patients. Notably there was improvement on the Buschke selective reminding task. Unfortunately, physostigmine has a short half-life, and clinical improvement was not striking (Blass & Weksler, 1983). Recent reports suggest that oral physostigmine given in combination with lecithin has a longer half-life and may have longer-lasting effects on long-term recall (Thal et al, 1983). Other cholinergic agents which have been variably but briefly effective include the anticholinesterase tetrahydroacridine and the direct agonist arecoline (Blass & Weksler, 1983).

Treatment attempts have also been directed to other neurotransmitter systems in Alzheimer's disease. Amantadine, which liberates dopamine in the brain, reportedly increased alertness and decreased agitation in 7 out of 19 patients with senile dementia. However, 6 of these patients had toxic side effects including hyperactivity, anxiety, and visual hallucinations, and withdrawal symptoms of lethargy and unsteadiness were seen when the drug was discontinued (Muller et al, 1979). Similarly, dextroamphetamine and other adrenergic agents may improve alertness but at the cost of side effects (Hollister, 1975). The acetams, a group of γ-aminobutyric acid derivatives, have not had striking effects on performance (Gaitz & Varner, 1979).

Since hypophysectomised animals lose their ability to learn conditioned tasks, neuropeptides secreted by the pituitary may play some role in cognitive function. Adrenocorticotrophic hormone-melanocytic stimulating hormone fragments given to demented patients did not improve memory or cognitive tasks. Vasopressin given to head trauma patients caused no improvement on cognitive testing or functional peformance (Reichert et al, 1979).

Since cerebral blood flow and oxygen consumption are decreased in dementias, reversing this process might theoretically improve cognitive function. There has been no evidence of long-lasting improvement in demented patients given hyperbaric oxygen. Similarly anticoagulants and antiatherogenic drugs, which might theoretically increase cerebral blood flow, have no effect on established dementia, although they might prevent further strokes in patients with multi-infarct dementia.

Vasodilators have also been given in dementia in an attempt to increase cerebral blood flow. Different types of vasodilators have different sites of action, such as papaverine which acts directly on vascular smooth muscle, hydergine which acts on adrenoreceptors, and betahistine which acts on histamine receptors (Cook & James, 1981). The effect of these drugs on cognitive functions in dementia has not been impressive, and the limited improvements seen with hydergine might actually be due to its inhibition of cerebral phosphodiesterase, which might stimulate new protein synthesis (Hollister, 1975). Since decreased cerebral blood flow in dementia is most likely the effect and not the cause of decreased metabolism it is not surprising that this class of drugs has been largely ineffective.

CONCLUSIONS

Increase in the senescent population and in costs of institutionalisation necessitate efficient but effective evaluation and management of the cognitively impaired patient. Geriatric evaluation must be geared toward detecting treatable factors impairing cognitive function.

Neurologic evaluation can help in assessing whether cognitive impairment actually exists and whether the dementia is focal, multifocal, diffuse cortical, or subcortical in nature. Laboratory tests can further narrow down possible aetiologies. In the absence of effective therapy, there is no need to be in a hurry to make the diagnosis of Alzheimer's disease until the clinical picture is so clear cut that one can be certain. Over-diagnosis can harm the patients and their families; slow diagnosis does not.

Appropriate management of the demented patient includes treatment of exacerbating factors, medical management of agitation, depression and other symptoms, environmental manipulation to decrease disorientation and safety hazards, and behavioural techniques to promote awareness and psychological well-being. Counselling should be directed at helping the family deal with their feelings toward the demented patient, and social intervention should help obtain needed services. Although effective biological treatment of Alzheimer's disease is not yet possible, research in this area is accelerating. Evidence implicating cholinergic mechanisms provides a solid lead for therapeutic research.

REFERENCES

Barclay L L, Blass J P, Kopp V, Hanin I 1982 Red cell plasma choline ratio in dementia. New England Journal of Medicine 307: 501

Bird T D, Koerker R M, Leaird B J et al 1983 Lipomembranous polycystic osteodysplasia (brain, bone, and fat disease): a genetic cause of presenile dementia. Neurology 33: 81–86

Blass J P 1980 Metabolic dementias. In: Amaducci L (ed) Aging Raven Press

Blass J P, Weksler M E 1983 Approaches to the treatment of Alzheimer dementias. Annals of Internal Medicine 98: 251–3

Blessed G, Tomlinson B E, Roth M 1968 The association between quantitative measures of dementia and of senile change in the cerebral grey matter of elderly subjects. British Journal of Psychiatry 114: 797–811

Bondareff W, Mountjoy C Q, Roth M 1982 Loss of neurons of origin of the adrenergic projection to cerebral cortex (nucleus locus ceruleus) in senile dementia. Neurology 32: 164–168

Brain L, Adams R D 1965 In: Brain W R, Norris F H (eds) The Remote Effects of Cancer on the Nervous System. Grune and Stratton, New York

Carrol B J, Feinberg M, Greden J F et al 1981 A specific laboratory test for the diagnosis of melancholia: standardization, validation, and clinical utility. Archives of General Psychiatry 38: 15–22

Cassel C K, Jameton A L 1981 Dementia in the elderly: an analysis of medical responsibility. Annals of Internal Medicine 94: 802–807

Cook P, James I 1981 Cerebral vasodilators. New England Journal of Medicine 305: 1508–1513 & 1560–1564

Dobyns W B, Goldstein N P, Gordon H 1979 Clinical spectrum of Wilson's disease (hepatolenticular degeneration). Mayo Clinic Proceedings 54: 35–42

Folstein M F, Folstein S E, McHugh P R 1975 'Mini-mental status.' A practical method for grading the cognitive state of patients for the clinician. Journal of Psychiatric Research 12: 189–198

Gaitz G M, Varner R V 1979 Pharmacotherapy of age-associated brain syndromes. Interdisciplinary Topics in Gerontology 15: 169–178

Garcia C A, Reding M J, Blass J P 1981 Overdiagnosis of dementia. Journal of American Geriatrics Society 29: 407–410

Goodin D S, Squires K C, Starr A 1978 Long latency event-related components of the auditory evoked potential in dementia. Brain 101: 635–48

Hachinski V C, Lassen N A, Marshall J 1974 Multi-infarct dementia: a cause of mental deterioration in the elderly. Lancet 2: 207–210

Hakim S, Adams R D 1965 The special clinical problem of symptomatic hydrocephalus with normal CSF pressure: observation on CSF hydrodynamics. Journal of Neurological Sciences 2: 307–327

Hakim A M, Mathieson G 1979 Dementia in Parkinson disease: a neuropathological study. Neurology 29: 1209–14

Herbst K G, Humphrey C 1980 Hearing impairment and mental state in the elderly living at home. British Medical Journal 281: 903–11

Hollister L E 1975 Drugs for mental disorders of old age. Journal of the American Medical Association 234: 195–8

Jackson J A, Jankovic J, Ford J 1983 Progressive supranuclear palsy: clinical features and response to treatment in 16 patients. Annals of Neurology 13: 273–8

Kahn R L, Goldfarb A I, Pollack M, Peck A 1960 Brief objective measures for the determination of mental status in the aged. American Journal of Psychiatry 117: 326–29

Kral V A 1978 Benign senescent forgetfulness. In: Katzman R, Terry R D, Bick K L (eds) Alzheimer's Disease: Senile Dementia and Related Disorders. Raven Press, New York

Kurucz J, Charbonneau R, Kurucz A, Ramsey P 1981 Quantitative clincopathological study of senile dementia. Journal of American Geriatrics Society 29: 158–163

LaRue A 1982 Memory loss and aging. Distinguishing dementia from benign senescent forgetfulness and depressive pseudodementia. Psychiatry Clinic of North America 5: 89–103

Malletta G J, Pirozollo F J (eds) 1980 The Aging Nervous System. Praeger, New York

Marsden C D, Harrison M J G 1972 Outcome of investigation of patients with presenile dementia. British Medical Journal 2: 249–252

Mayeux R, Stern Y, Rosen J, Benson D F 1983 Is 'subcortical dementia' a recognisable clinical entity. Annals of Neurology 14: 278–283

Muller H F, Dastoor D P, Klingner M A, Cole M, Boillat J 1979 Amantadine in senile dementia: electroencephalographic and clinical effects. Journal of American Geriatrics Society 27: 9–16

Naeser M A, Gebhardt C, Levine H L 1980 Decreased computerized tomography numbers in patients with presenile dementia. Detection in patients with otherwise normal scans. Archives of Neurology 37: 401–409

Okazaki H, Reagan T J, Campbell R J 1979 Clinico-pathologic studies of primary cerebral amyloid angiopathy. Mayo Clinic Proceedings 54: 22–31

Ouslander J G 1981 Drug therapy in the elderly. Annals of Internal Medicine 95: 711–22

Perry E K, Tomlinson B E, Blessed G, Bergmann K, Gibson P H, Perry R H 1978 Correlation of cholinergic abnormalities with senile plaques and mental scores in senile dementia. British Medical Journal 2: 1457–9

Rabins P V 1981 Management of irreversible dementia. Psychosomatics 22: 591–97

Reisberg B, Ferris S H, Gershon S 1979 Psychopharmacologic aspects of cognitive research in the elderly: some current perspectives. Interdisciplinary Topics in Gerontology 15: 132–52

Ron M A, Toone B K, Garralda M E, Lishman W A 1979 Diagnostic accuracy in presenile dementia. British Journal of Psychiatry 143: 161–168

Roos R, Gajdusek D C, Gibbs C J 1973 The clinical characteristics of transmissible Creutzfeld-Jakob disease. Brain 96: 1–20

Rosen W G, Terry R D, Fuld P A et al 1980 Pathological verification of ischemic score in differentiation of dementias. Annals of Neurology 7: 486–488

Skomer C, Stears J, Austin J 1983 Metachromatic leukodystrophy (MLD). XV. Adult MLD with focal lesions by computed tomography. Archives of Neurology 40: 354–355

Smith J S, Kiloh L G 1981 The investigation of dementia: results in 200 consecutive admissisons. Lancet 1: 824–7

Thal L J, Fuld P A, Masur D M, Sharpless N S 1983 Oral physostigmine and lecithin improve memory in Alzheimer disease. Annals of Neurology 13: 491–496

Terry R D, Davies P 1980 Dementia of the Alzheimer type. Annual Review of Neuroscience 3: 77–95

Wells C E 1970 Pseudodementia. American Journal of Psychiatry 136: 895

Whitehead A 1973 Verbal learning and memory in elderly depressives. British Journal of Psychiatry 123: 203

Whitehouse P J, Price D L, Clark A W, Coyle J T, DeLong M R 1981 Alzheimer disease: evidence for selective loss of cholinergic neurons in the nucleus basalis. Annals of Neurology 10: 122–126

Wikkelso C, Andersson H, Blomstrand C, Lindqvist G 1982 The clinical effect of lumbar puncture in normal pressure hydrocephalus. Journal of Neurology, Neurosurgery and Psychiatry 45: 64–69

Wilkins R H, Brody I A 1969 Neurological classics. XX. Alzheimer's disease. Archives of Neurology 21: 109

Zarit S H, Miller N E, Kahn R L 1978 Brain function, intellectual impairment, and education in the aged. Journal of American Geriatrics Society 26: 58–67

Zemcov A, Barclay L, Vitale V, Blass J P 1983 Measurement of cerebral blood flow in the diagnosis of dementia. Journal of Cerebral Blood Flow and Metabolism 3: S512–513

12

The acutely confused patient

R. Jones & T. Arie

'Leave me alone!' A hand smacks against the doctor's enquiring face. Papers and clothes litter the floor and drawers askew complete the disorderly picture. An ammoniacal hint in the cold air suggests more urgent calls than the walking frame could competently aid. Provocative behaviour in a chaotic setting often characterises the confused elderly patient, and the inexperienced may find their reactions quick, uncharitable and hard to contain.

The problems of acute confusion closely concern modern medical services but they have been well known since ancient times. Clinical descriptions of confusion appear first in Hippocrates (born c.460 B.C.) who called it 'phrenitis', the seat of the disorder being placed in the brain (Chadwick & Mann, 1950). The clarity and precision of observation is impressive, and there is reference to visual hallucinations, changing mood, relationship to physical illness and particularly to pyrexial states; to sleep disturbance, restlessness, variable clear periods and worsening at night. Hippocrates also observed that a patient could one day be 'well behaved and silent' and later could show 'much tossing about'. 'Phrenitis' occurring in an already ill and weakened individual was regarded as a poor prognostic omen, especially when the patient became quiescent and 'insensible'. The groping and picking movements of some profoundly ill people were referred to as 'carphologia' (straw collecting) and this is reminiscent of the later Aretaeus of Cappodicia's reference to 'crocydismos' (plucking the blankets).

By around 2000 years ago the main clinical features of acute confusional states had been well described, as had some principles of management which would still be accepted now. The historical development of the concepts of 'confusion' and 'delirium' has recently been critically reviewed by Berrios (1981) who has shown how important they have been in the evolution of psychiatric thinking, particularly at the end of the last century. Three twentieth century contributions are especially relevant to the contemporary practitioner.

First Bonhoeffer's careful clinical observations of the mental states of patients exposed to a wide variety of physical diseases showed that the mental states encountered were not specific to any particular physical disease (Bonhoeffer, 1909). The reverse of this is that no physical disease gives rise to a uniquely specific abnormal mental state. Characteristic of the 'exogenous reactions' which he found was disturbance of consciousness.

The second major contribution was from Wolff and Curran (1935) who gave a careful clinical description of the features found in patients known to be physically ill, and on account of this mentally disturbed and admitted to psychiatric hospitals. Their work may be criticised as selective, reflecting a severely ill population. Nevertheless their findings have been influential in confirming the lack of a specific relationship between 'a particular noxious agent and the form and content' of the mental disturbance.

The third major contribution was from Engel and Romano (1959), who applied electro-encephalography and standardised psychological testing to the study of delirium. They demonstrated that disturbances of the level of consciousness established by characteristic responses on standardised cognitive tests was accompanied by slowing on the electro-encephalogram (EEG). Their ratings of cognitive impairment correlated with their graded EEG characteristics.

Acute confusional (or delirious) states can thus be produced by a wide variety of different physical disturbances, and the nature of the provoking condition cannot be inferred from the presence of confusion alone. But one can identify a characteristic series of features, some or all of which will always be present, and 'clouding of consciousness' is central.

DEFINITIONS

'Confusion' means 'lack of clarity of thinking' (Lishman, 1978). Thus 'the acutely confused patient' in the context of the elderly is an old person unable to think with their 'customary clarity and coherence'. Sometimes this may simply be a reflection of fatigue or other transient factors, and certainly confusion is often seen in old people with functional psychiatric disorder. But people often use 'confusion' to mean mental disturbance due to 'organic' cause and mean primarily the confusion of dementing states (chronic organic reactions) and of acute confusional states. Dementia is dealt with in chapter 11, and we here will concern ourselves with acute confusional states.

'Acute confusional state' is the term most commonly used by British psychiatrists; synonyms include acute psycho-organic syndrome (World Health Organisation, 1978), acute organic reaction, acute organic brain syndrome (Diagnostic and Statistical Manual II, 1968) and delirium (Diagnostic and Statistical Manual III, 1980). Lipowski (1980) defines this state (which he prefers to term 'delirium') as an episode of 'acute onset and transient duration, characterised by global cognitive impairment and due to widespread disturbance of cerebral metabolism'.

Most people would link such states to the concept of 'clouding of consciousness' but here again there are problems of definition, detection and measurement. Clouding of consciousness is a state of diminished alertness and diminished awareness, often with drowsiness. Characteristically it fluctuates with more lucid intervals. It seems sensible to think of a continuum, with coma at one end and at the other the hyperaroused concentrated expectancy of the sprinter under the starting pistol. Clouding of consciousness is a recognisable phase, though not necessarily an easily defined one, on this continuum. Although usually regarded as the hallmark of acute confusional states, mild degrees may be difficult to detect with confidence. There are no accepted instruments for measuring clouding and some studies of acute confusion in the elderly neither define clouding nor attempt to measure it, for instance, the important multicentre survey of Hodkinson (1973). Experience suggests that clouding is often much less prominent in the elderly. The intensity and abruptness of the onset of underlying physical noxae may be important in determining the prominence of clouding. With the elderly a multiplicity of factors may together give rise to an acute confusional state, perhaps insidiously over a period, leading to clouding being little evident.

HOW COMMON AND HOW SERIOUS IS ACUTE CONFUSION?

The very young and the aged are particularly prone to acute confusional states. The febrile deliria of childhood are commonplace and usually self-limiting. The incidence of acute confusional states amongst the elderly is difficult to measure, for we cannot tell how much of the morbidity comes to medical services. It seems likely that many episodes are either self-limiting, or are coped with by families or by social work agencies. Certainly general practitioners often deal with such problems without referral to specialist services. Even in hospital the condition may, especially when associated with other specific conditions (for example a fractured femur) be either not remarked on or not recorded, or often both. The problems

of epidemiological research in this field are therefore obvious. Bergmann & Eastham (1974) looking at elderly patients admitted to an acute general medical ward found that more than half had a morbid mental state and of these the most common was delirium.

Two recent studies describe the changing incidence and outcome of acute confusion among elderly people admitted to particular psychiatric units. Between 1974 and 1976, more than 20% of admissions aged 70 years and over to Crichton Royal Hospital were admitted with acute confusional states (Christie, 1982). Of all admissions of persons aged 65 and over to a psychiatric hospital in Newcastle-upon-Tyne in 1976 some 16% were for acute confusional states (Blessed & Wilson, 1982).

These two studies were designed to compare outcome in the case of various old age mental disorders with that reported by Roth (1955) for the 1930s and 1940s. Roth found around 8% of admissions aged over 60 years to be suffering from acute confusion, of whom some 40% were dead after six months. At two years this figure rose to some 50%. The remaining 50% had been discharged from hospital. The more recent surveys have broadly confirmed this picture, but in Blessed's study the mortality rate at two years had risen beyond 50% and, whilst most of the survivors had been discharged, a substantial minority were in residential care rather than living at home.

An acute confusional state in an elderly person is thus potentially a very serious event; depending on both the cause and the management, the outcome may be recovery, continuing dependency or death. Since the management is, of course, likely to differ between different types of services (e.g. specialised psychogeriatric units, general hospital units, mental hospitals) further outcome studies are needed. Certainly some residual brain damage may well be the consequence of an acute episode. Clinical experience suggests that the outcome is worse if treatment is inadequate or late. But how far can early and effective management reduce ultimate damage? Are particular regimes of treatment demonstrably successful in this respect? Are certain drugs demonstrably better at minimising ultimate damage? At present there are still only incomplete answers to these questions.

CLINICAL ASPECTS — SIGNS AND SYMPTOMS

Many of the clinical features of acute confusional states have already been mentioned and are summarised in Table 12.1.

Some points are worthy of further emphasis. A 'short' history will generally be of weeks at most but a 'subacute' state can go on for months and this must be considered when an individual has apparently developed a dementing state over a period of less than about a year, especially if there are atypical features.

Table 12.1 Signs and symptoms in acute confusional states

Short history
Clouding of consciousness
Reduced wakefulness
Disorientation in time and space
Increased motor activity — restlessness
                          — plucking, picking
Impaired attention, impaired concentration
Impaired memory (especially registration and recall)
Anxiety, suspicion, agitation
Variability
Worse at night
Misinterpretations, illusions, hallucinations
Disrupted thinking
Delusions (most transitory, primitive)
Speech abnormalities
Usually diffuse EEG slowing

Mood, whilst it often is anxious or apprehensive may instead be depressed and even, rarely, elated. Disturbance of mood is not typical. The greater the level of arousal the greater will be the degree of general disturbance. Such arousal may in great measure derive from the patient's environment and the stimulation that comes from it.

The aroused patient will be more likely to experience illusions, hallucinations and delusions and so to be more disturbed, restless and aggressive. Indeed Lipowski distinguishes between two varieties of delirium which he calls hyper-active and hypo-active respectively. This highlights the variability, both between patients or indeed in an individual, but these subtypes probably represent descriptive rather than nosological entities.

CLINICAL ASPECTS — TRACING THE CAUSE

There is generally an important physical cause of confusion, but often a multiplicity of factors may contribute. In the demented patient confusional states are common, seeming to arise with little to provoke them, and often with no clearly demonstrable cause; indeed failure to find a specific cause in the absence of a history of previous dementia is grounds for again seeking such a history. Confusion of unknown origin should be as unsatisfactory as a diagnosis as 'pyrexia of unknown origin'. It is fruitless to list all the possible physical causes, and such a list would in any case embrace most of medicine. A framework of possible categories of cause may however be useful (Table 12.2).

Various causes could be picked out as being particularly important in the elderly — urinary tract and chest infections, heart failure, and cerebro-vascular disease. Epilepsy is a cause sometimes overlooked. But the importance of unwanted effects of drugs, both intoxication and withdrawal states, cannot be too strongly stressed.

Figure 12.1 shows diagrammatically factors involved in the maintenance of consciousness. This is useful for thinking about causes but it also serves as a framework for

Table 12.2 A framework for tracing the cause

Intracranial	Space occupying lesions — e.g. tumours
	Trauma — e.g. subdural haematoma
	Infections — e.g. meningitis
	Cerebrovascular accidents
	Epilepsy
Extracranial	Infectious — e.g. pneumonia
	Metabolic — e.g. liver failure
	Anoxic — e.g. cardiac or respiratory failure
	Vascular — e.g. giant cell arteritis
	Endocrine — e.g. hypoglycaemia
	Vitamin deficiency — e.g. thiamine
	Intoxication/Withdrawal — alcohol, drugs
	Physical agents — e.g. hypothermia
	Psychological/Environmental

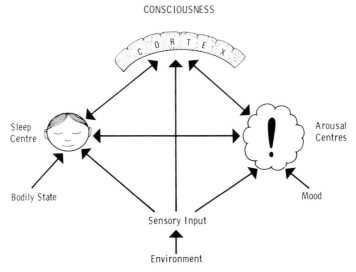

Fig. 12.1 Factors involved in the maintenance of consciousness (Jolley, 1981).

management and to this background we return below. Three particular systems are shown. First, the cerebral cortex, secondly, the arousal centres in the reticular activating system of the brain stem, and third the sleep-waking centre in the hypothalamus. All three appear to interact in the maintenance of normal consciousness, and indeed in the production and maintenance of normal sleep. Additionally there is a constant flow of sensory data from the external world, and from the internal world of the individual. It is well known that the normal conscious mental state becomes disrupted in individuals deprived of external sensory input (political torturers in our time have come to put this to sadly widespread use). The high prevalence of auditory and visual impairment in old age makes this obviously relevant. 'Over-loading' with excessive sensory stimulation, for example pain, may be disruptive and may contribute to an acute confusional state; a painful fracture may provoke such problems or sometimes even simple but painful constipation may be important.

On this diagram we also indicate a contribution from the state of emotional arousal and from the mood state of the individual. It is a matter of common observation that anxiety can disrupt the efficient performance of the individual. In confusional states a vicious circle of loss of control — anxiety — loss of control probably often obtains.

Depressed mood can play an important part in vulnerability to confusion, presumably through arousal effects (Cawley et al, 1973) and depression as the basis of acute confusion is not uncommon (though more commonly when depression presents with marked cognitive impairment it is as a 'pseudodementia' rather than as delirium).

Although confusional states are likely to be caused by a number of different factors working together, often only one of these factors is recognisably 'medical', and it may appear relatively minor in degree. Unravelling of all the various strands combining together to produce the acute confusional state is essential to the proper assessment of such patients.

In this perspective the history of the development of the state is of prime importance. Proper gathering of information is crucial. Sometimes in the busy general hospital ward an elderly confused patient seems marooned, giving every appearance of having arrived without trace from outer space. Usually there are friends, relatives or neighbours and they must be interviewed at the earliest opportunity. Too often they seem to have a way of disappearing or becoming unavailable; this is part of the process whereby the 'hole' left in the community by the hospitalised elderly person closes behind her. The necessity to obtain a reliable history is part of the case for home assessment.

The clinical examination, the next important step in assessment, needs to be informed by such a full history.

Then physical disorders giving rise to the state will often be substantially established simply on physical examination, though this must be meticulous and patient. Frequently the examination will have to be taken in parts, according to the patient's co-operativeness, and in order to avoid both fatigue and over-arousal. The results of the history and examination will determine investigations, which according to circumstances range from a simple blood count to highly sophisticated techniques. However the aim must be to elucidate the individual's disorder, rather than simply to apply routinely a predetermined battery of investigations.

MANAGEMENT

Management can be summarised under the following headings:—

1. Initial home assessment whenever feasible.
2. Examination and investigation.
3. Treatment of the main causative factors.
4. Nursing measures, rehabilitation where necessary, and promotion of normality and good health.
5. Use of symptomatic drugs.
6. Follow-up and after care.

1. Initial home assessment. This is now so widely accepted as good practice that the point need not be laboured. The value is obvious of observing the patient in her normal surroundings, of collecting information from relatives and neighbours and of avoiding a premature decision to move the patient which may subsequently be proven unnecessary, unwise and irreversible. These and other aspects, as well as some of the difficulties, have recently been comprehensively reviewed by Arie & Jolley (1982).

2 & 3. Our approach to examination and investigation has already been dealt with. With treatment the aim will be to reverse those features which are reversible and to ameliorate those which are not. This ranges from surgical procedures, the treatment of infections with antibiotics, or the correction of cardiac arrhythmias to 'simple' tasks such as removal of ear wax or enemas for constipation.

4. Good nursing is essential. Nurses, unlike doctors, are continuously with the patient and their observations are vital. Certain important themes can be derived from the principles which we described above.

Lighting needs to be clear, or the patient should be nursed in darkness. Ambiguous lighting and strange shadows may cause misinterpretations, illusions and even hallucinations.

As far as possible the nurses themselves should be few, familiar and regular in their appearances. Often this is very difficult on a busy general ward, but it must be the aim. Visitors can be reassuring, but a constant flow of changing faces may overtax the patient's comprehension and compound confusion. All who deal with the patient must be reassuring, and be willing to take their time, speaking clearly and being willing to repeat themselves if this is necessary, as it often is. Use of the patient's name is not only a courtesy, but provides reassurance that not everything has gone wrong; at least people know who she is. There is rarely need for raised voices: old people's deafness, where it exists, is of the sort that is more helped by clarity of phrase and articulation than by shouting. Provision of a secluded side room will often be appropriate and helpful to the rest of the ward. But there may be a cost in difficulties of observation and access.

Nurses will need to attend both to specific medical problems and to the patient's general condition, of which a crucial aspect is hydration. Such patients should be on fluid balance charts. Their electrolytes need to be monitored with results obtained promptly and taken note of.

Nursing observations may be of great importance. If depression is suspected behind a confusional presentation, the nurses must be instructed to record any utterances that might reflect this, and to note the patient's demeanour and facial expression. In other words whether (often transiently) she looks or seems depressed.

If things go well, the promotion of normality and good health soon become important. The nurse helps the patient to return as far as possible and as quickly as possible — without excessive stress — to the normal pattern and rhythm of healthy life, for instance, a pattern of activity during the day with rest and sleep at night time. Fluid balance has been emphasised and nutrition is important too, as is attention to bowel and bladder habit. The nurses may need to help the patient to become upright and to start to walk. Resumption of normal motor activity probably plays an important part in helping the patient to reassert a grip on normality. Here is an important role for physiotherapists, who happily are increasingly becoming part of the team working with mentally ill and old people. They should be influential both through direct therapy and by teaching and supporting other members of the team.

Restoration of normality to the patient's confused perception can be helped by ensuring that items are brought from home which are recognisable and familiar, such as small ornaments, photographs or pictures. Sometimes the switching on of a regularly followed radio or T.V. programme may aid in this process of restoration. There is great scope here for imagination and ingenuity in all members of the team, and relatives and friends often have excellent suggestions.

5. The use of drugs is deliberately placed low on our list, for it is too often the first line of response. Of course, drugs for specific disorders — e.g. antibiotics — are essential. Symptomatic drugs are a potent arm of management, but not an invariable one. The restless patient may well need calming medication to enable her to benefit from other approaches, or even to overcome possibly life-threatening resistance to attempts at hydration etc. The right dose is the minimum necessary to produce a reasonable response. This must be tailored to suit the patient and often the regime will need to be 'titrated' to a patient's diurnal pattern of disturbance. Regimes should be individually set up in this way and frequently reviewed; they must not be allowed to fossilise, and accretion of multiple medicaments is a common danger. All tranquillising drugs may themselves cause confusion as well as many other unwanted side effects, high among which is liability to fall. There is often only a thin line between harm and benefit.

Pharmacokinetics are dealt with in Chapter 7; they have obvious relevance to drug regimes. It is wise to have only a small repertoire of drugs, tranquillising and sedative, and to become accustomed to their benefits and limitations.

This repertoire will include phenothiazines and, amongst these, promazine is a useful drug which can be built up from low levels to higher dosages as necessary. Neither liver damage nor dystonias are a problem. Thioridazine is a more powerful drug, and dystonias are common at higher dosage. Thioridazine is a sedative tranquilliser; haloperidol, a butyrophenone, is a less sedative drug though more prone to cause dystonias but cautious use in low dosage often avoids these problems. The objective is to reduce arousal whilst avoiding over sedation and depressed consciousness.

The benzodiazepines tend to linger, accumulating in the system; even the short acting benzodiazepines have longer half-lives in the elderly. We use them only rarely, often finding that they have contributed — perhaps as sleeping tablets — to causing confusion in the first place. If night time sedation is necessary chloral or its derivatives are useful, or chlormethiazole which is quickly excreted and generally safe, though a few patients are intolerant of this drug, becoming dopey on even small doses. A combination of chloral with a small dose of phenothiazine will often ensure a quiet night — though sometimes at the price of a wet bed.

6. When the patient recovers and is discharged it is vital that there should be effective communication, both about what has been done and about future arrangements, with all those concerned outside hospital. This means the family doctor, the family or other supporters and, of course, the patient; and often other services such as social services and nursing services who are providing help. It is a waste of resources if all the effort in hospital lapses after the patient returns home. Often the patient has residual impairments of mind and body, and the acute hospital episode is merely a phase in a continuing process of care.

PREVENTION

Not everything that can cause confusion in the elderly is preventable, though much is. But prevention here begins with identifying those at special risk and providing effective and responsive services for surveillance and intervention (see Chapter 5). Here family practices with age/sex registers are at a special advantage. Old people with dementia, or with marked special sense impairment, or others who are socially isolated and depressed, are at special risk and the very aged most of all. The family doctor may see ways to ameliorate important factors in those at risk, or he may provide early intervention when illness threatens to usher in confusion.

Secondary and tertiary prevention aim to limit effects of illness once it has already started, and to minimise the resultant disabilities. A responsive service able to mobilise resources to the patient's home (we have already described the importance of initial home assessment) can avoid the further challenge of moving the patient to an unfamiliar setting; and if the illness is not too serious or the necessary treatment or investigations not too specialised, the elderly patient will very often have a better prospect of recovery in familiar home surroundings.

Above all, open-minded, and positive attitudes on the part of those involved with the patient will achieve vastly better results than the all too common rejection or defeatism that characterises much of the handling of confused old people. Elsewhere the necessary services have been described in detail (Arie & Jolley, 1982). Their essence is collaboration between professions, access to the full facilities of a general hospital and prompt availability. The recent rapid development of such services in many countries and the creation of the educational framework needed to sustain them, is a heartening feature of the professional response to the needs of confused old people.

REFERENCES

Arie T, Jolley D 1982 Making services work: Organisation and style of psychogeriatric services. In: Levy R, Post F (eds) The Psychiatry of Late Life, Blackwell Scientific Publications, Oxford, ch 8, p 222

Bergmann K, Eastham E J 1974 Psychogeriatric ascertainment and assessment for treatment in an acute medical ward setting. Age and Ageing 132: 441–447

Berrios G E 1981 Delirium and confusion in the 19th century: A conceptual history. British Journal of Psychiatry 139: 439–449

Blessed G, Wilson I D 1982 The contemporary natural history of mental disorder in old age. British Journal of Psychiatry 141: 59–67

Bonhoeffer K 1909 Zur frage der exogenen psychosen. Zentral Nervenheilkunde 32: 499–505

Cawley R H, Post F, Whitehead A 1973 Barbiturate tolerance and psychological functioning in elderly depressed patients. Psychological Medicine 3: 39–52

Chadwick J, Mann W N 1950 The medical works of Hippocrates. Blackwell, Oxford

Christie A B 1982 Changing patterns in mental illness in the elderly. British Journal of Psychiatry 140: 154–159

Diagnostic and Statistical Manual of Mental Disorders, 2nd edn. 1968. The American Psychiatric Association, Washington D.C.

Diagnostic and Statistical Manual of Mental Disorders, 3rd edn. 1980. The American Psychiatric Association, Washington D.C.

Engel G L, Romano J 1959 Delirium, a syndrome of cerebral insufficiency. Journal of Chronic Diseases 9: 260–277

Hodkinson H M 1973 Mental impairment in the elderly: Journal of the Royal College of Physicians, London 7: 305–317

Jolley D 1981 Acute confusional states in the elderly. In: Coakley D (ed) Acute Geriatric Medicine, Croom Helm, London

Lipowski Z L 1980 Delirium. Charles C Thomas, Springfield

Lishman A 1978 Organic Psychiatry. Blackwell Scientific Publications, Oxford

Roth M 1955 The natural history of mental disorder in old age. Journal of Mental Science 101: 281–301

Wolff H G, Curran D 1935 Nature of delirium and allied states. Archives of Neurology and Psychiatry 33: 1175–1215

World Health Organisation 1978 Mental disorders: glossary and guide to their classification in accordance with the ninth revision of the International Classification of Diseases. WHO, Geneva

13

Depressive disorders

D. Cohen & C. Eisdorfer

INTRODUCTION

Hippocrates, *circa* 460–370 included depression in his classification of mental illness, attributing its cause to an excessive amount of black-bile, melan chole (or melancholia) in the body (Adams, 1939). Since the lifetime prevalence of major depressive disorders is estimated to be 26% (Weissman & Meyers, 1978), depression has been called 'the common cold of psychiatry', with symptoms ranging from sadness associated with an adjustment reaction to a major psychotic depressive episode. Depressive disorders are generally regarded as the most common psychiatric problem among the aged, but relatively little empirical data exists to describe the etiology and phenomenology of late life depressions, to clarify standards for accurate differential diagnosis, to identify the efficacy of various treatment modalities, and to identify risk factors for late-life depression.

Although the point prevalence of major depressive disorders diagnosed in the aged (8.2/100 000 persons) appears to be the same as other age groups, depressive symptoms appear to be more prevalent in the aged ranging from 15–65% (Blazer, 1982 a & b; Cohen & Eisdorfer, in press). This variance may reflect methodological differences in community surveys as well as the existence of a significant community population with atypical and transient depressions caused by physical disorder, economic and social circumstances, multiple losses and personal distress. The high suicide rate in men over 60 argues for the existence of significant latent depression in this age group. More people over 60 make successful suicide attempts than at any other stage of life. Although representing only 12.5% of the population, persons 60 and older commit nearly a quarter of all suicides in the US (Vital Statistics, 1978). This figure may actually be higher due to failure to identify many deaths as actual suicides.

DIFFERENTIAL DIAGNOSIS OF DEPRESSIVE FORMS IN THE AGED

Although most clinicians and investigators agree about most of the basic signs and symptoms of significant depression, accurate diagnosis of the depressed older

patient may be complicated by concurrent physical illness, drug side-effects, co-existing psychiatric conditions, social isolation, cognitive impairment and sensory losses, as well as other medical, behavioural and social factors. Theories of depression and late-life depression will not be reviewed here since they are well represented in other sources (Blazer, 1982a). The differential diagnosis of depressive disorders will be presented using a descriptive framework adapted from the Diagnostic and Statistical Manual-Third Edition (DSM-III) and the clinical literature (Table 13.1).

Table 13.1 Differential diagnosis of forms of depression in the aged (Cohen & Eisdorfer, in press).

I. Affective disorders
   A. major depression (single episode or recurrent)
   B. Bipolar disorder
   C. Dysthumic disorder (or depressive neurosis)
II. Depression-anxiety disorder (Depressive symptoms are likely to accompany an anxiety disorder)
III. Depressive-somatoform disorder
   A. Psychogenic pain disorder
   B. Hypochondriasis or high bodily concern
IV. Depressive paranoid states (Paranoid states in later life may have a significant depressive impact)
V. Schizoaffective disorder (Uncommon in later life)
VI. Depression associated with physical illness (Depressed affect may be associated with almost all acute and Chronic Illnesses in the aged)
VII. Depression accompanying a psychiatric disorder
   A. Late-life dementia
      1. Alzheimer's dementia
      2. Multi-infarct dementia
   B. Substance related dementia
      1. Alcohol
      2. Drugs (Antihypertensive, antiarrhythmic agents)
   C. Affective syndrome secondary to:
      1. Cushing's syndrome
      2. Hypothyroidism
      3. Malignancy e.g. carcinoma of pancreas
      4. Vitamin deficiencies (especially B complex and folic acid)
      5. Brain lesions
VIII. Adjustment disorder with depressed mood
IX. Phase of life reaction
   A. Bereavement
   B. Marital problems
   C. Family problems
   D. Parent-child problems
X. Existential sadness

A diagnostic and statistical manual which adequately describes the characteristics, frequency and symptom distribution of the psychiatric and behavioural problems of the aged remains to be written when more empirical data are available. Although it will be used as a framework here, it should be noted that there are difficulties with the use of DSM-III for the aged, for example the symptoms of depression may be somewhat different in older persons. Although anxiety and depression often co-exist in the aged, symptoms of anxiety are not listed as criteria for any type of depressive disorder in DSM-III (Crook, 1982). Older persons may also manifest atypical depressive disorders, e.g. significant vegetative symptoms with dysphoria or sadness without major somatic signs. Some clinicians have also suggested that older persons are more likely to 'mask' their depression compared to younger persons (Goldfarb, 1974; Salzman & Shader, 1978).

The major affective disorders, which include major depressive disorders and bipolar depressive disorders or manic-depressive disorders, are currently differentiated by clinical symptoms and course of illness, family genetic history and drug response. The limited epidemiological data from early studies in Europe indicate that the prevalence of manic-depressive disorders in the community is between 1–2% while unipolar depression is well above 2% (Neilsen, 1963; Kay et al, 1964).

The American Psychiatric Association (1980) outlined the diagnostic criteria for major depressive disorders (DSM III) as follows:

A. Dysphoric mood, loss of interest or pleasure in all or almost all usual activities is present. Dysphoric mood is characterised by depressed symptoms such as sadness, blue feelings, hopelessness, and irritability. The disturbance must be prominent and relatively persistent but not necessarily the most dominant symptom. It does not include momentary shifts from one dysphoric mood to another e.g. anxiety to depression to anger, such as are seen in states of acute psychotic turmoil.

B. The illness must have a duration of at least two weeks during which, for most of the time, at least four of the following symptoms have persisted and been present to a significant degree.

(1) Poor appetite or significant weight loss (when not dieting), or increased appetite or significant weight gain.

(2) Insomnia or hypersomnia.

(3) Loss of energy, fatigability, or tiredness.

(4) Psychomotor agitation or retardation (but not subjective feelings of restlessness or being slowed down).

(5) Loss of interest or pleasure in usual activities, or decrease in sexual drive (not included if limited to a period when delusional or hallucinating).

(6) Feelings of self-reproach or excessive or inappropriate guilt (either may be delusional).

(7) Complaints or evidence of diminished ability to think or concentrate such as slowed thinking, or indecisiveness (not associated with obvious formal thought disorder).

(8) Suicidal ideation, desire to die, or any suicide attempt.

C. The depressive symptoms cannot be superimposed on either Schizophrenia, Schizophreniform Disorder, or a Paranoid Disorder.

D. None of the following should predominate the clinical picture for more than three months after the onset of the Depressive Episode.

(1) Preoccupation with a delusion or hallucination.

(2) Marked formal thought disorder.

(3) Bizarre or grossly disorganised behaviour.

Although Blazer & Williams (1980) observed that 1.8% of an aged community met DSM-III criteria for major unipolar depression, 4.5% of the community population had dysphoric symptoms, 3.7% had symptoms of a major depressive disorder, 1.9% had symptoms of a secondary depressive disorder and 6.5% had depressive symptoms secondary to poor physical health. Thus DSM-III clearly provides operational criteria for comparison across populations, but a broader set of precise criteria would appear to be necessary to deal with depressive problems which impair a significant proportion of the aged. Approximately half of the depressed subjects in Blazer & Williams' (1980) survey had impaired physical health, and the authors suggest that grief over loss of health, physical pain and loss of independence may contribute to depressive symptoms. Although many of the depressed individuals were socially isolated and economically deprived, the role of social and economic distress in the etiology of late life depression has not been well studied.

Little is also known about bipolar affective illness in the aged, which includes patients with repeated depressive episodes and infrequent manic periods as well as patients with alternating manic and depressive episodes. Pitt (1974) has estimated that only 1 in 20 psychogeriatric admissions are individuals with manic disorder. Manic episodes are often atypical in the aged (Langley, 1975). Overactivity is not usually prominent in the older patient, and the mania can be confused with agitated depression. Manic and depressive affect often appear together in the same patient, and anger and irritability are often seen rather than the euphoria of younger patients. Though patterns are often obsessive and speech circumstantial in contrast to the wild flight of ideas of a younger manic-depressive. Paranoid delusions are frequently seen in the older manic, and the patient may appear confused and be inaccurately classified with mild dementia.

There is controversy about the relative merits of differentiating neurotic depression (dysthmic disorder) from recurrent unipolar depression (Blazer, 1982). Furthermore, among the aged abnormal bereavement reactions to multiple losses are implicated in the precipitation of depressive disorders, or dysthymic disorder (Goldfarb, 1974; Verwoerdt, 1976). Bergmann (1978) studied two groups of older persons with neurotic symptoms (long-standing and late-onset) and one sample without them. Older patients with late-onset neurotic conditions were more functionally impaired, had few hobbies or outside activities and suffered from loneliness. A discriminant analysis of life-event stresses and personality traits showed that physical health and personal vulnerability were the most powerful predictors of late-life neurosis.

Dysthymic disorders are challenges for treatment. Although biological therapies may successfully resolve certain vegetative symptoms, most symptoms of the disorder persist. Diagnostic criteria for a depressive neurosis include persistent symptoms of depression over at least two years but not severe enough to be classified as unipolar depressive, absence of psychosis, and at least three of thirteen symptoms i.e. irritability or anger, social withdrawal, inability to respond to praise, decreased productivity, crying spells and so on (American Psychiatric Association, 1980). Indeed many of these symptoms are chronic and entwined with the individual's complicated non-adaptive relationship with their world.

Depression and anxiety often co-exist in individuals of all ages. A 1979 national community survey (Mellinger & Balter, 1982) revealed that among persons aged 65–79, significant psychic distress was experienced by 5.7% as the result of anxiety, but 3.8% from depression and by 9.5% as the result of mixed anxiety-depression. The relationship of anxiety states and depressive neuroses has long been controversial and distinguishing between the two is generally difficult (McNair & Fisher, 1978). One study by Sir Martin Roth and his colleagues (Roth et al, 1972) reported that 13 factors e.g. panic attacks or early waking, significantly discriminated between anxiety and depressive neuroses.

High bodily concern is frequently seen in older patients (Busse & Blazer, 1980) and the differential between hypochondriasis and depression may be difficult. Pain and hypochondriacal complaints may mask a real depression (Lesse, 1979). However, a number of clinical features may help differentiate between the two (Blazer & Siegler, 1981). The older depressed people appear to suffer from their symptoms in contrast to the hypochondriacal patient. Social withdrawal is prominent and suicidal thoughts are common in depression, whereas the hypochondriacal older adult seldom talks of suicide, and although social activities may be decreased, the patient is not socially withdrawn and dysfunctional. In general, the quality and degree of the patient's complaints are the most useful clues to identify the hypochondriacal patient.

Paranoid states may be accompanied by significant depressive symptoms in older persons. Schizo-affective disorders characterised by mixed depressive, paranoid or schizophrenic-like symptoms are reported to be uncommon in later life (Blazer, 1982).

The relationship between physical illness and depression is important for successful treatment (Blazer, 1982; Ouslander, 1982). Depression may be a significant symptom of a wide spectrum of many prescribed disorders as well as appearing as a side-effect of many prescribed and non-prescribed drugs (Eisdorfer et al, 1981b). Depression has been associated with cardiovascular disease, hormonal disturbances, cancer and many other diseases. Furthermore depression can result as a side-effect of many drugs or the abuse of alcohol. Schuckit & Pastor (1978) suggest that depression exists in all active alcoholics.

A significant proportion of patients with the dementias of later life manifest depressive symptoms (Eisdorfer et al, 1981a; Reifler et al, 1982). Furthermore, depression occurs in one third to one half of patients with Parkinson's disease (Mayeux et al, 1981) and in a substantial number of stroke victims (Robinson & Price, 1982).

It is often difficult to assess where sadness appropriate to situational losses merges into more serious symptoms of depression. It is particularly difficult to distinguish symptoms of an atypical grief reaction from a more profound depressive episode in the older population who suffer multiple and profound losses (Himmelhoch et al, 1982). Unfortunately aging in modern society is accompanied by decreased usefulness and prestige, reduced income, loss of family and friends, social isolation, loss of autonomy and loss of opportunities to thrive. The distinction between an adjustment disorder with depressed mood, phase of life reaction and existential sadness may well be a matter of severity and duration of symptoms as well as their impact on functional effectiveness.

Common symptoms of depression in the older population may include apathy and withdrawal instead of clear dysphoria, as well as memory impairment, attentional disturbances and significant cognitive deterioration. Without a comprehensive biomedical and cognitive evaluation these symptoms may be falsely attributed to Alzheimer's disease or a related disorder. Approximately 35% of older persons presenting with cognitive dysfunction have a depression or physical illness, sometimes inappropriately called 'pseudodementia', which is treatable and reversible (National Institute on Aging Task Force, 1980). Several factors may emerge from the history and clinical evaluation of the patient to clarify the diagnosis. The history may reveal a previous episode of depression which is not the case with Alzheimer's disease and related disorders. The course of depressive illness usually progresses rapidly with a definite date of onset, whereas there is a more insidious and variable course in dementia. Furthermore, during formal mental status testing, depressed patients tend not to respond or answer with 'don't know' responses.

THE CLINICAL EVALUATION

The clinical evaluation for depression should be comprehensive enough to evaluate the full range of potential biomedical, psychosocial and environmental factors which may contribute to the clinical manifestations (Finestone & Blazer, 1982). The diagnosis is often complicated by the presence of co-existing medical disorders which frequently are accompanied by depression as well as the effects of multiple medications. Polypharmacy, high doses of medications, altered pharmacokinetics, changes in the aging body and drug side-effects may all contribute to a depressive-like syndrome. Thus the evaluation must include an examination with a review of all medications and complete laboratory studies. The latter should include a complete blood count to rule out anemias contributing to weakness and apathy, serum chemistries and thyroid function tests to exclude metabolic and endocrine disorders, and an electrocardiogram to exclude cardiac pathology. Complete neurological, psychiatric and cognitive examinations should be carried out to provide information to make the differential between non-reversible dementias and depression (Wells, 1979).

A dexamethasone suppression test (DST) may help distinguish a major depressive disorder from dysthymic-related disorders and bipolar depression. Between 40 and 60% of patients with a major depressive disorder have an abnormal response to dexamethasone, i.e. they do not suppress their cortisol production during the 24 hours after the dexamethasone. Dexamethasone (1–2 mg.) is given to a patient at 11 pm, and plasma cortisol levels are assayed at 4pm and 11pm the following day for inpatients and at 4pm for outpatients. A plasma cortisol level of more than 5 mg/dl is usually positive, reflecting an abnormality in cortisol secretion (Brown, 1979; Schlesser et al, 1980; Carroll et al, 1981; Schatzberg et al, 1982). Unfortunately, most studies have included relatively few patients over age 60, and further research is required to clarify the relationship between age, results on the DST and forms of depression.

TREATMENT ISSUES IN DEPRESSION

Although depression is regarded as the most common disorder among the aging population, persons over age 60 have not usually been included in controlled studies of treatment outcome (Weissman & Meyers, 1979; Mintz et al, 1981). The treatment of depression may include several therapeutic modalities depending on the severity of the depression, the presence of co-exising physical illnesses and the availability of family and social supports. Treatment may consist of one of many psychotherapies either on an individual or group basis, pharmacotherapy, electroconvulsive therapy (ECT) or some combination thereof. A combination of psychotherapy and active drug treatment may be the optimal treatment plan for major depressive disorder (Weissman, 1979). Treatment may take place in an inpatient or outpatient setting. The severity of

the depression is usually the decisive factor. However, older patients tend to deteriorate in inpatient settings, and if they are not in a life-threatening or medically complicated situation, every effort should be made to maintain them in their home environment.

Selection of the therapeutic modality depends, at least in part on the type of depression. Usually mild adjustment depressive reactions without vegetative symptoms (gastrointestinal symptoms, severe anhedonia, sleep problems, diurnal variations) are related to an obvious precipitating event, and they are usually responsive to inter-personal contact and environmental changes. Brief supportive psychotherapy and realignment of social supports are the treatment of choice. More severe and prolonged depression characterised by psychological and physical deterioration usually require psychopharmacological intervention in conjunction with either group or individual supportive psychotherapy. Unfortunately in the aged a fine line often exists between the point where a longstanding psychosocial stressor of longstanding, for example a chronic debilitating illness, transforms an adjustment depressive reaction or phase of life reaction into a subsequent major depressive illness.

PSYCHOTHERAPY

Despite nihilistic beliefs of psychiatrists and patients alike, older persons may benefit from formal psychotherapy (Steuer, 1982). Unfortunately, empirical psychotherapy studies have not included many older persons. A recently published study compared the effectiveness of cognitive-behavioural group therapy (Beck et al, 1979) and psychodynamic group therapy (Grotjahn, 1977) over a 22 week period in older persons aged 55–80 years (Jarvik et al, 1982). There were no differences in outcome between the two groups. The outcomes were distributed as a bell-shaped curve with an average improvement of 30%. Most patients showed modest improvement, but remained symptomatic.

In the frail aged, the therapeutic objective is to provide the fastest possible symptom relief with a minimum number of sessions adjusted to the physical capabilites of the patient. The therapist should be active and instrumental in the treatment process (Yesavage & Karasu, 1982; Blum & Tross, 1980). Sharing personal life experiences with patients often enhances the therapeutic process when the therapist is younger than the patient. When possible the patient's family should be involved in the treatment process by educating them about many aspects of depressive illness, discussing their expectations of treatment, and explaining the side-effects of prescribed medications.

The therapist must be willing to utilise the services of other professional disciplines (Cohen et al, 1983). Referral to visiting nurse services, homemaker and health aids, telephone reassurance services, meals-on wheels, widow and self-help groups are important to reintegrate the individual into their social world and the greater community. Senior citizen centres are one of the few referral sources which give old people an opportunity to learn new coping skills and enhance their self-esteem.

Although short-term treatment is often the treatment of choice for most older patients, some individuals are candidates for long-term therapy and even psychoanalysis. This decision should be made after a thorough evaluation by a psychiatrist. In 1919 Karl Abraham outlined the requirements for such a procedure, stating that older patients who have functioned well socially and sexually during their life may be suitable candidates for extended therapy (Abraham, 1919).

PHARMACOTHERAPY

When depression interferes with normal functioning and there is evidence of vegetative symptomatology, a trial of antidepressant medication should be considered. Table 13.2 lists the most commonly prescribed antidepressants. The selection of antidepressant medication is best determined by a knowledge of the nature of the depression, of any history of a positive response to a particular medication either in the patient or in blood relatives, and of the presence of concomitant physical illness.

In older patients who suffer from bipolar of manic-depressive illness, lithium carbonate is still the drug of

Table 13.2 Commonly prescribed tricyclic antidepressants (Modified from Eisdorfer et al, 1981b)

Tricyclic Antidepresant	Unusual Dose Range (mg/day)		Sedative Propety	Anticho-linergic Property
	Young Adult	Older Adult		
Tertiary Amines				
Amitriptyline (Evavil)	100–300	25–150	+ + +	+ + + +
Imipramine (Tofranil)	100–300	25–150	+ +	+ + +
Doxepin (Sinequan)	100–300	25–150	+ + +	+ + + +
Secondary Amines				
Nortriptyline (Aventyl)	50–100	10– 50	+	+ + +
Desipramine (Norpramin)	100–300	25–150	0	+ +
Protriptyline (Vivactil)	20– 60	5– 30	0	+ + +
Triazolopyridine				
Trazodone (Desyrel)	150–400	50–300	+ + +	+
Tetracyclic				
Maprotiline (Ludiomil)	100–300	25–150	+ +	+ + +

choice for mood stabilisation. Because of the slower metabolism of the drug in older persons, lower doses are often indicated to obtain a therapeutic blood level. Careful monitoring of blood levels is optimally done under a psychiatrist's control (Thompson et al, 1983).

Patients who are apathetic and withdrawn should be started with one of the less sedating medications e.g. imipramine or nortriptyline, but a positive response to a known medication takes precedence over this choice. Agitated patients should be started with more sedating medications e.g. doxepin, imipramine or trazodone. In patients who show severe agitation which is not ameliorated with antidepressants, low-dose high potency neuroleptics such as trifluoperazine, or short-acting benzodiazepines e.g. lorazepam and oxazepam, may be useful (Salzman, 1982). Whenever possible, drug combinations should be avoided since multiple drugs make it difficult to assess the effective agent and vary the dose. When patients manifest severe agitation, delusions and hallucinations, they are usually managed most effectively within inpatient settings.

In patients with life-long histories of characterological depression accompanied by high levels of anxiety, monoamine oxidase (MAO) inhibitors e.g. phenalizine or tranylcypromine, are potentially indicated. (Dally & Rhode, 1961; Sargent, 1962; Overall et al., 1966; Paykel et al, 1979). Phenelzine appears to be more effective in older persons than in younger persons and it is also more effective than amitriptyline in the aged (Robinson, 1981). This may be explained by the increased MAO activity in the aged (Robinson, 1975; Horita, 1978). Phenelzine and tranylcypromine appear to be efficacious in the treatment of depression in patients with dementia (Ashford & Ford, 1979).

Although dietary restrictions are necessary to minimise the potential for cardiovascular crises, MAO inhibitors are not absolutely contraindicated in older persons (Bethune et al, 1964). They make a radical difference in the lives of patients who have suffered for many years. These medications should be given in consultation with or by a psychiatrist (Ashford & Ford, 1979).

Stimulant drugs such as dextroamphetamine and methylphenidate have also been used to treat depression in the elderly, especially among the frail aged with severe physical illness. They may often produce immediate relief in selected patients. However they have rarely been found to be effective over a long period of time (Katon & Raskind, 1980).

Regardless of the medication used, it is essential that the patient as well as close family members, if available, be included in treatment planning. The physician has an important responsibility to inform them about the action of the medication and its possible side-effects. Furthermore, involving the patient may give him a sense of control which is vital in the treatment of depression.

As a general rule, antidepressant medication should be started at 25–50% of the normal adult dose, two hours before bedtime, and increased by 25% of the initial dose every five days until a therapeutic dosage is obtained and there is stabilisation of side-effects, particularly sedation (Conrad & Bresslor, 1982). Some patients will respond better to a total night-time dosage, while others will prefer a divided dose regimen to minimise side-effects. Although depressed mood will not return to normal until there has been a full therapeutic dose for about two to three weeks, most patients will begin to feel better within a week to ten days.

A suicidal patient is at the greatest risk for a successful attempt during the early 're-energising period' and requires careful observation during treatment. Tricyclic antidepressants can be toxic substances: 600 mg of imipramine or amitriptyline i.e. a four day supply at 150 mg/day, is a lethal amount (Conrad & Bresslor, 1982). If possible, a family member should ration the medication in daily doses, and if it is not possible, hospitalisation is appropriate.

After the patient improves, for example when there is a change in mood or sleeping and eating patterns return to normal with a gain in weight, the patient should be maintained on the same dose for a month. Medication may then be reduced gradually in 25 mg decrements weekly until the lowest possible maintenance dose, usually providing effective sleep, is obtained. The patient should be kept on this dose for at least 6–12 months, at which time the medication may be decreased gradually i.e. 25 mg per week. If symptoms do not recur, the drug may be stopped with strong encouragement for the patient to return should there be any change of symptoms, for example if minor agitation or increasing insomnia re-emerge. It may be necessary to place the patient on a maintenance dose for a longer period (Grof, 1980).

Antidepressant medications often produce non-compliance because of pronounced side-effects (Blackwell, 1982). In addition, the physician should be aware of both cardiovascular and anticholinergic effects (Conrad & Bresslor, 1982) which suggest caution. General guidelines exist for the safe utilisation of drugs in patients with cardiovascular pathology (Thompson et al, 1983). Tricyclics are absolutely contra-indicated during an acute myocardial infarction, crescendo angina, or decompensated congestive cardiac failure (Davidson & Wenger, 1982). When the cardiac condition has been stabilised, they may be used if the need for antidepressant medication is clearly indicated.

Among the more serious common side-effects of tricyclic medications and MAO inhibitor antidepressants is orthostatic hypotension. Glassman & Bigger (1981) reported that significant orthostatic hypotension occurred in 20% of all patients treated with antidepressants, but that only 3% of those patients on therapeutic doses sustained

fractures as a result of falls. The degree of orthostasis can usually be predicted by the amount of postural hypotension prior to the initiation of medication. It seems appropriate to perform, prior to initiating tricyclic medication, determination of both standing and sitting blood pressures. Such examinations should also be continued throughout treatment. Patients should also be educated about methods to reduce the possibility of dizziness and syncope, e.g. rising slowly and purposfully in stages, counting to ten between each stage (especially when getting out of bed). Lowering the dose of medication often helps to improve the situation if dizziness or falling continues to be a substantial risk.

Increasing doses of tricyclic medication may cause progressive atrio-ventricular prolongation of conduction by increasing PR, QRS and QT intervals on the electrocardiogram (ECG) (Glassman & Bigger, 1981). Patients with pre-existing conduction defects should be treated cautiously since their condition may deteriorate during treatment. Serial ECGs are essential in the management of the patient.

Although patients who have cardiac arrhythmias need to be carefully evaluated, there are no contra-indications to antidepressant medication when needed (Veith et al, 1982). Indeed, imipramine can clearly reduce ventricular ectopic beats by its quinidine-like membrane stabilising effect (Bigger et al, 1977; Kantor et al, 1981). Consequently under careful cardiac monitoring a patient may be treated both for depression and a cardiac arrhythmia with tricyclic medication.

The procedure for patients with cardiac pathology is to first carefully evaluate the absolute need for antidepressants, but then not to fear them. Continuing careful management with cardiac consultation, physical examinations and serial ECGs permit the patient to be treated successfully for depression without compromising cardiac pathology. Patients with pacemakers may be successfully treated with antidepressant medication when needed (Alexopoulos & Shamoian, 1982).

The anticholinergic effects of tricyclic medications frequently complicate their use in the aged. For example, patients will often complain about a dry mouth or report that their food tastes differently. Although this would seem a minor complaint, for many patients it can be sufficient for them to stop the medication. The use of hard sweets and chewing gum together with the encouragement of a sympathetic clinician is often effective to convince the patient to continue tricyclics. If the patient does not complain about a dry mouth it should raise the suspicion that the patient is not taking the medication as indicated. Monoamine oxidase inhibitors do not cause the anticholinergic effects associated with tricyclics (Robinson, 1981).

Both female and male patients alike, particularly men with enlarged prostates, are susceptible to symptoms of urinary obstruction. If urinary symptoms occur, they can be treated by either reducing the dose of medication, administering urecholine, or changing to a drug with less potential for anticholinergic side-effects before a major urinary obstruction occurs.

Tricyclics often cause constipation. Patients and their families should be educated about the daily use of natural laxatives such as prunes or bran, with laxatives only being used when necesary. Faecal impaction can be an incapacitating complication of unsupervised tricyclic medication use in older persons, requiring immediate medical intervention. Ophthalmologic status should also be evaluated before drug treatment. Patients with narrow angle glaucoma are at risk for an acute attack of glaucoma if they are inadvertently started on large doses of medication. Patients with wide-angle glaucoma should have no problems. Consultation with an ophthalmologist may be necessary to resolve pertinent questions prior to initiating and continuing drug treatment.

Another anticholinergic side effect of tricyclics is the induction of delirium, an acute change in mental status, confusion, agitation, and hallucinations, (Johnson et al, 1981). All medication should be stopped before reinstituting treatment. A lower drug dose with more gradual progression is usually indicated (Preskorn & Simpson, 1982).

Older persons are also particularly prone to the adrenergic side-effects of medication which may manifest as tremulousness and a subjective feeling of 'inner skin tightening'. This is best managed by reducing the dosage.

A rare but incapacitating side-effect in older persons is the development of Parkinsonian tremors. A reduction in dosage or change in the type of medication is indicated, not the introduction of anti-Parkinson drugs. Often neurological consultation is required and the use of ECT to avoid drug toxicity (Conrad & Bresslor, 1982).

NEW ANTIDEPRESSANTS

Two new antidepressants, maprofiline and trazodone, have recently been approved by the Federal Drug Administration. Maprofiline is a tetracyclic compound with moderate sedative properties. It is comparable in efficacy to the tricyclics but with reduced cardiovascular and anticholinergic effects (Loque et al, 1979). It has not been well studied in the older population.

Trazodone, a triazolopyridine compound, is reported to have minimal if any anticholinergic effects and greatly reduced cardiovascular effects in young adults (Gershon et al, 1981; Fabre et al, 1979; Goldberg et al, 1981; Kellams et al, 1979), as well as older adults (Branconnier & Cole, 1981). Only a few clinical studies have been published using older patients. Trazodone appears to be equivalent to imipramine in the treatment of depression in older patients,

but imipramine appears to be more effective in mixed anxiety-depression (Gerner et al, 1980). One study, an open trial, suggests the potential utility of trazodone for cognitively impaired patients with agitation (Nair et al, 1973).

A series of other compounds i.e. nomifensine bupropion, and mainserin (Feighner, 1983) are being tested in clinical trials. Their efficacy in older patients remains to be seen.

ELECTROCONVULSIVE THERAPY

ECT can be an effective treatment for older patients with biological depression (American Psychiatric Association 1979; Fink, 1981; Kendall, 1981). Indeed, it may be the treatment of choice in certain patients because of the multiple side-effects of antidepressant drugs and the long latency period before their initial antidepressant action. ECT should be considered in the following cases: the recurrence of depression in a patient who has responded well before to this kind of treatment; seriously depressed patients who are in imminent danger of dying and cannot tolerate the three to four week delay in antidepressant response; suicidal patients in the absence of adequately controlled environment; and patients who have not responded to other forms of treatment and who are incapacitated by drug side-effects (Fink, 1979).

In general ECT should be given on an inpatient basis, but it may be done in an outpatient service. Prior to treatment all serious systemic illness should be ruled out which could complicate the procedure. However in a dying anorectic patient these may be secondary considerations. ECT should be administered every three to five days until seven to eight treatments have been received (equivalent to 0.2 seconds of shock time). ECT should be given with muscle relaxants, general anesthesia and single electrode non-dominant electrode placements; under these conditions there are minimal side-effects reported (Fink & Johnson, 1982).

Post ECT confusion may occur in some patients. However, non-dominant electrode placement seems to be effective in reducing post-treatment confusion and the period of post-amnesia. Inpatient care provides a secure, supervised environment until there is a return to pre-ECT clarity.

CONCLUSION: CARING FOR THE OLDER PATIENT WITH DEPRESSION

A continuum of depressive disorders are prominent in the older population. If unrecognised and untreated, depression has many consequences, the most serious of which is suicide. The need is acute for health professionals to identify accurately the various forms of depression in older persons. Furthermore depression often co-exists with other medical, psychiatric and social problems. Accurate recognition of depressive illness and differentiation from other medical, psychiatric and social problems is necessary for successful treatment. Depression is a treatable disorder and many forms of psychotherapy and pharmacotherapy can be successfully used.

Major issues still require substantial research. What clinical laboratory tests are helpful in diagnosis and treatment prediction in the aged? What is the efficacy and safety of newer antidepressants? What specific psychotherapies are effective for various depressive illnesses? The phenomenology of depressive disorders remains to be clarified and operational criteria developed for classification. Little is known about risk factors for late life depression. The identification of antecedents of the various forms of depression in the community aged is an important area of investigation with profound implications for intervention and prevention.

REFERENCES

Abraham, K The applicability of psychoanalytic treatment to patients at an advanced age (1919). Selected papers on New York: Basic Books, 1953

Adams F 1939 The Genuine Works of Hippocrates. Williams and Wilkins, Baltimore

Alexopoulos G S, Shamoian C A 1982 Tricyclic antidepressants and cardiac patients with pacemakers. American Journal of Psychiatry. 139; 519–529

American Psychiatric Association 1980 Diagnostic and Statistical Manual, DSM III. American Psychiatric Association, Washington, DC

American Psychiatric Association Task Force on ECT 1979 No. 14 American Psychiatric Association: Washington DC

Ashford W Ford C V 1979 Use of MAO inhibitors in elderly patients. American Journal of Psychiatry 136: 1466–1467

Beck A T, Rush A J, Shaw B F, Beck A T, Rush A D, Shay B F, Emery G 1979 Cognitive Therapy of Depression. Guilford Press, New York

Bergmann K 1978 Neurosis and personality disorder in old age. In: Isaacs A D, Post F (eds) Studies in Geriatric Psychiatry. John Wiley & Sons, New York

Bethune H C, Burrell R H, Culpan R H, Ogg G B 1964 Vascular crises associated with monoamineoxidose inhibitors. American Journal of Psychiatry 121: 245–248

Bigger J T, Giardina E G V, Perel J M, Kantor S J, Glassman A H 1977 Cardiac anti-arrhythmia effects of imipramine hydrochloride. New England Journal of Medicine 296: 206–208

Blackwell B 1982 Antidepressant drugs: side effects and compliance. Journal of Clinical Psychiatry 43: 14–22

Blazer D 1982a Depression in Late Life. Mosby, St Louis

Blazer D 1982b The epidemiology of late life depression. Journal of the American Geriatrics Society 30: 587–592

Blazer D, Siegler I 1981 Working with the family of the older adult patient. Addison-Wesley, Menlo Park, California

Blazer D, Williams C 1968 Epidemiology of dysphoria and depression in an elderly population. American Journal of Psychiatry 114: 797–811

Blum J E, Tross S 1980 Psychodynamic treatment of the elderly: a review of issues in theory and practice. In: C. Eisdorfer (ed) Annual Review of Geriatrics and Gerontology. Springer, New York

Branconnier R J, Cole J O 1981 Effects of acute administration of trazodone and amitriptyline on cognition, cardiovascular function, and salivation in the usual geriatric subject. Journal of Clinical Psychopharmacology 1: 82–88

Brown W A, Johnston R, Mayfield D 1979 The 24—hour dexamethasone suppression test in a clinical setting: Relationship to diagnosis, symptoms, and response to treatment. American Journal of Psychiatry 136: 543–547

Busse E W, Blazer D G 1980 Disorders related to biological functioning. In: Busse, E. W., Blazer, D.G. (eds) Handbook of Geriatric Psychiatry. Van Nostrand Reinhold, New York

Carroll B J, Feinberg M, Greden J F, Tarika J, Albala A A, Haskett R F et al 1981 A specific laboratory test for the diagnosis of melancholia. Archives of General Psychiatry 38: 15–22

Cohen D, Eisdorfer C Major psychiatric and behavioral disorders. In: Andres A, Bierman E L, Hazzard W (eds) Principles of Geriatric Medicine. McGraw Hill, New York, in press

Cohen D, Hegarty J, Eisdorfer C 1983 The 'Social PDR' A physicians reference for social and community services for the aged. Journal of the American Geriatrics Society 31: 338–341

Conrad K, Bresslor R (eds) 1982 Drug Therapy for the Elderly Mosby, St Louis

Crook T 1982 Diagnosis and treatment of mixed anxiety-depression in the elderly. Journal of Clnical Psychiatry 43: 35–43

Dally P J, Rhode P 1961 Comparison of antidepressant drugs in depressive illnesses. Lancet 1: 18–20

Davidson J, Wenger M D 1982 Using antidepressants in patients with cardiovascular disease. Journal of Clinical Therapeutics 12: 655–64

Eisdorfer C, Cohen D Keckich W 1981a Depression and anxiety in the cognitively impaired aged. In: D Klein, J Rabkin (eds) Anxiety, New Research and Changing Concepts. Raven Press, New York

Eisdorfer C, Cohen D. Veith R 1981b Psychopathology of Aging. Scope, Kalamazoo, Michigan

Fabre L, McLendon D, Gainey A 1979 Trazodone efficacy in depression: A double-blind comparison with imipramine and placebo in day-hospital patients. Current Therapeutic Research 25: 825–834

Feighner J P 1981 Clinical efficacy of the newer antidepressants. Journal of Clinical Psychopharmacology 1: 23–26

Feighner J P 1983 Second and third generation antidepressants: A clinical overview. In: M R Zales (ed) Affective and Schizophrenic Disorders. Brunner/Mazel, New York

Finestone D H, Blazer D 1982 Clinical clues to depression in the elderly patient. Geriatric Medicine Today. 1: 87–94

Fink M 1979 Convulsive Therapy and Practice Raven Press, New York

Fink M 1981 Random thoughts about ECT American Journal of Psychiatry 138: 484–485

Fink M, Johnson L 1982 Monitoring the duration of electroconvulsive therapy seizure. Archives of Geriatric Psychiatry. 39: 1189–1191

Gerner R, Estabrook W, Steuer J et al 1980 Treatment of Geriatric depression with Trazodone, imipramine, and placebo: A double-blind study. Journal of Clinical Psychiatry 41: 216–220

Glassman A H, Bigger T 1981 Cardiovascular effects of therapeutic doses of tricyclic antidepressants. Archives of General Psychiatry 38: 815–820

Golberg H, Rickels K, Finnerty R 1981 Treatment of neurotic depression with a new antidepressant. Journal of Clinical Psychopharmacology 1: 35–38

Goldfarb A 1974 Masked depression in the elderly. In: Lesse S (ed) Masked Depression Jason Aronsons, New York

Grof P 1980 Continuation and maintenance antidepressant drug treatment. In: Ayd F J (ed) Depressions: Diagnositc and Therapeutic Challenges. Ayd Medical Communications

Grotjahn M 1977 The Art and Technique of Analytic Group Therapy Jason Aronson, New York

Himmelhoch J M, Auchenbach R, Fuchs C 1982 The dilemma of depression in the elderly. Journal of Clinical Psychiatry 43: 26–32

Horita A 1978 Neuropharmacology and Aging. In: Roberts J , Adelman R C, Cristofalo V J (eds) Pharmacological Intervention in the Aging Process. Plenum, New York

Jarvik L F, Mintz J, Steuer J, Gerner R I 1982 Treating geriatric depression: A 26-week interim analysis. Journal of the American Geriatric Society. 30: 713–717

Johnson A L, Hollister L E, Berger P A 1981 The anticholinergic intoxication syndrome, diagnosis and treatment. Journal of Clinical Psychiatry 42: 313–315

Kantor S J, Glassman A H, Bigger J T,Perel J M, Giardina E V 1978 The cardiac effects of therapeutic plasma concentrations of imipramine. American Journal of Psychiatry 135: 534–538

Katon W, Raskind M 1980 Treatment of depression in medically ill elderly with methylphenidate. American Journal of Psychiatry 137: 963–965

Kay D W K, Beamish P, Roth M 1964 Old age mental disorders in Newcastle-upon-Tyne. British Journal of Psychiatry 110: 146–158

Kellams J J, Klapper M H, Small J G 1979 Trazodone, a new antidepressant: Efficacy and safety in endogenous depression. Journal of Clinical Psychiatry 40: 390–395

Kendall R E 1981 The present status of electroconvulsive therapy. British Journal of Psychiatry. 139: 265–283

Langby G E 1975 Functional Psychosis. In: J.G. Howells (ed) Modern Perspectives in Psychiatry of Old Age. Brunner and Mazel, New York

Lesse S 1979 Behavioural problems masking depression — Cultural and Clinical Survey. American Journal of Psychotherapy. XXXIII: 41–48

Logne J, Sachais B, Feighner J 1979 Comparisons of maprotiline with imipramine in severe depression: A multi-center controlled trial. Journal of Clinical Pharmacology. 19: 64–74

Mann J J, Georgotas S, Newton R, Gershon S 1981 A controlled study of trazodone, imipramine, and placebo in outpatients with endogenous depression. Journal of Clinical Psychopharmavology 1: 75–80

Mayeux R, Stern Y, Rosen J, Leventhal J 1981 Depression, intellectual impairment and Parkinson's disease. Neurology 31: 645–650

McNair D M, Fisher S E 1978 Separating anxiety from depression. In: Lipton M A, DiMascio A, Killam K (eds) Psychopharmacology: A Generation of Progress. Raven Press, New York

Mellinger G D, Balter M B 1982 Prevalence of patterns of use of psychotherapeutic Drugs: Results from a 1979 national survey of American Adults. In: Tognoni G, Bellantuono C, Lader M (eds) Epidemiological Impact of Psychotropic Drugs: Proceedings of an International Seminar on Epidemiological Impact of Psychotropic Drugs. Elsevier, Amsterdam

Mintz J, Steuer J, Jarvik L F 1981 Psychotherapy with depressed elderly patients: Research considerations. Journal of Consulting and Clinical Psychology 49: 542–548

Nair N P V, Ban T A, Hontela S, Clarke R 1973 Trazadone in the treatment of organic brain syndromes, with special reference to psychogeriatrics. Current Therapeutic Research 15: 769–775

National Institute on Aging Task Force 1980 Senility reconsidered: Treatment possibilities for mental impairment in the elderly. Journal of the American Medical Associaton 244: 259–263

Nielson J 1963 Geronto-psychiatric period-prevalence investigation in a geographically delimited population. Acta Psychiatrica Scandinavica 38: 307–330

Ouslander J 1982 Physical illness and depression in the elderly. Journal of American Geriatrics Society 30: 593–599

Overall J E, Gorham D R 1967 The brief psychiatric rating scale. Psychological Reports 10: 779–812

Paykel E J, Parker R R, Penrose R J, Rassaby, E R 1979 Depressive classification and prediction of response to phenelzine. British Journal of Psychiatry 134: 572–581

Pitt B H 1974 Psychogeriatrics Churchill Livingstone, Edinburgh

Preskhorn S H, Simpson S 1982 Tricyclic antidepressant induced delirium and plasma drug concentration. American Journal of Psychiatry 139: 822–824

Reifler B V, Kethley A, O'Neill P, Hanley R, Lewis S, Stenchever D 1982 Five year experience of a community outreach program for the elderly. American Journal of Psychiatry 139: 2 220–223

Robinson D 1981 Monoamine oxidase inhibitors and the elderly. In: Raskind A, Robinson D, Levine J (eds) Age and Pharmacology of Psychoactive Drugs Elsevier, New York

Robinson D S 1975 Changes in monoamine oxidase and monoamines with human development and aging. Federation Proceedings 34: 103–107

Robinson R G, Price T R 1982 Post-stroke depressive disorder: A follow-up study of 103 patients. Stroke 13: 635–640

Roth M, Gurney C, Gorside R F et al 1972 Studies in the classification of affective disorders. The relationship between anxiety states and depressive illnesses. British Journal of Psychiatry 121: 147–161

Salzman C 1982 A primer on geriatric psychopharmacology. American Journal of Psychiatry 139: 67–74

Salzman C, Shader R I 1978 Clinical Evaluation of depression in the elderly. In: Raskin A, Jarvik C F, Jarvik L F (eds) Psychiatric Symptoms and Cognitive Loss in the Elderly. Hemisphere Washington, DC

Sargent W 1962 The treatment of anxiety states and atypical depressions by the monoamine oxidase inhibitor drugs. Journal of Neuropsychiatry 3: 96–102

Schatzberg A F, Rothschild M D, Stahl J B,Bond T C, Rosenbaum A H, Lofgren S B et al 1983 The dexamethasone suppression test: Identification of subtypes of depression. American Journal of Psychiatry 140: 88–90

Schlesser M A,Winokur A, Sherman B M 1980 Hypothalamic-pituitary-adrenal axis activity in depressive illness. Archives of Geriatric Psychiatry 37: 737–743

Schuckit M A, Pastor P A 1979 Alcohol-related psychopathology in the aged. In: Kaplan H I (ed) Psychopathology of Aging. Academic Press, New York

Steuer J 1982 Psychotherapy with depressed elders. In: Blazer D (ed) Depression in Late Life. Mosby, St. Louis

Thompson T, Moran M, Nies A 1983 Drug therapy. New England Journal of Medicine 308: 194–198

Veith R C, Raskind M, Caldwell J, Barnes R F, Gumbrecht G, Ritchie J L 1982 Cardiovascular effects of tricyclic antidepressants in depressed patients with chronic heart disease. New England Journal of Medicine. 306: 954–959

Verwoerdt A 1976 Clinical Geropsychiatry. Williams and Wilkins, Baltimore

Vital Statistics of the United States 1975. 1978 U.S. Department of Health Washington DC

Weissman M 1979 The psychological treatment of depression: Evidence for the efficacy of psychotherapy alone, in comparison with, and in combination with pharmacotherapy. Archives of General Psychiatry 36: 1261–1269

Weissman M M, Myers J K 1978 Affective disorders in a U.S. urban community: the use of research diagnostic criteria in an epidemiological survey. Archives of Geriatric Psychiatry. 35: 1304–1311

Weissman M M, Myers J K 1979 Depression in the elderly: Research directions in psychopathology, epidemiology, and treatment. Journal of Geriatric Psychiatry 12: 187–201

Wells C E 1979 Pseudodementia. American Journal of Psychiatry. 136: 895–900

Yesavage J A, Karasu T B 1982 Psychotherapy with elderly patients. American Journal of Psychotherapy XXXVI: 41–55

14

Sleep disorders

R. Pascualy

SLEEP AND AGING

Numerous surveys of sleep disturbance in the general population have established high correlations between advancing age and disturbed sleep. That these changes lead to physician intervention is reflected in recent drug surveys documenting the disproportionately large number of sedative hypnotic prescriptions written for patients over the age of sixty. A 1977 survey by the United States Public Health Service of physicians' prescribing practices in skilled nursing facilities showed that 92 833 prescriptions had been written for a staggering 94.2% of the 98 505 charts reviewed (Miles & Dement, 1980).

The clinical consensus of sleep specialists is that in the elderly specific sleep disorders, physical conditions, drugs and alcohol are collectively more significant aetiological factors than major psychiatric conditions. The neurotic elderly rarely come to the attention of sleep specialists and next to nothing is known about their sleep complaints (Miller & Barns, 1980). The collective experience of the Association of Sleep Disorders Centres (ASDC) (which has data from over 5000 patients with persistent sleep problems), suggests that a specific diagnosis can be made in over 90% of patients (Coleman et al).

It is well known that there are two physiologically distinct sleep states: rapid-eye-movement sleep or dreaming (REM) and non-REM sleep, deep sleep, slow wave sleep (NREM), the latter being subdivided into Stages 1–4. Although bodily movements are relatively infrequent in NREM sleep, the muscles continue to show electrical activity and reflex excitability is well maintained. In REM sleep the brain is very active and the electro-encephalogram (EEG) patterns are similar to the waking state. With the exception of eye movement activity, there is subsidence of muscle activity and spinal reflexes can no longer be elicited. When normal adults fall asleep they usually pass into NREM sleep. There is then a regular 90–100 minute alternation between NREM sleep and REM sleep. This 90–100 minute rhythm is sometimes referred to as the 'basic sleep cycle'.

Polysomnographic studies of the effects of age on sleep are woefully inadequate, but certain changes with age have been established that are important to the practicing clinician. Polysomnographic recordings may include measures of the EEG, electro-oculogram (EOG), chin electromyogram (EMG), respiratory movements and airflow, cardiac rhythm, blood oxygen saturation, leg movements and penile tumescence. The EEG activity is scored using the criteria of Rechtschaffen & Kales (1968).

Elderly people do seem to spend more time lying in bed at night without attempting to sleep, unsuccessfully attempting to sleep and resting in bed or napping. There also appears to be a tendency for individuals to advance their customary bedtime with age and to arise at an earlier hour.

The overall structure of nocturnal sleep changes with age. Total nocturnal sleep time decreases and the number of wake periods (Stage 0) becomes more frequent and prolonged. The number of stage shifts, particularly to Stage 1 and Stage 0 are increased, and this increase is considered a sign of disturbed sleep. Men have a higher percentage of Stage 1 than women from puberty onwards and the total amount of Stage 1 increases steadily throughout the lifespan in both groups. The mean percent of total sleep time spent in Stage 2 approximates a U-shaped curve throughout life with the levels in old age resembling those in early adult life. Stage 3 remains relatively unchanged but Stage 4 shows an absolute and relative reduction beginning in the second decade. By the sixth decade 25% of the population may show no Stage 4. The decline in slow wave sleep has been established in many studies and may be a sensitive biological marker of aging in the central nervous system (CNS). The relative amount of REM sleep remains stable throughout adult life with some decrease in the seventh and eighth decades. The length of each REM period becomes more constant with age, and the REM EEG is more fragmented by slow waves (Miles & Dement, 1980).

These changes in objective parameters correlate well with the typical complaints of less refreshing sleep, more frequent and prolonged wakes, less night-time sleep, and 'lighter' less sound sleep.

Central nervous system degeneration and sleep

Changes in sleep-wake patterns are one of many neurobiological alterations seen in healthy elderly and include decreased memory and cognitive function, decreased cerebral blood flow and metabolism, loss of cortical neurons and Alzheimer type neuronal degeneration (Prinz et al, 1982). Neurobiological changes contribute to changes in mental and physical function that result in reduced capacity for work, recreation and self-care. Decreased ability to perform skilled tasks rapidly, to resist fatigue, to make rapid judgements in changing situations and to learn new problem-solving methods are all cited by Pfeiffer as age-related changes (Pfeiffer & Busse, 1977). Webb's work suggests that older individuals also have a decreased response relative to sleep deprivation (Webb, 1981).

The vague complaints of the elderly of general fatigue, slowed mentation and aches and pains, are remarkably similar to the 'fibrositis syndrome' reported in young adults deprived of slow-wave sleep (Moldofksy & Scarisbrick, 1976). Fibrositis syndrome is a musculoskeletal disorder characterised by generalised periarticular pain, stiffness and exhaustion, with the majority of patients also complaining of a sleep disturbance (Smythe & Moldofsky, 1977; Yunis et al, 1981; Hester et al, 1982). This disorder affects approximately 15% of rheumatology patients and is felt to be underdiagnosed in a larger percentage of the general public. A specific sleep abnormality alpha-delta sleep, has been identified in these patients (Hauri & Hawkins, 1973; Moldofsky et al, 1975). Since fibrositis-like symptoms can be induced in young adults by selective deprivation of Stage 4 sleep, perhaps the loss of slow wave sleep with aging may be pathogenic in the development of non-specific somatic complaints in the elderly.

The Alzheimer's type changes in non-demented elderly may begin in the fourth decade and are seen in a similar anatomic distribution as in Alzheimer's type dementia. These changes involve the monoaminergic brain stem nuclei considered responsible for the regulation of sleep (Ishino & Otsuki, 1975). Prinz et al (1982) suggest that neuronal degeneration of these regulatory pathways may underlie the sleep-wake changes seen in Alzheimer's disease. Clinically advanced Alzheimer's patients show a polyphasic sleep cycle with numerous naps distributed evenly across the day. Night-time sleep is brief and fragmented by numerous wakes with markedly decreased slow wave and REM sleep.

Other studies suggest a relationship between diffuse CNS degeneration (defined as slowing of the dominant waking EEG frequency), cognitive deterioration and sleep-wake function. A Duke University group (Wang et al, 1970) followed healthy elderly subjects over three and a half years and found that those with the lowest waking dominant occipital frequencies showed the most deterioration on the performance scale of the Weschler Adult Intelligence Scale.

Another study demonstrated that in a group of intact elderly the faster learners on a verbal memory test had higher dominant occipital EEG rhythms (Thompson & Wilson, 1966). These studies are of particular interest in light of Hazemanns' work using portable telemetry to measure the EEG of elderly subjects in their normal waking environments as they followed their usual daytime routines. A total of 22 subjects ranging in age from 82 to 97 were studied. Behavioural measures of waking, somnolence and naps correlated with age and background EEG (Hazemann et al, 1977).

If decreases in the frequency of waking rhythm correlate with decreased function, preservation of REM sleep may be associated with preservation of intellectual function and higher background rhythm. In the Duke study the preservation of intellectual function in those elderly with relatively higher REM time held up over an 18 year period (Prinz, 1977).

Aging alone is not an adequate explanation for these changes as many elderly sleep soundly, show few signs of degeneration, or despite objective measure of disturbed sleep have no sleep complaints.

Sleep complaints and mortality

Data from 1 000 064 subjects surveyed under the auspices of the American Cancer Society indicated that men and women *without* a prior history of heart disease, high blood pressure, diabetes or stroke were more likely to die within six years if they reported and complained that they usually slept less than 7 hours or more than 7.9 hours (Hammond, 1964). Those men and women who reported sleeping more than 7.9 hours had an increased mortality rate from coronary artery disease, stroke and aortic aneurysm. Those individuals who reported using sleeping pills 'often' had one and a half times the mortality rate of those subjects who never used sleeping pills (Kripke et al, 1979).

These data also suggested a more complex relationship between sleep and mortality than the simple explanation that poor sleepers have more physical illness. There is, however, an established association between illness and sleep complaints.

Finally, death from any cause is most common during sleep with a peak just prior to morning arousal. Some authors have speculated that early morning REM-related events such as sleep apnea may be responsible for this phenomenon.

The need for sleep and daytime sleepiness

The image of an elderly person napping in an easy chair or on a sunny park bench is a compelling image of increasing daytime sleepiness with age. Observational studies of napping suggest that in men the number of daytime naps increases with age, while this is also true of women who are not employed full-time. Yet less than 2% of the elderly poor sleepers in McGhie & Russel's survey 1962 admitted to napping, and several authors have concluded that daytime napping does not compensate for impaired nocturnal sleep (Tune, 1969). Although there is no evidence to support changes in nocturnal sleep in countries observing the custom of a single afternoon nap, frequent or prolonged daytime naps may desynchronise the sleep-wake cycle.

Recent studies using the Multiple Sleep Latency Test (MSLT) have shown that with increasing age the physiological tendency to sleep also increases (Carskadon & Dement, 1982). The MSLT consists of five scheduled attempts by the subject to fall asleep under controlled circumstances in a sleep laboratory. Data from these studies show that the prepubescent child is optimally alert and rarely achieves sleep during these tests. There is a gradual increase in sleep tendency with age that is significantly different in adolescents, young adults and elderly patients. Because daytime sleepiness increases with age we can conclude that the need for sleep clearly does not decrease. Preliminary data also suggests that non-complaining healthy elderly subjects may be objectively sleepy because of disturbed sleep caused by respiratory disturbances of which they remain unaware (Carskadon et al, 1981).

Circadian rhythms and sleep

Animal studies and human data suggest that disruption of the circadian rhythms may accompany the aging process. Alterations of the phase relationship of certain rhythms in humans present clinically as sleep-wake disorders such as jet lag or delayed sleep phase syndrome (Weitzman et al, 1981). Bedrest in young volunteers resulted in desynchronisation of the sleep-wake cycle and body temperature and appeared to be postural effects unrelated to exercise and confinement (Winget et al, 1972). These data have obvious implications for the elderly in prolonged hospitalisations or enforced bedrest.

Organic central nervous system disease, endogenous depression and blindness all affect circadian rhythms. These disorders have a significant increasing prevalence with age. The prevalence of legal blindness doubles between the ages of 65 and 75 and triples by the age of 85. Many studies of the blind have documented significant abnormalities in the circadian rhythms and associated incapacitating sleep-wake disturbances (Miles & Wilson, 1977).

THE OFFICE EVALUATION OF SLEEP DISTURBANCE IN THE ELDERLY

General considerations

The office evaluation and management of sleep disorders is hampered by a variety of factors. Unless the physician requests a sleep questionnaire and a sleep diary prior to the visit the initial interview will be time consuming. A sleep questionnaire and sample sleep diary should be sent prior to the clinic visit. The savings in physician time makes this a valuable investment. The unreliability of subjective reports of sleep behaviour, the presence of occult disorders such as e.g., periodic leg movements in sleep, co-existing physical illness, multiple drug regimens and complex psychosocial stresses all combine to create a difficult diagnostic and treatment situation. Information from a sleeping partner is very important diagnostically but many elderly live alone or sleep alone.

The failure to recognise otherwise easily diagnosable sleep pathology is related to the common practice of focusing on a sleep complaint as if it were a diagnosis thereby bypassing the careful review that will elicit other signs and symptoms. The widespread notion that sleep disturbances are primarily of psychological origin may have some merit in the young adult but is not applicable to the elderly individual. Even the expert somnologist will in a significant number of cases find the history equivocal and require polysomnographic evaluation to reach a conclusion. The expense and scarcity of polysomnography, absence of well-trained sleep specialists and the inability or refusal of many elderly to travel great distances for evaluations all further complicate the situation.

Treatment itself may be frustrated by patients' wishes for a 'pill solution', poor compliance with behavioural treatment and lack of efficacious treatments for disorders such as periodic leg movements in sleep, restless legs, neuropathic pain and some of the chronic insomnias. Despite these obstacles many insomnias will yield to thorough office care and provide unusual patient gratitude and professional satisfaction.

Taking a sleep history

1. Establish the onset of the complaint and any associated changes in health or psychosocial function that occurred at that time. Attempt to characterise the difficulty in falling asleep, maintaining sleep and awakening at the desired hour. General daytime function and its relationship to nocturnal sleep should clearly describe the possible contrast to function prior to the sleep disturbance.

2. Attempt to characterise the presence and quality of excessive daytime sleepiness. This may be described as lethargy, fatigue, tiredness, dull mentation, low energy or sluggishness. These are common complaints in many elderly and may or may not be sleep-related. Non-complaining elderly may be objectively sleepy yet minimise or deny their symptoms. However, for office screening purposes certain clinical clues will identify the seriously sleepy patient. These patients are persistently sleepy day in and out, report needing to fight sleep throughout the day, will frequently fall asleep spontaneously in most quiet situations such as reading, watching T.V. or travelling by the train or bus. They may take frequent daily naps.

Clearly pathologic sleepiness is indicated by a history of falling asleep while driving reasonable distances, while eating, during a conversation or while waiting on the phone.

3. Inquire about the patient's night-time routine and bedroom environment including the pattern of wake and bedtime, timing of evening meals and liquids, use of caffeine products and the presence of environmental noise. Caffeine appears to disrupt nocturnal sleep to a great extent with advancing age (Brezinova, 1974). Environmental noise is more disturbing with age, and decreases in the auditory awakening threshold have been documented in aged men (Zepelin et al, 1980). Noise, anxiety and arousals related to an ill spouse may also contribute to the sleep disturbance.

4. A review of organ system function during nocturnal hours should be performed including specifically colon pain, muscular or skeletal discomfort, urinary urgency, cramps, breathing difficulties, proctalgia, dyspepsia, palpitations, cough, temperature discomfort, nightmares and anxiety. Episodes of confusion, falling out of bed, falls and near falls at night should also be specifically sought for.

5. A thorough review of current medications, over-the-counter drug use, use of alcohol and illicit drugs is essential. Attempt to establish previous treatments as carefully as possible including drug dosages and regimens, duration, side effects and the patient's general response to them. Inquire specifically about rebound insomnia or a history suggestive of drug habituation or abuse. If suspected attempt to corroborate a history of alcoholism. Home remedies and treatments performed by various other professionals should be specifically requested.

6. A thorough psychiatric review is essential including any past history of depression, anxiety, suicidal behaviour, panic, phobia and previous use of psychotropics. A review of endogenous symptoms of depression easily follows from open-ended questions regarding family life, socio-economic concerns, diet and daily activity. Dementia may be associated with nocturnal sleep disturbance and daytime sleepiness, therefore memory function should also be investigated.

7. The presence of snoring and respiratory pauses observed by a sleeping partner should be established, and the associated symptoms of sleep apnea sought for.

8. A sleeping partner if available should be interviewed and ideally should have helped in the completion of the sleep questionnaire. As a general rule, the partner should be interviewed separately to allow a candid discussion of psychological factors, sexual behaviour, drug and alcohol use. If no bed partner is available, a family member or friend may have had the opportunity to observe the patient's sleep during a holiday or vacation. The informant should be questioned particularly on the presence of snoring, sleepiness, respiratory disturbance, excessive leg or body motion and changes in cognitive or emotional functioning.

THE DIAGNOSTIC APPROACH TO SLEEP COMPLAINTS IN THE ELDERLY

By reviewing the following six categories the physician can organise his evaluation in a systematic manner and consequently devise a multimodal treatment plan: 1. Undiagnosed major physical or psychiatric illness, 2. suboptimal management or exacerbation of pre-existing conditions, 3. organic sleep disorders, 4. drug related sleep disturbances, 5. psycho-physiologic insomnia and 6. miscellaneous conditions including sleep-wake disturbances, poor sleep hygiene and parasomnias.

1. Undiagnosed major physical and psychiatric illness

It cannot be overemphasised that insomnia and daytime sleepiness are symptoms that require a thorough differential diagnosis. In the elderly a sleep complaint should lead to a thorough general medical history and a physical examination. The presence of a long-standing complaint should neither be discouraging nor imply a functional problem. Individuals with sleep disorders often see many physicians over many years before a definitive evaluation is performed.

That non-psychiatric physicians have difficulty diagnosing affective illness and fail to treat or treat inadequately when it is diagnosed, has been established in several studies (Zung et al, 1983). Depression in the elderly may be masked by somatic complaints, anxiety symptoms, denial of depressed mood and minimisation of loss of function. Vegetative symptoms may be attributed to age or concommitant physical illness. In questionable cases further history from family, friends, health workers or home visit will usually clarify the change in function and mood.

2. Suboptimal management or exacerbation of a pre-existing condition

The review of organ function systems will identify any specific symptoms present during the sleep period. The sleep diary is invaluable in pin-pointing the relative frequency and importance of various physical and psychologic stimuli associated with sleep disruption. Memory alone or a general impression can often be misleading.

Suboptimal management may be related to poor compliance with a good medication regimen. Intentional non-compliance with treatment in the elderly is more common than suspected and is often erroneously attributed to forgetfulness or a complex drug regimen (Cooper et al, 1982). Although these are certainly important factors they may be polite excuses for avoiding direct conflict over treatment with the physician. If forgetfulness is out of keeping with the patient's general independent function and mental status, sympathetic questioning regarding unpleasant side effects, therapeutic scepticism, and fear of multiple drug regimens may clarify the reasons for non-compliance.

The treatment of specific symptoms of known diseases may restore the normal sleep pattern. Huskisson & Grayson's study (1974) showed indomethacin to be superior to a hypnotic alone or in combination with indomethacin in improving insomnia in rheumatoid arthritis. Giulleminault's case report (in press) demonstrates how altering the medication schedule of a Parkinson's patient resulted in decreased night-time stiffness and resolved his insomnia. The popularity of salicylates as sleep aids in drug surveys probably relates to the improvement of musculoskeletal discomfort in sleep and may be of particular signficance in the elderly.

3. Organic sleep disorders

The ASDC established a comprehensive Diagnostic Classification of Sleep and Arousal Disorders in 1979. The first large case series using this system included over 5000 patients, with the elderly underrepresented. This is probably related to many factors including inadequate insurance coverage, high cost of polysomnography, patient and physician unawareness of sleep disorders in the elderly and scarcity of qualified somnologists and sleep clinics. Two polysomnographic case series are available examining a total of 110 elderly patients.

Reynolds examined 27 patients, aged 55 or older, and identified insomnia associated with affective disorders (30%) and sleep apnea (18.5%) as the most common diagnoses (Reynolds et al, 1979). This high prevalence of affective illness is not in keeping with the clinical experience of other centres. Nevertheless obstructive sleep apnea and affective illness are the two sleep disorders that have both very effective treatments and significant morbidity and mortality if misdiagnosed and untreated. Thus high diagnostic suspicion should be exercised towards these two problems and 'false positive' consultations with geropsychiatrists and somnologists in questionable cases can be justified.

A larger study by Coleman et al (1981) examined 83 patients aged 60 or older who received psychiatric and polysomnographic evaluations. These patients were almost evenly divided between the disorders of initiating and maintaining sleep (DIMS) and the disorders of excessive somnolence (DOES). Overall, sleep apnea (39%) and periodic leg movements (18%) were the most common diagnoses. Of practical importance is that the largest group complaining of DIMS had a disgnosis of psychophysiologic insomnia. By definition no major psychopathology is found in these patients. Psychiatric disorders are the most common diagnoses in the younger population complaining of chronic insomnia.

Sleep apnea

Sleep apnea is a fascinating and complex disorder that has been thoroughly reviewed in recent publications (Guilleminault et al, 1980). It consists of a nocturnal sleep disturbance resulting in cessation of air flow with subsequent arousal and disturbance of sleep. It is subdivided into central and obstructive types, although in practice a mixed picture with obstructive predominance is most common. Recent work by Carskadon et al (1982) suggests that undiagnosed apnea and very brief arousals may be significant causes of sleep disturbance in non-complaining elderly.

In obstructive apnea respiratory effort is present but the airway is occluded by the soft tissue of the oropharynx resulting in decreased or absent air exchange. Partial occlusion of the airway produces snoring and partial decreases in air exchange, termed hypopneas. Total occlusion is heard as a silent pause with increasing respiratory effort, body movement and a snort heralding the overcoming of the obstruction with an associated arousal. In central apnea there is no respiratory effort due to the absence of CNS respiratory stimulus so there is no air exchange despite a patent airway.

These respiratory events may be associated with major oxygen desaturation, cardiac arrhythmias and asystoles, gross body movements, significant diaphragmatic fatigue and alteration of homeostatic respiratory mechanisms. There is gross disruption of sleep cycles and growing daytime sleepiness. It is believed that apnea may result in insomnia with complaints of disturbed night-time sleep (Guilleminault et al, 1981). This was diagnosed in 6% of the insomnia cases in the ASDC series.

The cardinal symptoms of sleep apnea are excessive daytime somnolence and snoring. Snoring indicates some impairment of upper airway function and heavy snoring has been associated with hypertension (Pollak et al, 1978), and nocturnal hemodynamic abnormalities (Lugaresi et al, 1980). As more than half of people over 60 snore and may be variably sleepy for a variety of reasons in questionable cases, some attempt to screen for apnea is necessary. A volunteer health aide may be instructed to observe and time snores and respiratory pause in the home environment. A nurse or paramedic accustomed to the night shift is an ideal observer. Alternately a cassette recorder turned on at bedtime may also confirm the suspicion. The patient may also complain of disturbed sleep and choking or gasping for breath. Family members may describe respiratory pauses, snorts and excessive body motion during sleep. Patient and family may also complain of early morning confusion and deterioration of memory and judgment, automatic or irrelevant behaviours and changes in personality such as jealousy, suspicion, anxiety or depressive outlook. Recurrent morning headaches and nausea are also seen. Impairment may be variable, ranging from sleepiness only in quiet sedentary moments to debilitating daytime somnolence. In mild cases the apneic events may be intermittent and may vary according to night-time alcohol use, exhaustion, upper respiratory infection, increases in air pollution, and seasonal allergies.

On physical examination, recent weight gain, obesity, a short thick neck, dental malocclusion, large soft palate and large uvula, large tongue, prominent tonsils and fat pharyngeal folds may be noted. Normal weight individuals without obvious oropharyngeal changes may also present with this syndrome.

If this syndrome is suspected overnight polysomnography is required. Daytime studies may confirm the presence of apnea, but will underestimate the severity of the illness in many cases. Furthermore, objective haemodynamic improvement following treatment requires a full study that can be compared to post-treatment results.

The differential diagnosis of sleep apnea syndrome includes alveolar hypoventilation, Cheyne-Stokes respiration, intracranial tumour, nocturnal seizures, acromegaly and myotonic dystrophy, hypothyroidism, Prader-Willi syndrome, the periodic hypersomnias and other conditions presenting with awakenings associated with choking or suffocation (Guilleminault & Miles, 1980).

The management of severe apnea requiring tracheostomy has been recently reviewed (Guilleminault et al, 1981). Conservative measures in milder cases include uvalopalatopharyngoplasty (Fujita et al, 1981), weight loss (Harman et al, 1982), protriptyline (Brownell et al, 1982) and progestational agents (Orr et al, 1979).

Periodic leg movement (Nocturnal myoclonus)
Of patients referred to sleep clinics this was the second largest cause of sleep complaints. It leads more frequently to a complaint of DIMS (79%), than of daytime somnolence (11%). The movements are most frequently limited to unilateral or bilateral extension of the big toe and commonly can include flexion of the foot at the ankle and partial flexion of the knee and hip. These movements have a periodic occurence and may occur throughout the night in severe cases. Periodic leg movements may be present in asymptomatic individuals and there is controversy as to its relationship with insomnia. However ASDC clinical consensus is that periodic leg movements that result in frequent wakes and arousals are commonly related to insomnia. There is no etiological explanation for the syndrome and further experimental work is necessary to clarify its role in disturbed sleep.

The ASDC case series shows a marked increase in the prevalence of periodic leg movements in sleep with advancing age, particularly in the fifth decade. A small case series followed for over eight years has shown a progressive increase in movements and arousals in advanced old age. A history from a bed partner of excessive nocturnal motion,

repetitive leg jerks or disheveled bed covers may suggest this entity.

Periodic leg movements may be clinically difficult to distinguish from chronic psychophysiologic insomnia and this should be considered in chronic insomniacs who are unimproved with a behavioural treatment programme after six months. Although direct observation of sleep might establish the presence of periodic movement in sleep (PMS) the relationships of these events to arousals and brief wakes cannot be established without polysomnography. Because periodic leg movements may be seen without symptomatic expression, polysomnographic evaluation is required.

There is no uniformly effective treatment for the problem although clonazepam at bedtime has been used with varying success. Anecdotal reports suggest clonazepam may have significant problems in the elderly with confusion, disorientation and sedation so slow, dose changes are necessary. Equivocal success has been claimed for diazepam, baclofen, gamma-hydroxybutyrate, valproic acid, and phenoxybenzamine (Guilleminault, 1982).

Restless legs syndrome
Patients with this disorder usually have periodic leg movements in addition. It is described as uncomfortable creeping crawling dysesthesias in the calves whenever the legs are at rest. The almost irresistable urge to keep the legs in motion disturbs sleep. The syndrome progresses with age and may be seen in chronic uremia, iron deficiency anemia, primary amyloidosis with peripheral neuropathy, carcinoma, diabetic neuropathy and pregnancy. About one third of patients show a familial incidence.

The differential should include painful cramps, akathisia secondary to neuroleptics and nervous agitation. There is no effective treatment and severe emotional disturbance including suicide may develop secondarily. Oxycodone and tegretol have been of benefit in some cases. Clinical success has been claimed for 5-hydroxytryptophan, folic acid, vitamin E and caffeine withdrawal (Frankel et al, 1974; Guilleminault, in press).

Delayed sleep phase syndrome (DSPS)
DSPS may be seen in the institutionalised elderly, older patients returning from foreign travel unable to readjust their sleep schedule or as a result of hospitalisations for any reason disrupt the day/night rhythm. This syndrome is characterised by the inability to fall asleep until the early hours of the morning, then sleeping a normal amount of time and awakening in the late morning or early afternoon. The patient may complain of night-time boredom and insomnia but is not usually sleepy or fatigued as total sleep time is unchanged. A third party may bring medical attention on the subject if he is disrupting others at night, missing breakfast and lunch or generally falling out of step with an institutional schedule. These subjects have shifted

their circadian rhythms including core body temperature and are unable to shift their pattern even with the use of sedative hypnotics.

Weitzman et al (1979) have shown that delaying the bedtime by two to three hours a day will bring the subject back to normal within a week or two.

Sundown syndrome
This is a common and difficult management problem characterised by confusion and disorientation often associated with nocturnal wandering between short naps. Activity during these times may appear purposeful but is usually without a reasonable goal. Hypnogogic hallucinations may result in aggressive or paranoid behaviour. Darkness and decreased stimuli may trigger or enhance the problem. This syndrome is usually seen in patients with some degree of dementia or other neurologic illness such as Parkinson's. The overall therapeutic success is poor unless a drug reaction or reversible somatic illness is responsible. Environmental changes such as night-lights, strict routine, familiar bedroom furnishings are often used and are believed to be helpful. Pharmocotherapy with barbiturates and long-acting benzodiacepines are not useful. Short-acting benzodiazepines, Haldol, thorazine, and chloral hydrate are used with variable results.

Although high potency neuroleptics such as Haldol are popular in this syndrome there is no definitive evidence of their efficacy. Despite its reputation in young adults for minimal side effects such as sedation and postural hypotension, both of these effects may be seen in the elderly. Bradykinesia and rigidity may impair mobility and be mistaken for apathy or withdrawal. The sedating phenothiazines such as thorazine should be avoided as associated anticholinergic side effects and significant postural hypotension are major problems. Further work in the management of this disorder is sorely needed.

4. Drug related sleep disturbance
Kales and others (1974) have established that chronic use of sedative hypnotics may disrupt nocturnal sleep. Habituation leads some patients to increase the dose to restore the therapeutic effect and the subsequent development of tolerance and physical and psychological dependence occurs. Sleep continuity is disrupted particularly in the second half of the night because the drug rapidly loses its sedative effect in a tolerant individual. Sleep latency may be gradually prolonged and unpredictable so night to night variability ensues. During gradual supervised withdrawal of sedative hypnotics many individuals will improve but may not return to normal for several weeks after discontinuation of treatment. At that time the sleep complaint, if it persists, can be investigated.

In the elderly physical dependence on sedative hypnotics can pose a tremendous difficulty particularly if barbiturates are involved. In younger patients it is estimated that as

many as nine out of ten patients refuse to discontinue these drugs (Cliet, 1975). An elderly individual who is physically dependent on barbiturates should be withdrawn in a hospital setting where the staff is familiar with the procedures and its complications. If therapeutic doses are involved gradual withdrawal not exceeding one therapeutic dose per week may be effective with limited side effects. Emotional support and reassurance that they will receive alternate treatment is required. Weekly brief office visits will provide close follow-up, encouragement and develop the trust that will be of great value in further treatment.

Some individuals who claim sedative hypnotic dependence related to DIMS are actually drug abusers and will be unable or unwilling to withdraw. Psychiatric evaluation and appropriate referral are indicated. Of clinical importance is Clift's data indicating that 21.6% of his sedative hypnotic drug patients had started their medications in the hospital (Clift, 1975). Psychiatric difficulties such as depression were over-represented in this group. This is consistent with other observations that the drug dependent individual is more likely to be concurrently depressed. The routine prescription of sedative hypnotics in the hospital should be questioned.

The difficulties in the identification of depression in the elderly also apply to the abuse of alcohol. Nocturnal alcohol use may bring on sleep rapidly but results in fragmented sleep and is known to induce or worsen sleep apnea. If alcoholism is suspected further history from family members or close workers may be necessary particularly in the isolated elderly person.

Sustained use or withdrawal from other drugs
This group of drugs includes those that have a direct effect on the sleep process, mild CNS depressants, and over-the-counter drugs (OTC). The first type includes aminophylline, sympathomimetic brochodilators, antimetabolites, chemotherapeutic agents, thyroid preparations, anticonvulsants, MAOIs, adrenocorticotropic hormone, oral contraceptives, alpha-methyldopa, anti-Parkinson's drugs, propanolol and many others. Propanolol and quinidine-like anti-arrhythmics have also been reported to produce nocturnal disturbances of nightmares and night terrors. Guilleminault emphasises the development of obstructive apnea in chronic steroid treatment and he has reported several cases of a 27 case series as yet unpublished (Guilleminault, in press).

While the Parkinsonian patient may present sleep problems directly related to their illness, the medications used to treat them may worsen the problem. Psychosis is a common problem in the long-term management of these patients and it is reliably preceded by the presence of vivid nocturnal disorientation, disturbed sleep or increased activity at or following sleep onset. The commonly used medications such as amantidine, bromocryptine, l-dopa and dopa-decarboxylase inhibitors may induce nightmares and night terrors along with mild toxic reactions presenting as nocturnal confusion and wandering. Terrifying hypnagogic hallucinations in association with panic reactions may also be seen. Inadequate night-time coverage may result in exacerbation of symptoms and insomnia that is best treated with alteration of the drug's schedule. Parkinsonian patients may also present another type of nocturnal sleep disturbance marked by a complete loss of circadian rhythms. This may well be related to development of progressive dementia and isolation from environmental and social contact due to their illness.

Tricyclic antidepressants may induce significant nightmares, sleep-related periodic leg movements, and sleep disturbance with abrupt discontinuation perhaps related to REM rebound or resetting of cholinergic mechanisms. Although tricyclic antidepressants are routinely believed to suppress REM, studies suggest that it is better described as a disorganisation of the three basic components: EEG, EOG and EMG (Passouant et al, 1972). These medications resulted in a near or complete disappearance of the tonic muscle atonia usually seen during REM sleep. This increase in muscle activity may be responsible for the appearance of periodic leg movements and the nocturnal sleep disruption (Guilleminault et al, 1976).

Mild CNS depressants. This group includes the common anti-anxiety drugs such as Valium and Librium, marijuana, opiates and opiate analgesics. During the use of these drugs sleep may be enhanced. Abrupt discontinuance may present a variable ranging from frank withdrawal to insomnia. Gradual tapering and patient education will minimise these effects.

OTC medications. Of particular interest to the geriatrician are sleep aids containing scopolamine and antihistamines, antidiarrheal preparations containing belladonna alkaloids, cold and allergy preparations containing sympathomimetics such as pseudoephedrine and phenylpropanolamine, and analgesics containing salcyilates. Scopolamine and belladonna alkaloids may produce an anticholinergic toxic psychosis initially manifest by agitation and presenting an acute organic brain syndrome. Sympathomimetics and the early stages of salicylism are associated with high arousal and insomnia. The signs and symptoms of OTC drug abuse and toxicity have been recently reviewed (Gardner & Hall, 1982).

5. Psychophysiologic insomnia

Psychophysiologic insomnia is a heterogenous condition seen in all age groups and in the available case series is an important type of insomnia in the elderly. This group of patients is well known to the physician and best represents the 'chronic insomniac' who is without major physical or psychiatric pathology yet has persistent sleep complaints. These patients often strike the physician as a worried, tense

and hypochondriacal lot. The young chronic insomniac may differ from the older person complaining of chronic sleep disturbance. Convincing studies demonstrate that over 80% of chronic insomniacs show elevated neuroticism scores (Kales et al, 1976). Less than one in five will have objective laboratory evidence of their subjective complaint of short-sleep or long-sleep latency, a third or more will have no objective sleepiness, and less than 10% will have pathologic sleepiness (Carskadon et al, 1976).

Comparable data are not available for the elderly, but preliminary evidence suggests that the older insomniac has more objective sleep disturbance, increased sleepiness and little psychometric evidence of psychologic abnormality (Roehrs et al, 1982). In patients seen in sleep clinics, psychiatric etiologies comprise the largest group of insomnias at 32%. In Coleman's series of 83 elderly patients, psychiatric illness accounts for less than 20% of insomniacs and is the third most frequent diagnosis after periodic movements in sleep and psychophysiologic insomnia.

The term 'psychophysiologic' refers to the process by which external stress and internal psychologic conflict produce tension and anxiety that is discharged through somatic channels. The somatisation of this tension/anxiety results in physiologic arousal that continues into the sleep period and has been measured by increased heart rate, increased basal body temperature, increased phasic vaso-construction and increased galvanic skin response (Monroe, 1967). A psychologic sketch of these patients drawn from several thorough studies shows them to be introverted individuals whose anxieties are turned inward with prominent chronic low-grade depression. Fearfulness and anxious worrying with ruminative thinking characterise their congnitive style. They may appear hypochondriacal due to multiple tension-related complaints such as headaches, back pains, and palpitations but psychiatric studies suggest this is not the case. Kales suggests that insomniacs general distress and readiness to complain is more directly a function of their chronic depression (Kales et al, 1976). This is particularly important in the elderly in view of the prominence of somatic complaints in the presentation of major depression or psychologic distress.

Almost everyone has experienced a transient or situational insomnia resulting from psychophysiologic overarousal. Sleepless excited children on Christmas Eve, the anxious groom on his wedding night, the grieving widow, the surgical patient awaiting a routine elective procedure are all well known examples of this type of insomnia. In some cases however, the insomnia persists beyond the period of the acute stress and becomes a persistent conditioned behaviour. From the foregoing discussion it may appear that certain personality types are more vulnerable to the development of this condition but prospective data are lacking. A recent retrospective study confirms the presence of increased negative life events, particularly related to health, just prior to the onset of a chronic insomnia (Healey et al, 1981).

Persistent psychophysiologic insomnia is maintained by a combination of mutually reinforcing internal and external conditioned factors. An internal conditioned factor is the anxious apprehension at bedtime that develops from repeated failed attempts to achieve sleep. Conscious attempts to fall asleep only result in further CNS arousal and a loss of confidence in a normal physiologic process develops. External conditioned factors refers to the association of miserable sleeplessness with familiar bedtime routines, the smells, sounds and feel of the bedroom environment.

The role of tension is suggested by the variability of the insomnia in relation to pleasant or stressful life events. Internal conditioned factors are suggested by the patient who falls asleep readily while watching T.V. or reading in bed yet is unable to sleep once they turn out the light and 'try to sleep'. External conditioned factors may be present if the patient sleeps well on the living room couch, the spare guest bed or away from home. Only a careful interview and knowledge of the patient's makeup can clarify these factors. Of clinical importance in some elderly insomniacs is their ability to fall asleep readily in contrast to their younger counterparts who commonly complain of prolonged sleep latency. Physical exhausation may bring on sleep in the elderly and long wakes throughout the latter part of night may be their chief complaint. Finally, chronic psychophysiologic insomnia may be impossible to distinguish from periodic leg movements with frequent wakes and non-restorative sleep. Those patients with long sleep latencies may also resemble the patients with delayed sleep phase syndrome.

Treatment of psychophysiologic insomnia

Transient psychophysiologic insomnia. The clearest indication for a brief trial of benzodiazepines is a situational insomnia associated with a traumatic event. The associated sleep deprivation may further impair the patient's coping ability at a time when the need to function at their best. A week's prescription will minimise overdose potential and provide a clear reason for a follow-up visit that will allow time for physician counselling and close monitoring of efficacy and side effects. If daytime anxiety and arousal are high this may be a situation where the daytime sedation of a long acting benzodiazepine may be therapeutic. The attending risks, particularly with driving, need to be considered.

Chronic psychophysiologic insomnia. Chronic psychophysiologic insomnia (CPI) is a heterogeneous condition and future research will allow specification of subsyndromes and improved treatment results. Sedative hypnotics have no established role in the treatment of this problem, although they may be used with care in certain

circumstances. Behavioural programmes (Coates & Thoresen, 1977), psychotherapy (Moldofksy & Scarisbrick, 1976), and intermittent treatment with L-tryptophan (Schneider-Helmient, 1981) have been recommended as treatment for this condition. There are no significant studies evaluating the efficacy of these treatments in the elderly population, although clinical experience in younger patients indicates they may be of significant value. To succeed in the management of these patients the physician must overcome any prejudice against the use of psychologic techniques, including psychotherapy, in the elderly.

The general goal in the behavioural treatment of psychophysiologic insomnia is to change the patient's focus from night-time sleep to improving daytime well-being and changing the daytime behaviours contributing to their poor sleep. Consolidating the total sleep time by setting a firm waketime and eliminating naps is necessary in many insomniacs as they prolong the total bed-time hoping to get a full night of broken sleep. However, the long bed-time produces much of the discomfort, worry, and conditioning that contributes to the cycle of negative reinforcement. The patient should be educated regarding the following points using specific examples from their individual history: nature of psychophysiologic insomnia, changes in sleep with aging, lack of efficacy of hypnotics, toxicity of hypnotics and related sleep disturbance, need for patience and persistent compliance with treatment programme if recovery is to be expected.

The following general hygiene rules should be established: 1. Establish a set wake-up time to be maintained, including on weekends and holidays. 2. Daytime naps should be eliminated or consolidated into one mid-afternoon nap not to exceed 30 minutes. 3. Discontinue or diminish the use of caffeine and alcohol particularly in the evening. If urinary urgency is causing regular wakes the patient should avoid liquids three hours before bedtime and should void before retiring. 4. Late evening activities including books, movies, conversations and home projects should not include content which can be stimulating or disturbing. 5. Increased daytime socialisation and activity should be encouraged and noted in the diary. 6. Bedroom environment should be optimised for sound sleep to be as dark and quiet as possible. A small night light will prevent accidents and if placed appropriately will not disturb sleep. 7. The bed and bedroom, as far as possible, should be reserved for sleeping i.e. no reading in bed, watching T.V. in bed etc. These rules are best implemented by maintaining a daily sleep/wake diary to be reviewed with the physician.

Patients should be specifically instructed to avoid attempting to sleep when they are not sleepy as this is a common problem. Furthermore, they should be instructed to get out of bed if they are not able to achieve sleep within 20 minutes of lights out. This may result in considerable sitting time at first, but the habit of tossing and turning and the concommitant arousal and conditioning will eventually be broken. If external conditioning factors are identified simple redecoration, room deodorisers, and rearrangement of the furniture may be necessary.

Deep muscle relaxation techniques when learned from a competent instructor over several sessions with appropriate feedback can be a beneficial technique. These may be free or inexpensive when offered through a senior citizens or local community group. Expecting results from manuals, handouts or one-shot sessions is unreasonable despite claims to the contrary.

A stress reduction programme that will help the patient identify chronic sources of stress and negative thinking patterns may be prescribed. While the source of stress may not be altered in many cases it is as important to identify them and to consciously establish strategies for managing the discomfort. The self observation skills will enhance the value of the sleep diary and allow the patient to compare good and bad nights in relation to the day's events. Over time most patients will identify certain patterns and be able to make significant changes. The importance of socialisation and daily contact with others, participating in enjoyable activities however limited, should be promoted in whatever way possible.

It is clear that some of the above suggestions may be inappropriate in particular instances due to infirmity, sensory deficits, or rigid scepticism. Non-compliance with various aspects of this regimen may be a problem and is best handled by further education with specific concrete examples, and re-explanation of the underlying principles.

In the best of circumstances the above behavioural programme should be instituted by a sleep clinic with experience in the area or by an individual trained in these techniques. Given the clinical realities this is not usually possible and furthermore, many cases of moderate insomnia will yield to these simple techniques. If after six months of following the above recommendations the insomnia persists with significant daytime consequences, referral should be considered.

6. Parasomnias and other sleep related conditions

Sleep walking and night terrors are part of the differential in the evaluation of nocturnal confusional episodes. These symptoms may appear together or separately. Classifiable night terrors are associated with a vague terrifying image and sudden arousal with autonomic discharge and panic. The abrupt appearance of nocturnal wanderings should also suggest temporal lobe pathology, either epilepsy or infarction (Boller et al, 1975; Pedley & Guilleminault, 1977). Night terrors and nocturnal wandering may also represent typical non-REM dysomnias as seen in children. If they follow clear-cut psychological trauma, psychotherapy should be the initial approach. Diazepam 5-10 mg at night may be helpful in some severe cases by suppressing Stages 3 and 4. A full description of various unusual nocturnal syndromes are listed in the ASDC nosology.

Sleep and associated medical conditions

Recent articles have confirmed that significant hypoxemia is present during sleep in patients with chronic obstructive airflow disease (Wynne et al, 1979). Borderline ventilation while awake will present significant desaturation during sleep and has been polygraphically confirmed in kyphoscoliosis muscular dystrophy, hemidiaphragmatic paresis, multiple sclerosis, amyotrophic lateral sclerosis and ablation of bilaterial carotid glomi. Airway obstruction with impaired nocturnal ventilation has been seen in Shy-Dragger syndrome, and the chronic lymphadenopathy of chronic leukaemia (Guilleminault, in press).

The effects of sleep on cardiovascular function remain to be elucidated. Significant arrhythmias have been reported with obstructive sleep apnea but the effect of sleep states on cardiac disease, myocardial infarction, and the recovery from these disorders is unknown. Peripheral nocturnal dyspnea secondary to heart failure may disrupt sleep and the rapid eye movement state may present in increase in arrhythmias.

The loss of pharingo-pharyngeal reflexes, the supine position, and decreased esophageal peristalsis in sleep may explain the worsening of gastroesophageal reflux (GER) at night (Guilleminault, 1982). Unexplained nocturnal cough associated with awakening, heartburn and a sour taste in the mouth should suggest this syndrome. The complications of aspiration such as pneumonitis, aspiration pneumonia, and bronchiectasis are a significant factor in the morbidity associated with GER.

Sleep states and sexual function

Penile tumescence during REM sleep shows a gradual decline with aging although REM itself changes little until advanced age. Kahn & Fischer (1969) found full moderate erections in 45% of REM periods in 18 healthy subjects ranging from 71 to 96 years of age. This is significantly less than the 80–95% reported for young males. Of importance is that 5 subjects aged from 71 to 80 had erections similar in frequency and quality to young adult males. Correlation between REM penile tumescence and sexual activity just fail to reach significance. This may be explained by cultural inhibition of sexual expression in the aged, inhibition of REM erections by anxiety or the absence of a partner.

Available data suggest that in the older man without obvious cause for importance, aging may be accepted as the cause without evaluation and thus treatment of psychosocial factors avoided.

Sleep and thermal regulation

Hypothermia is a recognised problem in the elderly, particularly the poor and malnourished. These factors combined with poikilothermic mechanisms in REM sleep may result in hypothermic events in the morning hours in poorly heated housing. Hypothermia has also been listed as a cause contributing to sleep deprivation in intensive care units (Dlin et al, 1971).

Sleep and hospitalisation

Little is known about the effects of hospitalisation on sleep in any age group. That intensive care settings result in significant sleep deprivation is accepted clinical experience and supported by several studies on post-cardiotomy psychosis (Dlin et al, 1971). Their observational study concluded that the chief deterrents to sleep in order of decreasing significance were: activity and noise, pain and physical conditions, nursing procedures, lights, vapour tents and hypothermia. Fabisan & Gosselin (1982) suggest realistic and practical intensive care nursing orders that maximise potential sleep time. Their suggestions and others include: turn off the maximum number of lights, provide eye-shades, keep noise at a minimum by providing earplugs, preparing medications away from the bed, turning off unnecessary sound monitors, placing ventilator bellows as far away from the head as possible, enforcing quiet on staff and visitors at night except for necessary communication, proper quiet footware, judge the need for hourly assessment especially when patients' vital functions are available from various monitors, consolidate nursing tasks into one prolonged wake, use of PRN analgesics, charting of uninterrupted sleep and accumulating sleep deprivation and continuing the education of staff to the importance of maintaining a regular sleep/wake schedule.

PRESCRIBING SEDATIVE HYPNOTICS IN THE ELDERLY

From a practical point of view the only purpose of sleep is to allow us to function in an alert and refreshed state of well being. When evaluating a complaint of insomnia and devising a treatment, daytime function rather than night-time sleep should be the uppermost consideration. Many an elderly individual complaining of insomnia will deny daytime sleepiness, naps, fatigue or other consequence of sleep deprivation. Their primary problem is the discomfort of a long restless night or a concern that they are not getting the sleep they 'should' that leads to worry about some unspecified ill effect. Reassurance and education may be all that is necessary.

The Stanford group has emphasized the illogical practice of altering night-time sleep with hypnotics without investigating its daytime consequences (Carskadon, 1982). Presumably the goal of treating an insomnia is to improve daytime alertness and well being. Use of the multiple sleep

latency test on flurazepam has demonstrated that in short-term use subjects are demonstrably sleepier on the days following ingestion as compared to baseline. The improvement of daytime alertness following the use of triazolam, a short-acting benzodiazepine, suggests that it is the long half-life of many sedative hypnotics which results in daytime sleepiness (Mitler et al, 1984). Long-acting sedative hypnotics should not be selected unless daytime sedation is a desired therapeutic effect.

Night-time sedation also has significant adverse effects by increasing the arousal threshold, impairing balance, and with benzodiazepines producing anterograde amnesia for night-time events. These effects may produce decreased ability to respond to emergency situations, worsening of sleep apnea and increased nocturnal falls and hip fractures (Institute of Medicine, 1979; Mendelson et al, 1981).

The toxicity profile of a given sedative hypnotic may be very different in the young adult compared to the elderly, yet most of the toxicity data are derived from studies on young adults. For example both flurazepam (Marttila et al, 1977) and chloral hydrate (Kramer, 1967), which enjoy reputations for mild side effects in young adults, may produce confusion and hallucinations in a significant number of nursing home patients. Nitrazepam has also been shown in several reports to have significant toxicity in the elderly (Greenblatt & Allen, 1978). Although many sedative hypnotics have been shown to be effective in some measure in the elderly, the absence of comprehensive studies of these drugs makes it impossible to make definitive statements about their relative merits. However established toxicities of some compounds and inadequate data on the efficacy of others, allows for recommendations to be made against particular classes of sedative hypnotics and certain specific compounds in the elderly.

L-tryptophan, a precursor of serotonin available in health food stores, may be an effective hypnotic in chronic insomnia with minimal side effects in doses of 2–5 g at bedtime when used on an intermittent basis (Schneider-Helmert, 1981). Its role in clinical medicine has yet to be established but deserves further evaluation in the elderly.

The use of phenothiazines as sedative hypnotics in the elderly should be condemned. There is no convincing evidence supporting their use as sedative hypnotics and the development of tardive dyskinesia, significant postural hypotension and anticholinergic effects are all well known complications of these medications. The toxicity of gluthetamide overdose and its weak and variable efficacy do not recommend its use as a sedative hypnotic in this age group. Methaqualone is a drug of widespread abuse and in EEG studies its effects have been inconsistent and disruptive of sleep stages during and after treatment. Methaqualone has also been associated with paresthesias and other symptoms of peripheral neuropathy (Goodman & Gilman, 1975). Although ethchlorvinyl constituted 7% of the prescriptions for sedative hypnotics in 1977 in the United States, its superiority over placebo has not been effectively established. Ethchlorovinyl may have considerable toxicity in therapeutic doses as well. Chloral hydrate at the commonly prescribed dose of 500 mg is a weakly effective drug at best in comparison to placebo. Evidence supporting its efficacy in well documented insomniacs is lacking (Piccione et al, 1980).

The efficacy of low dose tricyclic antidepressants as sedative hypnotics has not been established. In practice it is not uncommon to have adverse effects with dosages as low as 25 mg of imipramine. Unless a clinical depression has been diagnosed, convincing arguments for this practice are not available.

Although barbiturates may have comparable efficacy to the benzodiazepines in short-term use, their low therapeutic/toxic ratio, induction of liver enzymes, severe problems with withdrawal and the rapid development of tolerance are all strong arguments against their use. The current concern with interaction of respiratory depressants in elderly patients with occult or mild sleep apnea is the final argument against the use of barbiturates. It is well known that dose for dose barbiturates are stronger respiratory depressants than benzodiazepines.

Benzodiazepines

Benzodiazepines are not innocuous medications. Potentially hazardous attributes of the long-acting benzodiazepines such as flurazepam and nitrazepam include the accumulation of long-lived active metabolites, the increasing likelihood of adverse drug reactions with advancing age of the patient and the increasing likelihood of adverse drug reactions in patients with diminished kidney function. Benzodiazepines have a high therapeutic/toxicity ratio but do present an additive risk when used with other CNS depressants in suicidal or accidental overdoses. On tests of visual motor co-ordination and balance these medications have been shown to impair performance. With nightly reliance on a sedative hypnotic, dependency is just as likely to develop with a benzodiazepine as it is with many other sedative hypnotics (Institute of Medicine, 1979).

Safe effective treatment with hypnotics depends on thorough patient education prior to initiating treatment as much as on selecting the proper drug. In selecting a specific benzodiazepine the physician should be familar with its rate of absorption, elimination half-life in the elderly, and its metabolic degradation pathway (Greenblatt et al, 1974). A short-acting non-accumulating drug should always be chosen unless daytime sedation is specifically indicated. If a long-acting compound that accumulates such as flurazepam is prescribed, the patient should be advised that optimal therapeutic effects will not be seen for several nights and daytime sedation may increase throughout the first week.

When difficulty falling asleep is present rapid absorption is a desired property. Benzodiazepines metabolised by conjugation are preferable as this process is far less influenced by age than oxidative degradation. Fortunately the short-acting compounds such as trizolam and oxazepam are predominately metabolised by conjugation in contrast to the major metabolites of flurazepam.

Treatment may be complicated by demands for dose increases and routine prescriptions for chronic use. Complaints of renewed insomnia after stabilisation on an effective dose usually represents the development of tolerance. A previously effective dose should never be increased. The patient should be gradually withdrawn and the previous effective dose reinstituted. Reluctance to discontinue medication or patients already on chronic therapeutic doses pose common difficult clinical problems. The absence of any data on the safety and efficacy of prolonged nightly use or intermittent chronic use does not exist. That many responsible physicians report satisfied patients with years of hypnotic treatment as therapeutic doses does not change the current consensus that this practice should be avoided (Institute of Medicine, 1979). Polysomnographic evaluation, close follow-up and periodic office visits are necessary in those cases where it appears that this is the only therapeutic alternative available.

Physicians should rarely prescribe hypnotics for periods exceeding two to four weeks. Upon discontinuation of therapy sleep may be disrupted for several nights. In clinical situations it may be difficult to differentiate 'rebound insomnia' from re-emergence of the origianl complaint. Patient education prior to withdrawal will minimise this problem and allow a reasonable observation period to determine the need for further treatment. Rebound insomnia is more commonly seen with the shorter-acting compounds because the long-acting preparations provide a built in tapering effect. Unfortunately in the elderly this may also mean prolonged sedation persisting for up to two weeks with flurazepam (Salzman et al, 1983).

REFERRAL

Treatment of undiagnosed medical and psychiatric conditions, improved management of pre-existing medical problems, elimination of drug toxicity or abuse, management of acute emotional upsets and behavioural treatment for the chronic insomniac will improve many patients. There will remain a sizeable group with persistent complaints whose etiology remains obscure or remains unimproved after several months of treatment. In these and other cases of persistent insomnia, referral is indicated.

Referral will often lead to an appropriate diagnosis and specific treatment, or to reasonable resignation on the part of patient and physician.

SUMMARY

The principal causes of daytime sleepiness, together with the main points relevant to sleep hygiene and the treatment of sleep apnea syndrome are summarised in Table 14.1.

There are several processes that affect the sleep process of the aging individual. Certain changes such as the decrease in slow wake sleep and more frequent awakenings appear to be intrinsic to the aging process itself.

Pathological processes including organic sleep disorders become more significant etiologies of sleep disturbance with age. Sleeping pills have a very limited role in the management of sleep disorders in the elderly. Short-acting benzodiazepines are the drugs of choice when hypnotics are indicated.

Many older people suffer more from erroneous beliefs about their altered sleep patterns than from the actual ill effects of these changes. This is particularly true of the increase in nocturnal wake time and daytime napping. Cultural beliefs that normal people are awake all day and asleep all night may reflect a bias against children and the elderly.

Table 14.1 Summary of points relating to sleep disorders in the elderly

Some causes of daytime sleepiness:
Insufficient sleep
Sleep apnea
Periodic leg movements
Restless legs syndrome
Circadian rhythm disorders
Psychophysiologic insomnia
Psychiatric insomnia
Drugs and alcohol
Klein-Levin syndrome
Narcolepsy
Idiopathic CNS hypersomnolence

Sleep hygiene:
Fixed bedtime and waketime
Avoid caffeine and alcohol
Regular bedtime routine
Avoid exercise before bedtime
Avoid stimulating audio-visual material at bedtime
Void before retiring
No liquids three hours before bed-time
Use bed only for sleeping and sex

Sleep apnea syndrome — treatments:
tracheostomy
uvalopalatopharyngoplasty
mandibular advancement
protriptylene
progesterone
weight loss
C-Pap (continuous positive airway pressure)

REFERENCES

Association of sleep disorders centers 1979 Diagnostic classification of sleep and arousal disorders. Sleep 2: 1–137

Boller F, Wright D G, Cavalieri R, Mitsumoto H 1975 Paroxysmal 'nightmares'. Sequel of a stroke responsive to diphenylhydantoin. Neurology 25: 1026–1028

Brezinova V 1974 Effect of caffeine on sleep: EEG study in late middle age people. British Journal of Clinical Pharmacology. 1: 203–208

Brownell L G, West P, Sweatman P, Acres J C, Kruger M H 1982 Protriptyline in obstructive sleep apnea. New England Journal of Medicine 307: 1037–1042

Carskadon M (ed) 1982 Current perspectives on daytime sleepiness. Sleep 5

Carskadon M, Dement W 1982 The Multiple Sleep Latency Test: what does it measure? Sleep 5

Carskadon M, Dement W, Mitler M, Guilleminault C, Zarcone V, Spiegel R 1976 Self-report vs sleep laboratory findings in 122 drug-free subjects with complaints of chronic insomnia. American Journal of Psychiatry 133: 1382–1388

Carskadon M, van den Hoed J, Dement W 1981 Sleep and daytime sleepiness in the elderly. Journal of Geriatric Psychiatry 13: 135–151

Carskadon M A, Brown E P, Dement W C 1982 Sleep fragmentation in the elderly: relationship to daytime sleep tendency. Neurobiolgoy of Aging 3: 321–327

Clift A (ed) 1975 Sleep Disturbance and Hypnotic Drug Dependence. Excerpta Medical, Amsterdam

Coates T J, Thoresen C E 1977 How to sleep better. Prentice Hall, New Jersey

Coleman R, Miles L, Guilleminault C, Zarcone V, van den Hoed J, Dement W 1981 Sleep-wake disorders in the elderly: a case series analysis. Journal of the American Geriatrics Society

Coleman R, Roffwarg H, Kennedy S, Guilleminault C, Cinque J, Cohn M, Karacan I, Kupfer D, Lemmi H, Miles L, Orr W, Phillips E, Roth T, Sassin J, Schmidt H, Weitzman E, Dement W Sleep wake disorders based on a polysomnographic diagnosis. A national co-operative study. Journal of the American Medical Association 247(7): 997–1003

Cooper J K, Love D W, Raffoul P R 1982 Intentional prescription nonadherence (non-compliance) by the elderly. Journal of the American Geriatrics Soceity 5: 329–333

Dlin B M, Rosen H, Dickstein K, Lyons J W, Fischer H K 1971 The problems of sleep and rest in the intensive care unit. Psychosomatics 12: 155–163

Fabisan L, Gosselin M 1982 How to recognize sleep deprivation in your ICU patient and what to do about it. Canadian Nurse 4: 21–23

Frankel B L, Pattern B M, Gillin J C 1974 Restless legs syndrome: sleep electroencephalographic and neurologic findings. Journal of the American Medical Association 230: 1302–1303

Fujita S, Conway W, Zorick F, Roth T 1981 Surgical correction of anatomic abnormalities in obstructive sleep apnea syndrome: uvulopalatopharyngoplasty. Otolaryngology and Head and Neck Surgery 89: 923–934

Gardner E R, Hall R C W 1982 Psychiatric symptoms produced by the over-the-counter drugs. Psychosomatics 232: 186–199

Goodman L, Gilman A 1975 The pharmacological basis of therapeutics. MacMillan, New York

Greenblatt D, Allen M 1978 Toxicity of nitrazepam in the elderly: A report from the Boston Collaborative Drug Surveillance Program. British Journal of Clinical Pharmacology 5: 407–413

Greenblatt D J, Divoll M, Abernethy D R, Shader R I 1974, 1982 Benzodiazepine hypnotics: kinetic and therapeutic options. Sleep 5: S18–S27; Journal of the American Medical Association 227: 513–517

Guilleminault C Sleep and sleep disordes in the elderly. In: Cassel C, Walsh J (eds). Geriatric medicine principles and practice. Springer-Verlag, New York. In press

Guilleminault C Drug induced sleep disorders. In: Manzo L, Blum K Neurotoxicology (eds). Marcel Dekker, New York. In press

Guilleminault C (ed) 1982 Sleeping and waking disorders: indications and techniques. Addison-Wesley, Menlo Park

Guilleminault C, Cummiskey J, Dement W 1980 Sleep apnea syndromes: recent advances. Advances in internal medicine. 26: 347–372

Guilleminault C, Eldridge F, Dement W 1973 Insomina with sleep apnea: A new syndrome. Science 181: 856–858

Guilleminault C, Miles L E 1980 Differential diagnosis of obstructive sleep apnea syndrome: the abnormal esophageal reflux and laryngospasm during sleep. Sleep 9: 200

Guilleminault C, Raynal D, Takahashi S, Carskadon M, Dement W C 1976 Evaluation of short and long term treatment of the narcolepsy syndrome with clomipramine and hydrochloride. Acta Neurologica Scandinavica 54: 71–87

Guilleminault C, Simmons F B, Motta J, Cummiskey J, Rosekind M, Schroeder J S, Dement W C 1981 Obstructive sleep apnea syndrome and tracheostomy. Archives of Internal Medicine 141: 985–988

Hammond E 1964 Some preliminary findings on physical complaints from a prospective study of 1 064 004 men and women. American Journal of Public Health 54: 11–23

Harman E M, Wynne J W, Block A J 1982 The effect of weight loss on sleep disordered breathing and oxygen desaturation in morbidly obese men. Chest 82: 291–294

Hauri P, Hawkins D R 1973 Alpha-delta sleep. Electroencephalography and Clinical Neurophysiology 34: 233–237

Hazemann P, Laffort F, Lille F 1977 Elucidation of vigilance level in aged persons. Revenue D Electroencephalographic et de Neurophysiologie Clinique 7: 203–209

Healey E S, Kales A, Monroe L J, Bixler E O, Chamberlain K, Soldatos C R 1981 Onset of insomnia: Role of life stress events. Psychomatic Medicine 43: 439–451

Hester G, Grant A D, Russell I J 1982 Psychological evaluation and behavior treatment of patients with fibrositis. Arthritis and Rheumatism 25: 148

Huskisson E C, Grayson M P 1974 Indomethacin or amylobarbitone sodium for sleep in rheumatoid arthritis, with some observations on the use of sequential analysis. British Journal of Clinical Pharmcology 1: 151–154

Institute of Medicine 1979 Report of a study: sleeping pills, insomnia, and medical practice. National Academy of Science, Washington

Ishino H, Otsuki S 1975 Frequency of Alzheimer's neurofibrillary changes in the basal ganglia and brainstem of Alzheimer's disease, senile dementia and the aged. Folia Psychiatrica et Neurologica Japonica 29: 279–285

Kahn E, Fisher C 1969 REM sleep and sexuality int he aged. Journal of Geriatric Psychiatry 2: 189–199

Kales A, Bixler E O, Tan T L, Scherf M B, Kales J D 1974 Chronic hypnotic use: ineffectiveness, drug withdrawal insomnia, and dependence. Journal of the American Medical Association 227: 513–517

Kales A, Caldwell A, Preston T, Lealy S, Kales J 1976 Personality patterns in insomnia: Theoretical implications. Archives of General Psychiatry 33: 1128–1134

Kramer C 1967 Methaqualone and chloral hydrate: Preliminary comparison in geriatric patients. Journal of the American Geriatrics Soceity 1979 15: 455–461

Kripke D, Simons R, Garfinkel L, Hammond E 1979 Short and long sleep and sleeping pills. Archives of General Psychiatry 36: 103

Lugaresi E, Cirignotta F, Coccagna G, Piana C 1980 Some epidemiological data on snoring and cardiocirculatory disturbances. Sleep 3: 221–224

McGhie A, Russel S 1962 The subjective assessment of normal sleep patterns. Journal of Mental Science 108: 642–654

Marttila J K, Hammel R J, Alexander B, Zustiak R 1977 Potential untoward effects of long-term use of flurazepam in geriatric patients. Journal of the American Pharmaceutical Association 17: 692–695

Mendelson W, Garnett D, Gillin J 1981 Flurazepam-induced sleep apnea syndrome in a patient with insomnia and mild sleep-related respiratory changes. Journal of Nervous and Mental Disease 169: 261–264

Miles L, Dement W 1980 Sleep and aging. Sleep 3: 119–120

Miles L, Wilson M 1977 High incidence of cyclic sleep/wake disorders in the blind. Sleep 6: 192

Miller N E, Barns R T 1980 Sleep, sleep pathology, and psychopathology in later life: a new research frontier. Neurobiology of Aging 3: 283–286

Mitler M, Seidel W, van den Hoed J, Greenblatt D, Dement W 1984 Comparative hypnotic effects of flurazepam, triazolam, and placebo: A long-term simultaneous nighttime and daytime study. Journal of Clinical Psychopharmacology 4: 2–13

Moldofksy H, Scarisbrick P 1976 Induction of neurasthenic musculoskeletal pain syndromes by selective sleep stage deprivation. Psychosomatic Medicine 38: 35–44

Moldofsky H, Scarisbrick P, England R, Smythe H 1975 Musculoskeletal symptoms and non-REM sleep disturbances in patients with 'fibrositis symptoms' in healthy subjects. Psychosomatic Medicine 37: 341–351

Monroe K 1967 Psychological and physiological differences between good and poor sleepers. Journal of Abnormal Psychology 72: 255–264

Orr W C, Imes N K, Martin R J 1979 Progesterone therapy in obese patients with sleep apnea. Archives of Internal Medicine 139: 109–111

Passouant P, Cadilhac J, Ribstein M 1972 Les privations de sommeil avec mouvement occulaires par les antidepresseurs. Revue Neurologique 127: 173–192

Pedley T A, Guilleminault C 1977 Episodic nocturnal wanderings responsive to anticonvulsant drug therapy. Annals of Neurology 2: 30–35

Pfeiffer E, Busse E 1977 Behavior and adaptation in late life. 2nd edn. Little, Brown & Co, Boston

Piccione P, Zouck F, Lutz T, Grissom T, Kramer M, Roth T 1980 The efficacy of triazolam and chloral hydrate in geriatric insomniacs. Journal of International Medical Research 8: 361–367

Pollak C, Brodlow H, Spielman A, Weitzman E 1978 A pilot survey of the symptoms of hypersomnia-sleep apnea syndrome as possible risk factors for hypertension. 18th Annual Meeting of APSS: 289

Prinz P 1977 Sleep patterns in the healthy aged: Relationship with intellectual function. Journal of Gerontology 32: 179–186

Prinz P, Peskind E R, Vitaliano P P, Raskind M A, Eisdorfer C, Zemcuznikov N, Gerber C J 1982 Changes in the sleep and waking EEG of non demented and demented elderly subjects. Journal of Geriatric Psychiatry 30: 86–92

Rechtshaffen A, Kales A D 1968 A manual of standardized terminology, techniques and scoring system for sleep stages of human subjects. Brain Research Institute, Los Angeles

Reynolds C, Coble P, Black R, Holzer B, Carroll R, Kupfer D 1979 Sleep disturbances in a series of elderly patients: Polysomnographic findings. Journal of the American Geriatrics Society 28: 164–170

Roehrs T, Lineback W, Zorick F, Roth T 1982 Relationship of psychopathology to insomnia in the elderly. Journal of Geriatric Psychiatry 5: 312–315

Salzman C, Shader R I, Greenblatt D G, Harmatz J S 1983 Long vs short half-life benzodiazepines in the elderly Archives of General Psychiatry 3: 293–297

Schneider-Helmert 1981 L-Tryptophan interval therapy with severe chronic insomniacs. International Pahrmacopsychiatry 16: 162–173

Smythe H A, Moldofsky H 1977 Two contributions to the understanding of fibrositis syndrome. Bulletin on the Rheumatic Diseases 28: 928–931

Thompson L W, Wilson S 1966 Electrocortical reactivity and learning in the elderly. Journal of Gerontology 21: 45–51

Tune G 1969 Sleep and wakefulness in 509 normal adults. British Journal of Medical Psychology 42: 75–80

Wang H S, Obrist W D, Busse E W 1970 Neurophysiological correlates of intellectual function of elderly persons living in the community. American Journal of Psychiatry 126: 1205–1212

Webb W B 1981 Sleep state responses of older and younger subjects after sleep deprivation. Electroencephalography and Clinical Neurophysiology 52: 368–371

Weitzman E, Czeiesler C, Coleman R, Dement W, Richardson G, Pollak C 1979 Delayed sleep phase syndrome: a biological rhythm disorder. Sleep 8: 221

Weitzman E O, Czeisler C A, Coleman R, Spielman A, Zimmerman J, Dement W 1981 Delayed sleep phase syndrome: A chronobiological disorder with sleep onset insomnia. Archives of General Psychiatry 38: 737–746

Winget C, Vernikos-Danellis J, Cronin S, Leach C, Rambaut P, Mack P 1972 Circadian rhythm asynchrony in man during hypokinesis. Journal of Applied Physiology 33: 640–643

Wynne J W, Block A J, Hemenwa J, Hunt L A, Flick M R 1979 Disordered breathing and oxygen desaturation during sleep in patients with chronic obstructive lung disease. American Journal of Medicine 66: 573–579

Yunis M, Masi A T, Calabro J J, Miller K A, Feigenbaum S L 1981 Primary fibromyalgia (fibrositis): Clinical study of 30 patients with matched controls. Seminars in Arthritis and Rheumatism 11: 151–171

Zepelin H, McDonald K, Wanzie F, Zammit G 1980 Age differences in auditory awakening threshholds during sleep. Sleep: 109

Zung W W, Magill M, Moore J, George D T 1983 Recognition and treatment of depression in a family medicine practice. Journal of Clinical Psychiatry 1: 3–6

15

Transient ischaemic attacks and stroke

J. Marshall

A stroke is always a calamity, more so than a myocardial infarction. Recovery from a myocardial infarction may leave a patient with angina or limited exercise tolerance but he can communicate with others and care for his bodily functions This may not be the case for a stroke survivor who may be heavily dependent on others with all the loss of human dignity that this entails. For this reason emphasis must always be on prevention. To prevent is always better than to treat but this is particularly so in the case of stroke where even the best treatment is unlikely to produce a good end-result.

RISK FACTORS

Hypertension

A number of risk factors for stroke are now well established first among which is hypertension. There are many community and natural history studies attesting to this, perhaps the best known being the Framingham study (Kannel et al, 1970). Not only is the frequency of cerebral haemorrhage increased, but cerebral infarction is four times as common in hypertensives as non-hypertensives. That this risk can be reduced by the efficient treatment of high blood pressure is well documented (Veterans Administration Cooperative Study Group on Antihypertensive Agents 1967 & 1970). The main responsibility for detection and treatment of hypertension must fall on those charged with the care of the middle-aged population but even in the early years of the geriatric range there is scope for intervention. This is a more exacting task because older people are less tolerant of blood pressure reduction than are the middle aged. This reduced tolerance is not matched by a reduced risk of stroke from untreated hypertension, hence the task of reducing blood pressure should be tackled, more difficult though it is.

Cardiac disease

A second risk factor for stroke is cardiac disease. Cardiac embolism as a cause of stroke was always recognised but its frequency was greatly underestimated. The pathological studies of Blackwood et al (1969) and of Jorgensen & Torvik (1966) have shown that as many as one half of cerebral infarcts may be the result of cardiac emboli. In particular lone atrial fibrillation, that is fibrillation without clinical evidence of cardiovascular disease, has emerged as a risk factor with a 30% incidence of cerebrovascular incidents (Wolf et al, 1978; Kannel et al, 1982).

Other risk factors

Other risk factors include of course diabetes mellitus, hyperlipidaemia, cigarette smoking and less well recognised raised haematocrit. The increased frequency of vascular lesions including strokes in polycythaemia rubra vera is widely appreciated, but awareness that a haematocrit at the upper end of the normal range has been shown by the Framingham study (Kannel et al, 1972) to be a risk factor, is not so well known. Reducing the haematocrit by the simple process of venesection reduces the risk of vascular complications in polycythaemia rubra vera and may well do so in the high normal haematocrit situation.

It should be noted that all these risk factors, hypertension, cardiac diseases, diabetes mellitus, hyperlipidaemia and raised haematocrit are treatable. Though the treatment of strokes may be difficult the treatment of their predisposing causes is not so difficult which is all the more reason for placing emphasis on prevention.

TRANSIENT ISCHAEMIC ATTACKS

Recognition of the significance of a transient ischaemic attack (TIA) has been one of the most important developments in the field of cerebrovascular disease. TIAs provide a unique opportunity to study the mechanism of cerebrovascular episodes and, because they frequently give warning of an impending stroke, enlarge the scope for prevention.

Definition

A TIA is defined as a focal disturbance of neurological function lasting less than 24 hours, and attributable to cerebrovascular disease. The limit of 24 hours is arbitrary but has proved very useful in ensuring comparability between reported studies. Most TIAs do not in fact approach the time limit; they usually last five minutes to an hour or two. When signs and symptoms last longer than 24 hours the episode is referred to as a reversible ischaemic neurological deficit (RIND), the upper limit for this category being three weeks. Thereafter the term completed stroke is used.

Significance

The focal nature of a TIA implies that a single vascular territory is involved. It is important to try and determine which it is because the prognosis for the later development of a stroke differs beween territories (Ziegler & Hassanein, 1973). A TIA in the internal carotid territory is much more likely to be followed by a stroke than is a TIA in the vertebrobasilar territory. There is often confusion on this point. Vertebrobasilar TIAs tend to recur with considerable frequency but it is uncommon for them to lead to a stroke; the prognosis for recurrence is worse but for stroke is better than in the carotid territory. With carotid TIAs prognosis for continued recurrence is better but for stroke is worse.

TIAs are not simply indicators of vascular disease in general; they are territory specific. This is shown by the high correlation between the site of a TIA and the site of any subsequent stroke. Another important feature is the time relationship between the first TIA and a subsequent stroke. The first two months after the first TIA is the time of greatest risk; this subsequently declines so that by six months the risk is not appreciably greater than in the general population (Whisnant et al, 1971).

Clinical features

TIAs in the carotid territory are characterised by transient hemiparesis, hemisensory disturbance or dysphasia. Attacks of amaurosis fugax are not uncommon. The patient suddenly loses vision in one eye for a few minutes, usually not more than five. This may involve the whole field or only the upper or lower half. On the rare occasion when it is possible to examine a patient during an attack, ophthalmoscopy may reveal an embolus in the form of a small white body in the central retinal artery or one of its branches.

The symptomatology of vertebrobasilar TIAs is protean and more difficult to assess. Episodes of diplopia, facial numbness or paraesthesiae, especially around the mouth, vertigo, dysarthria and ataxia in various combinations are common. Vertigo is especially difficult to assess. The patient complains, not of vertigo, but of dizziness which may mean many things. Even if there is true vertigo in the sense of a subjective disturbance of equilibrium which may be rotatory or non-rotatory, it may be caused by disease of the end-organ. If however it occurs in conjuction with other brain stem symptoms the diagnosis of TIA can be made with more confidence.

Other manifestations of vertebrobasilar TIAs are alternating or bilateral hemipareses or hemisensory disturbance. Drop attacks may also occur and again pose a diagnostic problem as there are many other causes besides TIAs. The syndrome of transient global amnesia, seen largely in older patients, may also be seen. The site of the disturbance is believed to be the medial part of the temporal lobe which is supplied from the vertebrobasilar territory via branches of the posterior cerebral artery.

Ischaemia in the territory of the posterior cerebral artery may also cause visual field disturbance in the form of flashing lights or field loss.

Differential diagnosis

TIAs must be distinguished from other transitory disturbance of neurological function. Migraine and focal epilepsy are among these. It is uncommon for migraine to start late in life; there is usually a previous history but as the pattern of attacks may change, the patient may present as though with a new condition. Focal epilepsy is characterised by positive phenomena, that is jerking of the limbs or in the case of sensory epilepsy paraesthesiae. The symptoms of a TIA are more likely to be negative, weakness in the case of a motor disturbance and numbness in a sensory attack.

Management

Having decided that the patient is experiencing TIAs and in which vascular territory they are happening, the next step is to determine the cause. Clearly as by definition the disturbance is focal, there must be a focal vascular lesion. This may be giving rise to emboli as for example from an internal carotid stenosis. On the other hand, the focal vascular lesion may not in itself by symptomatic but become so when some general circulatory disturbance supervenes. Athough there are no good epidemiological studies of the question, clinical impression suggests that the latter happens more frequently in the older age groups.

Apart from following clues which may be in the history, a practical approach is to eliminate possible causes not in the order of frequency but in accordance with the ease with which this can be done. Anaemia and polycythaemia have both been shown to cause TIAs. They can be diagnosed by a simple blood count and readily treated.

Hypotension following the injudicious prescription of hypotensive drugs is particularly common in older people. The problem has already been discussed in the section on prevention. It should not be met by suddenly withdrawing hypotensives from patients who were definitely hypertensive prior to treatment as this may lead to cerebral haemorrhage. Careful adjustment of treatment is what is required.

Hypertension when severe can cause transient disturbance of neurological function particularly in the brain stem. This demands control of blood pressure without which hypertensive encephalopathy may supervene.

Abnormalities of cardiac function are particularly common as a cause of cerebral TIAs in older people. This may be because the heart is a source of emboli. Lone atrial fibrillation presumably on an ischaemic basis has been increasingly incriminated as a risk factor for stroke. The significance of other forms of dysrhythmia is less certain. Ambulant electrocardiographic monitoring has shown that unsuspected episodic abnormalites are frequent in older people. The difficulty has been to relate them to clinical events. Patients often have electrocardiographic abnormalities during a period free from clinical events. Equally, they may press the clinical event button on a monitor at a time when the tracing shows no disturbance. Despite these difficulties there can be no doubt that cardiac dysfunction is a common concomitant of cerebral TIAs and should be treated.

Cervical spondylosis may play a role in vertebrobasilar TIAs. Osteophytes deform the vertebral artery and may during neck turning cause temporary interruption of blood flow (Fig. 15.1). A history of the TIAs being clearly related to neck movement provides the clue. Wearing a soft collar to discourage and limit neck movement reduces the frequency of the attacks.

When none of these causes can be identified there remains the possibility that the TIAs are associated with a stenosis (Fig. 15.2). This is particularly so in the case of carotid TIAs. The stenosis may be a source of emboli or, less frequently, is interrupting flow. Evidence of a stenosis may be found by Doppler studies but this is reliable only when the stenosis is 50% or more of the lumen. Lesser degrees of stenosis, which may nevertheless be important as a source of emboli, are often missed. Nevertheless Doppler examination of the neck arteries when available is an important first step.

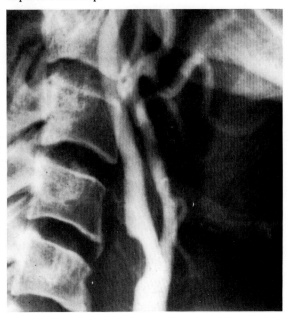

Fig. 15.2 Carotid angiogram showing a stenosis at the orign of the internal carotid artery.

There remains the question as to whether or not to proceed to angiography. The difficulty is that the procedure is not without hazard, there being a risk of stroke of about 1%. Moreover there is little point in doing angiography unless endarterectomy is being seriously considered, which raises a further difficulty in that available evidence does not permit a firm conclusion as to whether endarterectomy, warfarin or aspirin is best for TIAs associated with carotid stenosis. As a general guide, in patients under the age of 70 in whom a carotid stenosis seems likely, because they have experienced amaurosis fugax, or have a bruit or a positive Doppler examination, angiography should be undertaken with a view to endarterectomy. Patients over the age of 70 should not have angiography. If their TIAs are frequent they should be given warfarin for three to six months followed by aspirin. If their attacks are infrequent aspirin may be given from the outset. The ideal dose remains uncertain. The controlled

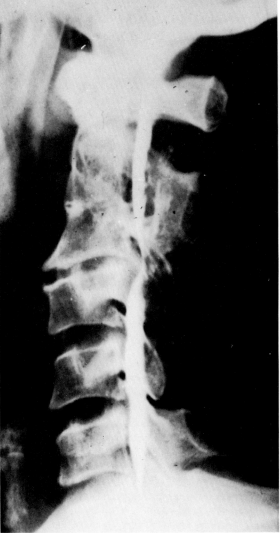

Fig. 15.1 Vertebral angiogram showing indentation of the artery by an osteophyte at one level.

trials of aspirin in TIAs (Fields et al, 1978; Canadian Cooperative Study Group, 1978) used large doses (600 mg b.d.). Smaller doses (300 mg b.d.) may suffice and are currently being tested in a United Kingdom trial; this dose would reduce the incidence of gastro-intestinal side effects. Meantime in older people it would seem reasonable to give the smaller dose.

Angiography is not indicated for vertebrobasilar TIAs except when a difference in the radial pulses, and blood pressure in the upper limbs and a supraclavicular bruit, point to a subclavian stenosis as the cause. Moreover because of the better prognosis of vertebrobasilar TIAs aspirin rather than warfarin should be given. The exception to this is when a crescendo of TIAs over hours or days indicates a brain stem infarct is threatened; heparin infusion is required until the attacks have ceased.

STROKES

Incidence
Stroke is very much a disease of old age. The incidence rises from under 0.25 per 1000 per annum in the 35–44 age group to 20 in the 75–84 decade (Whisnant et al, 1971). Mortality likewise rises with age. In western industrial nations stroke constitutes the third most common cause of death, being outstripped only by cardiovascular disease and cancer.

The close correlation with age makes it essential to have an accurate knowledge of the age structure of the population to be served when planning services. Overall prevalence rates have been estimated at 7–12 per 1000 but in those aged 65 years and over its prevalence rises to 50–70 per 1000 (Baum & Robins, 1981). Because social factors can produce marked differences between the age structure of geographically related communities, national prevalence figures are too crude to provide a basis for planning. The age structure of the community to be served must be ascertained.

Cause
A stroke is a clnical entity, being the focal neurological signs and symptoms produced by a vascular lesion of the brain. The commonest presentation is hemiplegia to the extent that the terms stroke and hemiplegia are sometimes used synonymously. This is a mistake because almost any combination of neurological signs and symptoms may be encountered, all of which may be properly called a stroke. This is particularly important in the older age groups where disorientation, ataxia, speech problems and other disturbance of higher cerebral function may be the main manifestation of a cerebrovascular lesion with little or noting in the way of a hemiplegia.

The two main pathological causes are haemorrhage and infarction. Massive haemorrhage is much less frequent

than it used to be presumably as a result of better treatment of hypertension. On the other hand, the advent of computed tomography (CT) scanning has shown that some strokes which on clinical grounds would hitherto have been attributed to infarction are the result of a small haemorrhage (Fig. 15.3).

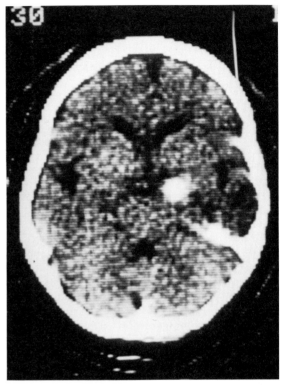

Fig. 15.3 Small discrete haemorrhage in the right hemisphere producing a hemiplegia.

There has also been a change of emphasis with regard to the cause of infarction. As mentioned in the section on risk factors, clinicopathological studies have shown that embolism is much more common than hitherto believed, accounting for almost one-half of cerebral infarcts. The source of the emboli varies; some come from the great vessels, in particular from atheroma at the origin of the internal carotid artery; many come from the heart, the range of cardiac conditions which may give rise to emboli being much wider than it used to be.

It is not in every case of stroke in older people that a haemorrhage or infarct can be found pathologically. Ischaemia, insufficient in degree to produce frank infarction, may give rise to clinical manifestations. The basis for this has been well demonstrated in the experimental stroke model in the baboon by Symon and his colleagues (1977). Levels of cerebral blood flow at which electrical activity, energy metabolism and ionic flux fail have been established. These are reached before infarction occurs and are compatible with recovery provided the blood flow does not remain below the threshold level for too long.

Diagnosis

The diagnosis of the classical hemiplegia presents little problem; it is less well recognised, though by no means infrequent, manifestations of a stroke which will cause difficulty. A lesion of the non-dominant perietal lobe is notorious in this respect. If the damage does not extend forward as far as the post-central gyrus there will be neither loss of primary sensory modalities nor weakness. The patient may have difficulty dressing, putting garments on back to front or in the wrong order. He may lose his way in familiar surroundings. All this may be written off as 'confusion' whereas close observation shows there is no clouding of consciousness or impairment of other higher cerebral functions.

Similarly a discrete lesion in the dominant temporal lobe may produce language difficulty without hemiplegia. If the dysphasia is mainly receptive, the inappropriated response of the patient to what is said to him may again be attributed to confusion or dementia. Likewise if an expressive dysphasia is of the fluent type, the stream of meaningless words may be misinterpreted.

A discrete occipital lobe lesion may give rise to a hemianopia which may be overlooked. The patient demands new spectacles whereas in the case of a left homonymous hemianopia, careful observation shows that it is words at the beginning of a line that he is missing. Alternatively he may complain of bumping into things or falling which again can be shown to be related to objects in part of the field of vision. Testing the visual fields by simple confrontation methods suffices to reveal the real nature of the deficit.

Brain stem leions may pose a problem particularly if the anterior part of the stem through which the pyramidal tracts pass is spared. Diplopia, vertigo, dysarthria or ataxia in varying degrees and combinations with or without long tracts signs may occur. Competent examination of the nervous system combined with a working knowledge of the anatomy of the brain stem is necessary if strokes from brain stem lesions are not to be missed.

Differential diagnosis

The onset of a major stroke is often associated with loss of consciousness so that the first and most pressing task is the differential diagnosis of the loss of consciousness. Head injury, neoplasm, an unwitnessed fit and the biochemical disturbances of hypoglycaemia, ketosis, uraemia and hepatic failure must be borne in mind. Endocrine disorders such as myxoedema and pituitary failure and coma caused by drugs and hypothermia must also be considered. Some of these causes will have had previous manifestations of the underlying condition, but with old people living alone a history of these may not always be forthcoming. Keeping alive to possibilities other than a vascular lesion is the most important factor in avoiding error coupled with appropriate investigations where indicated.

Perhaps the commonest difficulty in cases in which consciousness is not lost is subdural haematoma giving rise to a hemiplegia. A history of past head injury may not always be obtainable and in any case the trauma is often so trivial as to have been forgotten. An important feature is that though consciousness may not be lost it is usually clouded. It is very unusual for there to be an appreciable hemiparesis from a subdural haematoma without some clouding of consciousness.

Another difficulty arises from tumours which present as strokes. The general rule that symptoms from a tumour develop gradually is not always observed. Acute onset, usually the result of vascular events within the tumour, does occur. This may be so in as many as 5% of any series of acute strokes. A past history of increasing headache or gradual impairment of cerebral function should arouse suspicion but is not always forthcoming.

Investigation

Investigation of a patient with a stroke falls into two parts: the first is concerned with confirming the diagnosis of cerebral vasclar lesion; the second seeks to discover why the lesion occurred. CT scanning offers a non-invasive and reliable means of confirming the presence of a crebral vascular lesion and of excluding alternatives such as a neoplasm. Moreover, it will make the all important differentiation between a haemorrhage and an infarct (Fig. 15.4). The difficulty of distinguishing clinically between haemorrhage and infarction has long been recognised. Dalsgaard-Neilsen (1956) found that the clinical diagnosis of haemorrhage was confirmed at autopsy in only 65% of cases and that of infarction in only 58%. CT scanning provides an answer but there are often problems about its availability. If a stroke is to be treated only by general measures CT scanning cannot be said to be mandatory. But if specific therapy is being considered either for haemorrhage or for infarction, which if the diagnosis were to be wrong would be harmful, CT scanning must be carried out.

The timing of the scan is important. The high density of a haemorrhage can be seen almost immediately but the low density of an infarct will not become apparent before six hours. Not all infarcts can be detected even at this time as many are isodense with normal brain. However absence of the high density shadow of a haemorrhage enables one to infer that there is an infarct.

Having established that the stroke is the result of a cerebral vascular lesion the next problem is why it occurred. Here the history and examination may provide clues but in this situation it is worthwhile performing a

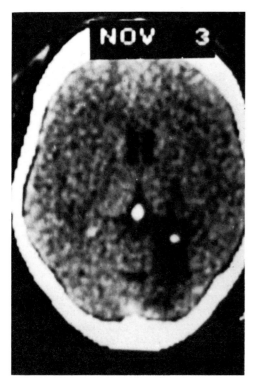 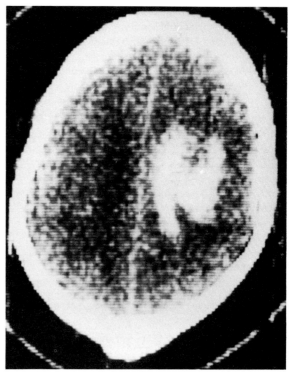

Fig. 15.4 CT scans showing a low density lesion due to an infarct in the right hemisphere (left) and a high density due to a haemorrhage in the right hemisphere (right).

series of screening tests as described in the section on TIAs to eliminate known risk factors.

Angiography has little place in the investigation of an acute stroke at any age. The pathology of the lesion is better established by CT scanning. Angiography only provides information about the vessels and even if an occlusion or stenosis were to be found, it would not be dealt with by surgery in the acute stage. There is therefore no indication for angiography on these grounds.

An exception to this is when there is reason to suspect that a haemorrhage is the result of a ruptured aneurysm. The frequency of a second bleed within the first two weeks is sufficient to necessitate surgery being carried out as soon as possible provided the well established criteria of fitness for aneurysm surgery are fulfilled. If therefore the clinical picture suggests that a stroke has been caused by a ruptured cerebral aneurysm, angiography should be carried out. In this context however the limitations of age must be obesrved, patients over 70 years being in general unsuitable for aneurysm surgery.

Doppler examination of the neck vessels may well be carried out. Though the results are unlikely to affect immediate management as the test is non-invasive and takes only a short time to perform, it can be done in the acute stage. In experienced hands it can identify occlusion or 50% stenosis of the carotid artery in the neck with a high degree of reliability. Lesser degrees of stenosis, which may nevertheless provide a source of emboli, are unlikely to be identified with confidence.

Treatment

The treatment of acute stroke is conveniently considered under two headings, general and specific. There can be no doubt that general measures have a profound effect and that the reduction in mortality from acute strokes which has taken place has been largely due to the vigorous application of such measures rather than to the development of specific therapy.

Maintaining the airway

Foremost among the general measures is the need to maintain the oxygen supply to the brain. This may be compromised by obstruction of the airway in patients who are drowsy or unconscious or are unable adequately to clear their secretions. The use of an airway or, in severe cases, of an endotracheal tube for a time combined with regular suction to clear secretions can be life saving. Cerebral anoxia may also be due to respiratory infection or cardiac failure both of which are more liable to be present in older stroke patients and demand urgent and vigorous treatment.

Water and electrolyte balance

Maintenance of water and electrolyte balance is the next most important consideration requiring a nicety of judgement. Cerebral infarction gives rise to oedema which might argue in favour of a degree of dehydration being maintained. Dehydration raises the haematocrit, thereby increasing blood viscosity which may reduce cerebral blood flow in the affected area in the likely event of the limits of vasodilatory compensation having been reached. Moreover many older people may have a degree of renal failure and are intolerant of dehydration. The aim therefore should be to keep them in water balance. This should receive early attention because after a stroke there is inevitably a delay whilst medical aid is called, the patient transported to hospital and examination and investigation carried out, a period which may extend to many hours during which no fluids may have been given.

Disturbance of the electrolyte balance, in particular hypernatraemia as a direct effect of the cerebral lesion rather than secondary to dehydration, must also be looked for and treated appropriately.

Temperature regulation
Temperature regulation is less efficient in older people and may in addition be specifically disturbed in brain stem strokes. Furthermore old people who live alone and suffer a stroke may well be exposed to a low environmental temperature for a considerable time before they are found. Measurement of the rectal temperature is required with appropriate steps in patients found to be hypothermic. Hyperpyrexia is usually caused by the lesion itself rather than by environmental conditions. It also requires vigorous treatment by tepid sponging, fans, covering the patient with a sheet rung out of ice-cold water, ice-packs or ice-water enemas.

Care of the bladder
Retention is common following a stroke giving way later to incontinence. Retention apart from causing discomfort and restlessness raises the blood pressure and may further damage an already diseased bladder. It should be treated by catheterisation under strictly aseptic conditions. The later phase of incontinence is best dealt with in men by use of a sterile condom, tube and collecting bag. Incontinence in women is more difficult to manage and may necessitate the use of an indwelling catheter for a time.

Care of the skin and joints
Paralysis and sensory loss expose the patient to the risk of skin damage and pressure sores. Preventive measures should be instituted from the outset (see chapter 00). Likewise correct positioning and passive movement of joints will reduce the risk of later contractures and speed up the process of rehabilitation. The shoulder joint should receive particular attention because of the risk of development of a frozen shoulder or of the 'shoulder-arm' syndrome.

Specific therapy
A wide variety of specific treatments have been tried during the last two decades with conflicting claims as to their value. The aim has been either to deal with the thrombus or embolus (anticoagulants and fibrinolytic agents) or to dilate the blood vessels (vasodilator drugs) or to reduce oedema (steroids) or to improve flow by rheological measures (mannitol, glycerol and low molecular weight dextran). Other measures which have been tried include prolonged hyperventilation and barbiturates. Attention will be confined here to those measures for which there is some evidence as to their efficacy and are feasible in general geriatric practice.

Controlled trials of anticoagulant therapy with coumarin derivatives in acute infarction have failed to show benefit (Marshall & Shaw, 1960) with two exceptions. One is when the stroke is due to an embolus of which there is a continuing source (Carter, 1957). The danger here is of converting an ischaemic to a haemorrhagic infarct. For this reason some physicians prefer to wait for three weeks before starting therapy. The disadvantage of delaying is that further emboli may, indeed are likely, to occur during this period. The best compromise is to secure a CT scan and if there is no evidence of haemorrhage in the infarct to start anticoagulation immediately. If the scan shows evidence of haemorrhagic change, then anticoagulants should be delayed. If CT scanning is not available examination of the cerebrospinal fluid should be carried out and anticoagulants given to those in whom there is neither macro nor microscopic blood. Treatment should commence with heparin and warfarin, the former being discontinued as soon as the dose of the latter has been stabilized.

The other role for anticoagulant therapy is in the stroke-in-evolution which is defined as a stroke which takes more than six hours to evolve. It is on the whole uncommon, being most often seen in brain stem infarction. Anticoagulation by heparin infusion appears to arrest progression of the infarction (Carter, 1961; Baker et al, 1962).

For non-embolic infarcts low molecular weight dextran may be recommended for its effect in lowering blood viscosity and increasing cerebral blood flow. 500 ml dextran 40 is given intravenously within the first hour with 500 ml every 12 hours for 3-7 days. Controlled and uncontrolled trials have suggested this may lower immediate mortality (Gilroy et al, 1969; Spudis et al, 1973; Gottstein 1981); one trial confirming this suggested that by six months the gain has been lost (Matthews et al, 1976).

Because oedema is a major factor in haemorrhage and especially in infarcts, steroids have had a vogue. Though they have the advantage of being easier to administer than is an infusion, survey of the literature suggests there is little to indicate they are of value (Drug and Therepeutics Bulletin, 1983).

REFERENCES

Baker R N, Broward J A, Fang H C, Fisher C M, Groch S N, Heyman A, Karp H R, McDevitt E, Scheinberg P, Schwartz W, Toole J F 1962 Anticoagulant therapy in cerebral infarction. Report on co-operative study. Neurology (Minneap.) 12: 823–835

Baum H M, Robins M 1981 Survival and prevalence in the National Survey of Stroke. Stroke 12: Suppl. 1 59–68

Blackwood W, Hallpike J F, Kocen R S, Mair W G P 1969 Atheromatous disease of the carotid arterial system and embolism from the heart in cerebral infarction: a morbid anatomical study. Brain 92: 897–910

Canadian Cooperative Study Group 1978 A randomized trial of aspirin and sulfinpyrazone in threatened stroke. New England Journal of Medicine 299: 53–59

Carter A B 1957 The immediate treatment of cerebral embolism. Quarterly Journal of Medicine 26: 335–348

Carter A B 1961 Anticoagulant treatment in progressing stroke. British Medical Journal 2: 70–73

Dalsgaard-Neilsen T 1956 Some clinical experience in the treatment of cerebral apoplexy (1000 cases). Acta Psychiatrica Scandinavica Suppl 108: 101–119

Drug and Therapeutics Bulletin 1983 Treatment in the first 12 hours of a stroke. 21: 21–24

Fields W S, Lemak N A, Frankowski R F, Hardy R J 1978 Controlled trial of aspirin in cerebral ischaemia. Part II: Surgical group. Stroke 9: 309–317

Gilroy J, Barnhart M J, Meyer J S 1969 Treatment of acute stroke with dextran 40. Journal of the American Medical Association 210: 293–298

Gottstein U 1981 Normovolemic and hypervolemic hemodilution in cerebrovascular ischemia. Bibliotheca Haematologica (Basel) 47: 127–138

Jorgensen L, Torvik 1966 Ischaemic cerebrovascular diseases in an autopsy series. Part I. Prevalence, location and predisposing factors in verified thrombo-embolic occlusions, and their significance in the pathogenesis of cerebral infarction. Journal of the Neurological Sciences 3: 490–509

Kannel W B, Wolf P A, Verter J, McNamara P M 1970 Epidemiological assessment of the role of blood pressure in stroke. The Framingham study. Journal of the American Medical Association 214: 301&310

Kannel W B, Gordon T, Wolf P A, McNamara P 1972 Hemoglobin and the risk of cerebral infarction. Stroke 3: 409–420

Kannel W B, Abbott R D, Savage D D, McNamara P M 1982 Epidemiologic features of chronic atrial fibrillation. The Framingham study. New England Journal of Medicine 306: 1018–1022

Marshall J, Shaw D A 1960 Anticoagulant therapy in acute cerebrovascular accidents. A controlled trial. Lancet 1: 995–998

Matthews W B, Oxbury J M, Grainger K M R, Greenhall R C D 1976 A blind controlled trial of Dextran 40 in the treatment of ischaemic stroke. Brain 99: 193–206

Spudis E V, de la Torre E, Pikula L 1973 Management of completed strokes with dextran 40. A community hospital failure. Stroke 4: 895–897

Symon L, Lassen N A, Astrup J, Branston N M 1977 Thresholds of ischaemia in brain cortex. Advances in Experimental Medicine and Biology 94: 775–782

Veterans Administration Co-operative Study Group on Antihypertensive Agents 1967 Effects of treatment on morbidity in hypertension: Results in patients with diastolic blood pressures averaging 115 through 129 mmHg. Journal of the American Medical Association 202: 1028–1034

Veterans Administration Co-operative Study Group on Antihypertensive Agents 1970 Effects of treatment on morbidity in hypertension: II. Results in patients with diastolic pressure averaging 90 through 114 mmHg. Journal of the American Medical Association 213: 1143–1152

Whisnant J P, Fitzgibbons J P, Kurland L T, Sayre G P 1971 Natural history of stroke in Rochester, Minnesota 1945 through 1954. Stroke 2: 11–22

Wolf P A, Dawber T R, Thomas H E, Kannel W B 1978 Epidemiologic assessment of chronic atrial fibrillation and risk of stroke: The Framingham study. Neurology (Minneap.) 28: 973–977

Ziegler D K, Hassanein R S 1973 Prognosis in patients with transient ischemic attacks. Stroke 4: 666–673

16

Space-occupying intracranial lesions

F. I. Caird

Most space-occupying intracranial lesions increase in frequency with age up to at least 80 years (Table 16.1) (Twomey, 1978). This is true of primary malignant intracranial tumours, and of metastatic tumours (Gudmundsson, 1970). If intracranial tumours diagnosed only at autopsy are included, the continuing rise with age is even more striking (Annegers et al, 1980). In life, 35% of

Table 16.1 Age of 110 patients with intracranial tumour (Godfrey & Caird, 1984)

Age in years	< 70	70–79	> 80	Total
No	29	68	13	110

primary intracranial tumours are never diagnosed. Three-quarters of these are meningiomas, and almost all are found in people over the age of 60. Subdural haematoma also probably increases in frequency with age; approximately 35% of cases are in patients over 65 years of age. Intracranial abscess and primary intracerebral haemorrhage are less common in the elderly.

DIAGNOSIS

The symptoms of intracranial space-occupying lesions may be divided into those of raised intra-cranial pressure, and those of the causal lesion. In the elderly, the symptoms of raised intracranial pressure are vague and indefinite; they resemble those of many other conditions. Headache is relatively infrequent, occurring in perhaps 10% of patients with intracranial tumours (Godfrey & Caird, 1984), and distinctly fewer elderly than younger patients in the case of subdural haematoma (Luxon & Harrison, 1979). Vomiting is also uncommon. The predominant symptoms are apathy, lethargy, confusion and increasing immobility and incontinence (Turner & Caird, 1982). The signs of raised intracranial pressure are also few and nonspecific. Apathy, slowness of response and drowsiness are characteristic. Papilloedema is unusual; it was only certainly identified in approximately 5% of intracranial tumours in the elderly, and then mostly under the age of 75 (Godfrey & Caird,

1984). The age-related reduction in brain volume may well be responsible, and the consequent availability of more space within the cranium for tumour growth, whose main effect is thus distortion of the brain rather than increase of intracranial pressure. It is possible that there may be changes in the transmission of raised intracranial pressure to the optic nerve head as a result of local age changes there.

The cardinal symptoms of space-occupying intracranial lesions are those of a progressive focal cerebral disorder. A hemiparesis due to tumour is likely to be attributed in the first instance to stroke; this is much the commonest initial diagnosis (McLaurin & Helmer, 1962). In the great majority of patients with stroke, unless this is due to an intracerebral haemorrhage, mental state and usually motor power improve over a period of a few days or weeks. If the focal lesion is due to tumour there is no improvement, but rather a steady worsening. Repeated review and careful assessment are thus necessary if the correct diagnosis is to be suspected and made. Accurate documentation of physical signs is particularly important. The progression of the focal symptoms and signs is over at least a week. Many cases of cerebral infarction appear to progress or actually do so over shorter periods of 2–3 days, but rarely over a longer period. In general a shorter history (of under 3–4 months) will be found to be due to malignant tumour and longer periods to benign lesions. Fluctuation in some physical signs, particularly in mental state, undoubtedly occurs in some cases of meningioma (Daly et al, 1961), but steady progression is the rule. Epileptic seizures are a feature of between 15 and 30% of cases of hemisphere tumour in the elderly. Only 10–15% of seizures of all types developing for the first time in old age are due to intracranial tumour (Roberts et al, 1982), but the proportion may be higher in the case of partial seizures.

The essential diagnostic measures consist of establishing a possible primary site in the case of metastatic tumours (bronchial carcinoma being the commonest single primary) (Table 16.2), a scintiscan and perhaps an electro-encephalogram (EEG). The scintiscan will be normal in only a very small proportion of elderly patients with space-occupying lesions of whatever kind (MacDonald, 1981),

Table 16.2 Primary tumour in intracranial metastases in the elderly (Godfrey & Caird, 1984)

	Male	Female	Total
Lung, definite	16	2	
			23
Lung, probable	4	1	
Uncertain	3	4	7
Other	3*	3+	6
	26	10	36

* One each: rectum, kidney, melanoma
+ One each: breast, thyroid, melanoma

but is often abnormal in the first few weeks after cerebral infarction. This implies that false positive scintiscans will be much commoner than false negatives, which are virtually confined to cystic lesions. The EEG is also likely to be abnormal. The definitive investigation is the computed tomography (CT) scan, which in many cases can in addition indicate the probable pathology (Figs. 16.1–3).

Verification of the pathology of intracranial tumour by biopsy is still important in the elderly (Turner & Caird, 1982). Its principal purpose is to establish the diagnosis

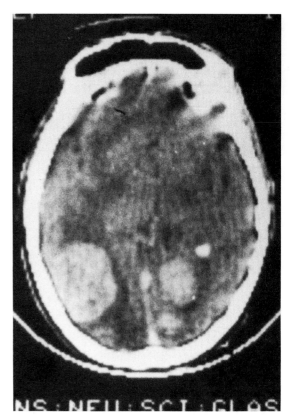

Fig. 16.2 Multiple lesions enhanced with contrast, and oedema of right hemisphere: metastases from carcinoma of colon.

beyond doubt. Biopsy should be undertaken if there remains uncertainty as to whether the lesion is a tumour (and not for instance an abscess), or any serious possibility that a known tumour may be benign, and so situated that surgical treatment is possible. If the tumour is in the dominant hemisphere and dysphasia might be worsened, biopsy is less desirable. It should be undertaken after at least 24 hours of steroid therapy, so as to lessen any surrounding oedema and decrease the immediate hazards of the procedure.

INTRACRANIAL TUMOURS

Malignant tumours

The numbers in the elderly of primary and secondary malignant tumours are approximately equal (Table 16.3). In the case of primary malignant tumours biopsy will establish the diagnosis, or the absence of any definite primary site, combined with the characteristic CT scan appearances of a malignant astrocytoma (Fig. 16.1), may make the diagnosis virtually certain. By contrast in secondary tumours, an obvious primary will usually be

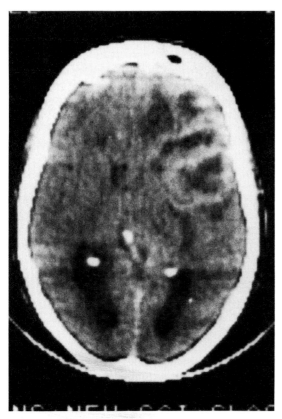

Fig. 16.1 Multicentric lesion in right frontal region, with surrounding oedema, displacement to right of septum and pineal and backwards of choroid plexus: astrocytoma.

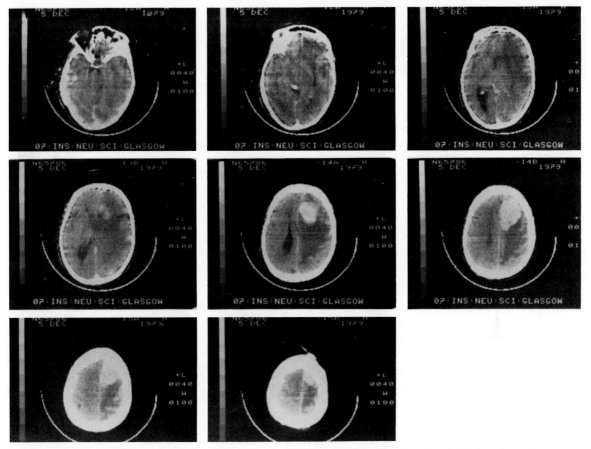

Fig. 16.3   Contrast-enhancing well defined uniform lesion of right frontal region, with obliteration of right lateral ventricle and massive oedema of right hemisphere: meningioma.

present (Table 16.3). There may be multiple tumours evident on the CT scan, but the metabolic consequences of malignant disease, in particular hyponatraemia and hypercalcaemia, may mimic multifocal metastatic intra-cranial disease. However, these complications do not in themselves produce focal neurological signs, while confusion, apathy and even drowsiness are essentially signs of diffuse intracranial disorder. The greatest difficulty in distinguishing multifocal from diffuse cerebral disease occurs when there are multiple metastases and much increase in intracranial pressure, but even then, there are usually signs indicating one or more focal lesions.

Other malignant lesions include lymphoma, and occasionally direct spread from lesions of the skull. Lymphomas will usually be diagnosed in the elderly as astrocytomas if no biopsy is done, and local invasion from skull lesions is usually evident on a combination of straight X-ray and CT scan appearances.

Table 16.3   110 intracranial tumours in the elderly (Godfrey & Caird, 1984)

Hemisphere		95
Astrocytoma	38	
Metastasis	36	
Meningioma	14	
Other	7	
Posterior Fossa		10
Primary	2	
Metastasis	5	
Acoustic neuroma	3	
Pituitary		5
Total		110

Meningioma

Meningiomas are the only common benign supratentorial tumours (see Table 16.3 & Fig. 16.3). They are relatively frequent and always worth looking for. A considerable number may not be the cause of symptoms, and such incidental tumours are increasingly found not at autopsy but on clinical investigation by scintiscan or CT scan. There must be then a careful review, to determine whether the tumour could possibly be related to the patient's complaints. In the case of surprisingly large tumours this may not be so; presumably they have grown extremely slowly, so that the underlying displaced brain has continued to function normally. Such cases should not be treated. Other cases should be treated surgically if at all possible. Surgical treatment may be preceded by external carotid embolisation of the tumour; this helps to reduce its size and to make the surgical procedure easier. Subtotal removal may be all that is technically possible, without compromise to vital structures such as the middle cerebral artery; as much as is possible of the tumour should be removed. The results are in general good, even when symptoms and signs are relatively far advanced.

Treatment of malignant intracranial tumours

Malignant intracranial tumours, whether primary of secondary, should be treated with high-dose steroid therapy. Some 60% may be expected to improve (especially metastases), increased alertness and reduced motor disability being evident within as little as 12 hours, and usually within 5 days; improvement may continue to increase for several weeks. This is due more to reduction in the mass effect of the oedema surrounding the tumour than of the tumour itself; it is thus more likely the greater the oedema evident on the CT scan. A satisfactory policy (Turner & Caird, 1982) is to begin with dexamethasone 12–16 mg daily, to continue for 5 days and then to review the situation. If there has been no response, the dose should be rapidly reduced, and the drug withdrawn after a further 7 days. If a response has occurred, the dose should be gradually reduced over 7–10 days to one at which symptoms are controlled. Some improvement will usually be maintained for some weeks or months. When there is the inevitable relapse, steroids should be withdrawn altogether; rapid and fatal deterioration is then likely over some days, for most of which the patient will be unaware.

Side-effects can be attributed to steroids in some 10% of cases. Minor adverse effects include insomnia and oral moniliasis. Steroid psychosis is much less common, as are diabetes, rapid increase in blood pressure and perforation of a viscus. Weight gain and a Cushingoid facies may occur after some weeks. There can be no doubt the benefits of treatment are much greater than the risks of its serious complications. Many patients are brought to a state where they can at the very least communicate with their relatives, who themselves do not doubt that treatment has been worthwhile.

Posterior fossa tumours

Tumours of the posterior fossa constitute approximately 10% of all intracranial tumours in the elderly (see Table 16.3). Primary tumours (astrocytoma etc) are relatively rare and metastatic lesions, often from bronchial carcinoma, constitute at least half. The usual presentation is with increasing symptoms and signs of raised intracranial pressure, combined with those of a unilateral cerebellar disorder or, if the metastasis is in the brainstem, with cranial nerve lesions. Investigation should be by CT scan in the first instance (Fig. 16.4), since the scintiscan may be misleadingly negative. Ventriculo-peritoneal shunting is the first line of treatment, while partial excision should be undertaken on some occasions, and radiotherapy on others. Posterior fossa lesions in general seem to respond poorly to steroids in the long term, but may do so at least in the short term. Benign posterior fossa lesions are rare and virtually confined to acoustic neuromas. The characteristic manifestations are of a cerebello-pontine angle lesion. Treatment should be surgical, preceded in some cases by reduction of increased intracranial pressure by ventriculo-peritoneal shunt.

Pituitary and parasellar tumours

Pituitary and parasellar lesions are even rarer (see Table 16.3). The diagnosis is often suggested by the finding of enlargement of the pituitary fossa on a skull X-ray taken for another purpose. In the elderly it is unusual for such lesions to act by occupying space, and the endocrine manifestations of pituitary failure are much commoner than those of pressure on the optic chiasm or of raised intracranial pressure. Careful charting of the visual fields is often difficult in elderly patients, and the visual evoked potentials are a more accurate diagnostic method (Halliday et al, 1976). If these are normal, the optic nerves and chiasm may be assumed to be intact. If they are abnormal, an ocular cause should be excluded before assuming that the pituitary lesion is responsible. Tests of pituitary endocrine function should be carried out and appropriate replacement therapy instituted.

INTRACRANIAL HAEMORRHAGE

Intracranial haemorrhage in the elderly occurs in four main forms. Massive intracerebral haemorrhage, originating usually from rupture of a perforating artery in the basal ganglia, with rupture into the ventricles and formation of a tentorial pressure cone, is fatal within a few days. As in younger patients, it is a complication of severe hypertension. After a short period of headache the patient rapidly lapses into coma, with hemiplegia, deviation of the head and eyes away from the paralysed side and often neck stiffness. The cerebrospinal fluid will be blood-stained, and other investigations are unnecessary. No treatment is of any avail, and proper management of high blood pressure is much the best prevention.

Localised intracerebral haemorrhage may be of two kinds. Since the introduction of CT scanning it has been realised that a small proportion of cases of what presents as

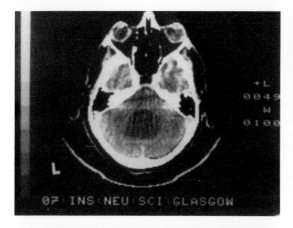
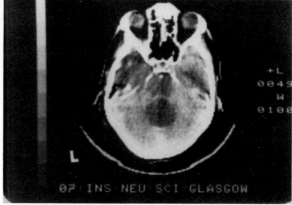
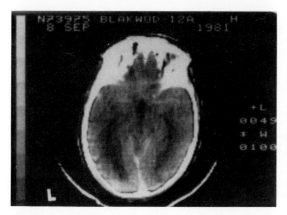
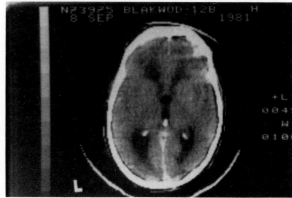

Fig. 16.4   Central cystic astrocytoma of cerebellum with large third and lateral ventricles of obstructive hydrocephalus.

cerebral infarction is due to deep or capsular haemorrhage (Fig. 16.5). The development of hemiplegia is usually rapid, and recovery may also be relatively rapid, over a period of a few weeks. Such haematomas resolve with the development of a haemorrhagic cyst. There is little to distinguish patients with this variety of intracranial haemorrhage from those with cerebral infarction, except that improvement in conscious level may be delayed (see below). Surgical treatment should not be undertaken, for fear of creating greater damage than that due to the haematoma itself. Improvement is due partly to reabsorption of the haematoma and partly to recovery of function in fibre tracts disrupted by surrounding oedema, which also resolves.

The second kind of localised intracranial haemorrhage is a spontaneous subcortical haematoma. This is also a complication of hypertension. It presents as the rapid development of focal supratentorial signs. The patient remains drowsy for several days. If pneumonia, metabolic disorder and inappropriate drug therapy (with hypotensive drugs such as methyldopa or with others) is excluded, such patients should have a CT scan. The indication for surgical

treatment is failure of improvement in consciousness. If consciousness improves, the natural course is also one of improvement, with a varying degree of residual disability due to destruction of brain tissue. However if there is no return of consciousness and there is evidence from the CT scan of a major space-occupying lesion, surgical evacuation should be undertaken. The results are surprisingly good, perhaps because the amount of destruction of brain substance is relatively small. The symptoms are due as much to disordered function of fibre tracts resulting from oedema and the pressure of the haematoma.

Subdural haematoma

Subdural haematoma is a relatively uncommon condition in elderly people, intracranial tumour being approximately five times commoner. A history of a head injury is present in at least 60% of cases, or a story of repeated falls. Headache is relatively common (about 20% of cases) but papilloedema is rare. The usual presentation is with increasing confusion and signs of focal cerebral disorder — a hemiparesis rather than a complete hemiplegia. On examination there may be a varying degree of impairment

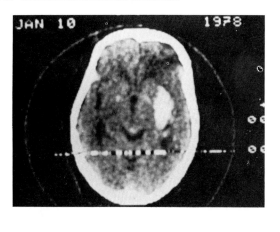
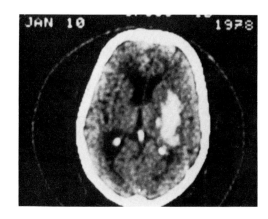
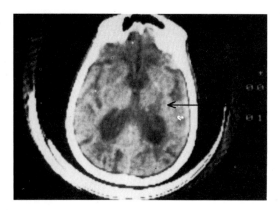
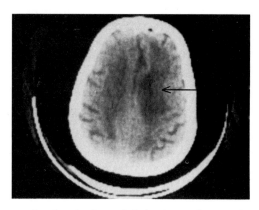

Fig. 16.5 Haemorrhage (high-density) in right capsular region. Lower scans show low density cystic lesion (arrowed) two weeks later.

of consciousness, often impairment of upward eye movements (Pennybacker, 1949) and some long tract signs. These may be motor and/or sensory (including sensory suppression), but a true hemianopia is most unusual. A skull X-ray may reveal pineal shift. The scintiscan in the elderly is almost always positive in chronic cases (those of over three weeks duration) (McDonald, 1981), probably because the haematoma in the elderly is large if it causes symptoms (Fogelholm et al, 1975). The CT scan shows shift of the midline structures such as the septum and the pineal, a peripheral lesion often of low density, and obliteration of the ventricle and of the cerebral sulci on the same side, giving rise to apparent unilateral cerebral atrophy (Fig. 16.6). Treatment should be by aspiration through burr-holes. Craniotomy is very rarely needed and there is no place for the medical management of symptomatic subdural haematoma. Early recurrence in the first week after drainage is relatively frequent; the patient should be closely observed, and the CT scan repeated, to show resolution of the shift in midline structures. The results of treatment are excellent, with a mortality now well under 5% (Nath et al, in press). If there is a history of

diffuse brain disorder preceding the subdural haematoma over a long period (of months or years), improvement is less likely, and the patient may well be left with a greater degree of brain failure than before the haematoma. However in previously mentally normal patients, complete and lasting recovery may be expected.

INTRACRANIAL ABSCESS

Intracranial abscess is unusual in the elderly, but may complicate septicaemias and head injuries where the integrity of the dura is breached. A raised white cell count and erythrocyte sedimentation rate may help to distinguish it from primary intracranial tumour (Harrison, 1982). In either case, the lesion may well be fatal, but treatment should be by aspiration and appropriate antibiotic therapy.

SUMMARY

Space-occupying lesions are not rare in the elderly and are well worth proper diagnosis and proper treatment. Proper diagnosis is essential so that benign lesions are not over-

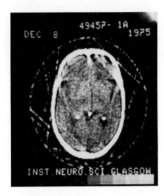
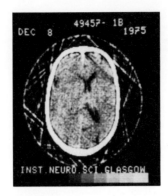
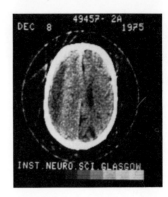
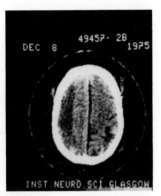
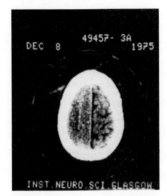
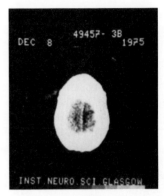

Fig. 16.6 Shift of third ventricle and septum to right, compression of left lateral ventricle, peripheral low density area with straight medial border, disappearance of cerebral sulci on left, and sulcal widening on right: chronic subdural haematoma.

looked, while a majority of malignant lesions respond at least temporarily to steroids. All malignant supratentorial lesions require accurate diagnosis so that a prognosis can be given to relatives, and so that scarce rehabilitation resources can be used on patients whose expectation of life is longer.

REFERENCES

Annegers J F, Schoenberg B S, Okazaki H, Kurland L T 1980 Primary intracranial neoplasms in Rochester, Minnesota, 1935–1977. In: Rose F C (ed) Clinical Neuroepidemiology, Pitman Medical, Tunbridge Wells, ch 37, p 366

Daly D D, Svien H J, Yoss R E 1961 Intermitent cerebral symptoms with meningioma. Archives of Neurology 5: 287–93

Fogelholm R, Heiskanen O, Waltimo O 1975 Chronic subdural haematoma in adults. Influence of patients' age on symptoms, signs, and thickness of the haematoma. Journal of Neurosurgery 42: 43–6

Godfrey J W, Caird F I 1984 Intracranial tumours in the elderly: diagnosis and treatment. Age and Ageing 13: 152–158

Gudmundsson K R 1970 A survey of tumours of the central nervous system in Iceland during the 10-year period 1954–63. Acta Neurologica Scandinavica 46: 538–52

Halliday A M, Halliday E, Kriss A, McDonald W I, Mushin Joan 1976 The pattern-effect potential in compression of the anterior visual pathways. Brain 99: 357–74

Harrison M J G 1982 The clinical presentation of intracranial abscesses. Quarterly Journal of Medicine 51: 461–8

Luxon L M, Harrison M J G 1979 Chronic subdural haematoma. Quarterly Journal of Medicine 48: 43–53

Macdonald J B 1981 The scintiscan In: Caird F I, Evans J G (eds) Advanced Geriatric Medicine 1, Pitman Medical, Tunbridge Well, ch 7, p 84–7

McLaurin R L, Helmer F A 1962 Errors in diagnosis of intracranial tumours. Journal of American Medical Association 180: 1011–16

Nath F, Mendelow A D, Wu C C, Hessett C, Caird F I, Jennett B, Chronic subdural haematoma in the CT scan era. Scottish Medical Journal. In press

Pennybacker J 1949 Intracranial tumours in the aged. Edinburgh Medical Journal 56: 590–600

Roberts M A, Godfrey J W, Caird F I 1982 Epileptic seizures in the elderly I: Aetiology and type of seizure. Age and Ageing 11: 24–8

Twomey C 1978 Brain tumours in the elderly. Age and Ageing 7: 138–45

Turner J W, Caird F I 1982 Other neurosurgical problems In: Caird F I (ed) Neurological Disorders in the Elderly, Wright PSG, Bristol, ch 4, p 231–41

17

Parkinsonism

M. Hildick-Smith

EPIDEMIOLOGY AND CHANGING NATURAL HISTORY

Parkinson's disease has been shown by workers in different countries (Brewis et al, 1962; Gudmundsson 1967) to affect 1–2% of those aged 60 or over. In one of the most complete studies, that of Kurland (1958) in the USA, the incidence was shown to rise further with increasing age.

The natural history of the condition seems to be changing. Since the advent of levodopa treatment patients are surviving longer (Sweet & McDowell, 1975; Rinne 1978). Birkmayer and his colleagues (1974) found that the increase in life-expectancy had a marked effect in the over-80 year olds, and some workers (Shaw et al, 1982) believe that expectation of life for the drug-responsive patient with Parkinsonism may now be virtually normal. The effect of these and other changes has been to shift the main incidence of Parkinsonism onwards from late middle-age, so that it is now largely a disease of the elderly. A recent epidemiological study (Godwin-Austen et al, 1982) has shown that 58% of sufferers in Britain are aged 70 or more.

The benefits of levodopa treatment particularly in increased mobility and independence, have been of great value to elderly sufferers. However as patients have lived longer there has been time for them to develop more advanced manifestations of the condition such as instability and variable performance, which have proved very difficult to treat. For example, Parkinsonism accompanied by dementia causes many difficulties in diagnosis and treatment. Overall the paradoxical result of successful treatment has been the unfolding of further and more difficult problems to solve.

CLASSIFICATION AND AETIOLOGY

Parkinson's disease may be a primary (idiopathic) or secondary condition.

Idiopathic

Idiopathic Parkinsonism shows wide variation both in onset and in progression, but is nonetheless believed to have a common though presently unknown aetiology.

Genetic

A widely-quoted study proposed a genetic element on some occasions, since up to 20% of the cases showed a positive family history (Gudmundsson, 1967). Later work (Yahr, 1982) denied a genetic component and suggested that the majority of family members in such studies when found and examined, proved to be suffering from benign essential tremor. This condition is four times as common in the elderly as Parkinson's disease and difficult to distinguish from it.

Vascular

In a recent study Godwin-Austen and his colleagues (1982) found a negative correlation between generalised vascular disease and true Parkinsonism, although the clinical effect of multiple cerebral infarcts could be to produce a confusing 'pseudo-Parkinsonism'.

Trauma

Repeated head trauma seemed, in this study, to increase the risk of developing Parkinson's disease three-fold, but it was not clear whether this effect occurred against a background of pre-existing subclinical disease.

Smoking

There was a lower incidence of smoking among those with Parkinson's disease in this and other studies, and this fact has not yet been explained.

Virus

A viral aetiology has been suggested, not only for post-encephalitic (see below), but also for idiopathic Parkinsonism, though no cases of viral transmission have yet been proved, and there is no definite confirmation from immunological studies. The last epidemic of encephalitis lethargica was in 1926, and so far there is not the decline in idiopathic Parkinsonism that one would expect if this virus were the main cause, however epidemiological studies over the next decade or two should clarify this.

Neuromelanin

A possible toxic role for neuromelanin (or its contents such as heavy metals or peroxides) has been suggested, and opens up further research possibilities into the cause of idiopathic Parkinson's disease.

Secondary Parkinsonism

Secondary Parkinsonism may be: post-encephalitic (with some characteristic features distinguishing these cases from those of idiopathic Parkinsonism; drug-induced, the main drugs involved in this increasingly common problem being those of the phenothiazine group, particularly chlorpromazine and prochlorperazine or butyrophenones such as haloperidol, or part of a generalised neurological condition such as senile dementia of Alzheimer type (SDAT) or Steele-Richardson syndrome.

PATHOLOGY AND NEUROCHEMISTRY

Although it is clear that Parkinson's disease is primarily a disorder of melanin-containing neurones in the brain, the exact site, extent and nature of the lesions is still not known. Degeneration and loss of neurones occurs most obviously in the substantia nigra and locus caeruleus but can also be seen in the globus pallidus, putamen and caudate nucleus. Less severe changes have been found in the dorsal nucleus of the vagus. The characteristic lesion is thought to be the Lewy body, an abnormal neurone occurring in the substantia nigra and containing a hyaline inclusion. Although this Lewy body is pathognomic of the disease, its precise significance is unknown.

Neuromelanin accumulates until middle-age as a waste product within neurones of the substantia nigra and locus caeruleus. It may accumulate to excess in Parkinsonian patients, leading to deterioration and death of the most heavily pigmented cells, leaving behind those less pigmented (Mann & Yates, 1982).

Overlap with SDAT

There is overlap in pathology between Parkinson's disease and SDAT. In one autopsy study (Boller et al, 1979), the prevalence of dementia and of Alzheimer changes (senile plaques and fibrillary tangles) among patients with Parkinsonism was over six times that of an age-matched population. Hakim & Mathieson (1979) confirmed the higher incidence of dementia in Parkinsonism (using clinical and histological data) and suggested the simultaneous presence of SDAT and Parkinsonism in a subgroup of elderly Parkinsonian patients who subsequently survived for a shorter period than those who were mentally alert.

Overlap with aging

There is overlap too, between the changes of Parkinsonism and those of normal aging. For example Lewy bodies are found in 4–6% of routine autopsies — perhaps these patients, if they had lived long enough, would have developed Parkinsonism?

NEUROCHEMISTRY

Despite much work over the last 20 years, our understanding of the neurochemical changes in Parkinson's disease is far from complete. The basic deficiency of dopamine in the substantia nigra was shown by Ehringer & Hornykiewicz (1960) and later correlated with the degree of cell loss (Bernheimer et al, 1965). The value of intravenous levodopa in treatment (Birkmayer & Hornykiewicz, 1961) appeared to confirm that the disease was a simple deficiency in dopamine (inhibitory) mechanisms, allowing the cholinergic (excitatory) mechanisms to predominate.

It was later found that the disease progressed despite levodopa replacement therapy, and that all the manifestations of the disease could not be explained by dopamine deficiency. The response to levodopa often failed after five years or so, for reasons which are still not clear. Hypersensitivity of the neurone has been suggested (Shaw et al, 1980), or alternatively the brain may lose the ability to synthesise and store the dopamine (Marsden, 1980). Mann & Yates (1982) have suggested that long-term levodopa treatment may lead to the formation of further excesses of neuromelanin, which may cause functional failure and death of neurones. This process accelerates the later stages of the disease and, perhaps by the adverse effects on the locus caeruleus, may promote the development of dementia.

Synaptic mechanisms and drug actions

Our present understanding of what happens at synaptic level is shown in Figure 17.1. Dopamine itself acts presynaptically, whereas the so-called dopamine agonists act either directly on the post-synaptic neurone or across the synapse by releasing adenyl cyclase, and can theoretically act when the pre-synaptic response has failed. Bromocriptine, the most successful of this latter group, is a partial dopamine agonist and may also stimulate adenyl cyclase. Lysuride may act by stimulating D_2 receptors. Deprenyl acts pre-synaptically by decreasing the degradation of dopamine, hence 'eking out' its effect. In

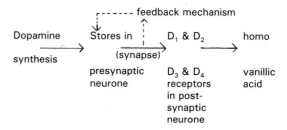

D_1 depends on adenyl cyclase
D_2 does not depend on adenyl cyclase
Symptoms of Parkinsonism probably relate to dysfunction of D_2 receptors.

Fig. 17.1 Dopaminergic synapse

drug-induced Parkinsonism the blockage is at post-synaptic level, hence dopamine drugs may be ineffective and anticholinergic treatment is often tried.

Other neurotransmitter changes

Although dopamine deficiency is the most important biochemical lesion in Parkinsonism (and it has been estimated that about 70–90% of brain dopamine must be lost before clinical features of the disease appear), the roles of other neurotransmitters may have some importance. As well as some loss of subcortical noradrenaline and of 5-Hydroxytryptamine, there may be loss of neuropeptides and metencephalins in some cases. It is difficult to clarify neurotransmitter changes because Parkinsonism often overlaps with SDAT or with the changes of normal aging.

Overlap with SDAT

Biochemical studies have pointed to a similarity between Parkinson's disease and SDAT in that they both show a loss of ascending projections (Rossor, 1981). The loss falls mainly on the dopaminergic striatal projection in Parkinson's disease, and on the cholinergic cortical projection (from septum and substantia innominata) in SDAT. Both diseases also show a loss of nor-adrenergic projection from the locus caeruleus resulting in a loss of subcortical nor-adrenaline.

The similarity is further emphasised by the fact that the cells of the locus caeruleus, substantia nigra, substantia innominata and septal nuclei all share a non-specialised isodendritic pattern (Fig. 17.2). The suggestion is made that the primary loss, in both conditions, is of cells in the isodendritic core. This leads in turn to loss of the relevant ascending projections, with some pathological, neurochemical and symptomatic overlap between the conditions according to whether the loss is predominantly on the dopaminergic (Parkinsonian) or cholinergic (SDAT) projections.

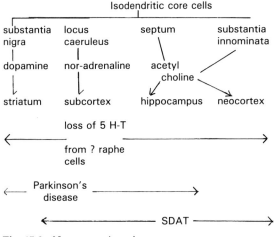

Fig. 17.2 Neurotransmitter changes

Overlap with aging

There is overlap between Parkinson's disease and normal aging (Carlsson et al, 1980) in which up to 50% of brain dopamine may be lost. It has been suggested that the cells of the isodendritic core may be vulnerable to a variety of environmental injuries, or may have a biochemical predisposition to premature aging.

In normal aging as in SDAT and sometimes in Parkinsonism, choline acetyl transferase (CAT) activity also declines (Bowen & Davison 1978) as may receptor binding of acetyl choline, perhaps enabling dopamine to be more effective in restoring the dopamine/acetyl choline balance in elderly Parkinsonian patients.

SIGNS AND SYMPTOMS

Although the diagnosis of Parkinsonism is often difficult in the old, many elderly patients will present with the classical signs and symptoms described by James Parkinson — rhythmic tremor, flexed posture, monotonous voice and tendency to fall. Many will have the characteristic rigidity (lead-pipe or cogwheel in type) and the immobile masklike face which did not feature in the original description, but which are now regarded as typical. The trunk rigidity may lead to difficulty in rolling over in bed. Rigidity of small hand muscles may lead to slowness in doing up buttons, writing a signature or cutting up meat.

Difficulty in initiating movement occurs in Parkinsonism, leading to problems in getting out of a chair or bed. Characteristic 'freezing' episodes may occur on encountering an obstacle (such as a doorway or the edge of a carpet), while the small steps, the loss of arm swing and turning 'all in one piece' may be diagnostic.

The physician should maintain a high 'index of suspicion' for this treatable condition, looking up as the patient enters the consulting room (when the instant diagnosis may be made) and confirming his suspicions by asking leading questions about the most characteristic disabilities.

DIAGNOSTIC DIFFICULTIES IN THE OLD

Parkinsonism often starts with non-specific symptoms and the patient may attribute the fact that he tires easily or needs frequent rests, to 'just old age'. Even in the later stages of the condition the symptoms of slowing, stooped posture etc are caricatures of the aging process, and may be missed by the patient. The doctor may also miss the diagnosis if he does not see enough elderly patients to be aware of the normal gait of an 80 year old and to contrast it with the Parkinsonian one. Conversely Parkinsonism may sometimes be overdiagnosed as the cause of stuttering gait, indistinct speech etc in patients who have, in fact, had a series of small strokes. Such patients may be kept for long periods on inappropriate anti-Parkinsonian drugs (White & Barnes, 1981).

When Parkinsonism starts unilaterally many doctors will misdiagnose the condition as a hemiplegia so that the chance of appropriate treatment will be lost. This is particularly likely to occur if the characteristic tremor is absent, as may frequently happen in elderly patients. On the other hand patients with benign essential tremor may be misdiagnosed as having Parkinsonism, and their medication may be increased to toxic levels in an attempt to control the tremor.

Muscle pain is a relatively common problem in Parkinson's disease, but may be attributed to cervical osteoarthritis (whose X-ray appearances are nearly always present in the old), or to polymyalgia. Arthritis in the hands may make movements slow and clumsy so that it is difficult to determine whether there is any bradykinesia. A hyperthyroid picture (of heat intolerance, flushing, seborrhoea and wide-eyed appearance) may occur if the main brunt of the Parkinsonism falls on the autonomic system. Hypothyroidism can produce a similar picture to that of a depressed patient with Parkinson's disease.

Dysphagic symptoms — similar to those of carcinoma of the oesophagus — may be produced when the Parkinsonism affects the vagal nucleus, leading to abnormal oesophageal contractions, however the Parkinsonian symptoms respond well to a levodopa preparation.

Falls in the elderly are almost as non-specific a symptom as fever in a child. Of the many causes, it is well worth thinking of Parkinsonism, as treatment may return an elderly patient to full independence.

MAIN CONDITIONS AFFECTING TREATMENT

It is more difficult to treat Parkinsonism in an elderly patient. Drug doses have to be watched (because of altered pharmacokinetics in the old), and problems of adverse reactions and of drug compliance faced (especially in confused patients). Multiple pathology is common, and the doctor may have to treat two or more conditions concurrently, risking problems of drug interation. Fortunately, combined preparations (containing levodopa and a decarboxylase inhibitor) give rise to less problems than levodopa alone. A patient with recent myocardial infarction may require caution with dosage. Persistent and severe postural hypotension may prompt the suspicion that the patient may have Shy-Drager syndrome and may be unlikely to respond well. Peptic ulcer and malignant melanoma may be activated by these drugs. Prostatism and glaucoma may be exacerbated by anti-cholinergic drugs which have only a small part to play in treatment of elderly patients, not least because they may cause or worsen confusion.

An acute confusional episode can occur in any elderly patient as a result of intercurrent infection or inappropriate medication etc and should subside with treatment of the cause. Long-term dementia (SDAT) may occur in one in three elderly patients with Parkinsonism (Loranger et al, 1972) and the clinical overlap has been repeatedly confirmed (Parkes et al, 1974; Martin et al, 1973; Pearce, 1974). An objective measure of the patient's mental state by questionnaire (Hodkinson, 1972) is probably the most important pre-treatment test. (It is important to check that the patient is not deaf, depressed, drowsy or dysphasic before accepting the mental score result). The confused patient will require smaller drug-doses on a trial basis (Broe & Caird, 1973; Hildick-Smith, 1976b) and the mental state will also affect compliance with both medication and exercise regimes.

Before treating for Parkinsonism it is also important to examine the patient for other neurological conditions. A history of small strokes together with signs of pyramidal tract damage (e.g. supranuclear palsy) will suggest a pseudo-Parkinsonian picture, which does not usually respond to drugs. Alternatively, the Parkinsonism may be part of a more relentless and intractable neurological condition. Examples are nigrostriatal degeneration (not diagnosable during life); the Steele-Richardson syndrome where there is progressive palsy of conjugate ocular movements; olivo-ponto cerebellar degeneration, where cerebellar signs may later appear; and Shy-Drager syndrome, where severe postural hypotension accompanies the Parkinsonism.

It is always worth asking whether the patient has taken phenothiazines drugs, as these are frequent causes of drug-induced Parkinsonism in the elderly. It may take months for the symptoms to subside after the offending drug is withdrawn, even with the help of anticholinergic treatment. Sometimes after drug-induced Parkinsonism has been treated and relieved idiopathic Parkinsonism will appear a year or two later. A useful objective measure of bradykinesia can be made before treatment by timing the patient as he signs his name and address in the clinical records. Functional assessment of his ability to dress, walk, get into and out of bed or chair, and to maintain continence, are useful in completing the pre-treatment picture.

TREATMENT

Non-disabling Parkinsonism

Modern teaching advises us to reserve levodopa drugs until the patient is disabled. In practice, the relevance of this changed approach is limited for the elderly, as the majority are disabled on first presenting for diagnosis. There is however, a small number of patients whose 'benign' Parkinsonism (Hoehn & Yahr, 1967) has continued for 10–20 years into old age without significant disability.

Secondly, there is a small group of patients whose minor rigidity or muscle pains can be relieved by orphenadrine 100–300 mg a day, or whose minor or stress-induced tremor can be treated by prophylactic propranolol.

Throughout all stages of the disease, the value of exercise and the dangers of excessive bed rest have long been known. Therapists have devised regimes of group exercise for leg, trunk and shoulder (Davis, 1977) but it is only recently that there have been any controlled trials of physiotherapy treatment (Flewitt et al, 1981; Steiner & Flewitt, 1981; Franklyn et al, 1981; Franklyn & Stern, 1981; Gibberd et al, 1981). There are many difficulties in standardising and evaluating this treatment, but attempts have been made using equipment of varying levels of sophistication. One hopeful line of treatment may be in video-recording and later analysing the gait disturbance and its alteration with treatment, which may be directed, for example, at improving 'heel-strike'. There is disagreement whether patients are best given physiotherapy at home (in districts where this service is available), or whether they benefit enough from the social contact and competition of group therapy in hospital to make up for the problems and expense of ambulance transport. When patients are in groups they may pass on to each other hints about how to start again when 'stuck'. Another advantage is that hospitals and gymnasia provide space for practice in using the valuable wheeled delta-aid.

The occupational therapist has a very useful and cost-effective role (either at home or in hospital) in advising, for example, how to raise the height of bed or chair, and in providing bathing or feeding aids (Beattie & Caird, 1980) to help the patient's independence. Only 3% of Parkinsonian patients (Oxtoby, 1981) in a survey of the Parkinson's Disease Society had seen a speech therapist, though speech disability causes embarassment and isolation throughout the disease. There may be evidence (Scott & Caird, 1981) of some benefit from speech therapy including tape-recording and play-back practice.

The Parkinson's Disease Society sponsors publications (Godwin-Austen, 1971; Godwin-Austen & Hildick-Smith, 1982) which are informative and up to date. Meetings of local branches are helpful in combating the social isolation which troubles many patients and families (Singer, 1973).

Disabling Parkinsonism

Once disability occurs most geriatricians (Sutcliffe, 1973; Vignalou & Beck, 1973; Caird & Williamson, 1978; Hildick-Smith 1976a) would agree that levodopa, now used in a combined preparation, is the treatment of choice. Up to 85% of patients have 50% objective improvement on these combined drugs.

Sinemet (a mixture of the dopa decarboxylase inhibitor carbidopa and levodopa) has been known since 1973 (Marsden et al, 1973) to be superior to levodopa alone. The carbidopa blocks the wasteful metabolism of levodopa outside the brain, enabling dosages to be reduced four or five fold, while side-effects on heart and gut are reduced. Sinemet is now available as:

Sinemet 275 (carbidopa 25 mg, levodopa 250 mg)
Sinemet 110 (carbidopa 10 mg, levodopa 100 mg)
Sinemet plus (carbidopa 25 mg, levodopa 100 mg)

An average daily dose for an elderly patient might contain 500 mg levodopa (Hildick-Smith, 1976a). Those taking less than 750 mg a day of Sinemet 110 or 275 might benefit from changing to Sinemet plus three times daily (Nibbelink et al, 1981; Hoehn, 1980). This latter preparation contains enough carbidopa to provide adequate decarboxylase inhibition and stop persistent nausea.

Madopar (a mixture of the dopa decarboxylase inhibitor benserazide with four parts of levodopa) is roughly equivalent to Sinemet in effectiveness (Barbeau et al, 1972; Diamond et al, 1978; Korten et al, 1975) and produces less initial nausea (Rinne and Molsa, 1975). It is available as:

Madopar 250 (benserazide 50 mg, levodopa 200 mg)
Madopar 125 (benserazide 25 mg, levodopa 100 mg)
Madopar 62.5 (benserazide 12.5 mg, levodopa 50 mg)

Policy on dosage of Sinemet and of Madopar has been changed in the last decade. At first, maximum tolerated dosages were given despite the resultant dyskinesias. Later it seemed that the levodopa benefit period (normally five years or so) depended partly on disease progress and partly on the accumulated levodopa dosage. The present tendency, therefore, is to give the lowest dosage acceptable to the patient. Timing of the dosage can be varied to fit in with physical and social needs. After a night's sleep the serum dopamine level is low, and many patients need their first dose on waking. After a short afternoon sleep, some patients wake refreshed and can wait an hour or two before needing the next tablet.

Depression frequently accompanies Parkinsonism (Mindham et al, 1976) and may need to be treated first. A tetracyclic preparation such as mianserin should be chosen if cardiac and anticholinergic side-effects are to be avoided. Alternatively a tricyclic such as amitryptilene may be given at night for its anticholinergic action if nocturnal incontinence is a problem. An alternative antidepressant nomifensine acts to inhibit dopamine uptake. It seems to have no significant effect on the Parkinsonism but could be useful for concurrent depression. Constipation is frequently a problem, and the patient will need to take bran, stool bulking agents (like Dorbanex), purgatives (Senokot) or enemas and suppositories as necessary.

Nausea and vomiting sometimes occur, even with the combined levodopa preparations. The phenothiazine metoclopramide is not a suitable treatment, as it can itself cause dyskinesias. The newer drug domperidone (20 mg tds) offers a non-phenothiazine alternative.

Decompensated Parkinson's disease

After some years the response of the patient to levodopa begins to fade (Hunter et al, 1973) and there is no agreed method for managing this difficult stage of the patient's illness. Anticholinergic drugs, helpful in younger patients, will probably worsen the situation in the elderly by causing confusion (Caird & Williamson, 1978). Loss of levodopa benefit may first show itself by 'end-of-dose deterioration'. A dose which was previously effective for 3–4 hours loses effect after 2–3 hours. The patient can try to combat this by altering drug timings within the same daily total, or can risk the dyskinesias and other problems which will arise if the total daily dose is increased. Shaw and his colleagues (1980) have shown that 80% of patients suffer from abnormal involuntary movements by this stage of their treatment. 'On-off' — sudden and unpredictable variation in resonse to levodopa — is less common, occurring in 10% of the patients in this study. The on-off complication is reported in up to 50% of patients in high-dose series (Sweet & McDowell, 1975; Marsden & Parkes, 1976) but in only 2.8% in low-dose series (Birkmayer, 1975). In elderly patients the problem appears to be uncommon, perhaps because they have received lower doses. Alternatively the elderly may have a more benign form of the disease, or may die before reaching this late stage of levodopa failure.

The present place of bromocriptine in treatment is in this stage of levodopa failure, since its longer half-life smooths out the uneven levodopa response. This enables the patient to regain benefit on a lower and less toxic levodopa dosage, and this benefit may continue for about two years (Calne et al, 1978). Dosage starts from 1.25 mg a day and increases to 10–20 mg in the elderly, the side-effects of confusion and infrequent dyskinesias being limiting factors. The role of bromocriptine as a first treatment for disabling Parkinsonism is being investigated at maximally-tolerated (Lees & Stern, 1981) and low doses (Teychenne et al, 1981). It may take 15–22 weeks to achieve 39% overall improvement in the patient's condition, and when bromocriptine fails after two years levodopa is ineffective.

Although bromocriptine is only partially successful, it is the most promising of the dopamine agonists now available, as many of those tried have shown unacceptable toxicity. Lisuride 0.6–4.8 a day (plus antiemetic) may prolong benefit for some months after bromocriptine has failed (Schachter et al, 1979). Pergolide (2–5 g a day) can enable toxic doses of levodopa to be reduced (Liebermann et al, 1979). Deprenyl is an inhibitor of monoamine oxidase (type B), which is the enzyme predominantly concerned in the degradation of dopamine. Deprenyl 5–10 mg a day can therefore be used to 'spare' levodopa dosage (Birkmayer, 1978), but benefit has not yet been maintained beyond a few months; the side-effect of confusion may limit its value in the elderly, but it may be a useful advance.

An alternative approach, pioneered by Sweet et al (1972) was the 'drug holiday'. By withdrawing all or part of the levodopa treatment for a week, it was hoped that the nigrostriatal neurones would regain normal sensitivity to the drug. Some workers (Weiner et al, 1981) reported benefit for 6–12 months, but others (Direnfeld et al, 1980) confirmed the dangers of prolonged immobility during the 'holiday'. As these dangers are of particular concern in the elderly, this method of treatment seems unlikely to be of benefit to them.

Terminal Parkinsonism

The excess mortality from Parkinsonism is decreasing (Hoehn & Yahr, 1967; Rinne, 1978) but patients are still dying of the condition, and the terminal stage requires the same care and skilled attention as was needed earlier. Multiple drug regimes should be critically assessed to see whether any medication can be removed, or reduced. All the anti-Parkinsonian drugs can cause confusion. Chlormethiazole is helpful for this, while the phenothiazine most effective (and least harmful) for the aggressive Parkinsonian patient is thioridazine.

While all essential treatment must be given for any condition causing the patient distress, overzealous treatment and investigation should be avoided and the patient given every help to enable him to die with dignity.

REFERENCES

Barbeau A, Mars H, Botez M I, Joubert M 1972 Levodopa combined with peripheral decarboxylase inhibition in Parkinson's disease. Canadian Medical Association Journal 106: 1169–1174

Beattie A, Caird F I 1980 The occupational therapist and the patient with Parkinson's disease. British Medical Journal 280: 1354–1355

Bernheimer H, Birkmayer W, Hornykiewicz O, Jellinger K, Seitelberger F 1965 Zur Differenzierung des Parkinsön-Syndroms. Proceedings of 8th International Congress of Neurology. Medical Academy, Vienna. 145–148

Birkmayer W 1975 Medical treatment of Parkinson's disease: General review past and present In: Birkmayer W, Hornykiewicz O (eds). Advances in Parkinsonism. Roche Scientific Press, Basel p 407–423

Birkmayer W 1978 Longterm treatment with L-deprenyl. Journal of Neural Transmission 43: 239–244

Birkmayer W, Ambrozi L, Neumayer E, Riederer P 1974 Longevity in Parkinson's disease treated with L-dopa. Clinical Neurology and Neurosurgery 1: 15–19

Birkmayer W, Hornykiewicz O 1961 Der L 3, 4 dioxyphenylalanin (=DOPA) Effekt bei der Parkinsonakinese. Wiener Klinische Wochenschrift 73: 787–788

Boller F, Mizutani T, Roessman U, Gambetti P 1979 Parkinson's disease, dementia and Alzheimer disease: clinico-pathological correlations. Annals of Neurology 7: 329–335

Bowen D M, Davison A N 1978 Biochemical changes in the normal ageing brain. In: Isaacs B (ed) Recent Advances in Geriatric Medicine 1. Churchill Livingstone, Edinburgh p 54–59

Brewis M, Poskanzer D C, Rolland C, Miller H 1962 Neurological disease in an English city. Acta Neurologica Scandanavica 42: 31–36

Broe G A, Caird F I 1973 Levodopa for Parkinsonism in elderly and demented patients. Medical Journal of Australia 1: 630–635

Caird F I, Williamson J 1978 Drugs for Parkinson's disease. Lancet 1: 986

Calne D B, Plotkin C, Williams A C, Nutt J G, Neophytides A, Teychenne P F 1978 Longterm treatment of Parkinsonism with bromocriptine. Lancet 1: 735–738

Carlsson A, Gottfries C-G, Svennerholm L, Adolfson R, Oreland L, Winblad B, Aquilonius S-M 1980 Neurotransmitters in human brain analysed post-mortem. In: Rinne U K, Klinger M, Stamm G (eds) Parkinson's Disease — current progress, problems and management. Elsevier North Holland Medical Press, Amsterdam, New York p 121–133

Davis J C 1977 Team management of Parkinson's disease. American Journal of Occupational Therapy 31: 300–308

Diamond S G, Markham C H, Treciokas L J 1978 A double-blind comparison of levodopa, madopar & sinemet in Parkinson's disease. Annals of Neurology 3: 267–272

Direnfeld L K, Feldman R G, Alexander M P, Kelly-Hayes M 1980 Is L-dopa drug holiday useful? Neurology 30: 785–788

Ehringer H, Hornykiewicz O 1960 Verteilung von Noradrenalin und Dopamin im Gehirn des Menschen und ihr Verhalten bei Erkrankungen des extrapyramidalen Systems. Klinische Wochenschrift 38: 1236–1239

Flewitt B, Capildeo R, Rose F C 1981 Physiotherapy and assessment in Parkinson's disease using the polarised light goniometer. In: Rose F C, Capildeo R (eds) Research Progress in Parkinson's Disease. Pitman, London p 404–413

Franklyn S, Kohout L J, Stern G M, Dunning M 1981 Physiotherapy in Parkinson's disease. In: Rose F C, Capildeo R (eds) Research Progress in Parkinson's Disease. Pitman, London p 397–400

Franklyn S, Stern G M 1981 Controlled trial of physiotherapy and occupational therapy for Parkinson's disease. British Medical Journal 282: 1969–1970

Gibberd F B, Page N G R, Spencer K M, Kinnear E, Hawksworth J B 1981 Controlled trial of physiotherapy and occupational therapy for Parkinson's disease. British Medical Journal 282: 1196

Godwin-Austen R B 1971 Parkinson's disease. Parkinson's Disease Society, London

Godwin-Austen R B, Hildick-Smith M 1982 Parkinson's Disease — a General Practitioner's Guide. Franklyn Scientific Publications, London

Godwin-Austen R B, Lee P N, Marmot M G, Stern G M 1982 Smoking and Parkinson's disease. Journal of Neurology. Neurosurgery and Psychiatry 45: 577–581

Gudmundsson K R 1967 A clinical survey of Parkinsonism in Iceland. Acta Neurologica Scandanavica 43: 1–61

Hakim A M, Mathieson G 1979 Dementia in Parkinson's disease: a neuropathologic study. Neurology 29: 1209–1214

Hildick-Smith M 1976a Alternatives to levodopa. British Medical Journal 1: 1406

Hildick-Smith M 1976b Assessing dementia in the older Parkinsonian patient. Modern Geriatrics 6: 33–39

Hodkinson H M 1972 Evaluation of a mental test score for assessment of mental impairment in the elderly. Age & Ageing 1: 233–238

Hoehn M M 1980 Increased dosage of carbidopa in patients with Parkinson's disease receiving low doses of levodopa. Archives of Neurology 37: 146–149

Hoehn M M, Yahr M D 1967 Parkinsonism: onset, progression and mortality. Neurology 17: 427–442

Hunter K R, Laurence D R, Shaw K M, Stern G M 1973 Sustained levodopa therapy in Parkinsonism. Lancet ii: 929–931

Korten J J, Keyser A, Joosten M G, Gabreels F J M 1975 Madopar vs. Sinemet. European Neurology 13: 65–71

Kurland L T 1958 In: W S Fields (ed) Pathogenesis and treatment of Parkinsonism. Charles C Thomas, Springfield, Illinois p 5–49

Lees A J, Stern G M 1981 Sustained bromocriptine therapy in previously untreated patients with Parkinson's disease. Research & Clinical Forums 3: 29–32

Liebermann A N, Liebowitz M, Neophytides A, Kupersmith M, Mehl S, Kleinberg D, Serby M, Goldstein M 1979 Pergolide and lisuride for Parkinson's disease. Lancet ii: 1129–1130

Loranger A W, Goodell H, McDowell F H, Lee J E, Sweet R D 1972 Intellectual impairment in Parkinson's syndrome. Brain 95: 405–412

Mann D M A, Yates P O 1982 Pathogenesis of Parkinson's disease. Archives of Neurology 39: 545–549

Marsden C D 1980 'On-off' phenomenon in Parkinson's disease. In: Rinne U K, Klinger M, Stamm G (eds) Parkinson's disease, current progress, problems and management. Elsevier North Holland Medical Press, Amsterdam, New York p 241–254

Marsden C D, Parkes J D, Rees J E 1973 A year's comparison of treatment of patients with Parkinson's disease with levodopa combined with carbidopa versus treatment with levodopa alone. Lancet ii: 1459–1462

Marsden C D, Parkes J D 1976 'On-off' effects in patients with Parkinson's disease on chronic levodopa therapy. Lancet i: 292–296

Martin W E, Loewenson R B, Resch J A, Baker A B 1973 Parkinson's disease. Clinical analysis of 100 patients. Neurology 23: 783–790

Mindham R H S, Marsden C D, Parkes J D 1976 Psychiatric symptoms during L-dopa therapy for Parkinson's disease and their relationship to physical disability. Psychological Medicine 6: 23–33

Nibbelink D W, Bauer R, Hoehn M, Muenter M, Stellar S, Berman R 1981 Sinemet 25:100 In: Rose F C, Capildeo R (eds) Research Progress in Parkinson's Disease. Pitman, London p 226–232

Oxtoby M 1981 Parkinson's Disease patients and their social needs. Parkinson's Disease Society, London

Parkes J D, Marsden C D, Rees J E, Curzon G, Katamaneni B D, Knill-Jones R, Akbar A, Das S, Kataria M 1974 Parkinson's disease, cerebral arteriosclerosis & senile dementia. Quartery Journal of Medicine 43: 49–61

Pearce J 1974 Mental changes in Parkinsonism. British Medical Journal 2: 445

Rinne U K 1978 Recent advances in research on Parkinsonism. Acta Neurologica Scandinavica 57: 77–113

Rinne U K, Molsa P 1979 Levodopa with benserazide or carbidopa in Parkinson's disease. Neurology 29: 1584–1589

Rossor M N 1981 Parkinson's disease and Alzheimer's disease as disorders of the isodendritic core. British Medical Journal 283: 1588–1590

Schachter M, Blackstock J, Dick J P E, George R J D, Marsden C D, Parkes J D 1979 Lisuride in Parkinson's disease. Lancet ii: 1129

Scott S, Caird F I 1981 Speech therapy for patients with Parkinson's disease. British Medical Journal 280: 1354–1355

Shaw K M, Lees A J, Stern G M 1980 The impact of treatment with levodopa on Parkinson's disease. Quarterly Journal of Medicine 49: 283–293

Singer E 1973 Social costs of Parkinson's disease. Journal of Chronic Diseases 26: 243–254

Steiner P, Flewitt B 1981 Controlled trial of physiotherapy and occupational therapy for Parkinson's disease. British Medical Journal 282: 1970

Sutcliffe R L G 1973 L-dopa therapy in elderly patients with Parkinsonism. Age & Ageing 2: 34–38

Sweet R D, Lee J E, Spiegel H E, McDowell F 1972 Enhanced response to low doses of levodopa after withdrawal from chronic treatment. Neurology 22: 520–525

Sweet R D, McDowell F H 1975 Five years' treatment of Parkinson's disease with levodopa: therapeutic results and survival of 100 patients. Annals of Internal Medicine 83: 456–463

Teychenne P F, Bergsrud D, Racy A, Vern B 1981 Low-dose bromocriptine therapy in Parkinson's disease. Research & Clinical Forums 3: 37–47

Vignalou J, Beck H 1973 La L-dopa chez 122 Parkinsoniens de plus de 70 ans. Gerontologia Clinica 15: 50–64

Weiner W J, Koller W C, Perlik S, Nausieda P A, Klawans H L 1981 The role of transient levodopa withdrawal (drug holiday) in the management of Parkinson's disease. In: Rose F C, Capildeo R (eds) Research Progress in Parkinson's Disease. Pitman, London p 275–281

White N J, Barnes T R E 1981 Senile Parkinsonism, a survey of current treatment. Age & Ageing 10: 81–86

Yahr M 1982 In Parkinsonism: recent advances. International Medicine supplement 3. Franklyn Scientific publications, London

18

Falls

B. Isaacs

The Giants of Geriatrics is the name given to the symptoms by which so much disease in advanced old age is manifest (Isaacs, 1976). These are immobility, instability, incontinence and intellectual impairment. Of these instability, the tendency to recurrent falls, is one of the commonest, the most frightening and the least understood.

In this chapter I shall present:

1. clinical and epidemiological information on falls in old people;

2. a discussion of causes and possible mechanisms;

3. some suggestions for prevention and management.

NATURE OF FALLS

A fall results when the vertical line which passes through the centre of mass of the human body comes to lie beyond the support base and correction does not take place in time.

Six stages of human development can be considered at which falls occur in different ways, reflecting changes in human behaviour with age; and a rise, a plateau and a decline in the efficiency of the correcting mechanism.

1. The *infant* exploring his environment falls frequently because he is unaware of the tolerable levels of displacement and his corrective mechanism is immature.

2. The *child* seeking adventure falls frequently because, through inexperience and imprudence, he exceeds the capacity of his corrective mechanism.

3. The *adolescent,* engaging in sport, falls infrequently despite large and rapid displacements and unstable support bases, because he has trained his corrective mechanism to a high pitch.

4. The *middle-aged* falls only in extremely hazardous environmental conditions because normally he keeps his displacing activity to within the limits of his well tested corrective ability.

5 The *young old person* falls occasionally because he imprudently indulges in activities involving large and rapid displacements, of which he was once capable but which now exceed the capacity of his corrective mechanisms.

(This was expressed by Lewis Carroll in his lines:

'And yet you persistantly stand on your head

Do you think at your age it is right?')

6 The *multiple disabled old* fall frequently because the efficiency of the balance mechanism has so declined that even small self-induced displacements cannot be corrected in time.

Results of falling

Most falls result in no injury or disability and are not reported to physicians. They are dismissed as trivial and they are not well recalled. The probability of sustaining injury depends substantially on the speed and force of the impact with the ground which in turn is affected by the speed of action preceding the fall. Paradoxically those most likely to suffer injury are those who were moving rapidly at the time of the fall and who are thus capable of rapid movement. Falls without injury may thus represent a graver disturbance of the balance mechanism than falls which result in fracture.

EPIDEMIOLOGY OF FALLS

Information is available about the number of fractures in the community as a whole and about the number of falls in isolated sections, such as patients in hospitals and residents in nursing homes. There is little acceptable information about the incidence of falls among elderly people living at home, but there are useful indications of who are the vulnerable population.

Fractures

Garraway (1979) provided complete figures for all fractures in the population of Rochester Minnesota. For fractures of the lower limb he demonstrated an exponential increase with age, with almost twice as many fractures occurring in females as in males. Similar findings were reported from the United Kingdom by Evans et al (1979), who showed that the incidence of fracture of the proximal femur doubled approximately every seven years after the age of 65, and that by the age of 90 one woman in four had already suffered this fracture. The incidence was twice as high in women as in men.

For fractures of the upper limb Garraway demonstrated a steady rise till the age of 75, after which the incidence dropped. This contrast between upper and lower limb fractures is intriguing and may well mean that in later life the falling subject is unable to put out a hand to protect himself in time because of slowing of the reflex, and in consequence strikes the ground first with the lower limb.

Hospital in-patients

Falls are of common occurrence in the very frail population of geriatric wards. Accident reports, required for insurance purposes, reveal that in 80% of these falls there is no injury, and the dreaded fracture of the femur occurs in only 1% (Morris & Isaacs, 1980). Falls in hospital are most likely to occur during the early stages of rehabilitation, particulary in stroke illness, when patients are anxious to retain independence and have not yet come to terms with their impaired balance. The lowest incidence of falls is in continuing care wards where patients have lost their sense of adventure. The incidence of falls in the geriatric hospital population is 422 per 1000 patient bed days. (Morris & Isaacs, 1980).

Nursing homes

The more active populations of Nursing Homes in the United States and Residential Homes in the United Kingdom have an incidence of falling of approximately twice this level (Gryfe et al, 1977, Wild & Isaacs, 1981). Contributing to the average is a small number of patients who fall frequently and who may be pre-terminal. Community studies show a somewhat lower incidence of falls than this (Overstall, 1978).

Falls as a cause of admission

In a study of emergency admissions to a geriatric unit, patients with recurrent falls comprised 16% and patients who were admitted immediately following a fall, usually having been found lying on the floor, accounted for 21% of admissions (O'Beirn, 1984; Wadwha, 1982). Amongst people admitted to Residential Homes in the United Kingdom (somewhat similar to American Nursing Homes) many were admitted because of anxiety about their sustaining falls at home, or because they had already fallen (Wild & Isaacs, 1981).

CAUSES AND MECHANISMS OF FALLS

All sorts of things can cause a fall, and invariably more than one factor is operating at a time. However, people with recurrent falls usually have a continuing cause or causes. A scheme for the elucidation of the causes of recurrent falls in old people is now presented (Fig. 18.1).

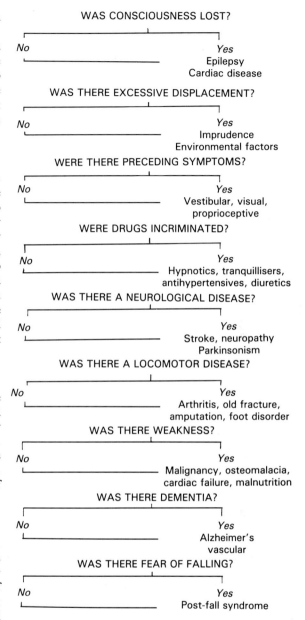

Fig. 18.1   Causation of recurrent falls

1. Was consciousness lost?

Did the patient lose consciousness? And if so, was this before or after the fall? A direct question may fail to give a clear answer but the following clues may be helpful:

(i) If the patient says 'I had a blackout' this usually means, in the United Kingdom anyway, loss of consciousness. Occasionally a 'blackout' is a visual experience of greying or obscurity of both visual fields, and is then attributable to focal ischaemia in basilar artery territory.

(ii) The phrases 'I was out' or 'I went out' usually signify loss of consciousness and, since retrograde amnesia is not a feature, the patient can usually describe what was happening immediately before the fall.

Causes of momentary loss of consciousness include:

Epilepsy

This is usually diagnosed from the history and from the statement of an observer. The electro-encephalogram (EEG) is not very helpful. Epilepsy originating in late life is not unusual and is seldom sinister.

Circulatory disturbances

The likeliest cause of transient loss of consciousness in old age is a transient disturbance of the cerebral circulation induced by a fall in cardiac output or an error in blood distribution. The causes are:

(i) cardiac dysrhythmia: heart block; sinus bradycardia; 'sick sinus' syndrome

(ii) obstruction of the cardiac outlet i.e. aortic stenosis; myxoma of the left atrium; hypertrophic cardiomyopathy

(iii) postural hypotension

(iv) carotid sinus hypersensitivity.

Cardiac dysrhythmia is diagnosed by finding sinus bradycardia, heart block or 'sick sinus' syndrome in an ordinary electrocardiogram (ECG). When these are not evident and a cardiac cause is suspected because of lack of any other explanation, it is usual to proceed to a 24 hour tape-recorded ECG. These are frequently rich with abnormalities (Rai, 1982) and it becomes a problem to determine the relationship between the abnormalities and the symptoms suffered by the patient (Zelois et al, 1980). If the patient registers symptoms at the same time as a dysrhythmia is evident the problem is solved, and it is usual to proceed to the insertion of a trial pacemaker. If, as is more usual, no such relationship can be demonstrated, 'significant' rhythm disturbances should be treated. These include periods of bradycardia; frequent multifocal ventricular extra systoles; ventricular tachycardia, and supra-ventricular tachycardia (McCarthy & Wollner, 1977). Atrial fibrillation alone does not cause transient loss of consciousness.

Cerebral ischaemia of cardiac origin causes general rather than focal symptoms. In doubtful cases medical management of a rhythm disturbance with appropriate arrhythmic drugs should be undertaken and may indeed relieve the patient of his disturbances of consciousness.

Postural hypotension. The autoregulatory mechanisms of the cardiovascular system, notably the baroreceptor, are inefficient in late life (Collins et al, 1980). Changing from the sitting to the standing position frequently results in a drop of systolic blood pressure in excess of 20 mm of mercury (Caird et al, 1973). This does not however as a rule cause a reduction in cerebral blood flow, and the mere demonstration of a drop of this magnitude is insufficient to attribute a fall on positional change to postural hypotension. Indeed falls of blood pressure much greater than this seem to occur during normal activity without causing symptoms. In a few patients however with jeopardised cerebral circulation a change of position causes postural hypotension with reduction in cerebral blood flow, loss of consciousness and a fall. Falls may also occur without loss of consciousness as a result of this condition. The fall does not necessarily occur at the time of positional change but may be delayed for a few moments so that the patient falls while walking after rising from the chair.

Loss of consciousness may also result from excessive sensitivity of the carotid sinus, which is a rare but definite phenomenon in old people attributed to the presence of atherosclerotic plaques adjacent to the receptor site. The fall may occur during shaving or by the rubbing of a collar against the appropriate part of the neck, but the condition must be rare.

Extra demand on the heart as a result of exercise may fail to elicit an adequate response. Cerebral circulation drops and a fall may then occur with or without loss of consciousness. A common example is when a patient with aortic stenosis climbs stairs and falls down the staircase while climbing up.

2. Was there excessive displacement?

Displacement is of two types – initiated and imposed – and can be thought of as *normal* or *excessive*.

Normal initiated displacements comprise the activities of daily living carried out at the subject's usual pace i.e. getting out of bed, rising from a chair, walking, dressing and sitting down. In all of these instability is induced but immediately corrected and falls are avoided.

Excessive initiated displacements occur when ordinary activities are conducted in haste or without preparation; or when actions are undertaken imprudently which exceed the reduced capacity of the balance system. Examples are suddenly turning the head in response to a sound signal or rising precipitately from a chair when the telephone or doorbell rings; or hanging out wet blankets on a high clothes line.

Normal imposed displacements refer to the unexpected events that pepper everyday activities but which are usually performed without falling. These include being jostled in a crowd, standing on a bus, tripping on a curb or being buffeted by the wind.

Excessive imposed displacements are those which are beyond the capacity of the normal balance system to correct, except when there has been special training or experience. The ordinary person might be exposed to an excessive displacement if the foot was placed on a treacherous surface during rapid movement.

The patient should always be asked where he was at the time of the fall and what he was doing. He will usually answer 'nothing' to the latter question, but persistent interrogation should reveal the type of displacement and this, together with an examination of the balance (see below) will permit apportionment of the cause of the fall between extrinsic and intrinsic factors.

3. Were there symptoms?

Questioners are required not to put words into the patient's mouth. Patients may have difficulty in recalling exactly what happened but they may feel obligated to devise an explanation and may be happy to say 'I must have tripped' or 'I must have been dizzy' even when they have no recollection of being so. It is difficult for the patient to accept that he might have fallen without adequate cause.

Despite this many patients emphatically state that they had no warning symptoms and 'just fell'. Others do however describe, with a variety of words and phrases, a sense of instability which preceded and may have been responsible for the fall. Sometimes it is as though they had been 'pushed from behind'. Others use words such as 'dizzy', 'giddy' (incidentally these words have opposite meanings in British and American English) to describe a sense of instability. What seems to be sensed is a relative movement between the subject and the environment, and it matters little whether this is described as a sense of rotation or a sense of the room spinning. The movement may be in any direction. It is frightening and it may be succeeded by the visual and proprioceptive sensation of falling. The patient often conveys more information by gesture than by words, representing a rotatory movement with a broad wave of the hand and a sense of instability by a horizontal sweep of the hand.

The cause of this sense of instability is speculative. It seems likely however to be due to a lack of congruity between information about the position and movement of the subject in space derived from the three major sources of vestibular, proprioceptive and visual receptors. Disease in any of these may produce conflict which creates this sense of unease.

Disturbance of proprioception may result from abnormalities in the mechanoreceptor system present in the capsule of the apophyseal joints of the cervical spine, which are frequently defective in old people (Wyke, 1979).

End-organ disease of the vestibule is a common occurrence in late life. The disease may affect the otoliths which become fragmented and detached, setting up abnormal signal patterns in the hair cells; or it may originate from other pathological changes in the vestibules.

In the moving subject visual orientation plays a major part in the control of balance, with the peripheral retinal field being particularly important. In elderly patients with visual disorder, especially chronic glaucoma, a defective visual input may contribute to the sense of instability.

Vertebral basilar ischaemia

Recurrent falls are sometimes attributed to this condition. The view that turning the head, in the presence of cervical spondylosis, may obstruct the flow of blood through the vertebral artery and cause the patient to fall has been exaggerated. It must be only very rarely that this mechanism causes falls. In any case, if the vertebral artery were to be occluded the patient would suffer symptoms of the lateral medullary syndrome which includes transient weakness of one or more limbs, paraesthesiae in the limbs, circum-oral paraesthesiae, transient dysarthria and perhaps ocular paresis. In the absence of these symptoms and signs, the diagnosis should not be supported.

4. Were drugs incriminated?

The ability to correct displacement is highly time-dependent. Any slowing of the flow of information from proprioceptors in the muscles, tendons and joints, from the vestibules and the eyes to the brain, their processing there and the dispatch of corrective instructions back to the muscles may delay the corrective movement until it is too late.

Unfortunately old people are exposed to many drugs which number among their effects the slowing of central conduction in the nervous system. These include not only hypnotics, sedatives and tranquillisers but also a group of drugs which are often prescribed for the symptom of 'dizziness'. Drugs used in Parkinsonism may also slow corrective mechanisms.

Another group of drugs which may be incriminated in falls are those which impair the circulatory adjustments to posture change. These include drugs with antihypertensive effects, both those given for the purpose of reducing the blood pressure and those in which a fall in blood pressure is a side effect. Prominent among these are diuretics and antidepressents.

As in all branches of geriatric medicine the removal of offending drugs is often the most efficacious and the most satisfying method of relieving symptoms.

6. Was there a neurological disease?

Most falls occur while walking. Locomotion is normally a sequence of regularly repeated and predictable movements which are modified slightly to conform to the perceived variations in the environment.

In a number of neurological diseases the rhythmicity and regularity of stepping is affected such that the legs make unplanned contact with one another or with the ground, thus perturbing the trunk and endangering stability. Stroke, recent and old, is thus a common accompaniment of falls, especially when there is a drop-foot deformity, or when proprioception is lost, as is commonly the case in a left hemiplegia. Weakness of the legs and failure to raise the feet is a factor also in peripheral neuropathy, multiple sclerosis and other neurological system diseases. In Parkinson's disease the stepping mechanism is wholly disordered. A feature of this condition is the sudden unexpected arrest of the stepping sequence. If, at the time of the arrest, the patient is about to make heel contact with the ground, he is liable to fall straight back; whereas if his stepping arrests while his forefeet are making contact he will rotate forwards. A good rule is that a patient with two black eyes has probably got Parkinsonism.

7. Was there a locomotor disease?

Stiff and painful joints modify the gait pattern and may cause a patient to place his foot on the ground in an inappropriate position and at an inappropriate stage of the walking cycle. Compounding this is the fact that arthritis destroys the proprioceptive mechanism of the joint and limits information about the position of the limb which reaches the brain. Stiffness also slows corrective responses to incorrect foot placement. Many people who fall and who have no other obvious cause are found to have arthritis of the hips and/or knees; and it is rather tempting, although there is no direct evidence, to attribute the falls to this abnormality.

Patients with gross structural abnormalities of the foot have an inefficient platform on which to support the body, and occasionally this may be responsible for falls.

8. Was there weakness?

A high proportion of old people who fall are ill, and those who fall experience an excess mortality in the year after the fall which cannot be a direct consequence of the fall itself (Wild et al, 1981b). Recurrent falling may thus be a signal of widespread impaired function and generalised weakness. This can be caused by any disease or combination of diseases common in late life, including malignant disease, malnutrition, cardiac failure and anaemia. The fairly common condition of osteomalacia, aggravated by remaining housebound, is believed to weaken the muscles and thereby cause falls.

9. Was there dementia?

Dementia is not in itself a cause of falling, indeed many demented patients wander large distances without coming to grief. Nonetheless, cerebral mechanisms may play a part in balance and their impairment in Alzheimer's disease may contribute to instability.

10. Was there fear of falling?

One of the commonest causes of falls is falls; that is to say that the experience of having fallen in the past generates anxiety, inhibits normal movement patterns and yields a picture of excessive anxiety and instability which has been called the post-fall syndrome (Murphy & Isaacs, 1982). The

patients with this syndrome characteristically grab and clutch at any object in sight and seem wholly incapable of independent progression when examined on the ward round. Characteristically, as the group of doctors moves on to the next patient, they can be seen to move smartly off independently in the direction of the bathroom or dayroom. The mechanism which inhibits normal gait performance has not been identified; but patients with this syndrome, at least in its more severe form, when independent walking is not at all posssible, suffer a very high mortality.

11. Did they just fall?

There remains a group of people who 'just fall' for no apparent reason and in whom no obvious cause can be detected. Investigation of this group has been entensive but entirely negative. Speculation that the mechanism might be transient ischaemia of the spinal cord with resultant transient paraparesis is unproven. Little is gained by calling these falls 'drop attacks' which conveys the spurious view that a diagnosis has been made. Prolonged follow-up may lead to elucidation of the cause but no studies have been reported.

EXAMINATION OF THE PATIENT

The examination of the patient with recurrent falls embraces, in addition to the clinical areas referred to above, the following special tests:

1. Static balance

The patient is observed standing, with legs apart then together, and with eyes open then closed. The observer should look for sway in the antero-posterior plane. This is just visible in normal subjects but is very obvious in those with impaired postural control.

A provocative test of static balance is to stand behind the subject and gently press on the sternum. In normal subjects this produces no response; but in those with balance disorder there is a marked sway backwards, and there may be corrective movements of the arm or staggering movements of the feet.

2. Posture

Patients with instability may stand with the knees and hips flexed, and especially with curvature of the upper dorsal spine accompanied by either an excessive cervical lordosis or by forward flexion of the head on to the trunk. The line joining the outer canthus of the eye to the external auditory meatus, which is usually a few degrees above the horizontal, becomes horizontal or even falls below the horizontal line.

3. Standing up

Observe the patient standing up from a chair. This is a good way of detecting patients whose falls are due to general weakness, and those who are unable to programme sequential movements properly. Many patients reveal instability when they attain the upright position.

4. Gait

Observation of gait aids greatly in the elucidation of the cause of the falls. As already stated it is the qualitative aspects of the gait which yield most information. Gait analysis in the laboratory reveals that the common associates of falling are increased variability of the length of successive steps, and an increase in the proportion of the total stride time that is spent in double support. However, simple gait speed seems to be as informative as any other observation, and it can easily be measured by recording with a stopwatch the time taken by the patient to walk betwen two marked points in the ward or physiotherapy department. In general gait speeds of less than 50 cm per second are indicative of gross disturbance of the balance mechanism.

The Get-Up-and-Go test gives a simple quantitative measure of efficiency of balance and walking, the result of which correlates well with gait speed and with outcome. The subject is simply asked to stand up out of a chair, to stand still for a few seconds, to walk two or three metres, to turn round, to return to the chair and sit down. The test is divided into five parts, for each of which a mark of two is awarded if the task if performed correctly, a mark of one if it is performed independently but incorrectly and a mark of nothing if it cannot be performed without help. The five elements are: rising; standing still; walking; turning and sitting down.

MANAGEMENT OF PATIENTS WITH RECURRENT FALLS

The establishment of a diagnosis and treatment of the causes are the most important factors in the management of the patient with recurrent falls; but in many cases specific treatment is unavailable and efforts must be made to improve the performance of the patient. A central need is to improve the patient's confidence in his own ability to remain upright throughout a range of daily activities.

Correction of the environment

Patients should be provided with well-fitting shoes with standard low heels. There are many simple sensible points about the type of floor surface, the arrangement of furniture, the lighting levels, the height of chairs, the types of upholstery and cushion, the height of the bed and the arrangement of floor coverings, which can be seen in almost any home to require correction. Experience indicates that relatives are very reluctant to change anything in the environment at the request of a visiting physician. Nonetheless attempts are always worth making to enlist allies to render the environment as safe and convenient as possible.

Some patients are addicted to walking frames or to clutching on to the furniture as they move around the house. However undesirable this may seem it is usually impossible to wean them from the habit, and in a sense they are safer progressing in this way and have to be allowed to do so.

For patients who have only recently fallen and whose balance system is still reasonably intact the use of walking frames is illogical. This alters the body posture and the pattern of walking, and prevents restoration of balance and proper locomotion.

Training the patient

Patients perform best in a large space with no object obstructing the visual field. They should be encouraged to walk with confidence and should be supported if at all necessary by a hand held lightly in front of them. Support from behind is not visible to the patient and more readily prevents falls should balance be lost. However, many patients when supported from the back will lean further backwards. Sometimes manoeuvres are required to bring the weight forward. Some patients behave as though they experience a sensation of falling forwards, and lean backwards to correct this. When they are straightened up they immediately feel as though they are again falling forwards and take further steps ostensibly to correct this, but in fact leading to a further leaning back syndrome. For the treatment of this mysterious phenomenon recourse is sometimes had to raising the heel of the shoe by two or three centimetres or placing weights in a belt or apron worn on the front of the body to try and move the centre of mass forwards. The condition is sometimes self-correcting.

The aim should be to increase walking speed because, as with cycling, the more rapidly the patient walks, within limits, the safer he appears to be. Stair climbing is no real problem for patients with balance disorders so long as they have the necessary movement and a bannister to hold on to.

Patients should practise transfers from bed to chair, from chair to tiolet and so on. Patients who are at risk of falling and who have demonstrated an inability to rise without assistance should unashamedly be taught how to get up in the event of a further fall. Far from this frightening them it gives them confidence. The technique is to train the patient, after falling, to turn on to the side and to bend up one knee. From this position they should be able to roll on to that knee and to bring up the second knee until they are kneeling. They may then be able to crawl or to reach out for a nearby chair and pull themselves towards it. It is then just a matter of rotating the trunk, pressing down with one foot and hoisting the bottom on to the chair. Relatives and nurses should be taught to use the same technique and should never haul a patient to his feet if he falls.

PROGNOSIS

Falls occurring outdoors in active people and not resulting in bone injury are trivial and have no adverse effect on function. Falls occuring outdoors which result in fracture present only a mechanical problem to the orthopaedic surgeon, and when the fracture has been repaired the patient himself is intact and able to function well.

Falls occurring indoors, with or without fracture, in a patient who was already disabled or housebound, carry serious significance. One-third of patients who fall in these circumstances die within the year. One-third of the remainder continue to have intermittent falls. The prognosis is particularly grave for patients who fall and lie on the floor all night, or even for more than one hour, without being able to rise or to attract attention. Patients of this type experience a 50% mortality within three months of the fall.

CONCLUSION

Falls range in severity from the trivial to the mortal; and in causation from a wet floor to an erratic heart. They become increasingly common in very advanced age and may at any time lead to that major disaster, a fractured neck of femur. A small but significant proportion of these falls need not have happened, and there are some opportunities for active intervention. As our knowledge grows of proprioceptive, vestibular and visual function in the elderly and their interrelationship in the control of balance, new diagnostic and therapeutic opportunities will present themselves.

REFERENCES

Caird F I, Andrews G R, Kennedy R D 1973 Effect of posture on blood pressure in the elderly. British Heart Journal 35: 527–530

Collins K J, Exton-Smith A N, James M H, Oliver D J 1980 Functional changes in autonomic nervous responses with ageing. Age and Ageing 9: 17–24

Evans J G, Prudham D, Wandless I 1979 A prospective study of fractured proximal femur: incidence and outcome. Public Health 93: 235–241

Garraway W M, Stauffer R N, Kurland L T, O'Fallon W M 1979 Limb fractures in a defined population. I – Frequency and distribution. Mayo Clinic Proceedings 54: 701–707

Gryfe C I, Amies A, Adhley M J 1977 A longitudinal study of falls in an elderly population: I Incidence and morbidity. Age and Ageing 6: 201–210

Isaacs B 1976 The giants of geriatrics: a review of symptoms in old age. University of Birmingham: Inaugural lecture

McCarthy S T, Wollner L 1979 Cardiac dysrhythmias: treatable causes of transient cerebral dysfunction in the elderly. Lancet 2: 202–203

Morris E V, Isaacs B 1980 The prevention of falls in a geriatric hospital. Age and Ageing 9: 181–185

Murphy J, Isaacs B 1982 The post-fall syndrome: a study of 36 elderly patients. Gerontology 28: 265–270

O'Beirn D 1984 Falls as a cause of admission to a geriatric unit. In press

Overstall P W 1978 Falls in the elderly: epidemiology, aetiology and management. In: Isaacs B (ed) Recent Advances in Geriatric Medicine I. Churchill Livingstone, Edinburgh

Rai G S 1982 Cardiac arrhythmias in the elderly. Age and Ageing 11: 113–115

Wild D, Nayak U S L, Isaacs B 1981a. How dangerous are falls in old people at home? British Medical Journal 282: 266–268

Wild D, Nayak U S L, Isaacs B 1981b. Prognosis of falls in old people at home. Journal of Epidemiology and Community Health 35: 200–204

Wild D, Isaacs B 1981 A prospective study of falls in Residential Homes. Report to the Department of Health and Social Services, University of Birmingham

Wyke B 1979 Cervical articular contribution to posture and gait: their relation to senile disequilibrium. Age and Ageing 8: 251–258

Zeldis S M, Levine B J, Michelson E L, Morganroth J 1980 Cardiovascular complaints, correlation with cardiac arrhythmia and 24-hour electrocardiographic monitoring. Chest 78: 456–462

19

Visual disorders

P. A. Gardiner

NORMAL AGING PROCESSES

Certain visual changes occur virtually universally in middle life and appear to be governed by a biological clock of considerable accuracy. Tales of the very aged with perfect vision at all distances in each eye are seldom true. Many may be satisfied with a degree of defect and are happy to be without glasses but adequacy is not perfection.

In Western races there are changes in everyone connected with near vision which occur between the ages of 40 and 65. These changes arise from gradual hardening of the lens making it less and less responsive to the ciliary muscle. As a result reading small print and other forms of near work are affected. In previously normal eyes glasses become necessary, in previously hypermetropic eyes glasses need to be strengthened and in previously myopic eyes (particularly in the lower degrees) glasses may have to be discarded for near work. This process is gradual and usually complete by the age of 65. Glasses in healthy eyes will provide total compensation.

Those who perform all visual tasks normally without glasses usually have 2–3 dioptres of myopia (sometimes more) in one eye only and have a normal refraction in the other. These people who seemingly retain visual youth do so by using their myopic eye for near work and their normal eye for everything else. Binocularity is sacrificed but is seldom a significant handicap.

Significant changes in vision after the age of 65 are no longer likely to have a predominantly optical cause and the equation 'Change in eyesight = Need for change in glasses' no longer holds good as often as in younger people. Pathological or degenerative processes of a more complicated kind are much more frequently associated with visual symptoms in this age group which cannot be so easily remedied by glasses. Deterioration is more likely to be continuous. For this reason trial and error selection of glasses is even more foolish than at younger ages. Many of the elderly cannot understand this fundamental change in the source of their visual disorder and search vainly for better glasses.

In addition to these normal optical changes, with advancing age there are changes in the pupil which commonly affect visual performance. Both its size and its agility change. There is a decrease in its diameter which reduces the amount of light reaching the retina. Therefore for a given task more illumination is needed than previously. The elderly often express this as failing vision towards the end of the day.

Secondly the pupil responds more slowly to changes in illumination so that the elderly are easily dazzled or confused by sudden changes (as in night driving). Adaptation from light to dark and vice versa is also impaired which has particular relevance to the lighting of hallways, stairs and passages in their homes (see page 168).

MAJOR PROBLEMS

These later changes occur in people whose cerebration and speed of general reflex response are likely to be diminished. Large numbers become visually handicapped and accident prone. The prevention of this state of affairs has many aspects but attention to the following factors is relevant. More than other sections of the population the elderly fail to report visual deterioration; fail to keep appointments (initially or on recall); fail to accept advice and fail to carry out treatment.

Attitudes to visual handicap
Blindness is the great fear amongst the elderly when visual deterioration is first noticed, whether expressed or not. It underlies all sorts of pointless change in use of the eyes such as using large print instead of small, curtailing T.V. viewing, giving up sewing and so on, in the mistaken belief that these are measures which conserve sight. It is well that the physician should recognise this and take every opportunity to encourage the patient and his relatives to abandon such restrictive ideas. However poor, every scrap of vision is there to be used as normally as possible. Relatives need to be forbidden to use the phrase 'You will ruin your eyes if . . .'. One component of the problem is the traditional attitude of the doctor as well as his patient's. If a patient does decide to seek advice about his vision he will normally consult an optician. He may well fail to report

this to his doctor, maybe in fear, maybe because he feels that visual changes are minor compared with his other complaints or even that it is no business of the doctor's! He may reason that failure by the optician to find effective glasses is in the nature of aging. Conversely the patient will often fail to report to the optician any physical disease or medical treatment. If he does report then the account is likely to be garbled resulting in an inadequate opinion. Doctors reinforce this if they adopt a disinterested role. To wait for a complaint of a specific disorder is, in this context, inadequate in terms of prevention of handicap. Preventable deterioration for these reasons may even occur in hospital if visual changes are not complained of by the patient whose major illness dominates his concern (Price, 1983). A particularly vulnerable group is the housebound amongst whom visual deterioration often passes unnoticed especially in its early stages.

Amelioration of the problem rests on the education of doctors and the public over a wide range of changed attitudes, one of these being that prevention requires detection.

SYMPTOMS OF REDUCED VISION

The diagnosis of deteriorating vision has to be based, very frequently, on indirect evidence.

Change in behaviour

Many a marked behaviour change may have a visual component as part cause. Anyone who gives up eating unfilleted fish because of inability to see the bones can understand this. More handicapping are restrictions on mobility such as giving up driving or using public transport because of difficulties in seeing route numbers, signposts etc. Handling money and seeing the price of goods in shops leads to fewer excursions outdoors and so on.

Accidents and falls

Changes in visual performance are often the cause of tripping or other accidents both in and out of the home. Not only are visual clues distorted but righting reflexes are inadequate. A common example in many people's lives occurs when they first wear bifocal glasses. Changes in acuity or in the field of vision may become dangerous. This particularly applies to driving (MacKeane & Elkington, 1982). The pedestrian victim of a road accident may be the cause of it. Impaired vision in the right eye or a restricted field on the right side (however good the vision in the left) may prevent his seeing an approaching car as he starts to cross the road. Where traffic keeps to the right the side of these conditions is reversed. It cannot be taken for granted that such a victim is aware of the defect either before or after the accident. Even if he is aware he may not take any steps other than to accept it and reduce his mobility

accordingly. It follows that the presenting symptoms of visual deterioration may be injury, going slow or a general restriction of activities rather than an open complaint.

This lacks of insight by the patient means that the doctor should perform an actual visual check in such people. The casualty officer is in a particularly responsible position especially if he discharges the patient. The admitting doctor or his successor should do a simple visual test on each eye and record it before the patient is discharged. Any defect found may be known to the patient but where this is uncertain an ophthalmological opinion should be sought.

The test required is the acuity *with glasses*, both for near and distance and simple field testing to peripheral finger movements. Each eye should be tested separately. Unaided vision is usually only relevant in those who do not possess glasses. Merely asking about vision is likely to be misleading if not useless.

PREVENTION

Screening

The section above takes account of the situation as it is. An effective improvement could be obtained by more regular screening of the eyesight of the elderly as has been the practice in the other section of the population who do not complain — namely the children. That this would be productive amongst those whose mental faculties are unimpaired is shown by the work of Fenton et al (1974) who examined all the inmates of a typical geriatric ward whose cerebration was good. He found all degrees of undiscovered and undisclosed visual handicap. He was able to produce improvement by surgery in some cases, by optical means (often simply spectacles) in others, and by mobilising the help of the social services so that those eligible obtained the benefits of registration as blind. In all some 30% of those examined had their lot improved and some functioned as normal instead of nearly blind. Outside hospital regular attention should be given in a similar fashion in old people's homes and should not be allowed to lapse or become haphazard.

The poor mobility of the aged, especially of the housebound makes local examination highly desirable. At a very simple but adequate level these examinations can be done in old people's homes, in day centres, in dispersed community clinics or, in remote rural areas, in a mobile caravan. Such a service is analogous to the community school service which is successfully carried out by school nurses or health visitors. It gets over the difficulty of transporting the infirm over exhausting long distances to eye centres and can be universally applied. Depending on local resources of professional skill and interest the service can be elaborated to include field testing, tonometry, or even testing for glasses and dispensing.

Those who have had recent competent advice or who are regularly attending hospital can be identified so that duplication of services can be avoided. By recent, in the healthy, two years is a reasonable limit for both eyes with good sight. However even amongst these people the result of the examinations are not always accessible to the doctor in charge, or they may be misunderstood by the patient or not acted upon. Screening of this kind can also be a follow-up of value, especially amongst defaulters from hospital clinics. Part of the difficulty is in the field of faulty communication.

Communication

All new defects found at any 'routine' examination for glasses which prevent the achievement of good acuity, whether for near or distance should be reported to the doctor. Experience has shown that when these reports are given they may be filed, perhaps unseen by him, and no action is taken until the patient attends and complains. This is especially unsatisfactory if the patient does neither. Many do. Delay in treating preventable deterioration can be caused producing unnecessary handicap, so the doctor needs to take the initiative when these are a possibility. If he refers a patient to *any* consultant, in whatever department at hospital, he should include a note on any eye disease known to be present. In particular this should note any therapy such as miotics for glaucoma, steroids, anticoagulants etc. This ensures continuity of treatment if the patient is admitted and prevents over-medication or conflicting advice (Davidson, 1975; Gardiner, 1979).

Particularly dangerous breakdowns of communications occur on admission or discharge from hospital or old people's home, or from one doctor's care to another's (Price, 1983). One of the essentials in the treatment of glaucoma for instance is continuity of treatment and if this is broken permanent harm can occur.

BASIC EXAMINATION

The kit required for home examination is simple and portable. The essential objective is the estimation of the visual acuity for near and distance *with glasses*. This can be measured for distance and near even in illiterates by a matching test such as the Sheridan-Gardiner. Folding test-types of the conventional Snellen standard are available, some which come with reversible letters so that they can be used at ten feet given a good mirror. There is no obligation to use standardised reading types, though for comparison they are desirable, as any small newspaper print will give all the necessary information. Central fields in co-operative patients can be assessed with an Amsler chart and peripheral fields by the reaction to finger movements between doctor and patient at varying distances from central fixation. The examiner controls this by his own peripheral vision, ensuring that the plane at the periphery is halfway between himself and the patient. The patient must maintain fixation on the bridge of the examiner's nose. These tests are best carried out in good daylight or bright artificial light, not in strong sunlight. The media and the retina can be examined with ophthalmoscope, if need be after dilatation of the pupil with a quick acting mydriatic aided by phenylephrine 10% (10 min). It is wise in all cases to ensure subsequent constriction of the pupil by pilocarpine (2–4%) or other miotic drops.

The pinhole test is a help in deciding whether a change of glasses is likely to be helpful. If a distance vision is greatly improved through the pinhole, say two Snellen lines or more, there is a good chance of improvement with new glasses. If not a search for glasses will be a waste of time.

Trial of a simple hand magnifier (see page 167) gives a clue to the ability of the patient to handle one and to the degree of improvement in reading likely to be achieved. An optician's help should be sought if these tests are promising but in doubtful instances it is wiser to start with an ophthalmologist.

One of the advantages of examination in the home is that the lighting needs (see page 162) and the reading tastes of the patient can be given practical attention rather than the academic guess emerging from a hospital clinic. There is evidence (Cullinan et al, 1979) that performance at home of all these tests varies by a large factor from that in a clinic.

THE MANAGEMENT OF SPECIFIC CONDITIONS

Cataract

Here we run into difficulties of terminology. Everyone develops some form of opacity in the lens by the time they reach great age. Only a proportion of these develop far enough to require surgery. Progression is intermittent in many eyes and not symmetrical between eyes. Since the term cataract is generally known and feared because of its potential for blindness, it is more desirable to call the early changes 'lens opacities' until there is evidence of definite and constant progression. There is no known method of preventing the formation of cataracts nor of influencing their rate of development.

Pre-operative management

In the last 20 years there has been a vast change in the technique of surgery for cataract but the public retains the myths of a bygone age still believing that the cataract has to be 'ripe', almost synonymous with blindness, before surgery can be performed, for instance. If they can be informed that the days of immobility are gone, double padding has gone, bedrest is minimal and that in many centres either a general or a local anaesthetic can be selected, many of their fears would dissolve. The T.V. stuns them with new technology without reassuring them about these simple facts. One of these is that cataract extraction can now be done on an out-patient basis in well organised centres provided they possess plenty of resources of skilled personnel and back-up.

No restrictions should be placed on reading, viewing T.V. or any form of visual activity however difficult it may be. The patient should be told to have regular checks of the visual acuity, say annually in the early stages, unless it is clear that visual changes of significance are occurring faster than this. Only when progress is unequivocal need the patient be told that he should see a consultant for advice. A loss of two lines in six months or four in a year would make reference essential though this would clearly be modified if at the first observation, the acuity with glasses was already seriously defective. If there appears to be definite handicap with either near or distance vision or the threat of it, further advice is needed. These guidelines are quoted at some length in the interest of saving the frail and the immobile unrewarding visits to hospital clinics.

As a general rule the lower the age at which opacities appear the more likely they are to be progressive but no two cases are identical and variability in the rate of change is characteristic. Retrogression can be discounted in practice.

Where hospital attendance is easy, early attendance is to be encouraged so that a favourable place on the waiting list can be obtained and so that the retina can be examined before dense opacities appear. Age in itself is no bar to successful surgery but in an elderly confused patient, cataract extraction will not improve the confusional state though it may help mobility and activities such as feeding. Glare is often a problem as cataracts develop and is better diminished by brimmed headgear rather than tinted glasses.

Post-operative management
It is useful to understand some of the common difficulties which arise post-operatively which may dismay the patient. Modern surgical practice solves the optical problem of the aphakic eye by employing one of the following:

(i) A lens implant
(ii) Various types of contact lenses
(iii) Traditional spectacles

Both (i) and (ii) provide the retina with normal sized visual images, (iii) does not. All three normally require additional glasses for near vision. In *unilateral* cases either (i) or (ii) is essential if the affected eye is to be used in effective combination with its normal fellow. If not the only immediate benefit to the patient is to increase the visual field to the affected side. There is in addition the gain of its immediate availability (saving a period of incapacity) should any deterioration occur in the good eye. This is not always explained, or understood by the patient who may become depressed at the seeming lack of restoration of his normal sight. Nearly all those who are given spectacles (iii) manage well after extraction but a few never come to terms with the magnified image they see. This particularly affects mobility and judgement of distances; sedentary vision remains excellent.

Spectacles are likely to be heavy and to become ill adjusted. Accurate and stable fitting are essential elements in their successful use. Self insertion of contact lenses is difficult for many and their loss a particular hazard in view of unaided vision being so poor (Hilbourne, 1975).

Glaucoma

Prevention
In theory glaucoma is a preventable disease. It needs to be prevented because reversal of the loss of field and of acuity that occurs is not possible after they have been present a relatively short time. The symptoms are often unnoticed or unreported in the common chronic forms until it is too late to prevent permanent handicap. Prevention therefore means the identification of susceptible eyes and of those in the early stages of the disease.

In general medical practice the family history is the best guide to finding those at risk. Any elderly person whose parents, grandparents or other close relatives suffered from glaucoma is more at risk than others. In these people, whether symptoms are present or not, the disease needs to be specifically excluded, say every 2 years, and all of them given the knowledge that the early symptoms of episodes of blurred vision or of coloured rings round light sources require immediate investigation. Only a minority of patients know the diagnosis of their relatives' eye disease and are also likely to misname it. Glaucoma can be deduced as a strong possibility if the relative attended hospital in late middle age or after and regularly used drops for treatment.

Tonometry of whole populations is not a fully satisfactory process, even when feasible, as it throws up a high proportion of false positives and equivocal cases. A discrepancy in the size and speed of reaction of the pupils can be an early indication. Central field estimation with the Amsler chart is quick and convenient in the surgery. Field defects require investigation on their own account and one eye acts as a control for the other. There are a number of drugs used systemically, mainly the anticholinergic group, or those with an atropine-like action which may precipitate or aggravate glaucomatous episodes. Steroids also raise intraocular pressure (Akingbehin, 1982).

Management
The following points are written with the problems in mind which the doctor in daily care may have to face.

Acute glaucoma
Characterised by a dilated pupil, a cloudy cornea and diminished acuity is usually accompanied by pain in and around the eye. However it quite often presents with vomiting and general prostration can mask its ocular source which dangerously delays specific treatment. Immediate treatment is sight-saving. A suitable programme is the instillation of a drop of 2–4% pilocarpine every minute for

5 minutes, followed by a drop every 5 minutes for a half-hour, and then each quarter-hour, until relief or help is obtained. Concurrently 500 mg acetazolamide should be given by mouth or 250 mg intravenously. Control is heralded by a reduction in the size of the pupil, by a brighter cornea and by relief from pain. Treatment should not be delayed while hospital admission or specialist help is being arranged. Emergency surgery is frequently necessary.

Chronic glaucoma

The treatment programme will be established by the ophthalmologist. Orthodox treatment comprises drops, tablets, slow-release conjunctival lamellae etc. Considerable numbers of elderly patients allow their treatment to lapse (Granstrom, 1982). Faulty instruction, faulty comprehension of the instructions, diverse fears, incapacity and spillage are among the reasons and need to be foreseen. Some common causes of lapse are sheer dislike of using drops, fear of putting in too many, or of putting them into the 'wrong' part of the eye. Therefore the instructions to the patient should include reassurance that overdosage is impossible merely a waste and that it is immaterial which area of the conjunctiva is selected to receive the drops. One current instruction can itself be misleading. This arises from the modern practice of putting an expiry date on drop bottles, without necessarily ensuring a continuity of supply. It is far less dangerous to use time-expired drops (except after recent surgery) than to go without. Spillage is another cause of a lapse in treatment. No patient should be without a reserve bottle. Holidays involve extra risks in this respect and so does admission to hospital or old people's homes. The latter arises from poor communication between professionals and from the patient's belief that cessation of treatment is intentional or from his inability to inform (Price, 1983). Instructions to patients should be written in large print and also be given to relatives and to staff in homes.

Ocular manifestations of systemic disease

As at previous ages temporary or permanent effects on vision occur associated with remote processes. These are too numerous to specify but in view of their increased prevalence in the elderly and their severity, certain features of their handling require emphasising. They derive from cardiovascular, circulatory, neurological metabolic or degenerative causes. Such multiple origins, if there is poor communication (see page 164) can sometimes lead to irrational or even dangerous therapy. For example an ophthalmologist may decide to treat, say, macular degeneration with some form of circulatory stimulant. Any side effects are of concern to the patient's general physician who may be treating him already for a related or different condition. The physician in charge is entitled to ask whether such treatment is essentially curative or speculative. Many elderly patients already pass much of the day watching the clock which governs their consumption of tablets and to add more could be needlessly burdensome. For this reason and diagnostically the ophthalmologist also needs to hear of any systemic therapy or disease in which the patient is involved.

Emergencies

Relative urgency can be a difficult assessment. Obviously sudden loss of vision (i.e. within minutes) in the better eye of a pair is more urgent than a similar event in an eye previously known to have poor vision, though in either case there may be implications for the second eye. This is one reason for the value of a visual record on every patient.

Of the treatable conditions glaucoma has already been dealt with (see page 165). Giant cell arteritis and central retinal artery (CRA) occlusion deserve special mention because emergency treatment can help. The period of time available is at most only a few hours in the case of CRA occlusion and may not be much more in giant cell arteritis. Of the two, giant cell arteritis is the more serious because blindness in both eyes can occur rapidly and irreversibly, rather than in only one which is the rule in CRA disease. There are no specific general symptoms associated with CRA occlusion but loss of sight in arteritis is usually associated with headache and tenderness in the scalp. These are sufficiently severe to interfere with sleep. A high erythrocyte sedimentation rate (ESR) confirms the need for immediate systemic administration of steroids in high doses. They not only preserve eyesight but usually have a dramatic effect on the pain. Treatment at a lower dose needs to be prolonged well beyond this relief.

Chronic and long-term disease

With few exceptions, notably in diabetes, little can be done specifically to prevent ocular complications in chronic or degenerative conditions. The rapidity with which changes in the treatment of diabetic retinopathy is occurring makes some form of joint medical/ophthalmic clinic the best arrangement for its handling, which is now highly specialised. The only general statement of value is that treatment of retinopathy is far more effective in the very early stages than later.

Other forms of untreatable retinal degeneration arising from artiosclerosis, ischaemia, hypertension, together with cerebro-vascular disorders, make up the majority of visual problems arising in old age. Specific ocular treatment is unlikely to be curative, but may prevent complications or further episodes. Supervision depends mainly on monitoring changes in acuity. It is questionable whether this requires as much hospital visiting as is customary once the diagnosis is made and if changes in acuity are slow or absent. Monitoring is necessary but can be carried out perfectly well in local surgeries, reducing the need for hospital visits to those whose acuity is found to be deteriorating. In one hospital clinic a 65 year old had visited the hospital at six-monthly intervals for 20 years after an initial episode of visual deterioration which subsequently remained unaltered (Personal observation). Many of these patients take matters into their own hands and default because 'the hospital does nothing for me'. This is not in their best interests but is understandable especially in the aged. The matron of an old people's home regularly sent a busload of handicapped old people on a 40 mile round-trip for routine review at an eye hospital. It was a rarity for anything practical to result from these visits but no alternative service was available to take its place and spare her charges the day or two's incapacity which many suffered as a result (Personal observation). It would be an advance if the local physician in charge decided whether these visits are productive, preventive or merely a formality for which he or his nursing assistants could substitute themselves. In the more severe cases of visual loss of known nature, he is in just as good a position to initiate registration procedures as is the hospital consultant (see below).

The patient's attitude to routine visits is often naive, being based on the idea that he would not be asked to return without good reason. On the other hand many seriously physically incapacitated will make superhuman efforts in order to obtain reassurance from a remote hospital clinic.

Registration as handicapped

At a certain stage of visual handicap (short of blindness) the patient will become eligible for registration as blind or 'partially sighted' in the system adopted in the United Kingdom. Neither of these terms are as precise as they sound and are based on complicated visual measurements of acuity and field, together with little recognition of the patient's general health and activities. Registration is voluntary not statutory. The system does little to reassure the patient about his visual future. In the first place only 5% of those on the blind register are totally without vision and most have useful vision in their accustomed surroundings, even if some activities have to be given up. The document is not available for medical scrutiny and is a poor guide to the patient's vision as it really is. The regulations concerning the partially sighted were drawn up many years ago with education in mind and have little relevance to the welfare of the elderly, though recently travel concessions have been granted.

Any person who is involved, including the doctor, can ask for an examination with a view to registration. This request would normally be addressed to the social services department or to the consultant ophthalmologist whose signature is obligatory anyway. Normally the request is not made by the patient because of the knowledge that he is not blind in the common meaning of the word so the initiative has to come from those around him.

Many, when they are introduced to the idea of registration, wrongly interpret it to mean that they are being told in a rather underhand way that they will become blind. The fact is that most elderly patients, after an initial decline whether fast or slow, reach a stationary state. There are not often any prognostic contents to registration, beyond the recognition that no improvement is expected.

The benefits

The rationale of early registration of those with visual handicap or of those who seem to be managing well perhaps with the help of a relative is not so much to obtain tangible benefits but more a policy of insurance. If the person is known to the social services, help in an emergency should be more speedy and more effective than otherwise. Such an emergency can arise for example if the responsible relative becomes ill. Few of the visually handicapped who are 'partially sighted' were registered in the past because of the absence of immediate benefit but such aids as special lighting modification, talking books and travel concessions are appropriate and available in very many cases.

The explanation of the desirability of registration needs to be simple and clear. It is often best done by an informed social worker. The benefits should include a visit to the patient's home, suggestions of suitable modifications to assist mobility, special cooking and telephone aids and so on. Self-consciousness prevents many from accepting the white stick but it may decide whether a handicapped person can leave the house in safety or not. There is nothing to stop anyone who feels insecure from painting a stick white which can be a sensible act. Once a person is registered he should be informed of the help that is obtainable from the institutes for the blind and other organisations concerned. These include the Royal National Institute for the Blind, the Partially Sighted Society, the Disabled Living Foundation and in the field of information the BBC publication 'In Touch'. Many localities provide local news on cassette. It can be seen that most of these aids are not optical or ophthalmic and are not provided or even thought of in a clinical setting. Few hospital clinics are equipped with a full range of magnifying equipment or the staff to provide such a service. Financial aid to the blind is confined to tax concessions, travel concessions and help toward a T.V. licence!

LOW VISION AIDS

Optical magnifiers

Reading

Reading vision falls much more often to a handicapping level than distance in the elderly. Low vision aids are those other than conventional spectacles. They include all forms of magnifiers, whether hand-held or on stands and those resembling watchmakers glasses assembled in spectacle frames. All restrict the field of vision so that rapid scanning becomes impossible. This puts great limitation on their use as does their critical focus and working distance. The hand that manipulates them therefore cannot be infirm. Their theoretical value is not matched by their practical application and many are bought or prescribed only to be neglected. However, with guidance at the time of their issue a good idea can be formed as to the likelihood of their use and they should always be considered. Left to their own choice the public will usually go for the bigger lenses in the mistaken idea that they are more powerful. In fact they are less powerful and less manageable than small-diameter lenses. The higher the power the smaller the field. If the field is already restricted as in hemianopia or some forms of macular degeneration magnifiers do nothing to enlarge it and in some cases enlarge the difficulty.

Distance

Telescopes of various specifications can fill a need in some people but again though good acuity can be obtained field restriction is extreme. For mobility, worn as spectacles, they are as useless as binoculars to the normally sighted. For the sedentary they can be of use for watching television, in the theatre or at sporting events. Monocular aids, hand-held and of pocket dimensions, have their uses in travel for identification of bus numbers, route indicators, street names and so on.

These limitations make it wise to obtain some sort of professional advice before ordering these aids, though the official National Health Service policy of confining their issue as a benefit to those willing and able to attend hospital is a hardship without justification. With the exception of closed-circuit television their cost is no more than that of many varieties of spectacles. Where centres can be set up they should be in every locality.

Closed-circuit television

These devices are more elaborate than magnifiers but give much greater magnification and up to a point greater field. Their price is a disadvantage but the elderly driver who can no longer see to drive and sells his car can afford one individually. They can be set up in public places such as libraries or council offices and in residential homes. Though many of the elderly do not read books or newspapers most receive letters, tax forms, social welfare and pension documents, bank statements and so on which they are embarrassed to show to others. Many of these form a challenge to all but the best eyes. Their legibility on a closed-circuit television screen, printed in colour or black and white, is no longer such a problem. Manipulation can soon be learnt by those with an incentive and is often easier than of a conventional magnifier. Charitable organisations and welfare services should be a source of information and expertise in handling and providing all these aids.

New instruments of this nature are being intensively developed so that cheaper, more compact and more manageable visual aids are likely to become available in the future.

Lighting

It is not inappropriate to conclude this chapter, especially the section on low vision aids, by stressing once more the importance of lighting. Light is the essential raw material — no light no sight — poor light poor sight. The elderly eye whether normal or not, requires more of it (see page 164) for all visual acts than the young one. With few exceptions the more defective the eye and the finer the visual task, the greater the aid given by more illumination. Fears that this can be harmful are groundless whatever the source of lighting. (Cullinan et al (1979) reported that quite simple improvements in domestic lighting would reduce the number of 'visually disabled' at home by nearly a half.)

The 'twilight years' is a misleading conception, though only too often an accurate one, of the style of life thought to be appropriate to the elderly.

REFERENCES

Akingbehin A O 1982 Corticosteroid induced ocular hypertension. British Journal of Ophthalmology 66: 536–541

Cullinan T, Gould E S, Irvine D, Silver J H 1979 Visual disability and home lighting. Lancet 1: 642–644

Davidson S I 1975 Drug interactions in ophthalmology. Transactions of the Ophthalmological Society of the United Kingdom 95: 277–281

Fenton P, Arnold R C, Wilkins P S W 1975 Vision in slow-stream wards. Age and Ageing 4: 43–48

Gardiner P A 1978 ABC of Ophthalmology. British Medical Association, London

Granstrom P 1982 Compliance of glaucoma patients with drug therapy. British Journal of Ophthalmology 66: 464–470

Hilbourne J F 1975 Social and other aspects of adjustment to cataract extraction in the elderly. Transactions of the Ophthalmological Society of the United Kingdom 95: 254–258

MacKean J M, Elkington A R 1982 Glaucoma and driving. British Medical Journal 285: 777–778

Price N C 1983 Importance of asking about glaucoma. British Medical Journal 286: 349–350

20

Hearing disorders

A. Glorig

INTRODUCTION

The fact that hearing is important to well-being cannot be disputed. The order of this importance is a relative matter, however. For example, the loss of hearing in early childhood is infinitely worse in its effects on well-being than when this loss occurs in late life.

It is well known that hearing disorders in the aged are a problem that is long overdue for attention. Numerous studies show that hearing loss increases with age to the extent that 30% of people over 65 years of age have enough loss to need assistance for everyday communication; that is, in the United States approximately 10 million people. It is further estimated that about 25 million people have enough hearing impairment to need amplification. About 40% of that group are over 65 years of age. Such statistics point out the enormity of the problem of hearing disorders in our aging population. A short discussion concerning these disorders is not out of place at this point (Glorig & Roberts, 1970). Perhaps the most important of these disorders is really not a disorder but a natural consequence of aging, i.e. presbyacusis.

The definition of presbyacusis is somewhat ambiguous in the general literature and in the mind of the clinician at this point. Because of this ambiguity, it is frequently used as a 'wastebasket diagnosis' for a hearing loss in someone over 60 that cannot be related to any specific disease or causative factor. In my opinion presbyacusis strictly defined should describe the effects of normal physiological aging on the auditory system from the external canal to the auditory cortex.

There are numerous studies of the effects of aging on the auditory threshold for pure tones, discrimination of speech, pitch perception, impedance changes in the middle ear and auditory brainstem responses. When studying the auditory effects of aging, we are confronted with an insurmountable problem. That environmental effects are present is indisputable and any attempt to separate normal physiological changes from changes due to auditory environment is doomed to failure.

There is evidence that when environment is controlled the effects of physiological aging appear to be measurably less. When various population studies are done, differences in hearing are found as a function of the environment from which the group came (Glorig & Nixon, 1962). Figure 20.1 shows a group of audiometric curves that can be used to estimate group mean hearing losses as a function of age.

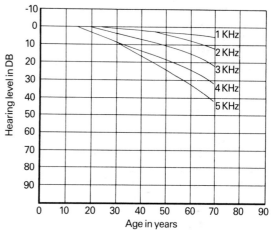

Fig. 20.1 Hearing level at .5, 1, 2, 3, 4 and 5 KHz as a function of age.

AUDITORY EFFECTS OF AGING

The auditory system sustains effects that follow the general changes of aging but are peculiar to the auditory system. This is not the place to discuss the basic pathophysiology of aging, however. We will confine our discussion to known effects on the performance of the auditory system and the coincident effects on the aged person.

In general the auditory system can be compared to an electronic device whose purpose is to receive sound waves, transmit them efficiently to a transducer, analyse them and convert them into meaning. Anatomically, the ear and its neural connections can be divided as follows: external, middle and inner ear, eighth nerve, mid-brain and auditory cortex.

The external and middle ear can be compared to a mechanical transformer whose purpose is to gather the sound waves and present them to the inner ear or electrical transducer properly matched, i.e. with the least loss of energy when the inner ear fluids are inserted into the circuit. The external and middle ear functions are strictly mechanical; they act to prevent a mismatch at the point where sound has to be transduced from mechanical energy or vibration to electrical energy or current. An analogy would be an audio device using a low impedance microphone with a high impedance amplifier (Ruben, 1971). The device would need an impedance matching transformer for the efficient transfer of mechanical energy to electrical energy. As sound continues through the auditory systems, it is transduced in the cochlea or inner ear and carried via the eighth nerve to the brain where analysis takes place. Another way of saying it is the inner ear codes the sounds into electrical pulses as a function of intensity, duration and time pattern and the brain decodes these pulses into meaningful messages. The effects of aging occur over the entire auditory system. I will discuss the principal components separately (Glorig & Davis, 1961).

Before discussing the auditory problems associated with aging, I should mention the types of hearing loss that may occur (Fig. 20.2). When difficulties occur that interfere with the mechanical transmission or conduction of sound, the hearing loss is called conductive. Usually, conductive hearing loss is associated with problems affecting the external and middle ear.

When problems arise in the inner ear, including the cochlea and the auditory nerve, they produce sensorineural hearing loss. That is a problem with the sensing organ (cochlea) and/or the acoustic nerve, including the mid-brain and cortex. If an audiogram shows a loss by air conduction i.e. earphone testing, but no loss by bone conduction i.e. by testing with a vibrator placed over the mastoid process, the person has a conductive loss. If the bone conduction test shows a loss equal to the air conduction loss, the person has a sensorineural loss. If bone conduction shows some loss but less loss than air conduction, the person has a mixed loss.

EXTERNAL EAR

There are many things that can happen to the external ear, but I will confine my discussion to those that effect hearing. Perhaps the most common of these is impacted cerumen. The amount of wax produced does not seem to change with age, but it appears to be more inspissated and consequently packs and becomes extremely dry and hard. It affects hearing only if the cerumen entirely blocks the canal and/or contacts the drumhead. The loss in hearing can be considerable if the canal is completely blocked. When the loss that accompanies impacted cerum is superimposed on the effects of presbyacusis, it is quite noticeable and, consequently, when the wax is removed the individual notices a distinct improvement. Removing the wax can be difficult, and, if not done expertly, it may damage the canal wall or even the drumhead itself.

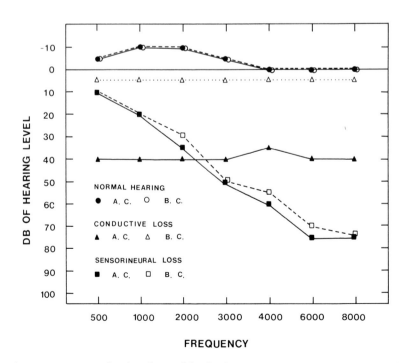

Fig. 20.2 Audiometric measurements as a function of type of hearing loss.

Another not uncommon problem is a collapsed canal. Frequently, as age increases, the cartilage of the pinna and outer third of the external auditory canal becomes soft and floppy and may partially close the external canal. This can produce a minor change in hearing, particularly when earphones are used for a hearing test. The pressure of the earphone collapses the canal and blocks the transmission of sound. Such cases need special care, especially when testing hearing.

Obviously, the external ear is subject to infection and tumours of the soft tissue and bone. Hearing loss is frequently the first symptom of a tumour of the ear and/or the upper nasopharynx. Anyone over 65 years of age with a unilateral hearing loss should be thoroughly studied before a final diagnosis is made.

There are changes in the drumhead and middle ear related to aging. Frequently, the drumhead thickens and loses its normal lustre and transparency. It also becomes stiffer and slightly less compliant. When the tissue of the middle ear is examined, microscopically the ossicular joints are somewhat arthritic and the ligaments show loss of elastic tissue. All these combine to make high frequency transmission less efficient and add to other changes to show the elevated high frequency thresholds in the older person.

Diseases of the middle ear in the aged are more or less the same as for middle age, i.e. infection, tumours, otosclerosis and trauma. Acute and chronic middle ear disease may result in acute or chronic mastoiditis which, if not treated properly, may result in a brain abscess, indeed this is the most common cause of brain abscess in the aged. Otosclerosis is primarily a disease of the middle ear but not exclusive to the middle ear. Its clinical manifestations are evident in the third decade but become troublesome in the fourth decade and it is more common in women than men (Beales, 1981). It is a hereditary disease that promotes bony changes in the oval window area which ossify and freeze the footplate of the stapes. As the stiffening increases, the air conduction threshold is elevated but the bone conduction threshold remains unchanged until years later when it also begins to become elevated. The mechanism that causes the sensorineural hearing loss after a period of time is not understood. Some think that during the otospongiotic period, a toxic material is released into the endolymph which damages hair cell function.

Hearing tests in patients with otosclerosis show what is called an air-bone gap. That is, the air conduction threshold is higher than the bone conduction threshold. Furthermore, the audiogram has a flat configuration showing nearly equal losses at all frequencies. People with otosclerosis usually have low, modulated voices and complain that they cannot hear well when chewing celery or other noisy food. Until a few years ago it was thought that otosclerosis did not affect the cochlea without first affecting the stapes. Recently, it has been shown that otosclerosis does affect the cochlea only and sometimes

produces a severe sensorineural hearing loss (Balle & Linthium, in press).

When an air-bone gap is found, surgery is the treatment of choice. On the other hand, when the loss is more severe than would be expected in uncomplicated presbyacusis, one should suspect cochlear otosclerosis. For sometime now, sodium fluoride has been used to arrest cochlear otosclerosis. There is real evidence to support this form of treatment. Temporal bone studies indicate that cochlear otosclerosis is not uncommon in the aged. Paget's disease and osteogenesis imperfecta may produce middle ear and cochlear changes. Unexplained progressive conductive hearing loss may indicate either of these diseases (Ruben, 1971).

INNER EAR

The aged inner ear is also subject to the same problems of middle age. Noise is a very important factor although, except when unusually loud, it can take years to produce a significant effect on the ear. Anyone who is over 50 years of age may suffer the effects of noise, This effect is principally on the hair cells population and produces mainly a high frequency (above 1000 Hz) loss (Fig. 20.3) (Glorig, 1980).

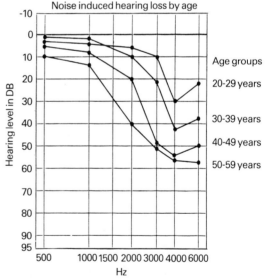

Fig. 20.3 Hearing level in a noise exposed population as a function of age groups.

Ototoxic drugs are a very important cause of sensorineural loss in the aged. Indiscriminate use of these drugs should be avoided. They can and do produce serious hearing losses. Acoustic neurinomas are not uncommon in the aged. If hearing tests show one ear to be significantly worse than the other, the physician should suspect a tumour. Recourse to surgery in the aged tumour patient depends on the size of the tumour and the severity of symptoms such as, hearing loss, tinnitus and dizziness. These tumours are usually slow-growing and surgery may not be indicated. Hearing loss, particularly unilateral loss in the aged patient, should alert the examiner to the possibility of a metastatic tumour as well (Brackmann, 1984).

CENTRAL NERVOUS SYSTEM

The central nervous system is the final component in the auditory system and it plays a very important role in the aged hearing-impaired person. It appears that the central nervous system, or the decoder of auditory imput, in the aged is not able to handle the complex information contained in speech and language. We know that there is a reduction in brain cell population, which could certainly be one explanation of this inability (Birren et al, 1959). Even when the pure tone audiogram shows only minor changes, aged people have difficulty understanding speech. Discrimination of speech, particularly in the situations with competing signals such as noise and group conversations, is very difficult for the older person (Jauhianen, 1983).

TREATMENT OF PRESBYACUSIS

If presbyacusis is accompanied by other specific problems such as tumour, infection or trauma, treatment is no different in the aged than in other persons. On the other hand if no treatable cause is present, then rehabilitation, including the use of a hearing aid, is considerably more complicated.

There is no doubt that hearing aids can be very helpful in the majority of subjects. However the success is directly proportionate to motivation. If the older person leads a busy, involved life and really needs to or wants to hear, a hearing aid can be highly successful. On the other hand, the person may be like the older man who was drinking heavily and when asked why, he answered, 'Because I can not hear'; and when asked why he didn't get a hearing aid, he replied 'Because I like what I drink better than what I hear.' Any attempt to get such older people to wear a hearing aid is often doomed to failure. If one can overcome their objection, modern hearing aids can be very useful, especially if properly fitted binaurally (Yarrington, 1976). Unilateral hearing aids should almost never be used, especially in the aged population. Until very recently, most doctors thought that a hearing aid was useless in the aging person. Nothing is further from the truth. However, fitting hearing aids to the older subject should not be treated lightly. It is important to do a complete hearing study and then evaluate the real ear performance with and without amplification before the examiner recommends a specific hearing aid. Only the most expert personnel should be involved. Furthermore, expert counselling is essential both before and after the hearing aid evaluation. The counselling team should include the professional as well as the hearing aid dispenser.

If counselling is slighted in any way, many hearing aids are relegated to the bureau drawer. It is also helpful to discuss the matter with the immediate family before a final decision about the hearing aid is made. The success of the hearing aid trial and use is highly dependent on motivation, and motivation of the patient should be cultivated by the family as well as the professional. The doctor is usually sought for problem solutions and he must take a sincere interest in the development or cultivation of motivation. It is a serious mistake for the doctor to turn this time-consuming process entirely over to the audiologist or the hearing aid dispenser.

It should be evident from this discussion that improving the communication performance of the elderly, particularly those over 60 years of age, is a complex problem that demands the use of highly trained personnel who are familiar with the needs as well as the limitations involved. It is firmly established that loss of sensitivity of the auditory periphery is not the important discrepancy. Many studies have shown that although the change in pure-tone threshold may be mild, there is still difficulty with everyday communication, even if the loss of sensitivity is compensated for by amplification. Remember that our primary goal is to establish communication. Getting sound to the individual is only a part of the process involved in human communication — albeit a very important one — but certainly not the whole of this very complex activity. We have mentioned motivation above, and perhaps when it is considered in its broadest aspect, motivation is the key to most of the communication problems of the aged. Many of our aged citizens are relegated to a lonely and isolated existence. Communication problems may be at the root of the isolation. It is well known that many aged people seek isolation because of their communication difficulties, which are usually due to hearing impairment. However, there are other factors that influence communication that must be recognised.

We have already stated that the capability of the aging brain to process information is reduced in many ways. Memory is certainly not the least. Compensating for a hearing loss does not really compensate for language problems related to comprehension, fluency of speech and vocabulary. Studies of these facets of communication are somewhat ambiguous but in the main do not show a lack of ability to comprehend, to speak fluently or to demonstrate a good vocabulary. Rather, the problem appears to be related to timing. Recall and processing are somewhat slower. Speech is more halting and, although the vocabulary might even be larger, there appears to be some difficulty recalling the proper words.

This is quite noticeable when other-than-routine subjects are discussed. There also appear to be noticeable problems with the receiving end when the talker speaks rapidly without pausing. Experiments have shown that if the speaker slows his speech and is more deliberate, the aged listener will do much better. A review of the literature shows definite evidence that as a whole language comprehension may be faulty; discourse, although elaborate in syntax, may be less fluent and vocabulary may be hesitant.

As far as remediation is concerned, it is not always good to focus attention on the elderly subject. Frequently, it is more rewarding to adjust the attitude of those who are associated with elderly subjects. For example, in a study of some of the communication needs of elderly residents of a nursing home, I found that training the personnel to recognise the communication problems of the elderly residents and to compensate appropriately, was far more successful than trying to get the residents to compensate for their own inabilities. Research has shown that many healthy, elderly subjects learn to re-route or reorder language-processing capacities that appear to bypass areas of reduced capacity, enhancing memory recall and timing functions. Some of us develop association ideas that help us compensate for inability to recall names. What person has not heard his older compatriots say from time to time, 'I guess I'm getting old — I can't remember names anymore.'

SUMMARY

It is quite evident that aging produces peripheral and central auditory changes that degrade communication ability. It is also evident that remediating these changes to improve communication ability in the aged is not simple. There are multivariate effects that demand and deserve the best in diagnostic procedures, counselling and rehabilitation. These needs are best met by a multidisciplinary team consisting of a physician, a psychologist, an audiologist, a hearing rehabilitation specialist and, when appropriate, a hearing aid dispenser. If a hearing aid is recommended, there is no one better qualified to handle the associated problems then an experienced hearing aid dispenser. The payoff to the older citizen, his family and friends, is a gratifying experience for everyone concerned, and if our senior citizens are to have a healthy and happy life, much more attention must be given to these problems.

REFERENCES

Balle V, Linthicum F H 1984 Histologically proven cochlear otosclerosis: sensorineural without conductive hearing loss. Annals of Otology, Rhinology & Laryngology 93: 105–111

Beales P H 1981 Otosclerosis. John Wright & Sons, Bristol

Birren J E, Imus H A, Windle W F 1959 The process of aging in the nervous system. Charles E Thomas, Ch 12

Brackmann D E 1984 A review of acoustic tumors: 1979–1982. American Journal of Otology 5: 233–244

Glorig A 1980 Noise — past, present and future. Ear and Hearing. 1: 1—18

Glorig A, Davis H 1961 Age, noise and hearing loss. Annals of Otology, Rhinology & Laryngology 70: 556

Glorig A, Nixon J 1962 Hearing loss as a function of age. Laryngoscope 72: 1596–1610

Glorig A, Roberts J 1970 Hearing levels of adults by age and sex — United States 1960–1962. Vital and Health Statistics

Jauhianen T 1983 Investigation of disorders of hearing In: Hinchcliffe R (ed) Hearing and balance in the elderly. Churchill Livingstone, Edinburgh, p 75–91

Ruben 1971 Aging and hearing In: Rossman I (ed) Clinical geriatrics. J B Lippincott Company, Philadelphia p 247–252

Yarrington C T 1976 Presbyacusis In: Northern J L (ed) Hearing disorders. Little Brown and Company, Boston, ch 16

21

Speech disorders

J. C. Meadows

Normal speech depends upon a co-ordinated flow of air from the lungs producing sound (phonation) by vibrating the vocal cords. Intrinsive laryngeal muscles supplied by the vagi alter the tautness of the cords and influence pitch. The sound is then modulated through continual alteration in the shape of the lips, tongue, pharynx and palate (articulation). The muscles of articulation are supplied by cranial nerves VII, IX, X, XI and XII These in turn discharge under the influence of descending pathways from the two motor cortices and ancillary structures including cerebellum and basal ganglia. The motor centres are controlled from the language areas. In 99% of right-handers and 60% of left-handers these are predominantly in the left cerebral hemisphere.

Speech may be disturbed in pathological processes affecting phonation (dysphonia and aphonia), articulation (dysarthria and anarthria) and language itself (dysphasia or aphasia).

DYSPHONIA

Dysphonia means disordered phonation (i.e. hoarseness) and aphonia absent phonation (i.e. whispering). Aphonia is usually hysterical but can occur with gross local disease of the larynx and also occasionally in extreme weakness, for example in terminal illness.

Dysphonia is most commonly due to local disorders of the vocal cords (inflammation, infiltration, tumours). The speech is then husky or hoarse. The patient can usually give a good cough. The common neurological cause of dysphonia is a lesion of the recurrent laryngeal branch of one or other vagus nerve (often the left because of its longer course, looping into the thorax around the aortic arch). Thyroid surgery or tumours of lung, thyroid, oesophagus and mediastinum may be responsible. Provided that only one recurrent laryngeal nerve is affected, mild hoarseness may be the only manifestation until the patient coughs; then, because the abnormal cord may not adduct satisfactorily to halt air flow at the beginning of a cough, the normal initial sound and quick decrescendo is replaced by a characteristically more prolonged hoarsely phonating exhalation. Bilateral vagal paralysis is rare and serious and

most commonly results from thyroid surgery. Dysphonia may be mild and stridor is the dominant symptom because the cords lie close to the midline and cannot be abducted; the reader is referred to specialised text books.

Strictly speaking some dysphonia accompanies many cases of dysarthria too. For example the volume is small and the variations in pitch limited in Parkinsonism, and phonation is rather explosive in cerebellar disease.

DYSARTHRIA

Dysarthria is disordered articulation and anarthria absence of articulation. Unless there is some obvious cause within mouth or pharynx, acquired dysarthria usually results from neurological disease. It may be due to bulbar palsy, to pseudobulbar palsy or to other disorders of motor function such as Parkinsonism and cerebellar dysfunction.

Bulbar Palsy
Bulbar palsy is the term given to paralysis of the muscles of speech and swallowing from damage to motor neurones whose cell bodies are in the medulla (originally called the 'bulb'). It is also used to include weakness due to rare cranial nerve neuropathies (idiopathic, diphtheritic) and myasthenia ('bulbar myasthenia'). Motor neurone disease and myasthenia are the commonest causes. Myasthenia is characterised by variability and fatiguability, and improvement with edrophonium or neostigmine.

Speech is weak and nasal (because of palatal weakness). There is usually associated facial weakness and there is dysphagia. In bulbar motor neurone disease wasting of face and tongue is present. The jaw jerk is absent in pure bulbar palsy but in motor neurone disease is commonly brisk because of concomitant pseudobulbar palsy. Weakness and fasciculation in trunk or limbs commonly makes the diagnosis obvious.

Pseudobulbar palsy
Pseudobulbar palsy is the term used for *bilateral* damage to the corticobulbar motor pathway (upper motor neurone damage). It causes slurring dysarthria, one word running into the next, sometimes delivered faster than normal.

There is accompanying dysphagia. The tongue is not wasted (unless there is accompanying bulbar palsy) but may be contracted and look small. Protrusion to command and movement of the tongue from side to side are both slow and limited in extent. The jaw jerk and pharyngeal gag reflex (response to touching the back of the pharynx with a swab stick) are both exaggerated. There may be lability of emotional expression, the patient breaking into laughter or, more commonly, tears at minor provocation.

If the onset is gradual, motor neurone disease is usually responsible and the pseudobulbar palsy is then comonly mixed with bulbar palsy. If the onset is sudden, vascular disease is responsible and the patient is frequently hypertensive. Bilateral infarcts are usual; sometimes there is a past history of transient hemiparesis and a second episode on the opposite side is enough to precipitate dysarthria and dysphagia. Sometimes there is no such history and one presumes a past possibly subclinical episode. Some degree of dysarthria may however accompany unilateral disorders of the central nervous system, for example Broca's aphasia (see below) or pontine infarcts ('dysarthria — clumsy hand syndrome').

Dysarthria in other neurological disorders
There are various degenerative disorders that may produce dysarthria by affecting ancillary neural structures (cerebellum, basal ganglia) concerned with motor function. Parkinson's disease is one of the commonest in older patients but cerebellar degenerations, Huntington's chorea and senile chorea may all cause dysarthria in the elderly. Wilson's disease, olivopontocerebellar degeneration and of course multiple sclerosis (the commonest of all in younger patients) are unlikely to present first in the elderly.

Parkinsonism causes mumbling, monotonous speech, often rapidly delivered and sometimes tailing off in a manner similar to Parkinsonian writing. Cerebellar disease causes clumsy, explosive scanning speech. In both cases the motor disturbance is usually more obvious in other parts of the body.

DYSPHASIA

Dysphasia (aphasia) is an abnormality of the symbolic function of speech caused usually by damage to the left cerebral hemisphere. Simply defined it is an acquired disturbance of language function. Generally it therefore affects written as well as spoken language, and in multilingual subjects all tongues are affected. By analogy with phonation and articulation the term aphasia should mean absence of language but in practice dysphasia and aphasia are used synonomously to describe any disturbance of spoken language. The former term is favoured in Britain, the latter in the US.

There are varying disturbances of word choice, grammatical structuring and comprehension and there have been many classifications. The simple terms expressive and receptive aphasia are in common use and can be helpful up to a point. They are not adequate for classification for they have limited significance in terms of neuroanatomical localisation. Moreover, pure receptive aphasia is a questionable entity and most aphasias are mixed receptive and expressive when properly assessed. This may not always be apparent to the untrained observer. It is extremely common to be told by nursing staff and even by close relatives of a patient that his understanding is intact. Yet one or two simple questions or commands reveal it to be grossly defective. Sometimes this is missed because of the patients ability to utilise non-linguistic cues, or cues that are peripheral to the main sense of the command. For example the command 'point to the pillow' may be successfully accomplished if the examiner glances inadvertently at it or if he says instead 'point to *your* pillow' which may give just sufficient additional information.

Nowadays the anatomically based classification popularised by the Boston school is used increasingly and is certainly the most rational from the neurological standpoint (Geschwind, 1970 & 1971; Benson, 1979a; Albert et al, 1981). But even with this there are patients who do not easily fit the classical syndromes. The classification is based on the known anatomical localisation of language areas within the dominant (left) hemisphere. The central structures (Fig. 21.1) are:

1. Wernicke's area which is placed appropriately next to left primary acoustic cortex. Acoustic cortex lies unseen within the Sylvian fissure on the upper surface of the temporal lobe.

2. Broca's area which is strategically placed in front of the lowest part of left primary motor cortex. This part of motor cortex represents articulatory movements of tongue, lips, pharynx and larynx.

3. The arcuate (superior longitudinal) fasciculus, a subcortical pathway connecting Broca's and Wernicke's areas. (There may also be connecting fibres traversing the insula, the flat oval island of surface cortex embedded deep within the Sylvian fissure).

Other areas of the left hemisphere play their part in language but are proportionally less important. Nevertheless, aphasia may complicate lesions of supplementary motor cortex, the angular gyrus, the inferior temporal region and other areas surrounding the central structures listed above.

The following clinical characteristics are examined in this classification (Goodglass & Kaplan, 1972; Meadows, 1975):

1. the character of spontaneous speech and particularly its fluency
2. the ability, when requested, to repeat words and sentences spoken by the examiner
3. comprehension
4. word finding

Spontaneous speech

For speech to be fluent the postero-inferior part of the left frontal lobe, including Broca's area and its connections with primary cortex must be intact. This area is responsible for the articulatory aspects of speech and grammatical structuring of sentences. Damage here leads to the non-fluent, effortful, poorly articulated and classically agrammatical speech of Broca's aphasia. There is some argument (Mohr et al, 1978) about whether damage confined to Broca's area, the posterior part of the inferior frontal gyrus, is sufficient or whether the lesion must be larger. Substantive meaningful content may be relatively preserved in spite of the lack of grammatical 'filler' words and verb, adjectival and adverb endings (e.g. -ed, -ing, -ly). Thus it may take on a telegrammatic quality. A poorly articulated effortful, slow '...me....home...' may convey the patient's wishes very well.

Contrasting with this picture, lesions further back in the brain damaging Wernicke's area produce speech which may be grossly aphasic but is nevertheless extremely fluent and well articulated. If such a patient were heard speaking in an unfamiliar language the observer would probably not detect an abnormality. But such speech lacks specific content and meaning since Wernicke's area is necessary for the semantic (meaningful) aspects of speech. In physiological terms Wernicke's area may be responsible for interrelating electrical patterns representing sounds and those representing 'meaning'. When damaged, false or inadequate information reaches the inferior frontal region (Broca's area). Specific nouns may be replaced in speech by non-specific substitutions such as 'thing' or 'the other' or 'the what's its name'. More abnormal substitutions (paraphasias) occur too and may be phonemic (e.g. 'cabbit' for rabbit), semantic (e.g. 'table' for rabbit) or frankly neologistic (e.g. 'pintoc' for rabbit), all well enunciated and grammatically structured within their sentences. The little filler words are preserved for these are programmed by the intact inferior frontal region. The speech may even be hyperfluent (logorrhea, or press of speech) with prolonged well articulated meaningless rambles delivered in response to a question that should require a simple two or three word answer. So-called jargon aphasia in an extreme form of Wernicke's aphasia.

Repetition

The ability to repeat accurately what the examiner says when requested is generally thought to depend upon the pathway:

acoustic cortex → Wernicke's area → arcuate fasciculus → Broca's area → inferior part of primary motor cortex

Damage to Broca's area, Wernicke's area or the left arcuate fasciculus will all produce aphasia with disturbed repetition. Arcuate fasciculus lesions produce a syndrome known as *conduction aphasia* (Benson et al, 1973) in which

comprehension is intact and speech fluent but interrupted by phonemic paraphasic errors of which the patient is aware so that he repeatedly tries to correct them. In one way the situation is like Wernicke's aphasia, with defective transmission of information forward to the inferior frontal region but the characteristic self-correcting efforts, some successful, help to distinguish it and of course depend upon self-monitoring by Wernicke's area itself.

Disturbances of repetition vary in severity and in mild aphasias single words or even short sentences may be repeated whilst longer or more complex ones are not. Little grammatical filler words structured into a meaningless sentence pose the greatest difficulty in repetition, the classical example being the nonsense 'no ifs, ands or buts'.

Comprehension

Disturbances of comprehension are often missed. A patient may give an affirmative response because he realises that one is required, from the intonation rather than the content of the question. Testing can be difficult if speech output is limited or it there is marked apraxia, but most patients can at least indicate yes or no or point to command. Some useful examples are:

1. Yes/no questions (for example 'are we on the ground floor of this nursing home?', 'do you put your shoes on before your socks?').

2. Pointing sequentially (for example 'point to the door, then the pillow, then the ceiling' — the normal person manages a sequence of three).

3. Relational manipulation of three objects (for example 'put the coin in the cup and the pencil on its right').

Comprehension is most grossly disturbed in Wernicke's aphasia, and almost normal in Broca's aphasia, though sequential pointing may sometimes be imperfect in the latter condition.

Word finding

The simplest and most useful way of testing this is by asking the patient to name objects shown to him.

Types of aphasia (Table 21.1)

Broca's aphasia, Wernicke's aphasia and conduction aphasia have been discussed and contrasted in the preceding paragraphs. The major additional point is that Broca's aphasia is nearly always accompanied by paralysis at least of the right arm and often of the entire right side, while significant paralysis is unusual in Wernicke's and conduction aphasia.

The best recognised of additional aphasic syndromes are:

Anomic aphasia

Word finding difficulty in spontaneous speech or on confrontation naming is a feature of most forms of aphasia. Where word finding is the predominant feature and speech is otherwise normal the term anomic aphasia is used.

Table 21.1 Main clinical featuers of aphasic types.

Aphasia type	Spontaneous speech	Repetition	Comprehension	Naming
Broca	Non-fluent	Impaired	Relatively normal	Impaired
Wernicke	Fluent	Impaired	Impaired	Impaired
Conduction	Fluent	Impaired	Intact	Variably impaired
Anomic	Fluent	Intact	Intact	Impaired
Global	Non-fluent	Impaired	Impaired	Impaired
Isolation of speech area	Non-fluent with echolalia	Intact	Impaired	Impaired
Transcortical motor	Non-Fluent	Intact	Intact	Impaired
Transcortical sensory	Fluent	Intact	Impaired	Impaired
Suppl. Motor Area	Minor differences only from transcortical motor aphasia			
Putamen	Minor differences only from Broca's Wernicke's & global aphasia depending upon lesion size			
Thalamus	Similar to anomic aphasia			

Comprehension and repetition are intact and speech is fluent without paraphasias though pauses occur when specific words cannot be brought to mind. In severe cases speech may be circumlocutary in an effort to substitute for a word that cannot be found.

Anomic aphasia may be the end result of a recovering aphasia of any type. It may also occur with lesions at the following two sites:

1. The angular gyrus region, where it may be associated with alexia, constructional apraxia and features of Gerstman's syndrome (agraphia, acalculia, right-left disorientation and finger agnosia).

2. The inferotemporal region, where for example mild word finding difficulty may be associated with right hemianopia in left posterior cerebral artery infarction (Benson et al, 1974).

Isolation of the speech area
This condition is seen when extensive infarction occurs in the ring shaped border zone between the middle cerebral artery on the one hand, and anterior and posterior cerebral arteries on the other (Fig. 21.1). The middle cerebral artery supplies the large central part of the lateral cerebral convexity and the other two arteries the margins of the hemisphere. In this syndrome (Geschwind et al, 1968), preservation of Wernicke's area, Broca'a area and arcuate fasciculus are held to be responsible for the patient's ability to repeat even quite complex sentences spoken to him (transcortical aphasia). This may amount to frank echolalia (compulsive repetition of anything heard). Comprehension and spontaneous speech are grossly defective because Broca's and Wernicke's area, though themselves intact, are disconnected from other areas of the brain. Severe hypotension, carbon monoxide poisoning or carotid occlusion may cause border zone infarction.

Transcortical motor aphasia and transcortical sensory aphasia
These are less global syndromes caused by border zone infarction confined to the anterior (frontal) or posterior

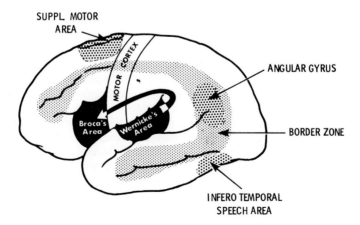

Fig. 21.1 Left cerebral convexity showing main speech areas, the heavy arrow representig the medial longitudinal (arcuate) fasciculus connecting Wernicke's and Broca's areas. Supplementary motor cortex is placed mainly on the medial aspect of the hemisphere. The large lightly stippled C–shaped area represents the border zone between arterial territories (see text) that may be damaged in the syndrome of isolation of the speech area.

(temporo-parietal) regions respectively and produce syndromes not too dissimilar from Broca's and Wernicke's aphasias but with notably preserved repetition.

Aphasia from supplementary motor area lesions
The supplementary motor area lies within anterior cerebral artery territory in front of the lower limb representation in motor cortex. Recent case studies suggest that its infarction may lead to initial mutism, with gradual improvement. Spontaneous speech is very limited at first, though there is good comprehension and repetition. The picture is similar to transcortical motor aphasia.

Aphasia from subcortical lesions
Lesion of deep structures within the left hemisphere may occasionally produce aphasia. Involvement of the anterior limb of internal capsule may affect language function particularly when adjacent putamen is involved. This is not very firmly established yet but it has been proposed that aphasias may resemble Broca's and Wernicke's aphasia (though with minor differences) depending upon whether damage is anteriorly or posteriorly placed. Left *thalamic* lesions can cause dysarthria and diminished speech volume, or some anomia if larger. Rarely more severe aphasia is claimed but it is not yet certain that the thalamic damage itself is responsible.

Global aphasia
This term is used to describe the syndrome that results from destruction of the whole central speech area, including Broca's and Wernicke's areas, frequently as a result of proximal occlusion of the middle cerebral artery. This vessel supplies most of the convexity of the hemisphere. The resulting infarction causes a non-fluent aphasia with grossly impaired comprehension and repetition.

Variability of aphasic syndromes
Although it is possible to recognise a predominant aphasic type in any patient, the syndromes are often atypical or show mixed features. There are several reasons for this. Firstly, pathological lesions rarely show any respect for the ill-defined boundaries of cerebral neuroanatomy. Secondly, tumours frequently produce effects remote from the main site of the lesion because of displacement and distortion of other parts of the brain. Thirdly, there may be some variability in the cerebral organisation of language from person to person. Left-handers in particular may produce atypical aphasias because of some bilateral representation. Even in right-handed aphasics it has been shown in research studies following injections of amylobarbitone into right and left carotids that residual aphasic speech sometimes arises in the right hemisphere (Kinsbourne, 1971), though in other cases it arises on the left. Fourthly, age has an effect, for very fluent aphasias simply do not occur in childhood and marked fluency (classical

hyperfluent Wernicke's aphasia for example) occurs predominantly in later middle life and beyond (Eslinger & Damasio, 1981). For these various reasons aphasias are often less easy to classify than this article might suggest.

Prognosis of Aphasia
Except where there has been a minor stroke or transient ischaemic attack, improvement from aphasia is slow. This is in keeping with recovery from other central disorders such as hemiplegia: most improvement occurs within the first three months and thereafter is much slower. However, unlike most other functions where a final level of function is reached is not much more than six months and often less, aphasia may occasionally continue to improve extremely slowly for a matter of years. On rare occasions the ultimate level of function may be remarkably good. Such late effects must result from adaptive change within the brain and they are unfortunatley less likely in the aged.

THERAPY

There has always been much more enthusiasm for speech therapy in aphasia than evidence that it works. What evidence there is suggests that the non-fluent aphasic with good comprehension does best. The subject has been positively reviewed by Benson (1979b). Elocution techniques, language exercises and conditioning procedures have been supplemented in recent years by additional techniques. The most promising is so-called Melodic Intonation Therapy (MIT) (Albert et al, 1973), which was developed from the early and well known observation that some aphasic patients can sing much better than they can speak. The essential point is that the patient is encouraged to impart a sense of rhythm and melody into his language output. By so doing verbalisation is improved.

In the case of the elderly aphasic there are special considerations. Patients need to be assessed individually to decide whether to undertake therapy, taking into account their general health, ability to co-operate and general attitude. Availability and geographical factors will also influence any decisions. Formal therapy may sometimes reap only modest benefit over what can be achieved by sympathetic family involvement. In a recent study of aphasic patients for example (David et al, 1982), untrained volunteers devoted two hours weekly to their patients after an initial explanation from the speech therapist of the patient's particular speech difficulty. When compared with patients treated by the trained therapists there were no differences overall in the amount of progress made. Such an approach might well prove fruitful in the elderly aphasic since it can be carried out in the home by relatives.

No therapist can substitute for the encouragement and understanding of those engaged in the patient's constant day to day management.

REFERENCES

Albert M L, Goodglass H, Helm N A, Rubens A B, Alexander M D 1981 Clinical aspects of dysphasia. Springer-Verlag, Wien, New York

Albert M L Sparks R W, Helm N A 1973 Melodic intonation therapy for aphasia. Archives of Neurology 29: 130–131

Alexander M, LoVerme S 1980 Aphasia after left intracerebral haemorrhage. Neurology 30: 1193–1202

Benson D F 1979a Aphasia, alexia and agraphia. Churchill Livingstone, Edinburgh

Benson D F 1979b Aphasia rehabilitation. Archives of Neurology 36: 187–189

Benson D F, Marsden C D, Meadows J C 1974 The amnesic syndrome of posterior cerebral artery thrombosis. Acta Neurologica Scandinavica 50: 133–145

Benson D F, Sheremata W A, Bouchard R, Segarra J M, Price D, Geschwind N 1973 Conduction aphasia. Archives of Neurology 28: 339–346

Damasio A R, Damasio H, Rizzo M, Varney N, Gersh F 1982 Aphasia with nonhaemorrhagic lesions in basal ganglia and internal capsule. Archives of Neurology 39: 15–20

David R, Enderby P, Bainton D 1982 Treatment of acquired aphasia: speech therapists and volunteers compared. Journal of Neurology, Neurosurgery and Psychiatry 45: 957–961

Eslinger P J, Damasio A R 1981 Age and type of aphasia in patients wih stroke. Journal of Neurology, Neurosurgery and Psychiatry 44: 377–381

Geschwind N 1970 The organization of language and the brain. Science 170: 940–944

Geschwind N 1971 Aphasia. New England Journal of Medicine 284: 654–656

Geschwind N, Quadfasel F A, Segarra J M 1968 Isolation of the speech area. Neuropsychologia 6: 327–340

Goodglass H, Kaplan E 1972 The assessment of aphasia and related disorders. Lea & Febiger, Philadelphia

Kinsbourne M 1971 The minor hemisphere as a source of aphasic speech. Archives of Neurology 25: 302–306

Masden J C, Schoene W C, Funkenstein H 1978 Aphasia following infarction of the left supplementary motor area. Neurology 28: 1220–1223

Meadows J C 1975 The clinical assessment of higher central function. British Journal of Hospital Medicine 14: 273–280

Mohr J P, Pessin M S, Finkelstein S, Funkenstein H H, Duncan G W, Davis K R 1978 Broca aphasia. Neurology 28: 311–324

Naeser M A, Alexander M P, Helm-Estabrooks N, Levine H L, Laughlin S A, Geschwind N 1982 Aphasia with predominantly subcortical lesion sites. Archives of Neurology 39: 2–14

Rubens A B 1975 Aphasia witn infarction in the territory of anterior cerebral artery. Cortex 11: 239–250

SECTION THREE
Vascular system

22

Cardiovascular disease, atherosclerosis and ischaemic heart disease

R. W. Stout

CARDIOVASCULAR DISEASE IN OLD AGE

Cardiovascular disease is both the commonest cause of death and the most important cause of ill health and disability in old age (Table 22.1). Atherosclerosis is the most important cause of cardiovascular disease in adults and the majority of deaths from diseases related to atherosclerosis occur in old people (Table 22.2). Other arterial diseases in old age include giant cell arteritis, while

Table 22.1a Impact of cardiovascular disease in old age: Distribution of leading causes of death — USA 1978 (Arteriosclerosis, 1981)

Coronary heart disease	33%
Cancer	21%
Cerebrovascular disease	9%
Respiratory disease	6%
Accidents	5%
Peripheral arterial disease	3%
(All cardiovascular disease	45%)

Table 22.1b Impact of cardiovascular disease in old age: Nature of illness reported by mobile elderly people in Great Britain (%) (Hunt, 1978)

	Men			Women		
Age (years)	65–74	75–84	85+	65–74	75–84	85+
Cardiac	13.5	12.5	15.2	10.3	16.1	10.0
Circulatory	3.0	4.5	13.0	4.4	4.6	3.3
Stroke	2.2	4.2		2.0	3.4	1.7
All cardio-vascular	18.5	21.2	28.2	16.7	24.1	15.0

Table 22.1c Impact of cardiovascular disease in old age: Cause of loss of mobility in people over 65 years old in Great Britain (Hunt, 1978).

Arthritis	36.2%
Pulmonary conditions	17.2%
Stroke, paralysis	14.9%
Visual impairment	14.4%
Circulatory conditions	13.8%
Cardiac conditions, blood pressure	13.2%
(All cardiovascular	41.7%)

Table 22.2 Age distribution of deaths from atherosclerosis-related diseases, (%) USA, 1978 (Arteriosclerosis, 1981)

Age	Coronary heart disease	Cerebrovascular disease	Peripheral arterial disease
Under 35	0.2	1.0	0.7
35–44	1.4	1.4	0.8
45–54	5.8	3.6	2.6
55–64	14.6	8.7	8.4
65–74	25.3	20.7	20.5
75–84	30.8	35.8	32.8
Over 84	21.8	28.6	34.1

the heart may be involved by amyloidosis or by degenerative disease of the aortic or mitral valves.

THE AGING CARDIOVASCULAR SYSTEM

The high prevalence of atherosclerosis and ischaemic heart disease in aging humans makes it difficult to separate age-related changes in the cardiovascular system from the effects of disease. Atherosclerosis, although considered to be a disease, is intimately related to aging. However, studies in disease-free humans and aging animals have revealed effects of age on the cardiovascular system (Gerstenblith et al, 1976; Kolata, 1977; Weisfeldt, 1980; Lakatta & Yin, 1982).

Morphological changes include myocardial hypertrophy, with increased stiffness of the ventricles and thickening of the endocardium and valves. Myocardial contraction is prolonged, due principally to slow relaxation, and the resting stroke volume and cardiac output are reduced. However, the contractile ability of the myocardium is unchanged and the reduction in cardiac output is mainly due to increased impedence to ejection. The larger vessels become thickened and stiff resulting in increased peripheral resistance and a rise in blood pressure, but also in a loss of adaptability to hypotension.

These changes are not severe enough to affect cardiac function at rest. It is when the heart is stressed that the effects of age become apparent. The maximal oxygen consumption and substrate oxidation rates in the myocardium appear to decline about 20% from adulthood to senescence and the cardiac response to exercise is diminished in old age. This appears to be related to a decreased response of both the heart and arteries to sympathetic stimulation. It is not clear if this is an intrinsic aging phenomenon and therefore irreversible, or if it is due to lack of conditioning resulting from, for example, decreased physical exertion in advancing age.

The age-related decline in the cardiovascular response to stress implies a diminished reserve capacity in the cardiovascular system. Maintenance of cardiovascular function in the presence of disease will be impaired in old age, and the response of the cardiovascular system to drugs will also differ.

ATHEROSCLEROSIS IN OLD AGE

Atherosclerosis is a universal disease in older people. It begins to develop in early adult life but it is only when it impairs the circulation that clinical effects appear. The important clinical syndromes related to atherosclerosis are ischaemic heart disease, cerebrovascular disease, arterial insufficiency of the lower limbs and aortic aneurysm. When considering these serious and often fatal conditions it is important to realise that they are the end stages of a chronic and progressive disease which has developed over many years.

The pathogenesis of atherosclerosis

Atherosclerosis is a disease of the intima and inner media of the artery and results from the interaction of the artery with the constituents of the blood (Ross, 1981). Four cells appear to have important roles in the pathogenesis of atherosclerosis — from the artery, endothelial and smooth muscle cells, and from the circulation, platelets and monocyte-macrophages.

The *endothelium* acts as a barrier, preventing the entry of circulating constituents into the inner part of the arterial wall. A current theory suggests that the earliest stage of the development of atherosclerosis is an injury or alteration to the endothelial barrier. *Platelets* adhere to the exposed sub-endothelial collagen and aggregate on the injured surface of the artery. Among substances released from the alpha-granules of the platelets is a potent mitogen, the platelet-derived growth factor (PDGF). The targets for PDGF and other circulating mitogens are smooth muscle cells which proliferate in the intima. The smooth muscle cells synthesise connective tissue and take up lipoproteins, becoming foam cells. Foam cells also originate from circulating monocyte-macrophages.

In its earliest stages the proliferation of arterial smooth muscle cells probably represents a repair process responding to endothelial injury. If endothelial integrity is

restored the lesion regresses and the artery returns to normal. However if endothelial injury is sustained or repeated, or if the composition of the circulation is abnormal, the process progresses. Aging may influence the development of atherosclerosis in two ways (Stout, 1981). Aging endothelial cells proliferate less readily than younger cells and hence injury will be less readily repaired in old age. Aging smooth muscle cells lose control of growth and hence proliferation will occur more readily.

The epidemiology of atherosclerosis

Prospective epidemiological studies, where characteristics are associated with the subsequent development of cardiovascular disease, have identified a number of 'risk factors' for atherosclerosis (Arteriosclerosis, 1981). Risk factors are not necessarily causative: they may be markers of another underlying abnormality, or may represent the earliest stage of the disease itself. It is useful to consider risk factors as intrinsic or extrinsic and to subdivide the latter into those that are reversible with or without proven benefit. Reversible risk factors are more common in younger people with atherosclerosis.

Intrinsic
    Age
    Male sex
    Genetic and familial

Extrinsic
    (a) Reversible with demonstrated benefit
        Hypertension
        Cigarette smoking
    (b) Potentially reversible but benefit not demonstrated
        Abnormal lipids and lipoproteins
        Diabetes mellitus
    (c) Reversible with likely but undemonstrated and possibly indirect benefit
        Obesity
        Exercise
Others
    Diet
    Hardness of drinking water
    Personality type
    Uric acid

Intrinsic risk factors

Age. Atherosclerosis becomes progressively more severe with advancing age. It may be considered to be an age-related disease but one whose progress can be accelerated by the superimposition of other risk factors.

Sex. Although ischaemic heart disease is more common in young males than in young females, the sex incidence tends to equalise with advancing age and after about the age of 70 the incidence is the same in males and females. It is not clear whether this change results from an increasing frequency in aging females or a relative decrease in males. The sex difference in incidence does not occur in cerebrovascular disease.

Family history. A family history of premature atherosclerosis is associated with an increased risk of the disease. While some of the other risk factors have a genetic basis, it appears that there is also a familial element to atherosclerosis itself.

Extrinsic risk factors

(a) Reversible with demonstrable benefit

Blood pressure. Both systolic and diastolic blood pressure are related to atherosclerosis and the frequency of cardiovascular disease progressively increases with rising blood pressure.

Cigarette smoking is one of the most important risk factors for atherosclerosis as it is purely exogenous in origin and therefore can be totally eliminated.

(b) Potentially reversible but benefit not demonstrated

Abnormal lipid metabolism. Atherosclerosis is associated with a number of disorders of lipid and lipoprotein metabolism. The best known is the relationship between serum cholesterol and low density lipoprotein (LDL) levels and atherosclerosis, but atherosclerosis is also associated with raised triglyceride and very low density lipoprotein (VLDL) levels and inversely related to high density lipoprotein (HDL) levels. Lipoprotein abnormalities may be genetic or secondary to other metabolic changes including obesity, diabetes mellitus or diet.

Diabetes mellitus. Atherosclerosis is common in both insulin-dependent and non-insulin-dependent diabetes mellitus but is unrelated to the duration, severity or treatment of diabetes. Whether blood glucose itself is the link between diabetes and atherosclerosis or whether it may be linked by other factors such as insulin is unresolved.

(c) Reversible with likely but undemonstrated and possibly indirect benefit

Obesity. Obese people have a higher frequency of atherosclerosis than those who are normal weight. This may be because obesity is associated with an increased frequency of other risk factors including hyperlipidaemia, hyperglycaemia and hypertension.

Exercise. People who take regular physical exercise have a lower incidence of atherosclerosis than those of more sedentary habits. Exercise is known to lower serum lipids, glucose and insulin levels, and has other beneficial effects on cardiac and skeletal muscle performance.

Others

A number of other risk factors have been described but the relationships are less clear. These include elevated uric acid levels, personality type and hardness of the drinking water. Although the use of the contraceptive pill increases the risk of vascular disease in younger women, oestrogen replacement therapy following the menopause does not. Diet may be related to atherosclerosis by a number of mechanisms including obesity and the production of abnormalities in lipid and carbohydrate metabolism

Multiple risk factors

While individual risk factors have a potent influence on the development of atherosclerosis and its complications, combinations of risk factors often occur in the same individual. The combined risk is greater than the sum of the individual risks.

Prevention of atherosclerosis

The identification of risk factors raises the possibility of prevention. In a disease so closely related to aging a more realistic aim would be delay rather than prevention. The fact that well designed trials have not produced conclusive evidence that alteration of some risk factors reduces the incidence of atherosclerosis and its complications, does not necessarily prove that risk factors are not causative, nor that alteration of risk factors is without benefit. Problems within the trials themselves have often prevented the attainment of a positive result. The organisational and financial problems of mounting large scale trials on the prevention of atherosclerosis are immense and even if these are surmounted a clear result is not guaranteed. It is likely that some questions on the prevention of atherosclerosis will never be answered by rigorous scientific methods.

In the present state of knowledge it seems prudent to advise changes in life-style which on empirical grounds appear both beneficial and harmless — avoid smoking, obesity and excess consumption of saturated fat and take regular physical exercise. Pharmacological intervention is not recommended unless of proven benefit, for example the reduction of blood pressure, or indicated for other reasons, for example the teatment of diabetes.

For the older patient the evidence is even sparser and treatment aims may be different. It is difficult to justify major and perhaps uncomfortable changes in life-style for happy and healthy old people, and impractical and almost certainly futile in those who are already ill or disabled. The hope must be that delay in the onset and progression of atherosclerosis earlier in life will lead to a healthier old age.

ISCHAEMIC HEART DISEASE

Ischaemia is by far the commonest cause of heart disease in old age (Table 22.3). There are three major clinical syndromes of ischaemic heart disease — angina pectoris, myocardial infarction and chronic ischaemic heart disease. The latter, which may complicate the other two or may occur without any definite history of angina or myocardial infarction, causes cardiac failure. The clinical features and management of cardiac failure are discussed in chapter 00.

Table 22.3 Prevalence (%) of heart disease in the elderly (Kennedy et al, 1977)

Age Sex	65–74 Male	Female	75+ Male	Female
Ischaemic	21	17	25	20
Hypertensive	1	5	4	10
Valvular	0	5	4	7
Pulmonary	2	0	1	0
Others and unclassifiable	15	7	22	14
Total	38	34	56	51

ANGINA PECTORIS

Angina pectoris (angina) is pain or discomfort caused by an imbalance between myocardial oxygen demand and oxygen supply. When a coronary artery is partially occluded the circulation is adequate to maintain oxygenation and metabolism of the myocardium when the heart is at rest but when cardiac work increases the blood supply cannot keep pace with the increasing demands and ischaemia occurs.

The commonest cause of angina is atherosclerosis of the coronary arteries. The coronary ostia may be involved by other conditions including syphilitic aortitis or calcific aortic valve disease. Ischaemia may also occur if cardiac work is increased by mechanical or haemodynamic loads on the left ventricle, for example from aortic valve disease or hypertension, or if the blood itself is abnormal from, for example, anaemia. Angina is reported in about 10% of people over 65 years old (Table 22.4).

Table 22.4 Prevalance (%) of evidence of ischaemic heart disease by age in men (Kitchin et al, 1973)

Age	Angina	Myocardial infarction	Abnormal ECG
50–59	4.0	2.0	29
60–69	9.1	10.8	44
70+	11.8	10.7	67

Clinical features

The classical symptom of angina is central chest pain or discomfort precipitated by exertion and relieved by rest. The pain is usually described as 'tight', 'heavy' or 'crushing' in nature. It may radiate into one or both arms, to the lower jaw but not usually to the head, or less commonly to the epigastrium or back. Occasionally it may only be experienced in these sites. The pain is closely related to the severity of the exertion and its onset is predictable. It may be associated with dyspnoea if left ventricular failure is also induced by exertion. Sometimes the patient's description of the pain is difficult to interpret and in particular a 'tight' feeling in the chest may indicate either anginal pain or shortness of breath. Pain may also be precipitated by cold, a meal or emotion combined with exertion, or, if severe, by these factors alone. Often no abnormalities are found on physical examination when the patient is at rest. It is important to check for anaemia, hypertension, aortic valve disease or manifestations of syphilis. If the patient is seen shortly after an attack of angina a third or fourth heart sound or a soft apical mid-systolic murmur is often audible. Signs of cardiac failure may be present if this occurs in addition to the angina.

Diagnosis

The diagnosis is made principally on the history. Chest X-ray and electrocardiogram (ECG) may be entirely normal when the patient is seen at rest. Serum levels of intracellular enzymes are normal as angina does not cause necrosis of myocardial tissue. On the other hand, angina frequently occurs in the presence of severe ischaemic heart disease and the ECG and chest X-ray will be correspondingly abnormal.

More detailed investigation of angina involves graded exercise testing on a treadmill accompanied by ECG monitoring, and coronary angiography. These are usually only used if cardiac surgery is being considered.

Management

General measures

It is important that any factors that might precipitate or worsen angina are identified and removed. These include anaemia, cardiac failure, obesity, hypertension and smoking. The patient should be advised to reduce exertion as soon as pain occurs. Regular exercise will improve exercise tolerance and increase the amount of exertion that can be taken before pain occurs. With severe limitation of exertion the patient must adjust his lifestyle to his abilities, avoiding heavy exertion such as stairs or carrying heavy objects and perhaps moving to a more suitable home. Social support may have to be arranged if family support is not available. Patients should be advised to be cautious in cold or very windy weather and after a heavy meal.

Drugs

Nitrates. The best drug for angina is glyceryl trinitrate. This is chewed or dissolved in the mouth and is best taken prophylactically shortly before the patient predicts that pain will occur. When this treatment is started patients often complain of a sensation of fullness in the head due to vasodilatation but this symptom is temporary. Patients should be encouraged to carry glyceryl trinitrate at all times and to take it as often as necessary. They should be advised that the drug is not addictive and that tolerance to its effects does not occur. Although nitrates may also be applied to the skin no advantages have been demonstrated over sublingual administration, and this route is much more expensive. Longer acting nitrates, for example, isosorbide dinitrate, may be taken regularly by mouth as a prophylaxis against angina.

Beta adrenoceptor blocking drugs act on the sympathetic nerve supply to the heart and reduce cardiac work and heart rate. Their effects are additive to the nitrates. β-blockers should only be used in patients with severe and frequent angina which is not effectively controlled with nitrates. They are initially given in small doses, with the dose gradually increased until pain relief occurs or complete β-blockade has been achieved as evidenced by a resting pulse of around 60 beats per minute. β-blockers should be used with caution in patients who have cardiac failure or who have a history of bronchial asthma.

Calcium antagonists (e.g. nifedipine and verapamil) have similar effects to β-blockers but different modes of action. The hypotention that these drugs may cause limits their use in older patients.

Cardiac surgery

Coronary artery (by-pass graft) surgery has a low risk in properly evaluated patients but there is little experience of cardiac surgery in elderly patients. While cardiac surgery appears to improve prognosis as well as symptoms in younger patients, no trials have taken place in elderly patients.

Unstable angina

Unstable angina is a syndrome intermediate between typical angina and acute myocardial infarction (Editorial, 1980). It consists of a changing pattern of angina with a less regular relationship to exertion, or occurring at rest. It may be of recent onset or occur after a myocardial infarction. The patient with unstable angina is at high risk of developing a myocardial infarction or sudden death.

The patient with unstable angina should be admitted to hospital, preferably to a coronary care unit. Intensive treatment with nitrates and β-blockers should be administered (Russell et al, 1982). Coronary artery by-pass surgery is often used in unstable angina but it is unknown how the prognosis following surgery compares with intensive medical treatment. Coronary angioplasty may be useful in older patients as surgery is avoided, but this technique has still to be fully evaluated.

MYOCARDIAL INFARCTION

Myocardial infarction is the most serious cardiac complication of atherosclerosis. It is the result of a sudden cessation of blood supply to part of the left ventricular myocardium with necrosis of the ischaemic tissue and eventual replacement by a fibrous scar. The commonest cause is a thrombus superimposed on an atheromatous plaque, but haemorrhage into a plaque or ulceration from a plaque with embolisation of the released material may also occur. Infarction may occur in the absence of complete occlusion if the filling pressure of the coronary artery is reduced by hypotension. Rarer causes of myocardial infarction include emboli originating from the left atrium or from a diseased aortic valve, or inflammatory disease of the artery particularly giant cell arteritis.

Clinical features

The *typical presentation* of myocardial infarction is the sudden onset of severe central chest pain. The pain is usually described as 'crushing', 'tight' or 'like a tight band surrounding the chest'. It is similar to the pain of angina pectoris but more severe, more prolonged, not related to exertion, and unrelieved by glyceryl trinitrate. It often radiates to the left or both shoulders and arms, into the jaw but not usually into the head, into the epigastrium or into the back. Sometimes the pain only occurs in the arm of the jaw. The pain is not affected by respiration or by posture. It is often accompanied by sweating, nausea and vomiting, weakness, faintness and anxiety. It is not itself associated with respiratory symptoms but myocardial infarction frequently precipitates left ventricular failure in which case dyspnoea occurs. The pain usually lasts for at least one hour and the duration of the pain is related to the size and severity of the infarct (Ledwich & Mondragon, 1980).

Atypical presentations of myocardial infarction become progressively more common with advancing age (Table 22.5). Presentation without pain but with some of the other

Table 22.5 Clinical presentation of myocardial infarction in 387 patients aged 65 and over (Pathy, 1967)

Sudden dyspnoea or exacerbation of heart failure	20%
'Classical' onset	19%
Acute confusion	13%
Sudden death	8%
Syncopal attacks	7%
Strokes	7%
Giddiness, vertigo or faintness	6%
Peripheral gangrene or increased claudication	5%
Palpitation	4%
Renal failure	3%
Recurrent vomiting	3%
Weakness	3%
Pulmonary embolus	2%
Restlessness	1%
Sweating	1%

clinical features is a frequent occurrence. A non-specific feeling of being unwell, lack of energy, and disinclination to take part in normal activities may be the only symptoms. Sometimes no symptoms occur and it is only when the patient is seen later for some unrelated purpose that a retrospective diagnosis of myocardial infarction is made on electrocardiography.

Physical signs

The patient is usually pale, clammy, anxious and in pain which he may attempt to relieve by moving about. With an atypical presentation, pallor and sweating may occur without pain. The body temperature is slightly elevated. In the early stages signs of mild congestive cardiac failure are common. The pulse may be weak and irregular. The blood pressure is often low, heart sounds may be faint in the acute stage and a third or fourth heart sound and an apical mid-systolic murmur may be heard. Two to four days after the onset a pericardial rub may be heard if the myocardial infarction is transmural. If the myocardial infarction is mild physical examination may reveal no abnormalities.

Diagnosis

When the patient presents with the classical symptoms of myocardial infarction he should be treated as such while awaiting the results of special tests. However when the presentation is atypical the diagnosis is usually only made on the results of special investigations. A good clinical history and physical findings consistent with myocardial infarction are of more value than diagnostic tests and the physician must therefore be prepared to back his clinical judgement when this is appropriate.

A mild leucocytosis and moderately raised erythrocyte sedimentation rate (ESR) occur in the early stages of myocardial infarction but marked elevations of the ESR suggest an arteritic process. Chest X-ray may show signs of left ventricular failure before clinical features appear.

Electrocardiography

The classical ECG changes of myocardial infarction are a pathological Q or Qs wave of 0.04 s or more in two or more leads, elevation of the ST segments over the affected surface of the heart with depression over the opposite side, and symmetrical inversion of the T wave (Fig. 22.1). The Q waves are only present in transmural infarctions and appear a few hours after the infarct. T wave inversion is the last change to appear and persists longest. The ECG is most helpful if a previous record can be inspected. When, as so often happens in the elderly, the initial ECG is abnormal,

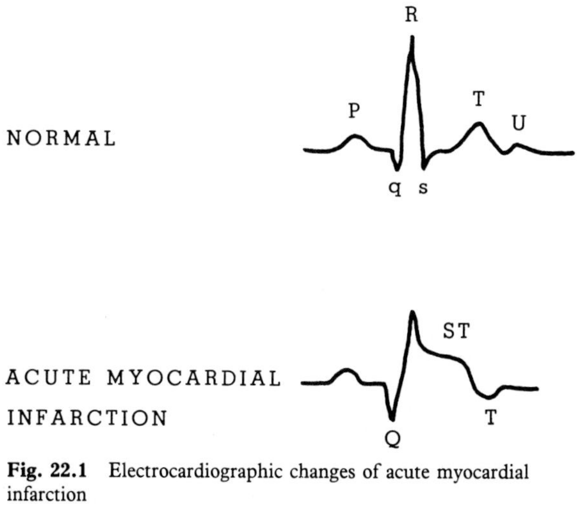

Fig. 22.1 Electrocardiographic changes of acute myocardial infarction

diagnosis is more difficult and comparison of present with past ECGs, and observation of serial changes in ECGs taken at daily or alternate day intervals is essential.

Serum enzymes

The three most commonly measured enzymes are the creatinine phosphokinase (CK), the aspartate amino-transferase (AST) and the lactate dehydrogenase (LD). The CK estimation can be made more specific by measuring the myocardial isoenzyme (CK-MB). Isoenzymes for LD can also be measured but are not performed in most clinical laboratories. Serial changes in the enzymes are most valuable (Fig. 22.2). The CK level may be raised by intramuscular injections, but this does not affect the CK-MB isoenzyme.

Other tests for myocardial infarction, including radio-isotope scanning with technetium or thallium and coronary angiography, involve sophisticated apparatus or invasive techniques and are rarely performed in elderly patients.

Management

Coronary care

Most of the deaths from myocardial infarction occur within the first four hours of symptoms. Many of these deaths are due to a disturbance of cardiac rhythm, especially ventricular fibrillation, which is often reversible. Thus if the patient is seen soon after the onset of typical symptoms of myocardial infarction he should be admitted to a coronary care unit without delay (Editorial, 1979). Although age probably has little influence on the results of coronary care, many coronary care units do not admit older patients. In these circumstances, the patient should be closely observed and attached to an ECG monitor if an experienced person is available to continually observe it. Resuscitation equipment should be close at hand. When the presentation is atypical it is unlikely that the diagnosis will be made soon after the onset of the condition. The most dangerous period will therefore have passed and coronary care is unnecessary. If the myocardial infarction is more than 24 hours old admission to hospital may be unnecessary.

Bedrest

The dangers and complications of bedrest, particularly in elderly patients, usually outweigh the benefits. Once pain has been relieved, and if there is no cardiac failure, hypotension or arrhythmias, the patient should be encouraged to be out of bed. Mobilisation should be gradual and limited if shortness of breath or pain occur. In the uncomplicated myocardial infarction, oxygen therapy is probably of little value but in the presence of left ventricular failure it is useful.

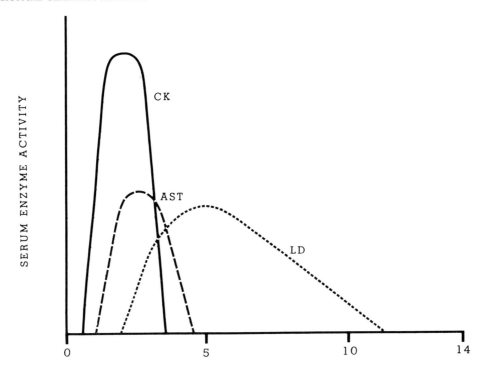

Fig. 22.2   Time course of serum enzyme changes after myocardial infarction. (CK — creatinine phosphokinase; AST — aspartate transaminase; LD — lactate dehydrogenase).

Pain relief
Pain should be relieved with intravenous morphine, 5–20 mg accompanied by an anti-emetic such as metoclopramide 10 mg or cyclizine 50 mg also given intravenously. These should be repeated as necessary but will usually only be needed for a few hours.

Anticoagulants
Anticoagulant therapy is of unproven benefit with respect to immediate mortality from myocardial infarction or in preventing further infarcts. However, anticoagulants prevent venous thrombo-embolism in immobilised patients. If early mobilisation is not possible, particularly if cardiac failure is present, 'low dose' heparin should be given — 5000 units subcutaneously two or three times daily (Mitchell, 1982).

Beta-adrenoceptor blocking drugs
There is evidence that β-blocking drugs prevent recurrence of myocardial infarction. However, the trials have not included elderly patients. The disadvantages of these drugs in old age mean that they cannot be recommended in older patients except for the treatment of severe angina or hypertension.

Rehabilitation
The older patient who has had a severe myocardial infarction will require skilled rehabilitation with a graded increase in activities under the supervision of the occupational therapist and physiotherapist. If the patient already has a chronic disease or disability, the degree of disability will be at least temporarily increased. Persistent chest pain, dyspnoea or congestive cardiac failure will limit activities of daily living. Anxiety followed by depression and psychological dependence on others may follow myocardial infarction. Patients should be encouraged to be as active as their symptoms and capabilities allow, and relatives should be discouraged from allowing or creating dependency. On return home the patient may be unable to fully resume all household tasks and if relatives are unable to provide help for a few weeks, support from social services should be arranged.

Complications
Major complications of myocardial infarction include arrhythmias, cardiac conduction disturbances and cardiac failure. These are described in chapters 23 and 24.

Cardiogenic shock
Cardiogenic shock is caused by very large myocardial

infarcts, usually involving more than 35% of the left ventricular myocardium. It is defined as hypotension (systolic blood pressure less than 90 mmHg), poor peripheral perfusion, with oliguria and metabolic acidosis. The mortality is more than 90%. Because the underlying disorder is lack of contracting left ventricular myocardium, treatment is frequently ineffective and in the aged patient should only be instituted after careful thought. Inotropic agents, such as dopamime, combined with vasodilators such as sodium nitroprusside and the usual treatment for cardiac failure may be tried.

Rupture of the ventricular septum or papillary muscle
These are catastrophic events resulting in rapid onset of severe left ventricular failure often with a fatal outcome. In both a loud pansystolic murmur is a prominent physical sign. Treatment should be for the cardiac failure. In favourable circumstances surgical repair of the defect may be life-saving.

Pericarditis
Pericarditis may occur as a result of a transmural infarct affecting the pericardial surface of the heart. In this case it occurs 2–4 days after the infarct and is usually associated with pain related to respiration and a pericardial rub. It settles in 1–2 days.

A pericardial rub with fever, pain, raised ESR and pleural involvement may occur 1–6 weeks after the infarct. This may be treated with aspirin, non-steroidal anti-inflammatory drugs or occasionally with steroids. Anticoagulants should be stopped immediately if a pericardial rub is detected as haemorrhage and pericardial tamponade may occur.

Shoulder hand syndrome
A painful stiff shoulder sometimes with vasomotor changes and oedema of the hand, usually on the left side, may occur several weeks after the myocardial infarction. This may be due to reflex vasomotor changes or to immobility of the shoulder. The stiff and frozen shoulder should be treated with heat or cold and exercise together with analgesics but

sometimes local injection of steroids may be required. The condition spontaneously resolves within about six months.

Left ventricular aneurysm
A large myocardial infarction may lead to aneurysm formation in the left ventricle. This leads to persistent cardiac failure, arrhythmias and the risk of systemic emboli from the thrombus in the aneurysm. The aneurysm may be suspected on a straight X-ray of the chest or from persistent ST-elevation on the ECG and confirmed by echocardiography. Treatment of choice is surgical removal of the aneurysm which is often combined with coronary artery by-pass grafting.

Mural thrombosis and systemic embolism
This usually happens within the first 48 hours of large myocardial infarctions. The patient should be anticoagulated.

Cardiac rupture
Rupture of the left ventricular myocardium through the infarct is rapidly fatal. It may be detected by the persistence of electrical activity of the heart in the presence of complete circulatory collapse.

Prognosis
The mortality from myocardial infarction is high in elderly patients although over 50% of those who reach hospital alive survive to be discharged. Myocardial infarction may be associated with chronic congestive cardiac failure or with recurrent attacks of chest pain but it may also be consistent with long and symptom-free survival. Decreased mobility, a decrease in the ability to undertake household or social activities, anxiety and depression are common in the first few months after acute myocardial infarction in the elderly (Peach & Pathy, 1979). Persistent physical or psychological disability is associated with a high mortality (Pathy & Peach, 1981). Those who are not disabled have a good prognosis and do not require long-term out-patient follow-up.

REFERENCES

Arteriosclerosis 1981 Report of the working group on arteriosclerosis of the National Heart Lung and Blood Institute. NIH Publication No 81–2034
Editorial 1979 Coronary-care-units — Where now? Lancet 1: 649–650
Editorial 1980 Unstable angina. Lancet 2: 569–570
Gerstenblith G, Lakatta E G, Weisfeldt M L 1976 Age changes in myocardial function and exercise response. Progress in Cardiovascular Diseases 19: 1–21
Hunt A 1978 The elderly at home. Her Majesty's Stationery Office, London
Kennedy R D, Andrews G R, Caird F I 1977 Ischaemic heart disease in the elderly. British Heart Journal 39: 1121–1127

Kitchin A H, Lowther C P, Milne J S 1973 Prevalence of clinical and electrocardiographic evidence of ischaemic heart disease in the older population. British Heart Journal 35: 946–953
Kolata G B 1977 The aging heart: changes in function and response to drugs. Science 195: 166–167
Lakatta E G, Yin F C P 1982 Myocardial aging: functional alterations and related cellular mechanisms. American Journal of Physiology 242: 927–942
Ledwich J R, Mondragon G A 1980 Chest pain duration in myocardial infarction. Journal of the American Medical Association 244: 2172–2174

Mitchell J R A 1982 'But will it help my patients with myocardial infarction?' The implication of recent trials for everyday country folk. British Medical Journal 285: 1140–1148

Pathy M S 1967 Clinical presentation of myocardial infarction in the elderly. British Heart Journal 29: 190–199

Pathy M S, Peach H 1981 Change in disability status as a predictor of long-term survival after myocardial infarction in the elderly. Age and Ageing 10: 174–178

Peach H, Pathy J 1979 Disability in the elderly after myocardial infarction. Journal of the Royal College of Physicians of London 13: 154–157

Ross R 1981 Atherosclerosis: a problem of the biology of arterial wall cells and their interactions with blood components. Arteriosclerosis 1: 293–311

Russell R O, Rackley C E, Kouchoukos N T 1982 Unstable angina pectoris: Management based on available information. Circulation 65: 72–77

Stout R W 1981 Atherosclerosis and the metabolism of the arterial wall. In: Caird F I, Evans J G (Eds) Advanced Geriatric Medicine 1, Pitman, London p 141–151

Weisfeldt M L 1980 Aging of the cardiovascular system. New England Journal of Medicine 303: 1172–1174

23

Cardiac failure

J. L. C. Dall

Heart disease is common in older patients and is the most frequent cause of death in those over 65 years. Heart failure is diagnosed by the appearance of clinical signs which indicate that the heart is unable to maintain a circulation required by the tissues. This may occur as a result of morbid change in the myocardium, its blood supply, the valves or the pericardial sac, or may be due to an excessive demand on the heart by other pathological circumstances which increase the ventricular work load. The heart may fail suddenly and abruptly as in the acute myocardial injury due to coronary artery disease with infarction, or more slowly and gradually after the compensatory mechanisms are exhausted in hypertensive disease and chronic valvular disease. In the acute situation, left ventricular failure, initial compensation may be achieved by increased release of catecholamines and an adrenergic response which will improve myocardial contractility for a short time. The Frank-Starling mechanism is the functional reserve capacity of the myocardium to respond to an overload by stretching the myofibrils and is again a relatively short lived attempt to achieve compensation. In the longer term less acute situation, hypertrophy of the ventricular muscle, and dilatation of chamber size will occur before the point arrives when one or other ventricle is unable to discharge a sufficient fraction of the end diastolic volume and there is no further reserve capacity to draw upon. There follows a series of haemodynamic changes, resulting in pulmonary congestion when the left ventricle has failed, or systemic congestion when the right ventricle, or both ventricles have failed which provide the clinical signs of heart failure. The inability to achieve end systolic emptying of the ventricle is quickly reflected in incomplete emptying of atrium during diastole, a rise in the pressure in the venous and capillary systems causing the transudation of fluid into the interstitial spaces of the lungs, the liver and the dependent subcutaneous tissues. This produces dyspnoea, hepatomegaly, juglar venous congestion and oedema as clinical signs of cardiac ailure. On the other hand, the reduced ventricular output results in impaired perfusion of the tissues so that confusion (brain), weakness and fatigue (skeletal muscle) become the symptoms in addition to shortness of breath arising from the changes in the lungs.

Reduced renal blood flow results in a compensatory increase in aldosterone production which in turn will cause increased sodium and water resorption from the renal tubules, thus expanding the extra-cellular fluid volume and increasing the circulatory burden on the heart and compounding the problem.

ROLE OF AGING

Few changes attributable to age alone are seen in the macroscopic appearances of the heart. Hearts of non-agenarians may be normal sized, have normal valves and have coronary arteries free from atheroma but these are exceptions and heart disease is common in the elderly because of the changes that relate to atherosclerosis and degeneration of collagen.

Endocardium
The endocardium of the atria thickens with an increase in collagen and elastic fibres (McMillan & Lev, 1959). Similar thickening occurs in the valves where haemodynamic factors are responsible for the appearance of lipid in the collagenous layers of both aortic and mitral cusps. This is seen as plaques on the aortic surface and these plaques increase in size with age (Pomerance, 1976). Ischaemic changes in myocardial pathology are found in about half of geriatric patients dying in heart failure whether there is a history of coronary incidents or not (Hodkinson and Pomerance, 1977). Amyloid change, mainly in the atria, is seen in about 42% of autopsy specimens from a geriatric unit, and although more common in the atria, is seen in the ventricles where there has been cardiac failure. Hypertrophic obstructive cardiomyopathy has been reported in several clinical series with an incidence of between 7 and 32% in patients over 60 years of age (Whiting et al, 1971).

Valves
Aging change in valve tissues may result in loss of pliability and therefore a degree of obstruction to flow. In the most part these changes are related to the mitral and aortic valves

and probably cause little haemodynamic effect 'per se'. Ballooning or 'parachute' type prolapse of the mitral valve is seen in the elderly, but not exclusively and arises from several morbid processes of which one or more may be present in the heart of an older patient (Barlow et al, 1981). Again the resultant haemodynamic effects may be relatively minor and only when associated with other factors does the likelihood of cardiac failure arise. Changes in the valve function and structure are more commonly a cause of signs and indeed symptoms when occurring as part of generalised atherosclerosis, with atheroma and calcification damaging the valve leaflets and so restricting movement and preventing complete opening and closing. This appears to happen in relation to the pressure changes across the valve and therefore is more common and more extensive at the aortic valve than the mitral and comparatively rare in the right side of the heart unless severe pulmonary hypertension has been present.

CAUSES OF HEART FAILURE

Primary heart disease

Ischaemic heart disease is the commonest single pathology but presents in two distinct ways. Atherosclerosis, degenerative arterial disease is a gradual process that may weaken the myocardium over many years and be detectable as multiple small areas of infarction or fibrotic change. This same process may attack the conducting tissues and result in progressive change in conduction culminating in complete heart block having passed through stages of bundle branch block to atrioventricular block. The latter is often associated with the development of bradycardia preceeding the recognition of atrioventricular dissociation and complete heart block.

These changes are gradual, usually without any significant clinical marker although cardiac failure may be precipitated by the fall in cardiac output associated with the bradyrhythmias. However insignificant the clinical features, changes in the electrocardiogram (ECG) occur and tend to be more frequent with advancing age. (Campbell et al, 1974). Complete heart block from this aetiology carries a relatively good prognosis and pacemaker implants are perfectly justified to correct cardiac failure, to increase exercise tolerance and to improve the quality of life.

Acute myocardial infarction does occur in the old, and may present with classical features of pain, dyspnoea, shock and heart failure and when it does so, the prognosis is poor. Semple & Williams (1976) compared the clinical features of presentation in a coronary care unit and showed that there was a significantly higher incidence of all the common clinical features they studied including shock, pericardial friction, pulmonary oedema and congestive heart failure and with the exception of pericarditis, the frequency increased with age. Early mortality in the old and very old was significantly higher than in younger subjects and was as likely to be due to dysrhythmias. The prognosis for defibrillation was unrelated to age, but the late onset of cardiac failure causes an excess of deaths among the very old, 11.5% compared with 5.7% among the younger group and this contributes to a higher overall mortality of 37.5% compared with 15.2% in those under 60 years of age.

Cardiac failure in this circumstance occurs because of the failure of adequate repair in the myocardium, and as early as the 10–14th day, a persistent tachycardia becomes complicated by increased jugular venous pressure, hepatomegaly and oedema. The progression is undramatic but the prognosis is poor and unless a prompt response accompanies the start of digoxin and diuretics, with a brisk diuresis, fall in the venous pressure and drop in the heart rate, the poor prognosis is likely to be borne out by the progression to increasing cardiac decompensation. Since the myocardial infarction in usually associated with a fall in blood pressure the attending physician is caught between the need to maintain an adequate pressure for cerebral and renal perfusion, and the use of vasodilator drugs to reduce the peripheral resistance. Further falls of systolic pressure in these circumstances are the rule, and rising blood urea signals the terminal phase of cardio-renal failure (Fig. 23.1).

'Painless' or atypical presentation of myocardial infarction is not confined to the older age group but occurs more commonly (Pathy, 1967). The reasons are not fully understood but old people report the pain of visceral disease (pleural friction, perforated peptic ulcer are other examples) less well and the ensuing complications may be the first clinical indication. In coronary disease this may be the onset of cardiac failure or an abrupt change in mental state. The prognosis is determined by the extent of the myocardial injury but confusion is not a welcome sign as it usually indicates a considerable fall in blood pressure.

Arrhythmias may precipitate cardiac failure and require urgent correction. When 'heart block' occurs as a complication of acute myocardial infarction the mortality is high if the infarct is anteroseptal and yet there is a good prognosis for survival and recovery of sinus rhythm if the infarct is of the inferior wall. Where bradycardia is marked, signs of cardiac failure will appear and temporary pacing will be required until sinus rhythm is restored. The outcome is usually determined within a few days.

Amyloid infiltration of the cardiac muscle becomes an increasingly important factor after the age of 80 years and has been found in 30% of hearts of patients greater than 90 years dying in a geriatric unit (Hodkinson & Pomerance, 1977). The clinical presentation is that of a large heart on X-ray, with small, or normal ECG complexes, the absence of appropriate left ventricular hypertrophy pattern, and a surprisingly quiet and docile heart on auscultation. Response to digitalisation is poor, only small doses of

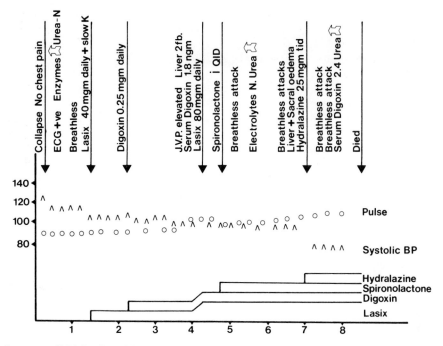

Fig. 23.1 Painless myocardial infarction with the onset of congestive cardiac failure in the third week despite treatment with diuretics and digoxin from the second week. Progress is shown in weeks from onset. (N — normal; J.V.P. — jugular venous pressure; arrow indicates an elevation)

digoxin may be required and there is an absence of hypertension or valvular murmurs to account for the cardiac size. Primary amyloid may occur only in the heart and cannot be confirmed without post mortem examination, but secondary amyloid occurs in association with long standing rheumatoid arthritis, chronic pyelonephritis, old pulmonary tuberculosis, affecting the heart, spleen and kidneys and a positive biopsy may be obtained from the gum or rectum during life. No treatment is of any consequence in affecting the amyloid change, but cardiac failure should be treated with diuretics and digoxin and vasodilator drugs.

Disease of the valves
Calcific aortic stenosis is usually associated with some degree of regurgitation heard clinically as an early diastolic murmur down the left sternal border but there may be some difficulty in differentiating the systolic ejection murmur of stenosis from the physiological bruit arising from sclerosis of the valve and thickening of the aorta. The presence of a bruit conducted into the carotid vessels is an important sign but equally important is the presence of left ventricular hypertrophy on the ECG. The presence of co-existent hypertension may mask the typical pulse contour and the characteristic blood pressure of aortic valve obstruction. When sufficiently severe to cause symptoms of fatigue, angina or cardiac failure, aortic valve disease is usually associated with enough calcification to be seen on a

lateral chest X-ray. As response to medication is poor, and the prognosis limited after the onset of severe anginal symptoms or the occurrence of cardiac failure, more experience is being gained of valve replacement (Copeland et al, 1977) as an alternative treatment.

Mitral valve disease in the elderly is occasionally a legacy of rheumatic mitral disease with stenosis of minor degree (Figs. 23.2 & 23.3) until the cusps thicken and calcify with aging, but more commonly calcification occurs in the mitral annulus inhibiting its normal contracting action during systole, and resulting in incompetence of the valve (Roberts & Perloff, 1972). The heart is enlarged, the apex beat is displaced to the anterior axillary line and a pan systolic murmur is heard all over the praecordium but is also conducted into the axilla. Cardiac failure is signaled by dilatation of the chambers on the left side of the heart which is seen to be considerably enlarged on the chest X-ray. Adequate response to treatment results in a reduction in size of the cardiac shadow on X-ray as well as clearing of the clinical signs. Atrial fibrillation frequently accompanies mitral valve disease, and responds well to management with cardiac glycosides.

Cardiomyopathy
An important differential diagnosis of aortic stenosis is a hypertrophic obstructive cardiomyopathy (idiopathic hypertrophic subaortic stenosis) which is no longer to be

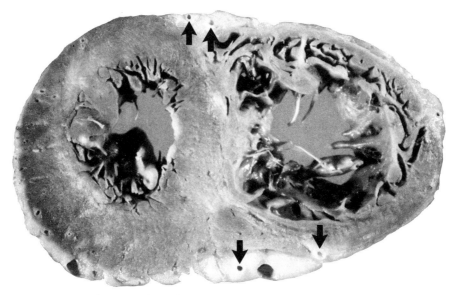

Fig. 23.2 From a male patient aged 92 years, the section shows right ventricular hypertrophy and widely patent coronary arteries (marked by arrows).

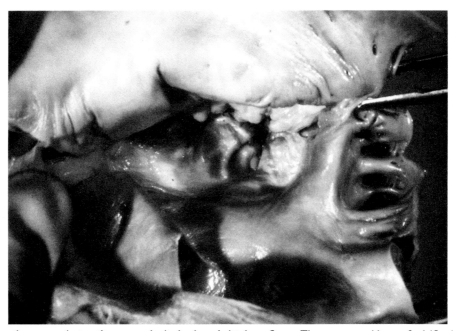

Fig. 23.3 From the same patient — the narrowed mitral valve admitted one finger. There was no evidence of calcification or atherosclerotic change on the valve.

regarded as a rare disease in the elderly (Whiting et al, 1971; Mintz & Kolter, 1981). A harsh ejection systolic murmur without a diastolic component and varying in intensity should raise clinical suspicion. Systemic hypertension (Petrin & Tavel, 1979) and calcification in the mitral annulus (Krozon & Glassman, 1978) occur in association with this form of cardiomyopathy, and when

present investigation by echocardiography is fully justified looking for evidence of assymetrical septal hypertrophy and abnormal movement during systole of the anterior mitral cusp (Rossen et al, 1974).

Secondary cardiac failure

Whereas primary heart failure results from the inability of a diseased heart to maintain an adequate circulation, secondary cardiac failure may arise when excessive demands are placed on a heart capable of functioning adequately in normal circumstances. Diagnosis is of fundamental importance as the standard treatment for cardiac failure is likely to fail and may even be dangerous. Treatment of the underlying cause is usually sufficient to restore the circulatory compensation and any treatment started to relieve cardiac failure should be withdrawn (Dall, 1970).

Anaemia
The classical combination of anaemia and heart failure would be in severe untreated pernicious anaemia, with haemoglobin values of 3 or 4 g; the whole clinical picture developing slowly and relentlessly in an old lady over a period of about a year. Iron deficiency to this level of anaemia is less common but can occur as a result of chronic bleeding haemorrhoids in embarassed old men and women. Treatment of the anaemia is all that is required but if transfusion is contemplated, diuretic therapy should be instituted to cover the period of the infusion as sudden expansion of the circulatory volume may aggravate heart failure.

Thyroid disease
Thyrotoxicosis is an important cause of rapid atrial fibrillation in old people. (Lazarus & Harden, 1969). The rate is unresponsive to standard doses of digoxin and this alone may be the diagnostic clue since eye signs, tremor or sweating of classical Graves' disease are rare. Even in the absence of atrial fibrillation, persistent tachycardia even at rest should be regarded as suspicious and thyroid function tests performed. Where cardiac failure has occurred, full doses of diuretics are indicated; digoxin appears of little value and may be pushed to toxic levels without benefit, but despite the apparent contraindication of cardiac failure, beta blockade with propranolol may rapidly relieve symptoms by slowing the heart rate and increasing the efficiency. Appropriate treatment of the hyperactive thyroid will restore cardiac compensation.

In myxoedema, the heart is slow and inefficient. The ECG may be diagnostic and the chest X-ray may show a diffuse cardiomegaly. The rapid response to thyroxine suggests the low voltage ECG is due to a pericardial effusion rather than myocardial infiltrate, and the same conclusion is supported by the rapid reduction in heart size on X-ray. If the diagnosis is overlooked, cardiac failure which appears to be 'resistant' to diuretics and digoxin results and this should be kept in mind where the response to therapy is inappropriately poor.

Paget's disease
Paget's disease of bone induces cardiac failure in those with extensive disease because of the great metabolic activity in the affected bones resulting in a functional A–V shunt. Heart failure is a cause of death in extensive Paget's disease. Digoxin and diuretics are ineffective and harmful and some treatment that will quickly reduce the metabolic activity in the bone is necessary. Calcitonin, mithramycin, or cyclophosphamide may be tried, but experience is lacking of their efficacy in this particular situation.

Chronic obstructive airways disease
In chronic obstructive airways disease, morbid change in the lungs cause the right side of the heart to fail. This may be a feature of chronic bronchitis, with cyanosis, cough and spit as major features of the clinical picture (blue bloater), or the problem may be due to emphysema (pink puffer) alone, in which case cough and spit are absent but dyspnoea is severe. In either event, improved respiratory performance with bronchodilators and antibiotics if necessary, reduce the obstruction, improve the oxygenation and in turn this will reduce pulmonary hypertension and thus the strain on the right ventricle is relieved. Where pulmonary disease is severe, and PO_2 levels of less than 55% are recorded, increased pulmonary artery pressures are found and this is reversed by adequate oxygenation and is one of the indications for continuous oxygen therapy (McNeill & Watson, 1966). Oxygen therapy is to be used with caution in the presence of severe cyanosis of this origin.

Pulmonary embolic disease
Pulmonary embolic disease does not occur in fit, active people but should be suspected when increasing breathlessness — out of proportion to the clinical signs in the chest or on the chest X-ray — is associated with signs of congestive cardiac failure. Obvious supportive ECG evidence of right ventricular hypertrophy or partial RBBB may be lacking if the problem arises as a result of multiple small emboli. A recent past history of dehydration, enforced bad rest, hip or pelvic fracture or retention of urine increase the clinical suspicion, and unilateral leg swelling in hemiplegia should not be ignored. Doppler scanning of the thigh veins in patients may be helpful but where suspicion is high even if leg swelling is absent, pelvic vein thrombosis may still be present and a trial of anticoagulant therapy may confirm the suspicion by relieving symptoms.

Maintenance therapy
In contrast to the relatively good prognosis for heart failure when this occurs as a secondary feature of another illness, heart failure in primary heart disease, due to myocardial ischaemia, hypertension, degenerative valvular disease or cardiomyopathies, usually requires some form of maintenance therapy even after compensation of the state of failure has been achieved. Nevertheless, in all cases an attempt should be made to withdraw digoxin at least once before the patient is committed to a long term therapy.

TREATMENT

The implied threat to life in the term 'cardiac failure' is fully justified, and despite the improvements in the last 20 years, heart failure remains the single most common cause of death in persons over 65 years of age (World Health Organisation, 1974). Advances in therapy have improved the quality of life but have made no difference to the underlying morbid processes from which the problem stems. Survival following a first episode of heart failure has probably been prolonged by the new diuretic agents and may be further altered by surgery of the coronary arteries or valve replacement, but even in these circumstances the relief is temporary as the damaged myocardium is not subject to a repair process and the morbid effects of the precipitating disease remain.

Bed rest is seldom recommended in the management of the older patient, but in acute cardiac failure associated with recent left ventricular decompensation and urgent dyspnoea, bed rest, or rest in a comfortable supporting chair is a necessary measure, and even minimal exertion like walking to the toilet should be avoided for 48 hours. A bedside commode should be provided if necessary and the patient prevailed upon to use it since at this critical stage even limited physical exertion may trigger further episodes of dyspnoea, or significantly reduce the renal blood flow thus reducing the effectiveness required even during the night. Sedation with small doses of morphine (10 mg) is helpful and allays anxiety, but by far the best is the relief of dyspnoea caused by pulmonary congestion. Persistent restlessness, like confusion is usually an index of impaired cardiac output and reduced cerebral perfusion; sedation may aggravate the situation, and the judicious use of oxygen may relieve it. Mobilisation from rest should be anticipated and gentle physiotherapy for the legs should be instituted to reduce the risk of venous emboli. The regression of dyspnoea and the control of the resting heart rate are the best guide to the timing of a graduated convalescence, but full mobility should not be attempted while a raised jugular venous pressure, hepatomegaly or persistent rales at the lung bases are still in evidence.

Salt restriction is an extreme measure, and since the appetite is already disturbed by hepatic and gastric congestion, it may make a misery out of meals. If a good diuresis is achieved with treatment, it is probably sufficient to forbid added salt to the cooked food. Where the regime is to be prolonged, as in the case of hypertensive heart failure, salt substitutes may be encouraged. Salt restriction should be limited to those cases where impaired renal function results in a poor diuresis, and in these circumstances it may also be necessary to restrict fluid (Braunwald, 1981).

Diuretic therapy

The advances in this area in the last 25 years are among the most striking achievements in clinical practice. Paracelsus in the sixteenth century is said to have recognised the ability of mercurous chloride (calomel) to cause a flow of urine (Hamdy, 1980), and the only sophistication achieved before 1950 was to give very toxic mercurial salts by injection in place of oral dosing. Renal damage was almost inevitable and cardio-renal failure common. In addition, a nephrotic syndrome due to tubular damage could add to the oedema and defeat the diuretic regimes. Cardiac beds, hugely swollen legs draining fluid from Southey's tubes inserted into the subcutaneous tissues are museum pieces, and it is difficult for the younger doctor to believe that such primitive methods of management were in daily use such a short time ago.

Oral diuretic therapy, with the thiazide (benzo-thiadiazines) group of drugs, beginning with hydrochlorothiazide in the late 1950s swept the toxic mercurials out of clinical use by their relative safety, the convenience of oral dosing, the prompt clinical response and the incomparably superior salt and water loss achieved. For treatment of the non-urgent situation or for maintenance therapy, they remain the drugs of first choice. More potent preparations which inhibit sodium resorption in the kidney, not only in the distal tubules but also in the proximal tubule and the loop of Henle, have been classified as the 'loop' type diuretics (furosemide, ethacrynic acid, butenamide), and are not only more potent in terms of sodium and water loss but act extremely rapidly when given by parenteral injection. In acute left ventricular failure, intravenous therapy with a 'loop' diuretic will initiate a diuresis within minutes and has assumed the central role in the management of this emergency. The same drugs given by mouth cause brisk response and effective diuresis in the early stages of cardiac failure, but are not necessary for maintenance regimes unless a significant level of renal damage has impaired the response to thiazides.

Side effects

All the drugs in these categories will cause a natriuresis as the primary effect, but all, to a varying degree, cause potassium loss and in the elderly patient, who may have a less than adequate dietary potassium content, the loss is both significant and clinically important (Dall et al, 1971; Judge et al, 1974). The clinical importance arises from the loss of muscle strength, the constipation and mental apathy that has been demonstrated to accompany hypokalaemia, as well as the increased sensitivity to digoxin that will occur. Potassium supplements are not always taken by patients in the quantity prescribed, and to be effective about 20 mmol of potassium needs to be provided each day. Most of the fixed combination preparations with added potassium are insufficient to correct depletion and barely enough to provide for loss in a maintenance situation where no real diuresis is taking place. Because of the problems of providing an acceptable form of potassium supplement, many physicians now prescribe a combination of a thiazide diuretic and one of the weak, potassium sparing diuretics (amiloride, triamterene, spironolactone). Here again the regime will maintain the status quo but not correct a deficit that has already occurred and in the first instance, potassium supplementation in adequate dosage (e.g. 600 mg slow K tid) is to be recommended. Other side effects of long term thiazide therapy have been carefully documented as part of the European Working Party on Hypertension in the Elderly (EWPHE) trial (Amery et al, 1978). This has shown that changes in glucose tolerance and in the serum uric acid excretion occur and are statistically significant when compared with controls, although clinical diabetes and clinical gout have not occurred. These changes are related to the therapy and return to normal when it is discontinued. Clinical gout will occur with bigger doses and may be a problem in the later stages of cardiac failure (Leading article, 1978). Diabetes can be aggravated, latent diabetes can be disclosed and diabetic ketosis have been recorded as complications of thiazide therapy (Hicks, 1973; Lavender & McGill, 1974). Skin rashes, so common and troublesome with mercurial diuretics, occur, but relatively infrequently with oral diuretic agents.

Cardiac glycosides

Digoxin and Digitoxin are the glycosides in common clinical use. Digoxin is poorly protein bound, well absorbed, with a good bio-availability and therefore prediction of dose should be reasonably accurate. Despite the ability to estimate serum levels, the management of digoxin therapy in the elderly remains one of the areas in which prescribing errors commonly occur. Many factors are involved including age, body weight, electrolyte status, and the cations, but most important in the older patient is the method of elimination. Digoxin is excreted almost completely unchanged by the kidney and therefore excretion may be impaired when renal function deteriorates from normal.

Digitoxin is 90% protein bound and is not excreted through the kidney but is metabolised in the liver and this would appear to be the drug of choice in renal failure. However the excretion is very slow and the fear of toxic effects if once induced lasting for several weeks in the elderly, has limited its popularity.

The role of the glycosides has been intensively studied since the estimation of serum levels became possible. The exact role of digoxin has not yet been clarified but it appears to shorten fibre length, increase the contractility of the muscle, reduce ventricular end-diastolic pressure, improve cardiac filling and cause a fall in the central venous pressure. This sequence of events is seen to best advantage where atrial fibrillation is associated with heart failure, but an effect, if less marked has been demonstrated in the heart in sinus rhythm, even when not in overt cardiac failure (Leading Article, 1979). The glycosides alter the cation content of the myocardial cell, or facilitate alterations across the membrane by an effect on sodium-potassium adenosine triphosphastase (Na+ K+ ATPase) receptors on the cell membrane (Glynn, 1969; Langer, 1971). The positive inotropic response induced is accompanied by a net loss of potassium and probably magnesium also from the myocardial cell and a net gain of sodium and calcium (Langer & Serena, 1970). Changes in the extracellular values of sodium, potassium, calcium and magnesium have all been shown to influence the effect of glycosides. Hypokalaemia and hypomagnesaemia increase the sensitivity to digoxin but high levels of potassium and low concentration of sodium in the extracellular compartment appear to inhibit the glycoside effects.

Ringer (1883) one hundred years ago appreciated the importance of calcium in myocardial function. It is known to influence excitation-contraction coupling and a small labile pool of calcium is closely linked with contractile activity (Langer & Serena, 1976). More recent studies suggest the excitability of cardiac muscle, the risk of digitalis induced automaticity and arrhythmias, is linked to a disturbance of the ratio of calcium and potassium. Where normal values exist, an appropriate therapeutic response to digoxin is achieved but where deficiency of calcium reduces the ratio, digoxin is relatively ineffective. By contrast, when Ca^{++} is normal and K^+ is reduced, the ratio is tilted in the opposite direction and increased sensitivity to digoxin will be more likely to occur even when the serum values of digoxin are not outside the accepted therapeutic range (Dall, 1980). It seems likely that detailed studies of the relationship between sodium and potassium, calcium and magnesium would demonstrate similar modifications of the expected therapeutic effects.

The clinical effects are best seen in the blocking of atrioventricular conduction. The slowing of conducting velocity in the conducting tissues results in a prolongation of the P.R. interval when in sinus rhythm and a reduced ventricular response rate in atrial fibrillation. The effect on the myocardial cell is to increase the force and velocity of contraction and a shortening of the refractory period which is seen as a shortening of the Q-T interval on the ECG tracing. The proper clinical use of digoxin depends not only on achieving satisfactory serum levels in the appropriate therapeutic range (usually 1–2.5 ng), but ensuring that due allowance is made for renal failure and resultant delay in excretion, and the corrections and supervision of the values of the other cations which manifestly alter response and sensitivity.

Dosage

Where renal function is normal, full doses of digoxin may be applied irrespective of age if the associated cation values are also normal. In practice there is little need for parenteral therapy. The response to a loading dosage of 0.5 mg, stat, is to reduce therapeutic levels within 48 hours.

This may be followed by maintenance regime of 0.25 mg daily.

When renal function is reduced to a creatinine clearance of less than 40 ml/min, smaller doses of digoxin, 0.25 mg, stat, and 0.125 mg daily will be adequate. Single doses of P–G digoxin (0.065 mg) do not achieve therapeutic serum levels unless there is gross renal failure (Caird & Kennedy, 1977).

Toxic effects are common because the therapeutic margin between effect, safety and toxicity is extremely attenuated in the old, by some of the factors already discussed and by the quality of the myocardium itself. Dangerous toxic effects are the arrhythmias which result from cardio-toxicity with hyperirritability. The use of atropine to slow a rapid dysrhythmia is an old remedy. It would now be more relevant to use a calcium blocker such as nifedipine to alter the Ca^{++}/K^+ ratio and reduce the effect of digoxin on the muscle cell. Central effects include confusion, nausea, vomiting and yellow vision and are associated with high serum levels rather than increased sensitivity as with the dysrhythmias. In excessive over-dosage, cholestyramine, kaopectate, maalox may reduce absorption from the gut and relieve nausea and confusion. Since digoxin increases the force of contraction it is best used to support heart failure in the absence of obstruction due to valvular disease. Heart failure in coronary disease especially when complicated by atrial fibrillation, and also in hypertensive disease. Where obstruction at a valve (aortic or mitral, or in the pulmonary vascular bed, in corpulmonale) is the cause of heart failure, it is unlikely that digoxin will have the same beneficial effect either in the acute stage or in a maintenance regime. The obstruction must be relieved if treatment is to succeed.

Where the myocardium is failing under the stress of a high output syndrome, a short lived improvement with the initial digitalisation may be followed by disaster if the dosage of digoxin is pushed too high in an attempt to reduce an associated tachycardia which is part of the compensatory mechanism.

It follows that accurate assessment of the underlying morbid disease in the heart is of utmost importance so that the clinican will know what can be achieved by digoxin, and more important, when the response will be limited. The frequent side effects reported with digoxin therapy are not due to the drugs but are entirely the responsibility of the prescribing physician. For this reason, digoxin should not be used in a maintenance regime without at least one attempt to discontinue, once compensation has been achieved.

Vasodilator drugs

Where cardiac failure persists despite adequate digoxin therapy and a significant response to diuretics, the use of vasodilator drugs (Table 23.1) to reduce the after-load on

Table 23.1 Vasodilator drugs in current clinical practice

Hydralazine	Oral 30–200 mg daily I.V.	Arterial
Prazosin	Oral	Arterial & Venous
Nitroprusside	I.V.	Arterial & Venous
Nitrates		
Nitroglycerin	Oral 5–20 mg	Venous
Isosorbide	Oral 10–60 mg	Venous
Captopril*	Oral 25–100 mg	Arterial & Venous

*(Converting Enzyme Inhibitor)

the left ventricle is a logical and attractive therapeutic concept. After-load is determined by the arterial impedence to be overcome by the left ventricle and systemic vascular resistance is the most important factor in arterial impedence. The objective is to reduce the after-load, allow the cardiac output to rise and in so doing relieve the clamant symptoms of fatigue, anorexia and mental confusion. The rise in cardiac output will also reduce the pulmonary artery pressure and relieve dyspnoea associated with pulmonary congestion. The response to nitroprusside is prompt but short lived and it is indicated only in the circumstances of acute left ventricular failure. The nitrates, prazosin, hydralazine and captopril have similar clinical effects but have slightly differing effects on the haemodynamics of heart failure. A comparative study of nitroprusside and captopril produced a similar reduction in the mean blood pressure in both regimes, but a greater decrease of the systemic vascular resistance with nitroprusside suggests that the overall augmentation of the cardiac stroke index is achieved by changes predominating in the after load with nitroprusside, and in the preload with the converting enzyme inhibitor captopril (Hermenovich et al, 1982). More detailed studies of the action of captopril (Powers et al, 1982) shows a fall in the mean arterial pressure and despite improved cardiac function, renal blood flow does not improve. Similar studies have been conducted with all the available drugs; hydralazine (Rubin et al, 1979), nitrates (Franciosa et al, 1977) and prazosin (Aronow et al, 1979) and benefit has been achieved in chronic heart failure.

While many authors have been able to demonstrate improved haemodynamics in short-term observations (Weber et al, 1980; Massie et al, 1981; Chatterjee et al, 1980) it has been more difficult to establish the role of this therapy in long-term treatment. Walsh & Greenberg (1979), Massie et al (1981) and Franciosa et al (1982) were unable to show any difference in body weight, clinical classification of dyspnoea, heart rate, blood pressure or heart size as estimated by X-ray and echocardiogram during and after 26 weeks of treatment with hydralazine or placebo. However successful results have been obtained in a similar trial using nitrates (Franciosa & Cohn, 1980).

The principal indication for vasodilator therapy is chronic left ventricular failure as in ischaemic heart disease, hypertensive disease or incompetence of the aortic and/or mitral valve, where the blood pressure is maintained or even raised. In other circumstances such as valve stenosis and cor pulmonale, the beneficial effect on the after-load component is reduced or eliminated and the adverse effects of falling mean arterial pressure may result in a further significant reduction in cerebral perfusion and renal blood flow. Where an effect is achieved and appropriate clinical improvement occurs, the opportunity should be taken to withdraw therapy if possible and introduce it again, short term, if the circumstances require it. In the present state of knowledge there is little justification for maintenance regimes.

The drugs available for the treatment of cardiac failure are potent and toxic. Where they are used appropriately, the response to therapy is good even in the very old. Toxic effects are likely to arise when the drugs are exhibited in higher dosage than usual because of impaired response. In these circumstances the need to re-examine the clinical information and to confirm the accuracy of the underlying pathology is fundamental. No amount of sophisticated therapy, with permutations of diuretics, digoxin or vasodilators justifies the failure to identify mitral stenosis or hypothyroidism as the cause of refractory failure. Finally, the clinician should remember that despite the improved management of heart failure, death from heart disease remains the most common terminal illness in the elderly.

REFERENCES

Amery A, Berthaux P, Birkenhager W et al 1978 Antihypertensive therapy in patients above 60 years. (Fourth Interim report of the European Working Party on high blood pressure in the elderly: EWPHE) Clinical Science and Molecular Medicine 55: 263–270

Aronow W S, Lurie M, Turbow M, Whittaker K, Van Camp S, Hughes D 1979 Effect of prazosin vs placebo on chronic left ventricular heart failure. Circulation 59: 344–348

Barlow J B, Pocock W A, Promund Obel I W 1981 Mitral valve prolapse; Primary secondary both or neither? American Heart Journal 102: 140–143

Braunwald E 1981 Heart Failure: Pathophysiology and treatment. American Heart Journal 102: 486–490

Caird F I, Kennedy R D 1977 Digitalisation and digitalis intoxication in the elderly. Age and Ageing 6: 21–28

Campbell A E, Caird F I, Jackson T F M 1974 Prevalence of abnormalities of the electrocardiogram in old people. British Heart Journal 36: 1105–1011

Chatterjee K, Ports T A, Brundage B H, Massie B, Holly A N, Parmley W W 1980 Oral hydralazine in chronic heart failure: Sustained beneficial effects. Annals of Internal Medicine 92: 600–604

Copeland J G, Griepp R B, Stinson E B, Slumway N E 1977 Isolated aortic valve replacement in patients older than 65 years. Journal of the American Medical Association 237: 1578–1581

Dall J L C 1970 Maintenance digoxin in elderly patients British Medical Journal i: 194–195

Dall J L C 1980 Observations on action of digoxin. In: Caird F I, Evans J G (eds) Advanced Geriatric Medicine. Pitman, London

Dall J L C, Paulose S, Ferguson J A 1971 Potassium intake of elderly patients in hospital. Gerontologia Clinica 13: 114–116

Franciosa J A, Pierpont G, Cohn J N 1977 Haemodynamic improvement after oral hydralazine in left ventricular failure. Annals of Internal Medicine 86: 389–391

Franciosa J D, Cohn J N 1980 Sustained haemodynamic effects without tolerance during long-term isosorbide dinitrate treatment of chronic left ventricular failure. American Journal of Cardiology 45: 648–653

Franciosa J A, Weber T, Levine B, Kinasewitz G T, Janicki J S, West J, Henis M M, Cohn J N 1982 Hydralazine in long term treatment of chronic heart failure. Lack of difference from placebo. American Heart Journal 104: 587–589

Glynn M 1969 In: Fisch C, Surawicz B (eds) Digitalis. Grune and Stratton, New York

Hamdy R C 1980 Diuretic Therapy in the Older Patient. Smith Kline and French, London

Hermenovich J, Awan N A, Lui H, Mason D T 1982 Comparative analysis of the haemodynamic actions of captopril and sodium nitroprusside in severe chronic congestive heart failure. American Heart Journal 104: 1211–1215

Hicks B H 1973 A controlled study of clopamide, clorexolone and hydrochlorothiazide in diabetics. Metabolism 22: 101–103

Hodkinson H M, Pomerance A 1977 The clinical significance of senile cardiac amyloidosis: a prospective clinics pathological study. Quarterly Journal of Medicine 46: 381–387

Judge T G, Caird F I, Leask R G S, MacLeod C 1974 Dietary intake and kidney excretion of potassium in the elderly. Age and Ageing 3: 158–161

Kitchin A H, Lowther C P, Milne J S 1973 Prevalence of clinical and electrocardiographic evidence of ischaemic heart disease in the older population. British Heart Journal 35: 946–955

Krozon I, Glassman E 1978 Mitral ring in idiopathic hypertrophic subaortic stenosis. American Journal of Cardiology 42: 60–66

Langer G H 1971 The intrinsic control of myocardial contraction. New England Journal of Medicine 285–1065

Langer G H, Serena S D 1970 Effects of strophanthin upon contractions and ionic exchange in rabbit ventricular myocardium. Journal of Molecular and Cellular Cardiology 1: 65

Lavender S, McGill R J 1974 Non ketotic hyperosmolar coma in furosemide therapy. Diabetes 23: 247–248

Lazarus J H, Harden R M 1969 thyrotoxicosis in the elderly. Gerontologia Clinica 11: 371–378

Leading Article 1978 Diuretics in the Elderly. British Medical Journal i 1092–1092

Leading Article 1979 Digoxin in Sinus Rhythm. British Medical Journal i 1103–1104

McMillan J B, Lev M 1959 The Aging Heart — Endocardium. Journal of Gerontology 14: 268

McNeill R S, Watson J M 1966 Oxygen therapy in the home British Medical Journal i 331–333

Massie B, Ports T, Chatterjee K, Parmley W, Ostland J, O'Young J, Haughom F 1981 Long term vasodilator therapy for heart failure. Clinical response and its relationship to haemodynamic measurements. Circulation 62: 269–275

Mintz G S, Kilte M N 1981 Are you overlooking I.H.S.S. in your elderly patients? Geriatrics 36: 95–102

Pathy M S 1967 Clinical presentation of myocardial infarction in elderly. British Heart Journal 29: 190–199

Petrin T E, Tavel M E 1979 Hypertrophic subaortic stenosis as observed in a large community hospital. Journal American Geriatrics Society 27: 43–46

Pomerance A 1976 Pathology of the myocardium and valves. In: Caird F I, Dall J L C, Kennedy R D (eds) Cardiology in Old Age. Plenum Press, New York & London, p 11–55

Powers E R, Bannerman K S, Stone J, Reison D S, Escala E L, Kalischer A, Weiss M B, Scacca R R, Cannon P J 1982 The effect of captopril on renal, coronary and sytemic haemodynamics in patients with severe congestive heart failure. 104: 1203–1206

Ringer S 1883 Journal of Physiology 4: 222–225

Roberts W C, Perloff J K 1972 Mitral valvular disease. A clinical pathological survey of the conditions causing the mitral valve to function abnormally. Annals of Internal Medicine 77: 939–975

Rossen R M, Goodman D J, Ingham R E, Popp R L 1974 Electrocardiographic criteria in the diagnosis of idiopathic subaortic stenosis. Circulation 50: 747–751

Rubin S A, Chatterjee K, Ports T A, Gelbert H J, Brundage B H, Parmley W W 1979 Influence of short term oral hydralazine therapy on exercise haemodynamics in patients with severe chronic heart failure. American Journal of Cardiology 44: 1183–1189

Semple T, Williams B O 1976 Coronary care for the elderly. In: Caird F I, Dall J L C, Kennedy R S (eds) Cardiology in Old Age. Plenum Press, New Tork and London, p 297–313

Walsh W, Greenberg B 1979 Late results of hydralazine in patients with refractory heart failure Circulation 60: Suppl ii 130

Weber K T, Kinasewitz G T, West J S, Jamickie J S, Reichek N, Fishman A P 1980 Long term vasodilator therapy with trimazosin in chronic cardiac failure. New England Journal of Medicine 303: 242–247

Whiting R B, Powell W J, Dunsmore R E, Sander C A 1971 Idiopathic hypertrophic subaortic stenosis in the elderly. New England Journal of Medicine 285: 196–200

World Health Organization 1974. World Health Statistics Report 27: 9–10

24

Disorders of cardiac rhythm and conduction

F. I. Caird

Disorders of cardiac rhythm and conduction are very common in the elderly. Their investigation depends initially upon a proper history. The sudden onset of palpitations, and their sudden offset should be apparent in episodic tachyarrhythmias. The relation of possible precipitating factors to the onset should be investigated. In the chronic cardiac dysrhythmias it is necessary to inquire into the occurrence of dyspnoea, of frank cardiac failure and of symptoms suggestive of thyrotoxicosis. Stokes Adams attacks in the elderly may be atypical and difficult to diagnose but their sudden onset, the occurrence of pallor at their beginning and more especially of generalised flushing on recovery, and the finding of an absent or very slow pulse during an attack are characteristic. They may require to be distinguished from the many other causes of loss of consciousness.

Clinical examination may reveal tachycardia, regular or irregular, or bradycardia (usually 40 beats per minute or less) in the case of complete heart block, but the pulse may be normal (e.g. in atrial flutter with a regular 4:1 block or bundle branch block). Irregularity of the pulse, the nature of the irregularity, variable intensity of the first heart sound and cannon waves in the venous pulse are important physical signs, as are those of any concomitant heart disease. The resting electrocardiogram is often crucial. Particular note should be taken of the frequency of any disturbance of rhythm. A longer duration of electrocardiogram may be obtained and may be extremely useful if the attacks are very frequent, occurring every few hours or so. It is now routine and popular to carry out 24 hour ambulatory electrocardiographic monitoring, but in geriatric practice is only useful if episodic arrhythmias or disorders of conduction are relatively frequent and occur at least several times per week. Only then will the investigation have any reasonable chance of detecting an episodic disorder. There are many difficulties, both technical and patient-derived. In particular the establishment of the elderly of a definite relationship between attacks of dysrhythmias and symptoms may be difficult or impossible (Rodriguez dos Santos & Lye, 1980). Tests of thyroid function may be needed, particularly in patients with atrial fibrillation, and serum levels of digoxin may confirm that a dysrhythmia is due to digitalis intoxication.

Investigations by Davies, Pomerance, Kulbertus and others have established the pathological basis of many disorders of rhythm and conduction. In the elderly each is superimposed on a background of age-related changes in the sino-atrial node, the atrial myocardium, and the bundle of His. There is a reduction in the number of pace-making cells as age advances (Davies & Pomerance, 1972; Thery et al, 1977), and the left bundle branch loses some of its size and many of its fibres (Hecht, 1980). The inter-atrial conduction system and the atrioventricular node are rarely much altered by aging (Davies, 1976). Other age-related diseases such as calcification of the mitral valve ring and of the aortic valve may involve the conduction system (Davies, 1976).

The haemodynamic effects of cardiac dysrhythmias in the elderly have been little studied, but may be best inferred from an examination of atrial fibrillation. In this dysrhythmia, the reduction in cardiac output is in the order of 20–30%, as established from the effects of converting the arrhythmia to sinus rhythm, and more directly from studies of its occurrence in the elderly (Caird, 1980; Caird & Williams, 1981). They are of the same magnitude as those of frank cardiac failure and sinus rhythm (Caird, 1980). Left ventricular performance as measured by the ejection fraction, on which many of the symptoms of arrhythmias depend, is reduced in atrial fibrillation if there is tachycardia or extreme bradycardia (Caird & Williams, 1981). The same is not the case in sinus rhythm, when the ejection fraction tends to increase during tachycardia. It follows that very fast ventricular rates are particularly deleterious, and the same may be true of extremely slow rates.

A useful classification of cardiac dysrhythmias is by site and duration. They may be supraventricular, atrioventricular or ventricular (Tables 24.1 & 24.2) and either brief, involving one or at most four or five beats, paroxysmal (of duration up to several days and often self-limiting) or sustained. They may occur in association with myocardial infarction or thyrotoxicosis. The implications for therapy are different in each case.

Table 24.1 Prevalence (%) of tachyarhythmia in 1171 institutionalised elderly people (Vaidya et al, 1976).

Sick sinus syndrome	0.3
Supreventricular tachycardia	2.5
Atrial flutter	1.8
Atrial fibrillation	14.7
Ventricular tachycardia	0.1
Ventricular fibrillation	0.2

Table 24.2 Prevalence (%) of conduction disorders in the elderly (Modified from Tammao, 1982).

	General elderly population	Institutionalised elderly
1° Atrioventricular block	1	2–10
2° Atrioventricular block		1–2
3° Atrioventricular block		0.2–0.9
RBBB	2–3.5	4–13
LBBB	0.6–2.5	4–5.7
LAH ('Left anterior hemiblock')	2	6–27
RBBB + LAH	1	0.5–9

In the elderly common brief arrhythmias include single and multiple atrial, nodal and ventricular ectopic beats, and single or at most a few dropped beats in second degree heart block. Common paroxysmal arrhythmias include multifocal atrial tachycardia, supraventricular tachycardia and atrial fibrillation, together with ventricular tachycardia and fibrillation in myocardial infarction. The common forms of heart block involve atrioventricular conduction and the right and left bundle branches. The patterns described as those of left anterior and posterior hemiblock (Rosenbaum et al, 1970) are evidence of abnormality of the left bundle, but not necessarily of the left anterior or posterior bundles as these have no real existence in man (Demoulin & Kulbertus, 1972). The so-called sick sinus syndrome occupies an intermediate position since the heart rate is usually slow and irregular, interspersed with occasional paroxysms of tachycardia.

Each disorder requires separate consideration and separate treatment.

DYSRHYTHMIAS

Ectopic beats

Ectopic beats are virtually universal in the elderly, being seen more often than one in ten beats in 3% of standard electrocardiograms (Table 24.1) and in almost all 24 hour ambulatory ECGs. In the resting ECG approximately 40% of ectopics are atrial and 40% ventricular (Campbell et al, 1974). Ectopic beats are very rarely symptomatic, and when they are it is the abnormal increase in size of the post-ectopic beat that produces the symptom of palpitation. They may be caused by such environmental factors as

excessive tea and coffee drinking or cigarette smoking, and if they are troublesome, attention to their cause is the first line of treatment. In general however they do not require treatment.

Multifocal atrial rhythm and tachycardia

Multifocal atrial rhythm is defined as a rhythm in which the ventricular rate is less than 100/min and there are at least three different atrial foci. In multifocal atrial tachyardia the heart rate is more than 100/min. Neither condition is uncommon in the elderly and the latter is particularly associated with chronic lung disease and other serious illness (Clark, 1977), so that the mortality is high. It is clinically indistinguishable from atrial fibrillation. Since it is most often due to exacerbations of bronchitis in chronic pulmonary disease, it usually disappears once the acute episode is brought under control. Treatment of heart failure, withdrawal of bronchodilator drugs, relief of hypoxia and correction of hypokalaemia are all important. If the dysrhythmia does not respond to these measures, it is best treated by cautious digitalisation (Clark, 1977).

Supraventricular tachycardia

This is a relatively common condition in the elderly and usually occurs following operations and myocardial infarction and during infections. It is rarely truly paroxysmal or recurrent, as in youth, though the variety associated with the Wolff-Parkinson-White syndrome may occasionally be seen. The heart rate is regular and rapid, and there is usually hypotension or cardiac failure if the arrhythmia is prolonged. It often remits spontaneously but if there are severe symptoms, it should be treated in the first instance with cautious carotid sinus pressure under electrocardiographic control, then by digitalis, verapamil, quinidine, procainamide or disopyramide, and only if phamacologically intractable by electroversion.

Atrial fibrillation

Atrial fibrillation is by far the commonest paroxysmal and persistent arrythmia in the elderly (Vaidya et al, 1976) (Table 24.1). It is for instance five times commoner than supraventricular tachycardia or atrial flutter. The pathology of the paroxysmal variety is uncertain, but when it is chronic and persistent, destruction of the pace-making cells in the sino-atrial node is often very severe (Davies & Pomerance, 1972). In about two-thirds of cases it is associated with other varieties of heart disease, in particular ischaemic, hypertensive, valvular, alcoholic and thyrotoxic. In the remainder there is no definite evidence of any structural heart disease, but tests of thyroid function should always be carried out to exclude a treatable and often occult cause. It may be associated with infections and occasionally with direct invasion of the heart by lung tumours.

The haemodynamic consequences of atrial fibrillation depend in part upon the ventricular rate. When this is rapid, left ventricular function is considerably compromised (Caird & Williams, 1981). When the ventricular rate is slow there is much less disturbance of cardiac output, but rates of less than approximately 50 beats/min are again associated with compromised ventricular function. It follows that there is an optimum ventricular rate at which treatment should aim. This is probably nearer 60 beats/min than the customary target of 80–85 beats/min.

The cardinal physical sign of atrial fibrillation is complete irregularity of the pulse, combined with the signs of any causative heart disease, and perhaps of cardiac failure, if the latter has been precipitated by the arrhythmia.

The prognosis of atrial fibrillation has been elucidated in several studies. It appears that it always worsens prognosis compared with sinus rhythm (Bedford & Caird, 1960), but in one large study (Martin, 1974) no effect on prognosis of atrial fibrillation in a group of geriatric patients was found. The rhythm may certainly persist for many years. The risk of systemic embolism is probably highest at and soon after the onset of fibrillation. If it occurs (and the diagnosis is difficult in the elderly (Bedford & Caird, 1960)), anticoagulation should be begun, with all its difficulties, but probably need not be continued longer than six months, at least in mitral valve disease (Adams et al, 1974).

Rapid atrial fibrillation should be treated by digitalisation. The combination of digoxin and a beta-blocker may give better control of ventricular rate especially during exercise (Wang et al, 1980). This form of treatment has not been extensively tried particularly as it may worsen cardiac failure, but may well be advocated in the future. A spontaneous ventricular rate of 60–70 beats/min is probably best also treated with digitalis. Conversion to sinus rhythm by quinidine, verapamil, or electroversion rarely results in permanent sinus thythm in the elderly, and is infrequently employed, despite the frequency of the dysrhythmia.

The treatment of paroxysmal atrial fibrillation is by an attempt to maintain permanent sinus rhythm. This frequently occurs spontaneously when the dysrhythmia has been caused by an infection which has resolved, and after treatment of thyrotoxicosis. The object of any treatment given is then to prevent recurrence of the arrhythmia with quinidine or verapamil, or to protect against the arrhythmia if it recurs with digitalis. It is uncertain what proportion of patients with paroxysmal atrial fibrillation develop permanent fibrillation, but clinical impression is that this is relatively frequent and perhaps occurs in about one-third of elderly patients within a year or so.

Atrial flutter

Atrial flutter is best considered as under the same heading as atrial fibrillation, though the cardiac rhythm may be regular, the rate depending on the degree of atrio-ventricular block. Atrial flutter may be either paroxysmal or permanent, and in either case the objective of treatment should be to control the ventricular rate. Digitalisation may produce atrial fibrillation, which is easier to control.

Sick sinus syndrome

In this condition, which appears to be associated with a combination of damage to the sino-atrial node and lesions of the atrial myocardium (Thery et al, 1977), the usual presenting syndrome is with chronic persistent sinus bradycardia, sometimes interspersed with episodes of atrial fibrillation or supraventricular tachycardia. In the elderly the condition is often asymptomatic, but if symptoms occur they are the result of the episodes of tachycardia or cardiac failure associated with bradycardia. The most satisfactory treatment is pacing.

Ventricular arrhythmias

These are uncommon in the elderly, ventricular tachycardia and fibrillation complicating myocardial infarction being the arrhythmias commonly seen. Both should be treated by cardioversion as an emergency, whatever the age of the patient. The prognosis is as good as in youth (Semple & Williams, 1976).

CONDUCTION DISORDERS

Atrioventricular block

First degree heart block is much the commonest single form of atrioventricular conduction disorder in the elderly. The P-R interval has been reported to increase with age at least up to the seventh decade (Harlan et al, 1967), though it does not appear that there is any increase over that age (Clark & Craven, 1981). First degree heart block is essentially an electrocardiographic diagnosis and has in itself no symptoms. The P-R interval may be variably prolonged (over 0.22 s). There is evidence that atrial disorder, presumably involving delayed conduction in the internodal tract, may be responsible (Caird et al, 1973). It requires no treatment.

Second degree atrioventricular block occurs when there is episodic irregular or regular frequent atrioventricular block. It may cause symptoms because of bradycardia. It is an indication for pacing following myocardial infarction, since symptoms are usually present.

Complete or third degree heart block may or may not cause symptoms in the elderly. Stokes Adams attacks or chronic congestive cardiac failure are frequent. It may be due to complete destruction of the atrioventricular node by fibrosis or ischaemia, or to fibrosis of the common bundle of His or of all its branches (Davies, 1976). The myocardium is usually anatomically and functionally normal.

The physical signs of complete heart block include

bradycardia, a high pulse pressure, cannon waves in the jugular venous pulse, variability of the first heart sound and an ejection systolic murmur due to an increase in stroke volume. These may assist in the differentiation between complete heart block and other causes of bradycardia such as beta-blockade (though this rarely produces such profound bradycardia).

If symptoms are present, and perhaps if they are not, permanent pacing should be instituted. The prognosis is then excellent (Amikam et al, 1976), the expectation of life of octogenarians for instance being restored to normal (Siddons, 1976). Temporary pacing may be indicated when complete heart block follows myocardial infarction, but spontaneous recovery almost always occurs when the infarct is inferior in site. Complete heart block complicating anterior myocardial infarction is usually an indication of bilateral bundle branch block associated with a large myocardial infarct involving much ventricular muscle and also the septum. It is often fatal despite temporary pacing (Davies, 1976).

Ventricular conduction disorders: left bundle branch disease

So-called left anterior hemiblock with pathological left axis deviation (of more than +30 degrees) is probably the commonest single disorder of conduction (see Table 24.2). It is by itself always symptomless and probably does not indicate serious heart disease in the elderly, since its prognosis is good (Caird et al, 1974).

Complete left bundle branch block has been shown to be of four types (Baragan et al, 1968). There may be prolongation of the initial period of conduction shown by the time between the Q-wave and the beginning of ventricular contraction on the apexcardiogram or the first sound on the phonocardiogram, or the later phase may be prolonged, with a delay between the beginning of left ventricular contraction and the beginning of ejection. In some cases both abnormalities are present, and in a small minority, neither. These four types are not distinguishable

clinically and they appear to have no different prognostic significance. The only clinical sign of left bundle branch block is reversed splitting of the second heart sound, which may be impossible to demonstrate clinically in an elderly patient unable to carry out the necessary respiratory gymnastics. Some haemodynamic abnormality is probably usually present, and certainly the left ventricular ejection fraction is often considerably reduced. It is often associated with serious cardiac disease, and this doubtless explains its effect in reducing life expectancy (Caird et al, 1974). As an isolated finding, it may be ignored, since it is not by itself a cause of symptoms.

Right bundle branch disease

Incomplete right bundle branch block is present in 1% of the general elderly population (Campbell et al, 1974), but is of no apparent significance since it carries no adverse prognosis (Caird et al, 1974).

Complete right bundle branch block remains somewhat of an enigma. Its pathology is poorly understood (Davies, 1976). Often there is no other evidence of heart disease, but it strongly suggests right ventricular hypertrophy when the latter is likely (as in cor pulmonale). Although systolic time intervals are normal, the right ventricular ejection fraction is variable, and sometimes reduced. Clinically it may be recognised by wide fixed splitting of the second heart sound.

When combined with so-called left anterior hemiblock, as is often the case, right bundle branch block has often been considered as an indication for pacing. Since such bifascicular block has no different a prognosis from right bundle branch block alone, it is not in the elderly an indication for pacing. In a study of such patients during operations for non-cardiac conditions, pacing precipitated more arrhythmias than it prevented (Pastore et al, 1978). Although there is a small chance of development of complete heart block (Tammaro, 1982), pacing should be confined to patients who have documented symptomatic arrhythmias (McAnulty et al, 1978).

REFERENCES

Adams G F, Merrett J D, Hutchinson W M, Pollock A M 1974 Cerebral embolism and mitral stenosis: survival with and without anticoagulants. Journal of Neurology, Neurosurgery and Psychiatry 37: 378–383

Amikam S, Lemer J, Rognia N, Peleg H, Riss E 1976 Long-term survival of elderly patients after pacemaker implantation. American Heart Journal 91: 445–449

Baragan J, Fernandez Caamano F, Sozutek Y, Coblence B, Lenegre J 1968 Chronic left complete bundle-branch block. British Heart Journal 30: 196–202

Bedford P D, Caird F I 1960 Valvular disease of the heart in old age. Churchill, London

Caird F I, Williams B O 1981 Left ventricular performance in atrial fibrillation in the elderly. Age and Ageing 10: 231–236

Caird F I 1980 Radionuclide studies of the circulation in the elderly. Journal of Clinical and Experimental Gerontology 2: 23–40

Caird F I, Kennedy R D, Kelly J C C 1973 Combined apexcardiography and phonocardiography in the investigation of heart disease in the elderly. Gerontologia Clinica 15: 366–377

Caird F I, Campbell A E, Jackson T F M 1974 Significance of abnormalities of electrocardiogram in old people. British Heart Journal 36: 1012–1018

Campbell A, Caird F I, Jackson T F M 1974 Prevalence of abnormalities of electrocardiogram in old people. British Heart Journal 36: 1005–1011

Clark A N G 1977 Multi-focal atrial tachycardia. Gerontology 23: 445–451

Clark A N G, Craven A S H 1981 P–R Interval in the aged. Age and Ageing 10: 157–164

Davies M J 1976 Pathology of the conduction system. In: Caird F I, Dall J L C, Kennedy R D (eds) Cardiology in Old Age. Plenum, New York, London, ch 3, p 57–80

Davies M J, Pomerance A 1972 Quantitative study of ageing changes in the human sinoatrial node and internodal tracts. British Heart Journal 40: 468–481

Demoulin J C, Kulbertus H E 1972 Histopathological examination of concept of left hemiblock. British Heart Journal 34: 807–814

Harlan W R, Craybiel A, Mitchell A E, Oberman A, Osborne R K 1967 Serial electrocardiograms: their reliability and prognostic validity during a 24-year period. Journal of Chronic Diseases 20: 853–867

Hecht F M 1980 Studie uber quantitative Altersvereranderungen am Hischen Bundel des Menschen. Virchows Archiv: A: Pathological Anatomy and Histology 386: 343–356

McAnulty J H, Rahimtoola S H, Murphy E S, Kaufmann S N, Ritzman L W, Kanarck P, et al 1978 A prospective study of sudden death in 'high risk' bundle branch block. New England Journal of Medicine 209–215

Martin A 1974 The natural history of atrial fibrillation in the elderly. Thesis, University of London

Pastore J O, Yurchak P M, Janis K M, Murphy J D, Zir L M 1978 The risk of advanced heart block in surgical patients with right bundle branch block and left axis deviation. Circulation 57: 677–680

Rodrigues dos Santos A G, Lye M 1980 Transient cardiac arrhythmias in healthy elderly individuals: how relevant are they? Journal of Clinical and Experimental Gerontology 2: 245–258

Rosenbaum M B, Elizari M V, Lazzari J O 1970 The hemiblocks. Tampa Tracings, Tampa, Florida

Semple T, Williams B O 1976 Coronary care for the elderly In: Caird F I, Dall J L C, Kennedy R D (eds) Cardiology in Old Age. Plenum, New York, London, ch 16, p 297–313

Siddons H 1976 Management of heart block. In: Caird F I, Dall J L C, Kennedy R D (eds) Cardiology in Old Age. Plenum, New York, London, ch 18, p 347–367

Tammaro A 1982 Heart block. In: Platt D (ed) Geriatrics 1. Springer, Berlin, Heidelberg, New York, p 139–160

Thery C, Gosselin B, Lekieffre J, Warembourg H 1977 Pathology of sinoatrial node: correlations with electrocardiographic findings in 111 patients. American Heart Journal 93: 735–740

Vaidya P N, Bhosley P N, Rao D B, Luisada A A 1976 Tachyarrhythmias in old age. Journal of American Geriatrics Society 24: 412–414

Wang R, Camm J, Ward D, Washington H, Martin A 1980 Treatment of chronic atrial fibrillation in the elderly, assessed by ambulatory electrocardiographic monitoring. Journal of the American Geriatrics Society 28: 529–234

25

Hypertension

M. H. Alderman & M. E. Stanback

Despite advances in science and medicine which have greatly increased life expectancy at birth in Western societies, life expectancy for those aged 65 and over has changed very little. This is because the disease problems of the elderly have been largely unimproved by medical progress. Of major importance among these is hypertension which, because of the progressive damage it inflicts on multiple organ systems, is a leading factor in both morbidity and mortality in the elderly.

Blood pressure increases with age in industrialised societies so that more than a third of those between the ages of 65 and 74 have pressures $\geqslant$ 160 mmHg systolic and/or 95 diastolic. This progressive rise in pressure is actually more accurately described as a persistent and continuing rise in systolic pressure. Diastolic values for the population as a whole tend to peak at about age 45–50 and then plateau. The overall diastolic increase is accounted for by the roughly one-third of the population in which pressures rise: in the U.S. Public Health Service — National Institute of Aging (N.I.A.) Longitudinal Study of Blood Pressure, where 254 male subjects were followed for a minimum of 10 years, 35% had a statistically significant rise in diastolic pressure, 11% a significant decline and 54% no change at all (Weksler, 1982).

The distribution of hypertension is not uniform across demographic lines — older black women tend to have the highest prevalence and white males the lowest (Tables 25.1 and 25.2) (Ostfeld, 1978). In the United States some geographic variation has also been demonstrated, with the highest prevalence of elevated pressure found among blacks for example in the south-eastern states.

Table 25.1 Prevalence of definite hypertension in the US National Health Survey for two time periods by sex and race (Ostfeld, 1978).

Sex	Ethnicity	1960 to 1962 Number per 1000	S.E.	1971 to 1974 Number per 1000	S.E.
Male	White	250	32.4	353	18.5
Male	Black	527	110.7	501	42.8
Female	White	466	41.9	423	22.6
Female	Black	641	128.2	588	47.3

Table 25.2 Proportion of hypertensive persons in the US National Health Survey age 65–74, by diagnostic status, race and sex, 1971–74 (Ostfeld, 1978).

Sex	Race	Number per 1000 Population Hypertensive	Previously Undiagnosed	% Previously Undiagnosed
Male	White	353	219	62
Male	Black	501	256	51
Female	White	423	174	41
Female	Black	588	230	39

The tendency of blood pressure to rise with age is not in fact inevitable. In many non-Western societies, generally those organised as hunting and gathering units, blood pressure tends to be low and remain so throughout life (Sever et al, 1980). The reasons for this apparent immunity to blood pressure rise are not known. Genetics do not provide the answer, since in all situations so far described, when residents of these societies migrate to metropolitan centres, their pressures tend to rise to at least the same extent as do those of individuals already living in the urban areas. The blacks of the Caribbean and the United States whose prevalence of hypertension is so very high are of course migrants from West Africa whose pressures are modest in their native rural Africa. Environmental factors, dietary and psychosocial, have been implicated as causes of the inexorable rise of pressure seen in Western societies. But as yet it is not possible to define with precision the exact cause of a phenomenon which occurs gradually over five to six decades.

IMPACT

The critical issue, of course, is not the prevalence of one or another level of pressure, but rather its associated prognostic implication. What is clear from a variety of sources is that elevated blood pressure is the most significant controllable risk factor for cardiovascular disease among the elderly (Kannel, 1976).

The frequently repeated clinical pearl that since blood pressure tends to rise with age, it can be well tolerated and in fact may be the physiological response to progressive vascular stenosis that maintains blood flow, is simply not supported by the facts. The Framingham data would suggest that cardiovascular disease risk actually increases with advancing age. A comparison of hypertensives aged between 65 and 74 with normotensives in that study over an 18 year follow-up reveals that risk of mortality overall is more than doubled among those with definite high blood pressure. Multiple regression analysis confirms that among possible factors the most powerful contributor to this risk is blood pressure. Analysis of attributable risk (hypertensive morbidity less normotensive morbidity) suggests that 69–75% of the morbidity in that population can be attributed to hypertension.

Nor is the common clinical impression that postmenopausal women tolerate elevated pressures well supported by these data. Despite the fact that risk associated with hypertension is twice as high in men as in women at all ages, the relative increase in risk with age due to hypertension is just as great for women as for men (Kannel, 1976).

These data from the Framingham study are confirmed by other studies. For example, Ostfeld et al (1971) reported that in a prospective study of 3400 members of a bi-racial community aged 65 to 74, the 43% with pressures ≥160/95 had twice the incidence of stroke of those with lower pressures (Ostfeld et al, 1971). Moreover the gradient of risk for those with only elevated systolic pressure but normal diastolic pressure was even steeper. Elevated blood pressure was also associated with an increased incidence of congestive heart failure and coronary heart disease, as well as chronic brain syndrome and senile dementia. In fact hypertension creates a six-fold increase in the occurrence of congestive heart failure among the elderly.

While in young people many other factors contribute to risk of cardiovascular disease, in the elderly hypertension is far and away the most important source of risk. Cigarette smoking has a more modest impact in this age group, as do glucose intolerance and left ventricular hypertrophy. High density lipoprotein levels continue to be positively related to protection but the adverse impact of total cholesterol elevation is muted in the elderly.

HYPERTENSION AND COGNITIVE PROCESSES

The impact of elevated blood pressure on the cerebral circulation, the extreme example of which is stroke, is well known. Moreover in many patients without clinical evidence of neurological deficit, post-mortem examination reveals substantial abnormality. Efforts to determine the functional significance of presumed pre-clinical cerebrovascular disease due to hypertension have so far yielded meagre results. Wilkie & Eisdorfer (1971) reported

that cognitive function showed a substantially greater decline over a ten year period after the age of 60 among elderly hypertensives with evidence of end organ disease and without treatment, than among normotensives. In addition antihypertensive therapy may impair mental acuity even further. Drug-related impairment of attention has been observed in animals and humans on reserpine, methyldopa and clonidine, on beta-blockers (although less consistently) (Light, 1980) and on diuretics (Francheschi et al, 1982). These observations must however be interpreted with caution, since many were made on animals or on normotensive subjects where drug effects may be different from effects on hypertensive patients, and since most of the human subjects tested were young adults, rather than elderly individuals.

SYSTOLIC HYPERTENSION

Generally speaking, systolic and diastolic pressures rise concommitantly at all ages. However after middle age the systolic pressure rise continues, while diastolic pressure in the aggregate may actually decline. Thus the phenomenon of isolated systolic pressure elevation, rarely occurring among young persons, becomes fairly common among the elderly. Typically, this condition is diagnosed when the diastolic pressure is less than 90 mmHg and the systolic exceeds 160 mmHg (Gifford, 1982). Table 25.3 reveals the

Table 25.3 Prevalence of isolated systolic hypertension in the US National Health Survey by age, race and sex, 1960–62 (Gifford, 1982)

| Age (years) | % With Pure Systolic Hypertension* | | | |
| | Men | | Women | |
	White	Black	White	Black
25–34	0.3	1.0	0.2	0.0
35–44	0.9	0.6	0.9	1.5
45–54	3.5	1.3	4.6	7.6
55–64	9.5	13.0	15.6	4.3
65–74	15.0	25.5	30.7	38.9
75–79	26.9	38.6	32.9	43.1

* Systolic pressure > 160 mmHg; diastolic pressure < 90 mmHG.

striking increase in incidence of systolic hypertension with advancing age so that, according to the U.S. National Health Survey, as many as one-third of those over 75 have isolated systolic hypertension. A variety of other studies are in reasonable agreement with these findings, although Colandrea et al (1970) have reported that the phenomenon is frequently evanescent and that an initial prevalence of 13.9% in a retirement community fell to 2.7% with repeated testing.

It has been argued that the systolic elevation of the aged is merely the result of reduced arterial elasticity. While this is clearly true in part, elevated systolic pressure has nevertheless been shown to be a strong signal of practical risk for cardiovascular myocardial infarction disease. Again through study of the Framingham population, Kannel et al (1971) prospectively assessed the predictive value of various components of blood pressure measurement in terms of myocardial infarction incidence among 5127 men and women over a period of 14 years. His findings were consistent and unequivocal. The risk of coronary artery disease was linearly related to the height of blood pressure in all its dimensions. However through the application of determinant analysis, he was also able to demonstrate that systolic pressure was actually the most powerful independent predictor of events among persons over the age of 45. This was true even in the setting of a normal diastolic pressure and was even more true in regard to stroke. Neither pulse pressure nor mean arterial pressure (diastolic plus one third the difference between systolic minus diastolic) was as powerfully associated with stroke or myocardial infarction as was systolic pressure. Thus in the older population systolic blood pressure elevation merits close attention, regardless of the diastolic level. The ability of antihypertensive therapy to reduce the risk of isolated systolic hypertension while a reasonable expectation has not yet been proven and is currently under study in a multi-centre project of the US Public Health Service-National Institutes of Health.

PSEUDOHYPERTENSION

This condition is defined as apparent arterial hypertension based on false perception of blood pressure when measured by the indirect sphygmomanometer method. Spence et al (1978) first reported a discrepancy between cuff pressure and nearly simultaneous intra-arterial pressures in 40 elderly subjects studied in London, Ontario, Canada. He found that cuff-obtained diastolic pressure was frequently falsely elevated — often by as much as 15–30 mmHg — while in contrast systolic pressure was more likely to be underestimated.

But while the actual prevalence of this discrepancy cannot be known, since the invasive technology required to determine the true pressure precludes such measurement on a routine basis, it is important in clinical practice to consider its possible presence, particularly where appropriate antihypertensive therapy produces postural or other symptoms in the face of apparently normal or even elevated pressure levels.

Another cause of artifactual distortion of blood pressure is the auscultatory gap. In elderly patients this is more frequently present and perhaps of greater span. To allow for this distortion, it is necessary to inflate the cuff 50 mmHg above any systolic pressure lower than 200 mmHg when measuring pressure in older patients.

PATHOPHYSIOLOGY OF HYPERTENSION IN THE ELDERLY

The interaction of vasoconstriction and volume explain the maintenance of blood pressure at any level and at all ages. Under normal circumstances a variety of negative feedback loops operate to defend blood pressure in the face of a variety of alterations of the body's internal environment. Thus a normal person may become dehydrated and reduce intravascular volume substantially but have pressure maintained by humorally controlled constriction of the vascular tree and retention of sodium and water by the kidneys. This is of course essential if blood flow to vital organs is to be sustained. The critical components of the interlocking feedback loops of blood pressure are plasma volume, vascular space, sympathetic nervous system activity and the renin-angiotensin-aldosterone system.

Not surprisingly, alterations in these systems occur in normal aging. Perhaps most dramatic is the increase in vascular resistance associated with a decrease in arterial elasticity. Renin activity, even in the face of unchanged or even reduced blood volume, seems to decrease with age and catecholamine activity to increase. Adrenoreceptor sensitivity and baroreceptor reflex function are both diminished, resulting in a dampened cardiovascular response to stress. It is clear that the homeostatic capacity of the older patient is somewhat compromised, perhaps permitting those factors such as increased arterial rigidity which tend to elevate blood pressure in Western societies at all ages to produce more hypertension in the elderly (Lakatta, 1979; Wiggers, 1932).

The special circumstances of blood pressure elevation in the elderly may require a definition beyond the usual systolic/diastolic to reflect hypertension accurately in this age group. In this group systolic pressure is particularly important as a measure of maximum cardiac effort. Any definition of hypertension based solely on diastolic pressure will miss many older patients whose mean arterial pressure and total peripheral resistance (TPR) are elevated. It should be recalled that TPR is generated in the small arterioles. Thus hemodynamically, in a young person with compliant arteries, cardiac contraction expresses a bolus of flow into the aorta which accommodates part of this through expansion. Only a part of each ejection of the heart is propelled directly to the pre-capillary arterioles. During diastole the young artery contracts to deliver the remainder of the cardiac output distally. The net result is a rather smooth flow of blood to the periphery throughout the cardiac cycle.

By contrast in the thickened, rigid, arteriosclerotic older aorta, the same cardiac output fails to distend the aorta, so that the total left ventricular ejection is transmitted directly to the small vessels during systole. There may even be no flow at all during diastole. Thus if the TPR of the young and old patient are the same, in the older subject the full burden of cardiac output is limited to systole.

Under the circumstances, it has been suggested that mean arterial pressure (MAP) might be a more satisfactory method for viewing blood pressure in the elderly, since it gives sufficient weight to the systolic pressure as well as the diastolic. Thus an older subject with a pressure of 220/70 and a younger subject with 140/110 will have the same MAP of 120 mmHg. Both may seek a goal MAP of 100, which would be 160/70 in the older and 120/90 in the younger subject. The vascular effect could be the same.

EVIDENCE OF EFFICACY OF ANTIHYPERTENSIVE THERAPY

Adequate data based on long-term prospective studies of antihypertensive drug therapy in representative populations of elderly subjects are not yet available. An ongoing European collaborative study should provide more definitive information within the next few years (Amery et al, 1977). For the present, while recommendations regarding treatment are still derived from studies not specifically designed to address the issue of therapy for the elderly, clinical decisions should be strongly influenced by the situation of the individual patient.

Perhaps the most powerful evidence that antihypertensive therapy can reduce morbidity and mortality derives from the Veterans Administration (VA) studies of the 1960's (Veterans Administration Cooperative Study Group on Antihypertensive Agents, 1967 & 1970). In all age groups, there was convincing evidence that treating patients with sustained diastolic blood pressure ⩾ 105 mmHg produced benefit. Moreover among patients over 60 in the VA study, drug therapy afforded protection even at pressures of 90–104 mmHg (Table 25.4) (Kirkendall & Hammond, 1980), although in contrast to patients with diastolic pressures over 105, the benefit at this level did not achieve statistical significance. While these results make a good case for the benefits of treatment, they can in no way be considered conclusive, since the elderly subjects in the VA study were few in number and, of course, were all males.

Table 25.4 Incidence of morbid events in patients age 60 and above in the Veterans Administration Co-operative Study (Kirkendall & Hammond, 1980).

Blood pressure prior to randomisation mmHg	n*	Control group Events	%	n	Treated group Events	%
90–104	21	13	61.9	19	8	42.1
105–114	22	14	63.6	19	3	15.8
Total	43	27	62.8	38	11	28.9

*Number of patients randomised.

In the Hypertension Detection and Follow-up Program (HDFP) trial (1979a & b) of stepped care treatment for mild hypertensives drawn from a general population, it was found that 2376 subjects aged 60–69 years were more likely than their younger confreres to achieve and maintain blood pressure control and had a greater decline in diastolic pressure. Fig. 25.1 shows that in comparison with the group referred to regular care in the community, there was

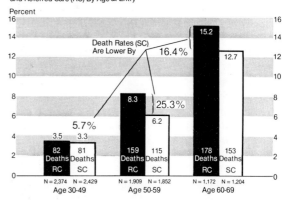

Mortality - All Causes by Age

5-Year Mortality Rates (%) From All Causes for Stepped Care (SC) and Referred Care (RC) By Age at Entry

Fig. 25.1 5 Year Mortality Rates (%) From All Causes for Stepped Care (SC) and Referred Care (RC) By Age at Entry, U.S. Hypertension Detection and Follow-Up Program (1979)

a substantial decline in mortality for those in systematic stepped care. Interpretation of this study must be guarded however, since the control group was in fact referred to community care and thus was not an untreated comparison group. Nevertheless these data are consistent with the VA findings and add further weight to the notion that hypotensive therapy can be efficacious. Moreover, the HDFP experience demonstrates that it is practical to reduce blood pressure in elderly subjects and maintain that reduction without substantial adverse consequences.

As for isolated systolic elevation, no prospective data exist to establish the benefit of therapy. A distressing recent report (Koch-Weser & Greenblatt, 1976) suggests however, that with standard stepped-care therapy it is not possible to achieve systolic normotension without provoking diastolic hypotension.

Studies of secondary prevention of stroke suggest that in some elderly hypertensives, blood pressure control exerts a protective effect. As for secondary prevention of myocardial infarction, Kannel used pre and post-event pressures in the Framingham data to demonstrate that blood pressure elevation after infarction carries adverse prognostic implications, but also that a marked fall in pressure in relation to pre-infarction levels may be of even greater negative impact. These findings suggest that any attempt to control blood pressure after infarction should be based on an awareness of pre-morbid levels.

THE EVALUATION OF THE ELDERLY HYPERTENSIVE

Most of the principles of patient evaluation that apply to the younger hypertensive apply to the older subject as well. The objectives of the work-up are to establish the diagnosis, uncover a correctable cause for the elevation of pressure if present, determine the extent of disease and establish baseline metabolic data to guide selection of therapy and follow-up. In the elderly patient certain additional issues become significant as well.

To establish the diagnosis of hypertension, repeated observations are necessary. In our programme, the diagnosis is made in the untreated patient only after a blood pressure $\geqslant 160$ and/or 95 mmHg is recorded on at least three occasions each separated by a week. The pressure at each encounter is actually the average of the last two of three measurements made after at least five minutes of sitting quietly. In the case of older patients, it is also important to obtain standing pressures because occasionally, particularly in patients with disproportionate systolic elevation, symptoms of postural hypotension occur associated with falls of as much as 30–40 mmHg systolic after one minute of standing. This fall on standing may be more common in subjects with either metabolic or neurologic disorders.

In the elderly, as in younger patients, most hypertension is of unknown etiology. Nevertheless the discovery of a curable cause of high blood pressure, while a rare event, offers a potential benefit to the patient which more than justifies a prudent search for such a condition. Modest blood pressure elevation over many years is a less likely setting in which to find a treatable cause than when blood pressure elevation can be documented to be of recent onset.

Primary aldosteronism and pheochromocytoma are both extraordinarily rare in the elderly. A pheochromocytoma can usually be suggested by history, and its presence in patients whose history raises the suspicion can be established by measurement of catecholamine excretion in the urine. Primary aldosteronism may be suggested by a low serum potassium without therapy, although modest hypokalemia (3.0–3.5 mmol/l) is not uncommon among hypertensives. A plunge in serum potassium after initiation of diuretic therapy should signal the need for assessment of the renin-angiotensin-aldosterone axis. This must be done under carefully controlled intake circumstances and after withdrawal of antihypertensive therapy for at least three weeks.

But whereas hypoparathyroidism (which is difficult to diagnose) is associated with hypertension, high output systolic elevation is rarely due to thyrotoxicosis, aortic insufficiency or an arteriovenous fistula. These conditions can generally be detected by appropriate physical examination.

Perhaps of greatest importance is the issue of renovascular disease. There are no hard data defining the prevalence or incidence of renovascular stenosis. In older patients where widespread arteriosclerosis is common, partial obstruction of a renal artery may be far more frequent than has been commonly believed. Clearly in patients with sudden onset of hypertension and/or the presence of an abnormal bruit, a thorough search for a vascular cause is warranted. To these indicators should be added any sudden acceleration in pressure in patients with long-standing but stable disease or in patients where control of pressure proves difficult. Since renovascular hypertension is mediated by excess renin secretion, the finding of relative hyper-reninaemia is further evidence for evaluation. Applying the nomogram developed by Laragh, a low renin classification is more common among the elderly (Brunner et al, 1972). If instead an ambulatory determination places the patient in the high category, the index of suspicion should rise. In addition, a failure to respond to diuretic therapy or a dramatic first dose response to angiotensinogen converting enzyme inhibitor (captopril) may also signal the presence of a renovascular lesion of functional significance.

Diagnosis of a renovascular lesion can be made by visualisation of the arteries in combination with a functional assessment of the renin system at the renal vein. This can be accomplished concurrently through digital subtraction angiography and sampling of bilateral renal venous and inferior vena caval blood to measure renin (Sos et al, 1982). Lateralised secretion of renin in the context of a vascular lesion establishes the diagnosis in advance of arteriography. The rapidly developing field of percutaneous transluminal angioplasty provides a non-surgical and highly effective therapeutic approach to the solution of this problem. Using this approach, arteriography will be done in advance of correction, but only after the diagnosis has been made. Certain lesions — particularly ostial lesions — are not amenable to this rather modest intervention, but require a surgical effort with its greater risk. In some cases, particularly where renal function is minimal or absent, nephrectomy may prove safe and highly efficacious.

In addition to the search for a correctable cause of elevated blood pressure, an important objective of the evaluation is to assess the overall status of the patient and identify relevant concurrent conditions which may influence the course of therapy.

More frequently than young persons, older patients are likely to suffer from multiple medical problems. The interactions of these conditions themselves adversely affect outcome. Of equal significance may be the interaction of individual therapies for the several conditions, or the adverse effect of one therapy on a separate underlying condition. Perhaps the most commonly found example of the latter is impaired glucose tolerance (IGT) (Amery et al, 1978). Its coincidence with hypertension is considerably higher than might be expected by the prevalence of the two conditions in the general population — 7.1% in one study of persons aged 26 to 78. In a study of patients attending a general medical clinic, fully 50% of those with IGT had co-existent hypertension, and the prognosis for those with both conditions was far worse than for those with IGT alone (Gerber et al, 1983). It is not surprising that these two relatively common conditions should be found in the same individuals since some of the same precursors are associated with both. It is not known whether control of blood glucose by itself would influence blood pressure control, but certainly weight reduction in the obese can favorably affect both blood sugar and blood pressure. Conversely of course, antihypertensive therapy, particularly with diuretics, can adversely influence glucose tolerance. Thus careful evaluation of the status of glucose metabolism in the elderly prior to initiation of therapy, as well as regularly during therapy, is necessary.

The pre-treatment work-up should also include, in addition to the routine history and physical examination, a careful assesment of the extent of disease, since the choice of treatment as well as the urgency with which treatment should be pursued is dependent to some extent on the degree of end organ involvement. Renal function assessed by serum creatinine, and cardiac status as revealed through ECG and echocardiography, are important components of the evaluation. Pulmonary function if impaired is another important complicating factor that may influence the selection of therapy. Plasma lipid levels, both total cholesterol and high density lipoprotein, may be adversely affected by diuretics or beta adrenergic blocking agents and thus pre-treatment levels should be established. Excess alcohol consumption may impair response to therapy and its intake should be quantified.

TREATMENT

Reduction of blood pressure, whatever the criteria used to establish eligibility for intervention, is probably more difficult to achieve in elderly than in younger subjects. The only type of intervention shown to be associated with a reduction in cardiovascular morbidity is drug therapy. For all patients however, drugs offer potential hazards as well as benefits and this is even more true for older subjects (Jackson et al, 1976). This group tends to have more medical problems and thus take more drugs, with a greater risk of adverse drug interaction. Altered liver and renal function may delay excretion, raising blood levels of antihypertensive compounds hazardously high. Syncope is more frequent in the elderly and neurogenic tone may be

higher and plasma volume lower, so that sensitivity to drugs affecting intravascular integrity may be more profound. Because of this blood pressure should always be monitored in the upright posture. A critical issue in the elderly is compliance, and in addition to the usual problems, older persons are more likely to have reduced intellectual acuity which may interfere with drug taking.

In view of all these potential hazards, it might seem wise to begin a blood pressure reduction effort with non-pharmacological measures. It must be kept in mind however, that these approaches have not been demonstrated to reduce morbidity. Moreover they demand lifestyle modifications which should be viewed as neither easy to accomplish nor unequivocally without risk in themselves. Nevertheless weight reduction in the obese and moderate restriction of sodium intake in individuals where intake is excessive, seem sensible first steps toward blood pressure control. The average American consumes roughly 140 mmol of sodium daily. Intakes of 70–90 mmol can be achieved without major intrusion on dietary patterns, and reductions of the magnitudue of 50–70 mmol have been shown to be efficacious in lowering blood pressure in some patients (Morgan et al, 1978).

Certainly if blood pressure remains above 105 mmHg diastolic or 160–170 mmHg systolic despite prescription of dietary changes, drug therapy is indicated. No empiric data exist to guide the physician in this area either. Current studies in England (mild hypertension in general) (Medical Research Council Working Party on Mild to Moderate Hypertension, 1977) and Europe (hypertension in the elderly) (Amery et al, 1977) are comparing alternate first step drugs, but the results of these trials will not be available for several years.

The drug invariably used first in all clinical trials has been the diuretic. Introduced in the late 1950s, the thiazides literally transformed hypertension from a condition whose treatment was almost as bad as the disease itself, to one for which tolerable and effective therapy could be simply provided on an outpatient basis. Thiazides act by increasing sodium excretion and reducing plasma volume, contributing to a lowering of cardiac output. Moreover, through total body sodium depletion they tend to reduce peripheral vascular resistance. Alone these agents, like their more potent conjoiners furosemide or ethacrynic acid, can successfully control pressure in probably half of all cases. Over time however it is not uncommon for a second agent to be required.

Hazards of diuretic therapy include hypokalaemia, hyperuricaemia and impaired glucose tolerance. Hypokalaemia can usually be avoided by initiating therapy with a small dose and slowly, over four to eight weeks, increasing it to a maximum of 100 mg of hydrochlorothiazide or its equivalent. Hypokalaemia is a particular hazard for those taking digitalis, in which case the addition of a potassium sparing agent such as triamterene or spironolactone or routine potassium supplementation might be wise. In any event monitoring of serum potassium and EKG is prudent. Gout is an infrequent complication and there is no indication that treatment of asymptomatic hyperuricaemia is of benefit. However our own practice is to prescribe allopurinol for patients with serum uric acid levels $\geqslant 12$ mg/dl. Recent reports of the British Medical Research Council trial indicate that impotence, rather commonly encountered with other antihypertensive agents, occurs with equal frequency among diuretic treated subjects.

An alternative first drug may be selected from the expanding array of beta adrenergic blocking agents. Some are water soluble and do not permeate the blood brain barrier; others are longer acting, or cardioselective, or metabolised by the liver. Each of these properties may be of value or detrimental and must be considered before choosing the appropriate agent. Contraindications to use of beta-blockers include congestive heart failure, A-V block, asthma and chronic obstructive pulmonary disease. These drugs are effective in controlling angina and have been shown to be cardioprotective — at least after myocardial infarction. They act by reducing cardiac output and inhibiting reflex autonomic activity and renin release from the kidneys. Theoretically in older patients where low renin hypertension is more common, these agents may not always be effective. Complications associated with the use of beta-blockers include bradycardia, possible reduction of high density lipoproteins, peripheral vasospasm and exacerbation of Raynaud's phenomenon, and some central nervous system effects including disturbing or vivid dreams.

If the first drug does not produce or maintain blood pressure control, the preferred second drug to be added should be either the diuretic or beta-blocker — whichever was not used first. If the addition of a diuretic to the beta-blocker (or vice versa) results in satisfactory control, an attempt to remove the beta-blocker should be made so that the lowest possible effective medication schedule can be achieved.

If on the other hand even two agents are not sufficient, a vasodilating agent, hydralazine for example, can be added. The direct action of hydralazine on the vessels produces a reflex sympathetic response that increases heart rate and cardiac output. The result, probably more common among the elderly, may be headache or angina, along with tachycardia. But experience has shown that pre-treatment with a beta-blocking agent will mute the sympathetic response to the vasodilator and prevent development of symptoms. In addition this combination seems to achieve a particularly potent hypotensive effect. Side effects of hydralazine are fairly rare, though a lupus-like syndrome

has been reported where high doses are used. This syndrome is reversible with discontinuation of the drug.

An alternate second or third drug is the alpha adrenergic blocker prazosin. As such it is primarily a vasodilator which has little cardiac effect and lacks the bronchospastic effect of beta-blockers. Prazosin may therefore be particularly attractive in patients with asthma or chronic obstructive pulmonary disease. It has proved equal in hypotensive effect to other second drugs and may have fewer side effects. Of these first dose syncope is the most distressing, but this can be avoided if the first few doses are small (1 mg) and are administered at bedtime, and the amounts of subsequent doses administered during the day are increased slowly. Unlike the beta-blockers and diuretics, prazosin has not been shown to adversely affect lipid metabolism.

Other agents commonly prescribed include the rauwolfia alkaloids, methyl dopa and clonidine. All are effective and have been well tolerated by great numbers of patients for many years. However, each of these has potential central nervous system depressant effects and therefore should be initiated cautiously in older subjects. There is no reason, however, to alter the regimen of those who are now successfully being treated with them.

SUMMARY

Among the risk factors that threaten older people hypertension plays a leading role. Effective therapy to reduce blood pressure is available, and for those with the highest levels of pressure, it promises significant benefit. For the vast majority of older persons with high blood pressure — those with mild elevations — treatment holds less promise and the indications for intervention are understandably less clear cut. Information soon to be forthcoming from prospective clinical trials now underway should help to define the benefit of treatment in the aggregate. However whatever the specific results of these studies, they cannot provide guidance for the management of any single patient. The proper management of the elderly hypertensive must be determined individually. The physician must consider all of the available data, including that derived from epidemiological studies, before arriving at a therapeutic plan. Any decision to treat should only be made after observation of the patient over time, and that treatment should be constantly under review to ensure that its cost, in human terms, does not exceed its potential benefit. The objective must always be to maintain the functional integrity of the hypertensive patient while attempting to reduce the risk of stroke and myocardial infarction through blood pressure reduction.

REFERENCES

Amery A, Berthaux P, Birkenhager W, Bulpitt C, Clement D, De Schaepdryver A 1977 Antihypertensive therapy in elderly patients. Pilot trial of the European Working Party on high blood pressure in the elderly. Geronotology 23: 426–437

Amery A, Berthaux P, Bulpitt C, Deruyttere M, De Schaepdryver A, Dollery C 1978 Glucose intolerance during diuretic therapy: Results of trial by the European Working Party on Hypertension in the Elderly. Lancet 1: 681–683

Brunner H R, Laragh J H, Baer L, Newton M A, Goodwin F T, Krakoff L R 1972 Essential hypertension: renin and aldosterone, heart attack and stroke. New England Journal of Medicine 286: 441–449

Colandrea M A, Friedman ç J, Nichaman M Z, Lynd C N 1970 Systolic hypertension in the elderly. Circulation 41: 239–245

Francheschi M, Tancredi O, Smirne S, Mercinelli A, Canal N 1982 Cognitive processes in hypertension. Hypertension 4: 226–229

Gerber L M, Madhavan S, Alderman M H 1983 The deleterious effects of coincident hypertension on patients with hyperglycemia. New York State Journal of Medicine 873: 693–696

Gifford R W 1982 Isolated systolic hypertension in the elderly. Some controversial issues. Journal of the American Medical Association 247: 781–785

Hypertension Detection and Follow-Up Program Cooperative Group 1979a Five-year findings of the Hypertension Detection and Follow-Up Program. I. Reduction in mortality of persons with high blood pressure including mild hypertension. Journal of the American Medical Association 242: 2562–2571

Hypertension Detection and Follow-Up Program Cooperative Group 1979b Five-year findings of the Hypertension Detection and Follow-Up Program. II. Mortality by race-sex and age. Journal of the American Medical Association 242: 2572–2577

Jackson G, Pierscianowski T A, Mahon W, Condon J 1976 Inappropriate antihypertensive therapy in the elderly. Lancet 2: 1317–1318

Kannel W B 1976 Some lessons in cardiovascular epidemiology from Framingham. American Journal of Cardiology 37: 269–282

Kannel W B, Gordon T, Schwartz J J 1971 Systolic versus diastolic blood pressure and risk of coronary heart disease: The Framingham Study. American Journal of Cardiology 27: 335–346

Kirkendall W M, Hammond J J 1980 Hypertension in the elderly. Archives of Internal Medicine 140: 1155–1161

Koch-Weser J, Greenblatt D J 1976 Pharmacotherapy of disproportionate systolic hypertension, abstracted. Clinical Pharmacology and Therapeutics 19: 109

Lakatta E 1979 Alterations in the cardiovascular system that occur in advanced age. Federation Proceedings 38: 163–167

Light K C 1980 Antihypertensive drugs and behavioural performance. In: Elias M F, Streeten D H P (eds) Hypertension and cognitive processes. Beech Hill, Maine, p 119–135

Medical Research Council Working Party on Mild to Moderate Hypertension 1977 Randomized controlled trial of treatment for mild hypertension: design and pilot trial. British Medical Journal i: 1437–1440

Morgan T, Gillies A, Morgan G 1978 Hypertension treated by salt restriction. Lancet 1: 227–230

Ostfeld A M 1978 Elderly hypertensive patient. Epidemiological review. New York State Journal of Medicine V: 1125–29

Ostfeld A M, Shekelle R B, Tufo H M, Wieland A M, Kilbridge J A, Drori J 1971 Cardiovascular and cerebrovascular disease in an elderly poor urban population. American Journal of Public Health 61: 19–29

Sever P S, Gordon D, Peart W J, Beighton P 1980 Blood pressure and its correlates in urban and tribal Africa. Lancet ii: 60–64

Sos T A, Vaughan E D, Pickering T G, Case D B, Snyderman K W, Sealey J 1982 Diagnosis of renovascular hypertension and evaluation of 'surgical' curability. Urologic Radiology 3: 199–203

Spence J D, Sibbold W J, Case R D 1978 Pseudo-hypertension in the elderly. Clinical Science and Molecular Medicine 55: 399–402

Veterans Administration Cooperative Study Group on Antihypertensive Agents 1967 Effects of treatment on morbidity in hypertension: I. Results in patients with diastolic blood pressures averaging 115 through 129 mm Hg. Journal of the American Medical Association 202: 1028–1034

Veterans Administration Cooperative Study Group on Antihypertensive Agents 1970 Effect of treatment on morbidity in hypertension: II. Results in patients with diastolic blood pressures averaging 90 through 114 mm Hg. Journal of the American Medical Association 212: 1143–1152

Weksler M E 1982 Personal communication

Wiggers C J 1932 Physical and physiological aspects of arteriosclerosis and hypertension. Annals of Internal Medicine 6: 12–30

Wilkie F, Eisdorfer C 1971 Intelligence and blood pressure in the aged. Science 172: 959–962

26

Peripheral vascular disorders

J. A. Spittell

The term 'peripheral vascular disease' is often incorrectly used to refer to occlusive arterial disease when it should more properly be used in reference to the totality of peripheral vascular disorders — whether arterial, venous or lymphatic in origin. In this chapter the specific peripheral vascular disorders commonly seen in older persons will be addressed. It is unfortunate that peripheral vascular disease is accorded so little attention in most medical school curricula and graduate training programmes since peripheral vascular diseases are common (particularly in the elderly). While not life threatening they do cause symptoms that may restrict the activity and thus adversely affect the patient's independence and quality of life. Fortunately with appropriate management and patient compliance many of the complications can be avoided.

Certainly occlusive arterial disease with its complications is the most common peripheral vascular disorder seen in geriatric practice since atherosclerosis is the most common cause of occlusive arterial disease. Another peripheral vascular problem related to atherosclerosis is arterial aneurysm and it, like atherosclerotic occlusive arterial disease, is more common in men and increases in frequency with age. Next in frequency of peripheral vascular disorders in the geriatric population is oedema which, with its multiple possible aetiologies, necessitates careful evaluation. Leg and foot ulcers are a significant problem in the elderly; their origin is fairly easily identified as due to venous or arterial (or arteriolar) disease or neuropathy secondary to diabetes — the usual causes. Rounding out the important vascular disorders seen in the elderly is giant cell arteritis, which with its variable and protean clinical manifestations is unique to persons more than 50 years in age and vital to recognise and treat early to avoid its possible, and serious, complications.

For the most part the peripheral vascular disorders seen in the geriatric age group affect the lower extremities. All of the conditions included in this chapter may cause symptoms that restrict the activity, interfere with sleep because of pain and thus jeopardise the patient's feeling of independence, enforce social isolation and create anxiety and/or depression because they may threaten the patient's digits or limbs. Most of the complications of the peripheral vascular disorders are preventable if only they are identified

and appropriately managed; this includes having the patient (or those responsible for care) fully informed about the nature of the problem and proper preventive measures (Spittell, 1982).

The diagnosis of the peripheral vascular disorders is not difficult since the extremities are easy to examine. Since peripheral vascular diseases are so common in older persons, examination of them should always include systematic observation of the extremities, the skin colour and texture and evaluation of all the peripheral arterial pulsations. Few other conditions offer so great an opportunity for secondary prevention, so that even asymptomatic and/or uncomplicated peripheral vascular disorders should be searched for aggressively.

Because older persons frequently have multiple health problems, treatment for non-vascular conditions that may have adverse effects on certain of the peripheral vascular diseases should be avoided or used with caution; this is particularly important in the patient with chronic atherosclerotic peripheral occlusive disease. Often also, because vascular disorders may be mimicked by, as well as associated with, non-vascular disorders, differentiation and evaluation of each is necessary if inappropriate management is to be avoided. It is important, too, that symptoms of neuropathy and nocturnal leg cramps not be ascribed to peripheral vascular disease lest the patient worry unnecessarily.

Another important general clinical aspect of certain peripheral vascular problems is that the vascular problem may at times be the first or dominant manifestation of an otherwise occult disease. Thus acute arterial occlusion, acute venous thrombosis or lymphatic obstruction can be valuable diagnostic clues.

An additional general point about vascular problems, as well as other painful disorders of the extremities that may require a period of bed rest, is awareness of flexion contracture of the knee and its prevention by regular active and/or passive extension of the knee.

OCCLUSIVE ARTERIAL DISEASE

Chronic

Arteriosclerosis obliterans is the cause of virtually all

chronic occlusive peripheral arterial disease in older persons.

When symptomatic, occlusive arterial disease causes pain, initially brought on by walking — intermittent claudication — and with occlusive disease that is severe enough to cause ischaemia at rest, pain at rest — ischaemic rest pain. Intermittent claudication may be described by various terms — cramping, tiredness, aching or weakness — and be located in the foot, calf, thigh or hip, but its occurrence with walking and relief with standing still are characteristic. Ischaemic rest pain often is worse at night, disturbing sleep and may lead the patient to try elevation or dependency of the limb to get relief. When ischaemia is severe, in addition to rest pain, there may also be an uncomfortable type of dysaesthesia of the foot and/or toes — so called ischaemic neuropathy — which the patient may try to relieve by gentle rubbing.

The amplitude of pulsation and quality of the carotid (best done with the patient supine), subclavian, brachial, radial and ulnar arteries as well as the abdominal aorta, femoral, popliteal, dorsal pedis and posterior tibial arteries should be determined in every patient. A system of grading and recording of each arterial pulsation — e.g. 0 to indicate absence and 4 to indicate normal amplitude with 1,2,3 indicating degrees of normal — is a worthwhile discipline. After palpating the arteries, listening for bruits over the carotid and subclavian arteries and the abdominal aorta, femoral and popliteal arteries can help to identify and localise the occlusive process (Carter, 1981).

Determination of pallor on elevation provides a rough but reliable estimate of the degree of ischaemia (Table 26.1). After determining elevation pallor additional confirmatory evidence can be obtained by having the patient move the feet to a dependent position and noting how long it takes for the skin colour to return and for the superficial veins to fill (Table 26.2).

A number of musculoskeletal and neurologic disorders may mimic occlusive arterial disease symptomatically, and of course, in the elderly patient both may be present. Differentiation of the non-vascular problems is usually

Table 26.1 Grading of elevation pallor (Spittell, 1981: With permission of the American Heart Association Inc)

Elevation of extremity at angle of 60° above the level	
Grade of pallor	Duration of elevation
0	No pallor in 60 seconds
1	Definite pallor in 60 seconds
2	Definite pallor in less than 60 seconds
3	Definite pallor in less than 30 seconds
4	Pallor on the level

Table 26.2 Colour return (CR) and venous filling time (VFT) (Spittell, 1981: With permission of the American Heart Association Inc)

	Time for CR (s)	VFT (s)
Normal	10	15
Moderate ischaemia	15–25	20–30
Severe ischaemia	40+	40+

possible with careful history and physical examination, but when they co-exist, non-invasive studies to evaluate the arterial circulation may be quite useful. Using a standard blood pressure cuff and a Doppler flow detector the systolic pressure at the ankle level can be determined and compared with that at the brachial level. Furthermore, when these determinations are made before and after standard exercise, an estimate of the functional impairment imposed by any occlusive arterial disease can be made in ambulatory persons (Table 26.3). Our standard exercise is walking on a treadmill at a 10% grade at a speed of 2 miles per hour for 5 minutes; the electrocardiogram of the patient is continuously monitored during and after the exercise because of the frequency of associated coronary artery disease in older persons.

Decisions about management of patients with chronic occlusive arterial disease should be based on the degree of disability it is imposing and/or the severity of ischaemia, the predictable natural history and the general health of the patient. In the non-diabetic person who has no symptoms or only intermittent claudication the prognosis for limb

Table 26.3 Non-invasive laboratory assessment of arterial insufficiency of the legs (Spittell, 1981: With permission of the American Heart Association Inc).

Degree of arterial insufficiency	Standard exercise		Systolic blood pressure index‡	
	claudication	duration (min)	Before exercise	After exercise
Minimal	0	5	Normal to mildly abnormal	Abnormal
Mild	+	5	>0.8	>0.5
Moderate	+	<5	<0.8	<
Severe*	+	<3	<0.5	<0.15

‡ systolic pressure index is obtained by dividing the systolic ankle blood pressure by the systolic brachial blood pressure, both taken in the supine position (normal 0.95 or greater)

* often have a systolic ankle blood pressure less than 50 mmHg in addition.

survival is favourable (about 95% over a 5 year period) (Juergens et al, 1960) so that any attempt to restore pulsatile flow by arterial surgery or balloon angioplasty is elective and designed only to relieve the patient's symptoms. When the ischaemia is more severe causing rest pain and/or ischaemic ulceration the prognosis for limb loss is worse (about 10% over a 5 year period) a more aggressive approach to restoration of pulsatile flow seems justified. When occlusive arterial disease develops in the person with diabetes, the prognosis for limb loss is much worse (about 25% over a 9 year period) (Schadt et al, 1961) so here also an aggressive approach to restoration of pulsatile flow is warranted.

Unless arterial surgery or percutaneous transluminal angioplasty is planned, arteriography is unnecessary for management.

For all patients with peripheral arterial disease a programme of conservative measures has much to offer. Smoking worsens the prognosis for limb loss so patients with occlusive arterial disease should abstain from tobacco completely. Since even trivial injuries heal poorly and may even lead to loss of an ischaemic limb, patients with occlusive arterial disease should be thoroughly instructed in protection of their limbs from all types of trauma. For geriatric patients, regular care of the feet and toe nails by a chiropodist, knowledgeable about peripheral arterial disease, is preferable to self care. Regular walking to the point of symptoms is encouraged in the hope of stimulating collateral circulation, increasing the walking distance (Jonason et al, 1979), and preventing 'age-acquired clubfoot' (Vega, 1982).

The usefulness of the many available vasodilator drugs is limited to those patients for whom cutaneous vasodilation is useful e.g. ischaemic ulceration. Since none of the currently available drugs has been shown to dilate the arterial circulation of extremity muscles, they are not recommended for the relief of intermittent claudication (Coffman, 1979). On the subject of drugs, an important point is to avoid agents that may aggravate ischaemia; since many older persons have coronary artery disease and/or hypertension, drugs such as the beta-adrenergic antagonists (Ingram et al, 1982) and clonidine are best avoided if the patient also has occlusive peripheral arterial disease. Likewise in the person with migraine, the ergot preparations are best avoided if occlusive arterial disease is present.

Lumbar sympathectomy is seldom advised with the advances in arterial surgery and angioplasty. Interruption of sympathetic nerve supply increases blood flow to the skin and not to muscle so the application of the procedure is the same as for vasodilator drugs.

Acute

Acute peripheral arterial occlusion can vary in its presentation from a dramatic picture of severe pain in the extremity with associated coldness, pallor, numbness and paralysis, to merely the abrupt appearance of intermittent claudication or shortening of the walking distance if claudication was already present.

On examination the findings are the same as those in chronic occlusive arterial disease, but in addition there is frequently tenderness over the occluded artery and commonly there is a level of temperature and sensation change distal to the level of the occlusion.

Since acute arterial occlusion may be either thrombotic or embolic it is desirable to try to make the distinction. In the patient with prior occlusive peripheral arterial disease, an acute arterial occlusion is usually thrombotic. In the person with cardiac disease on the other hand, particularly if atrial fibrillation is present, embolic arterial occlusion is likely. One other source of emboli is the thrombus that usually develops in an atherosclerotic aneurysm. In the older patient previously free of occlusive arterial disease it is important not to overlook the possibility of silent myocardial infarction, myeloproliferative disease and acute aortic dissection as causes of acute peripheral arterial occlusion.

Management of acute arterial occlusion should first be directed at preventing thrombosis in the collateral, arterial and distal venous circulation with heparin. It is important to avoid things which may have an adverse effect such as elevation of the ischaemic extremity and the application of either heat or cold to it. Thrombectomy or embolectomy using the Fogarty catheter is extremely useful in restoring arterial flow — it should not be delayed for even in seriously ill persons it can be carried out under local anaesthesia. In selected patients thrombolysis may be useful. When as much restoration of arterial flow as possible is completed, anticoagulant therapy is indicated to prevent rethrombosis or further embolisation. If the origin of an embolus is a proximally located arterial aneurysm then it should be resected.

Atheromatous plaques and the mural thrombus of aneurysms of the aorta or femoropopliteal arteries may shed atheromatous debris which occludes small (digital) arteries and/or dermal arterioles (atheroembolism; cholesterol embolisation) producing a characteristic picture of blue toes and livedo reticularis. It is important to recognise this syndrome since the only treatment is resection of the origin of the debris lest embolisation of the visceral and renal circulation, which also occurs, produces irreversible changes.

PERIPHERAL ARTERIAL ANEURYSMS

Since atherosclerosis is the most common cause of peripheral aneurysms they are usually seen in persons more than 50 years of age and they are far more common in men than in women. Hypertension appears to contribute to aneurysm formation (Spittell, 1983b). Once formed aneurysms tend to enlarge gradually and to develop laminated mural thrombus, features which account for some of the following complications of aneurysms:

1. Pressure on surrounding structures
2. Rupture
3. Thrombosis
4. Distal embolisation
5. Infection

Prior to developing complications, arterial aneurysms cause no symptoms or physical findings other than a localised pulsatile enlargement. Thus careful palpation of the abdominal aorta, the femoral and popliteal arteries is essential if these lesions are to be identified when uncomplicated, the ideal time to surgically resect them. Thoracic aortic aneurysms are often first discovered on chest roentgenogram. Differentiation from other mediastinal masses can be made by angiography and/or computed tomography (CT) scanning with or without contrast media. The prognosis for persons with thoracic aortic aneurysms is sufficiently poor (Fig. 26.1) (50% survival for 5 years and 30% survival for 10 years with

SURVIVAL RATES OF UNTREATED THORACIC AND ABDOMINAL AORTIC ANEURYSM

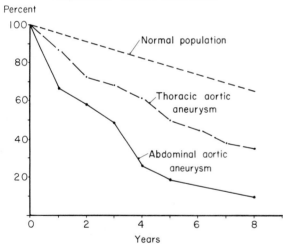

Fig. 26.1 Survival rates of patients with untreated thoracic aortic and abdominal aneurysms. (Pairolero & Bernatz, 1976: With the permission of Harper & Row Publishers)

death resulting from rupture of the aneurysm in about one-third of those dying) (Joyce et al, 1964) that surgical treatment is indicated except when associated disease or advanced age make the surgical risk too great.

Abdominal aortic aneurysms may be detected on physical examination unless the patient is obese. At times the aneurysm is first suspected by the finding of a curvilinear shadow of calcification or soft tissue mass to the right or left of the lumbar spine on a roentgenogram of the lumbar

spine (Fig. 26.2) or abdomen. The diagnosis and accurate determination of the size and extent of the aneurysm is best made by ultrasonography or CT scan. The prognosis for aneurysms more than 4.5 cm in diameter is grave (see Fig. 26.1). Studies have shown that if the patient with an abdominal aortic aneurysm does not have an associated malignancy or cardiac disease, death is more likely from rupture of the aneurysm than from anything else. Hence, surgical resection prior to complications is advisable unless associated disease or advanced age contraindicate it.

Aneurysms of the femoral and popliteal arteries are almost always seen in men (Wychulis et al, 1970). If the arteries are carefully examined in all patients these aneurysms are easily identified. In the popliteal space, aneurysm may be difficult to differentiate from a popliteal (Baker's) cyst but ultrasonography is excellent for this purpose (Fig. 26.3). Since these aneurysms usually contain laminated thrombus, (Fig. 26.4) thromboembolic complications may threaten the limb, so surgical resection is advisable before complications develop. Prior to surgery an arteriogram is necessary to make certain of the adequacy of the proximal and distal arterial circulation for successful grafting.

Since atherosclerosis affects multiple sites in the cardiovascular system it is wise to carefully assess the patient with an atherosclerotic aneurysm for associated coronary artery disease, cerebral vascular disease and aneurysms in other locations, because any or all of these may affect decisions about surgery.

OEDEMA

In the person with chronic oedema, particularly if it is bilateral, the systemic disorders — cardiac, renal, and hepatic — are usually the first consideration (Schirger, 1982). When systemic causes have been excluded, then oedema of the extremities in older persons may be venous, lymphatic or orthostatic in origin, or secondary to certain commonly prescribed drugs (Table 26.4), so the latter information should always be determined. The differential diagnosis of the usual types of chronic oedema in older patients is usually straightforward (Table 26.5). The oedema due to drugs is typically a soft pitting oedema that is bilateral, gradual in onset and subsides when the responsible drug is discontinued.

When differentiation of the type of oedema is in doubt, the non-invasive methodology using a handheld Doppler flow detector is reasonably reliable to determine deep venous patency and incompetence at the popliteal level and proximal. If doubt still exists contrast venography is the diagnostic procedure of choice.

Venous oedema

The oedema due to deep venous thrombosis is more acute, developing over hours. The swelling is soft, pitting and

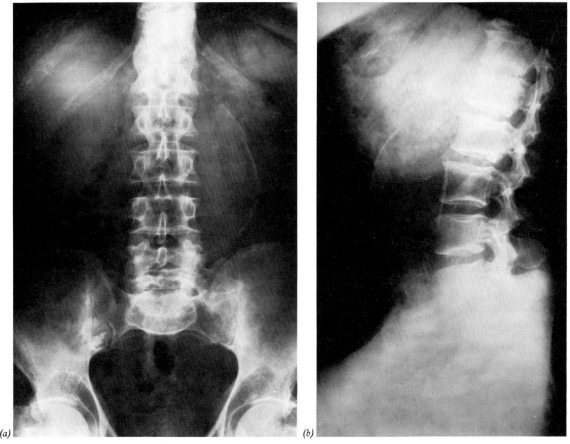

Fig. 26.2   Large aneurysm of abdominal aorta with calcification of aneurysmal wall. (a) Anteroposterior view (b) Lateral view. (Spittel & Wallace, 1980: With the permission of the Mayo Foundation)

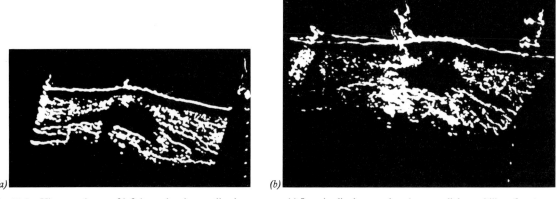

Fig. 26.3   Ultrasound scan of left knee showing popliteal aneurysm. (a) Longitudinal scan taken 1 cm medial to midline; foot is toward left. Communication with proximal portion of popliteal artery can be seen. (b) Longitudinal scan taken 1 cm lateral to midline, showing communication with distal portion of popliteal artery. (Carpenter et al, 1976: With the permission of the Mayo Foundation)

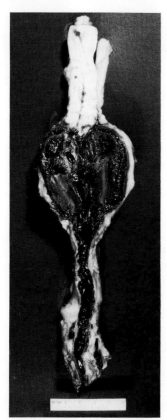

Fig. 26.4 Arteriosclerotic aneurysm of popliteal artery. Specimen opened; complete filling of aneurysm and portion of artery distal to aneurysm by thrombus may be noted. (Spittell & Wallace, 1980: With the permission of the Mayo Foundation)

variable in extent depending on the vein occluded. Typically the extremity is suffused in appearance with increased superficial venous pattern. Generally there is tenderness over the vein or veins involved and there may be a mild febrile reaction. Unexplained deep venous thrombosis in an older person always raises the possibility of an occult disease such as a myeloproliferative disorder or neoplasm.

Table 26.4 Drugs that may cause oedema of lower extremities (Fairbairn, 1980: With permission of the Mayo Foundation)

Hormones
    Corticosteroids and adrenocorticotropins
    Oestrogen
    Progesterone (including birth control agents)
    Testosterone
    Aldosterone-like substances
Antihypertensive drugs
    Guanethedine sulphate (Ismelin)
    Hydralazine hydrochloride (Apresoline)
    Rauwolfia preparations
    Monoamine oxidase inhibitors
    Methyldopa (Alodmet)
    Diazoxide
    Clinidine hydrochloride (Catapres)
    Minoxidil
Anti-inflammatory drugs
    Phenylbutazone
Others
    Carbenoxolone sodium
    Antidepressants (monoamine oxidase inhibitor type)
    Certain antibiotics (such as carbenicillin)

Chronic venous insufficiency is usually secondary to prior deep venous thrombosis but may also occur with chronic obstruction of a deep vein by a mass (e.g. Baker's cyst). The oedema is soft and pitting at first, but later may become more firm. Typically, increased superficial venous pattern develops along with stasis changes — pigmentation, dermatitis, ulceration — in the skin of the distal medial ankle.

The management of deep venous thrombosis is with antithrombotic therapy, bed rest with elevation of the involved extremity until the oedema and tenderness subside. With ambulation the use of adequate elastic support in the form of Ace bandages or an elastic stocking (30–40 mmHg compression) is advised for 1–2 months. If dependent oedema is still present without support after 1–2 months then the regular long-term use of an elastic stocking is advised. For chronic deep venous insufficiency due to obstruction from an extrinsic lesion, relief of the obstruction is, of course, the preferred management. For

Table 26.5 Distinguishing features of common types of regional oedema (Fairbairn, 1980: With permission of the Mayo Foundation).

Feature	Orthostatic oedema	Lymphoedema	Chronic venous insufficiency
Thickened skin	No*	Marked	Occasionally†
Ulceration	No	Rare	Common
Pigmented skin	No	No	Yes
Bilateral oedema	Always	Often	Occasionally
Soft, pitting oedema	Yes	Occasionally‡	Yes

* except rarely in severe, long-standing oedema
† if regional lymphoedema also present
‡ in lymphoedema of short duration

chronic postphlebitic oedema the regular use of adequate elastic support when ambulatory is advised.

Lymphoedema

In geriatric practice lymphoedema is uncommon but when it develops it is on an obstructive or inflammatory basis. While the oedema may be pitting and recede overnight with elevation early, as lymphoedema becomes chronic it is painless, progressive, firm with thickened skin and does not recede with elevation overnight. When it is due to inflammation (recurrent lymphangitis) the portal of infection is usually dermatophytosis. When obstructive, lymphoedema is most often secondary to neoplasm, usually arising in a pelvic organ.

Management of lymphoedema includes use of adequate elastic support, preferably with a fitted stocking of appropriate length and providing 40–50 mmHg compression. The support should be fitted after several days elevation of the extremity to gain maximum reduction of the lymphoedema. Weight reduction if the patient is obese and avoidance of salt in the diet are helpful adjuncts. At times periodic diuretic therapy is helpful also.

If recurring lymphangitis and/or cellulitis are problems, the first thing is to remove the portal of infection, usually dermatophytosis. Since streptococci are the usual cause of acute lymphangitis, treatment of the acute episode is with penicillin or for penicillin sensitive patients, erythromycin. For the patient with recurring attacks of lymphangitis, prophylaxis with oral penicillin V, 250 mg q.i.d. or erythromycin 250 mg q.i.d. the first seven to ten days of every month is effective.

Orthostatic oedema

In elderly people who are inactive particularly if they sit with their feet dependent, soft pitting oedema that recedes with elevation is common. It is always bilateral and unaccompanied by stasis change. The avoidance of extra salt in the diet and regular activity are useful measures to prevent orthostatic oedema. When the patient has associated lipoedema ('fat legs') elastic stockings may not be tolerated but otherwise they are useful.

LEG ULCER

Ulceration of the foot, toes or distal leg is common in older persons. The great majority are due to venous or arterial disease or to diabetic neuropathy (Spittell, 1983a).

With a careful history and a systematic examination the four common types of ulceration noted above are readily identified and differentiated one from another (Table 26.6).

The management of leg and foot ulcers is straightforward and includes correction of the basic cause (if possible), control of any infection with appropriate systemic antibiotics, local cleansing with non-irritating material (e.g. sterile gauze moistened three to five times a day with sterile water or isotonic saline) and control of pain.

For venous stasis ulceration (Fig. 26.5) elevation of the extremity to relieve venous congestion is basic. Moist

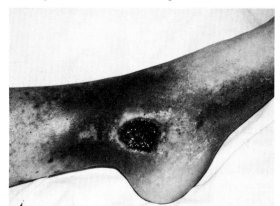

Fig. 26.5 Stasis ulceration (Spittell, 1983a: With the permission of Harcourt Brace Javanovich Inc)

Table 26.6 Leg ulcer — differential diagnosis (Spittell, 1983a: With Permission of Harcourt Brace Javanovich Inc).

	Stasis	Ischaemic Arterial	Neurotrophic	Ischaemic (Arteriolar)
Onset	Trauma ±	Trauma	Spontaneous	Spontaneous
Course	Chronic	Progressive	Progressive	Progressive
Pain ?	+ with infection	Severe	Absent	Severe
Location	Medial leg	Toe, heal, foot	Plantar	Lateral & posterior leg
Skin	Stasis change	Atrophic	Callous	Normal
Edges	Shaggy	Discrete	Discrete	Serpigenous
Base	Healthy	Eschar; pale	Healthy or pale	Eschar; ischaemic
Arterial	Normal	Abnormal	Normal or abnormal	Normal
Venous	Abnormal	Normal	Normal	Normal
Lymphatic	Normal	Normal	Normal	Normal

dressings for 30 minutes three to five times a day, with sterile dry gauze dressings between hasten the cleansing. Small ulcers will heal spontaneously but larger ulcers may require a skin graft when the ulcer base is clean and not infected. Long-term adequate elastic support is essential to prevent recurrent ulceration.

For ischaemic ulcers due to arteriosclerosis obliterans (Fig. 26.6) bed rest with elevation of the head of the bed is advised. Moist soaks or dressings, with sterile dry dressings between, are used to gently debride the ulcer. Any infection is treated with appropriate systemic antibiotics. The ideal therapy of course, is restoration of pulsatile arterial flow to the extremity; if this is not possible then use of one of the

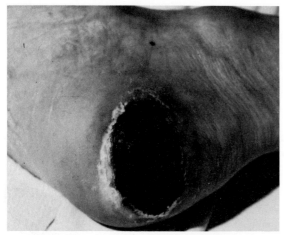

Fig. 26.6 Ischaemic ulceration of the heel. (Spittell, 1983a: With the permission of Harcourt Brace Javanovich Inc)

oral vasodilators to try to get cutaneous vasodilation, or lumbar sympathectomy may be tried.

The ischaemic type of ulceration due to arteriolar disease is the type most often incorrectly diagnosed. Its location on the leg, serpiginous borders and extreme pain are quite characteristic and most often these ulcers in geriatric patients are the 'hypertensive ischaemic ulcer' (Fig. 26.7). Management includes bed rest, elevation of the head of the bed, local moist dressing to the ulcer, control of pain and measures to effect cutaneous vasodilation — e.g. phenoxybenzamine hydrochloride 10 mg t.i.d. or q.i.d. or prazosin 1 mg b.i.d. to t.i.d. — are employed. If the ulceration does not improve on this programme then regional sympathectomy is advised. Skin grafting may be necessary for large ulcers.

Neurotrophic ulcers (Fig. 26.8) are usually due to diabetic neuropathy and typically develop in the callus on a weight bearing surface, usually the sole of the foot. Bed rest, control of any infection and removal of the callus are generally necessary for healing to occur. Adjustment of fotwear to redistribute the weight is advisable to prevent recurrences. Often, a moulded type of shoe is helpful for these patients.

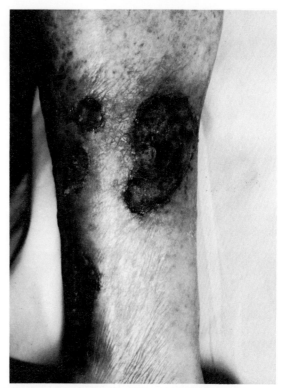

Fig. 26.7 Later stage of hypertensive ischaemic ulceration. (Spittell, 1983a: With the permission of Harcourt Brace Javanovich Inc)

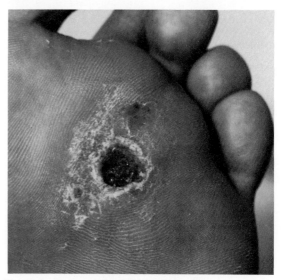

Fig. 26.8 Neurotrophic ulcer of the foot. (Spittell, 1983a: With the permission of Harcourt Brace Javanovich Inc)

GIANT CELL ARTERITIS

Giant cell arteritis (temporal arteritis; cranial arteritis) is an arteritis of uncertain aetiology with systemic manifestations (Hunder, 1983). It is unique to older persons seldom occurring before the age of 65, almost unheard of before the age of 50, and is slightly more common in women.

The disease may be insidious or sudden in onset with rather non-specific symptoms of malaise and myalgia. The most characteristic symptoms are headache, scalp tenderness and/or jaw pain with chewing. At times the patient or a member of the family will note prominent nodular, inflamed and tender temporal or other scalp arteries (Fig. 26.9). Laboratory studies typically show a mild anaemia and leukocytosis and an elevated sedimentation rate, often of 100 mm or more in one hour (Westergren).

Awareness of and early recognition of giant cell arteritis is important because prompt treatment with corticosteroids not only relieves the systemic symptoms but prevents the complication of visual loss that occurs in more than 40% of

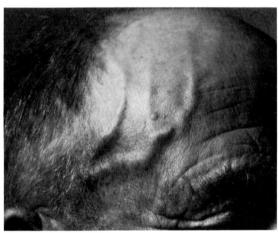

Fig. 26.9 Patient with temporal arteritis. (Sheps & McDuffie, 1980: With the permission of the Mayo Foundation)

untreated patients. Once visual loss has occurred however, it is not recovered, even with treatment. In the patient with partial visual loss treatment is vital to prevent further visual loss. It is essential for clinicians to be alert to the possibility of giant cell arteritis whenever older persons develop any of the symptoms or signs noted above and they are not readily explained otherwise.

When the disease is suspected, treatment with prednisone 45–60 mg per day or the equivalent dose of another corticosteroid is recommended. Histologic confirmation of the diagnosis is advisable for all patients suspected of having giant cell arteritis because of the high dose of corticosteroids and the problems of side effects and withdrawal associated with such therapy given over a period of several months. If the diagnosis is confirmed by biopsy, the dose of corticosteroids is maintained at the initial level for about a month. If symptoms subside and the sedimentation rate and blood counts return toward normal, gradual reduction of the corticosteroid dose can usually start after about one month at the initial dose. The dose of steroids must be decreased slowly, following the clinical response of the patient and the sedimentation rate. If recurrence of symptoms occurs during tapering, the dosage of steroids should be increased for several weeks before even more gradual tapering is begun. Most patients recover after several months to a year and steroid therapy can be discontinued but an occasional patient may require 5–10 mg of prednisone a day for several years to control the symptoms.

In older patients receiving such large doses of steroids, blood pressure and cardiac compensation should be closely watched. A diet with no extra salt is advisable and if elevation of blood pressure or oedema develops then the use of a thiazide diuretic is usually effective in their control.

REFERENCES

Carpenter J R, Hattery R R, Hunder G G et al 1976
 Ultrasound evaluation of the popliteal space: comparison
 with arthrography and physical examination. Mayo Clinic
 Proceedings 51: 498–503
Carter S A 1981 Arterial auscultation in peripheral vascular
 disease. Journal of the American Medical Association 246:
 1682–1686
Coffman J D 1979 Drug therapy: vasodilator drugs in peripheral
 vascular disease. New England Journal of Medicine 300:
 713–717
Fairbairn J F II 1980 Clinical manifestations of peripheral
 vascular disease. In: Juergens J L, Spittell J A Jr, Fairbairn J
 F (eds) Peripheral vascular diseases, 5th edn. W B Saunders,
 Philadelphia
Hunder G G 1983 Giant cell arteritis. Geriatrics. In press
Ingram D M, House A K, Thompson G H, Stacey M C,
 Castleden W M, Lovegrove F T 1982 Beta-adrenergic
 blockade and peripheral vascular disease. Medical Journal of
 Australia 1: 509–511

Jonason T, Jonzon B, Ringquist I, Oman-Rydberg A 1979 Effect
 of physical training on different categories of patients with
 intermittent claudication. Acta Med Scandinavica 206:
 253–258
Joyce J W, Fairbairn J F II, Kincaid O W, Juergens J L 1964
 Aneurysms of the thoracic aorta: a clinical study with special
 reference to prognosis. Circulation 29: 176–181
Juergens J L, Barker N W, Hines E A Jr 1960 Arteriosclerosis
 obliterans: review of 520 cases with special reference to
 pathogenic and prognostic factors. Circulation 21: 188–195
Pairolero P C, Bernatz P E 1976 Aneurysms. In: Lewis'
 Practice of Surgery. Harper & Row Publishers, Hagerstown,
 Maryland
Schadt D C, Hines E A Jr, Juergens J L, Barker N W 1961
 Chronic atherosclerotic occlusion of the femoral artery.
 Journal of the American Medical Association 175: 937–940
Schirger A 1982 Differential diagnosis and management of leg
 edema in the elderly. Geriatrics 37: 26–32
Sheps S G, McDuffie F C 1980 Vasculitis. In: Juergens J L,
 Spittell J A Jr, Fairbairn J F (eds) Peripheral Vascular
 Diseases, 5th edn. W B Saunders, Philadelphia

Spittell J A Jr 1981 Recognition and management of chronic atherosclerotic occlusive peripheral arterial disease. Modern Concepts of Cardiovascular Disease 50: 19–23

Spittell J A Jr 1982 Diagnosis and treatment of occlusive peripheral arterial disease. Geriatrics 37: 57–67

Spittell J A Jr 1983a Diagnosis and management of leg ulcer. Geriatrics 36: 57–65

Spittell J A Jr 1983b Hypertension and arterial aneurysm. Journal of the American College of Cardiology 1(2): 533–540

Spittell J A Jr, Wallace R B 1980 Aneurysms. In: Juergens J L, Spittell J A Jr, Fairbairn J F (eds) Peripheral Vascular Diseases, 5th edn. W B Saunders, Philadelphia

Vega R H 1982 Recognizing and treating age-acquired clubfoot. Geriatric Consultant 1: 16–17

Wychulis A R, Spittell J A Jr, Wallace R B 1970 Popliteal aneurysms. Surgery 68: 942–951

27

Chest diseases

J. E. Stark & R. G. Dent

With increasing age there is general atrophy of the tissues of the lung as with other organs and this is apparent as an increase in the size of the alveoli and thinning of their walls. Despite a superficial similarity to emphysema there are none of the clinical, physiological or radiographic features of emphysema. Thinning of the alveolar walls leads to a loss of elastic recoil and this allows the early closure of airways during expiration. Hence there is progressive decline of the vital capacity (VC) and of the volume of air expelled in the first second of a forced expiration (FEV1); the reduction of FEV1 is greater than that of vital capacity so that the ratio FEV1/VC falls to a mean of 65% at the age of 70 years compared to 85% at the age of 20 years and such a fall does not therefore reflect abnormal airflow obstruction. In parallel with the declining 'bellows' function of the lung there is a progressive fall in the partial pressure of oxygen in arterial blood from a mean of 95 mmHg at the age of 30, to 75 mmHg at the age of 60. The partial pressure of carbon dioxide is unchanged.

THE CHEST RADIOGRAPH

Kyphosis becomes increasingly common with advancing age and there is loss of height of the vertebrae; both of these may cause the lung fields to appear small and the transverse diameter of the normal sized heart to seem disproportionately large. A lateral film will establish the presence of kyphosis with vertebral thinning. The radiographic appearance of the lung fields in the elderly person superficially resembles that in emphysema because of an impression of radiolucency, but the other features of emphysema such as over inflation and the presence of bullae are not present. The lucency probably reflects loss of elastic tissue within the walls of alveoli and is reinforced by a loss of radioopacity of the ribs due to decalcification with age (Edge et al, 1964).

SOME PROBLEMS OF DIAGNOSIS IN THE ELDERLY

Breathlessness

The history and particularly the duration of symptoms will narrow the diagnostic possibilities. We will compare here the diagnostic approach to the extreme situations of breathlessness of at most a few days and that of longer duration.

Recent Breathlessness (Fig. 27.1)
Fine inspiratory crackles (crepitations) heard on auscultation will immediately suggest left ventricular failure. Except in the case of recent myocardial infarction, which has usually been associated with cardiac pain, examination will also reveal evidence of severe hypertension or of heart disease, with cardiac enlargement, triple rhythm, orthopnea or a rapid arrhythmia. Clinical signs alone may not allow a certain diagnosis of left heart failure but a chest radiograph will almost certainly show diagnostic features. Episodic or persistent breathlessness may be due to heart block with marked bradycardia, and if this is intermittent, diagnosis may be difficult at times of normal rhythm. 'Paroxysmal nocturnal dyspnoea', though a feature of left heart failure may equally occur due to nocturnal asthma or rarely episodes of aspiration from oesophageal reflux. In the absence of clear evidence of heart disease and severe hypertension and especially if the heart size is normal on a chest radiograph, a cardiac cause should not be presumed.

If inspiratory crackles are not heard on examination of the lungs evidence of airflow obstruction should be sought. Wheezing is as likely to be due to true asthma as to 'cardiac asthma'. A description of wheezing should be sought from the patient or from others near to him but cough may overshadow the wheeze. Quite severe airflow obstruction can occur in the absence of wheezing and can always be detected on spirometry. If wheeze is heard, stridor (a predominantly inspiratory noise best heard on rapid inhalation through the open mouth) suggests obstruction in the large airways at any level from the larynx to a main bronchus. Recent wheeze without stridor strongly suggests asthma. Chronic bronchitis and emphysema are chronic diseases and the absence of previous breathlessness virtually excludes these conditions.

In the absense of crackles, wheeze or evidence of airflow obstruction on spirometry, other causes of recent breathlessness must be sought. Non-respiratory causes such

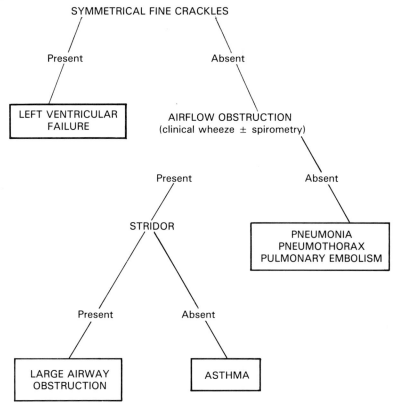

Fig. 27.1 The diagnosis of the cause of breathlessness of recent onset.

as anaemia will not be overlooked if actively considered. Pneumothorax or pleural effusion will normally be recognised on physical examination if large enough to cause breathlessness but may be overlooked in a breathless old person in whom examination is hampered by immobility. A chest radiograph is essential in these circumstances. Pulmonary thromboembolism is often difficult to recognise but must be considered in the breathless patient in whom no abnormal physical signs can be detected. A normal chest radiograph does not discount this diagnosis. The sequence of investigation on suspicion of pulmonary thrombo-embolism is outlined on page 230.

Pneumonia may cause breathlessness in the elderly with few of the 'typical' features of fever cough and sputum and with only sparse inspiratory crackles on examination of the chest.

Breathlessness of longer duration

This may be approached in a similar fashion but the likely causes are somewhat different (Fig. 27.2). Anaemia and hyperthyroidism are easily overlooked and must be considered before respiratory causes are sought.

By far the commonest respiratory cause of persistent breathlessness in the elderly is airflow obstruction. This can usually be suspected from a history of wheezing, by observing over-expansion of the chest and by hearing either wheeze or a prolonged phase of expiration. These features are not invariable and spirometry with measurement of FEV1 or peak expiratory flow rate is a more certain method of diagnosis.

Having listened carefully to exclude stridor the explanation for expiratory airflow obstruction lies between chronc bronchitis, emphysema, asthma and bronchiectasis. Bronchiectasis of sufficient extent to bring about breathlessness has nearly always produced cough with large quantities of purulent sputum for many years, and is usually accompanied by coarse inspiratory crackles and by clubbing of the fingers. Many years of smokers cough with mucoid sputum but exacerbations in which sputum is purulent suggests chronic bronchitis. Emphysema is uncommon in the absense of chronic bronchitis but may rarely be the cause of slowly worsening breathlessness on effort. It is unsafe to diagnose either chronic bronchitis or emphysema in the absence of many years of both cigarette smoking and of respiratory symptoms. An attempt must be made to distinguish the potentially reversible airflow obstruction of chronic asthma and the less reversible or irreversible obstruction of emphysema and chronic bronchitis. Failure to do so all too often leads to inadequate treatment of the asthmatic or, conversely, to unnecessarily

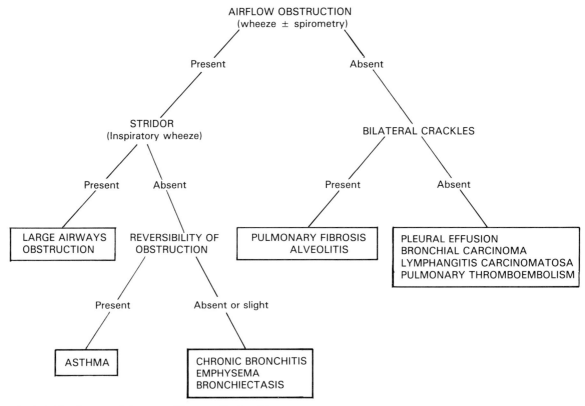

Fig. 27.2 The diagnosis of the cause of long-standing breathlessness.

hazardous treatment of the patient with chronic bronchitis or emphysema. It is important to realise that the physical signs on examination of the chest in these three conditions reflect over expansion of the lungs due to airflow obstruction and that no single sign or collection of signs distinguishes one from the other.

Features in the history which favour asthma include a fairly sudden onset (few patients with chronic bronchitis or emphysema can date the onset of their breathlessness whereas many asthmatics can), attacks of nocturnal breathlessness and cough (Lee & Stretton, 1972), and marked variation in the severity of breathlessness. Bouts of breathlessness at rest are uncommon in patients with chronic bronchitis or emphysema unless accompanied by frankly purulent sputum. The variability of airflow obstruction so characteristic of asthma can best be recognised by recording peak expiratory flow rate twice or more each day, and many elderly patients can keep such records at home if loaned a peak flow meter. The response of symptoms or measurements of airflow obstruction to inhaled bronchodilators is unfortunately not a reliable guide to diagnosis in this age group, as many chronic asthmatics fail to improve significantly on treatment with bronchodilator drugs alone. The distinction between chronic asthma and chronic bronchitis or emphysema may rest with a therapeutic trial of oral corticosteroids. After at

least a week of twice daily measurement of peak expiratory flow rate we prescribe 30 mg prednisolone daily for at least two weeks. A rise of peak flow readings of over 20% suggests that corticosteroids (but not necessarily by mouth) will be of value in therapy, which is probably the main practical advantage of reaching a diagnosis of asthma. The chest radiograph is of limited help in discovering the cause of chronic airflow obstruction, and all too often the over inflation of the lungs of an asthmatic is misinterpreted as emphysema with the disastrous outcome that potentially helpful treatment is not offered.

In the absence of severe airflow obstruction many less common conditions must be considered to account for persisting breathlessness. Bilateral inspiratory crackles are unlikely to be due to chronic left heart failure without easily recognisable and severe heart disease. Alveolitis whether of unknown cause (cryptogenic fibrosing alveolitis) or due to hypersensitivity to inhaled organic dusts (extrinsic allergic alveolitis) produces a similar clinical picture. Breathlessness on effort, with or without a dry cough is associated with symmetrical fine inspiratory crackles heard predominantly over the lower halves of the lungs. Cryptogenic fibrosing alveolitis may be associated with such connective tissue disorders as rheumatoid arthritis, systemic sclerosis or dermatomyositis and produces clubbing of the fingers in about 70% of sufferers.

The commonest cause of extrinsic allergic alveolitis in the elderly is hypersensitivity to inhaled protein dusts from a pet bird or its droppings. Many elderly people in the United Kingdom keep pet cage birds, usually budgerigars, which may be the cause of severe lung disease (Hendrick et al, 1978). The onset of symptoms may be acute with repeated bouts of breathlessness and cough, often with fever and therefore readily attributed to 'flu', but more often and more dangerously breathlessness may develop insidiously and be investigated only when irreversible fibrosis has developed. Suspicion will be aroused by the abnormal physical signs, and the chest radiograph usually provides confirmation of diffuse lung disease. Circulating precipitins against avian antigens can then be sought in the serum.

Pleural effusion of sufficient size to produce breathlessness should be detectable on clinical examination, but tumours of the lung, either primary or metastatic, may reach a considerable size and produce distressing breathlessness with few abnormal physical signs detected on examination of the lungs. A tumour which occludes a major bronchus causes collapse of the lobe, segment or lung beyond it but abnormal signs may not be easily recognised unless a large portion of lung has collapsed. Lymphatic spread of tumour may cause distressing breathlessness, sometimes with few abnormalities other than a rapid respiratory rate detectable on examination. In all these conditions a good chest radiograph may provide diagnostic help.

Cough

The commoner causes of cough, of recent onset and long-standing, are listed below.

Cough of recent onset
  Acute infection
  Asthma
  Lung tumour
  Tuberculosis
  Aspiration — foreign body

Long standing cough
  Chronic bronchitis
  Bronchiectasis
  Tuberculosis
  Lung tumour
  Aspiration of oesophageal contents

Cough of recent onset in the elderly, as at other ages is most commonly associated with respiratory infection. The overwhelming majority of such infections are viral but sadly they are the reason for much unnecessary and ineffective presciption of antibiotics. Bacterial infection of the lower respiratory tract in the previously healthy person is a less common cause but primary bacterial pneumonia in

the elderly may start with a distressing cough, although breathlessness and systemic symptoms usually follow quickly.

Recurring periods of distressing and often nocturnal cough, maybe after an upper respiratory infection, should suggest late onset asthma. Wheezing, if not the original complaint, will often have been noticed by the patient or a spouse. The lungs may appear normal when examined during the day but serial measurements of peak expiratory flow rate several times a day (and at night if woken by cough) will normally show the wide fluctuations characteristic of asthma.

Paroxysmal nocturnal cough in the elderly may also result from inhalation of oesophageal contents while recumbent. Achalasia of the oesophagus may cause this distressing symptom in the absense of troublesome dysphagia and some patients with oesophageal reflux associated with hiatus hernia have predominantly respiratory complaints, although the more typical symptoms of reflux can usually be elicited if sought.

The cough which is so often a feature of lung cancer may be sporadic and dry or may produce mucoid, purulent or blood-stained sputum depending on the size and site of the tumour, the degree of obstruction of the bronchus or trachea and the presence of secondary bacterial infection. A chest radiograph is essential for diagnosis but it is important to realise that a normal radiograph does not exclude the presence of a tumour in, but not completely obstructing, a central airway, and cough is a frequent symptom of tumours at this site.

Tuberculosis, although on the decline, remains an important cause of cough in the elderly, the more so because of the hazards of spread to others if the significance of the cough is not recognised. The patient with highly infectious tuberculosis may feel and look well and may have no symptoms or abnormal physical signs other than a cough. Tuberculosis is nearly always evident on a chest radiograph and now, as in the past, a chest radiograph is necessary in any elderly person with a persisting cough.

The long standing cough of chronic bronchitis will have been present for many years and the background of cigarette smoking, morning production of usually mucoid sputum and winter exacerbations with purulent sputum usually leaves little doubt of the diagnosis, especially if there are now features of airflow obstruction. It is a wise precaution to arrange a chest radiograph before finally making a diagnosis of chronic bronchitis. Changes in the pattern, frequency or character of the bronchitic's cough may signal the additional development of a carcinoma or indeed of tuberculosis.

The chronic cough of bronchiectasis can usually be distinguished from that due to chronic bronchitis by many years of persistent purulent sputum and the detection of coarse and often assymetrical crackles on auscultation as well as by clubbing of the fingers.

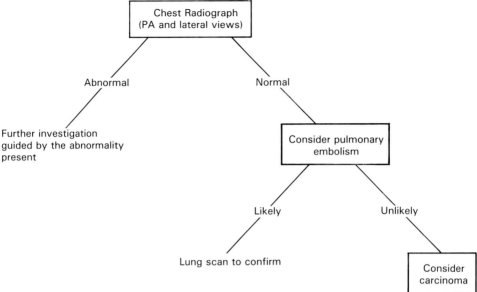

Fig. 27.3 The diagnosis of the cause of haemoptysis.

Haemoptysis (Fig. 27.3)

This is a frightening symptom which, unlike cough or even breathlessness, is usually reported soon after its occurence. This is important because a single haemoptysis may signify more important underlying disease than repeated blood spitting. It is important to consider at the outset whether the blood is likely to have originated from the upper respiratory tract and a history of previous epistaxis or of blood streaks on the handkerchief after nose blowing will justify careful examination of the nose and naso-pharynx. Even with such a history it is prudent to arrange a chest radiograph.

The radiograph is the first essential in seeking the cause of haemoptysis and the importance of a lateral view must be emphasised. Much of the lung is wholly or partially obscured on the posterior anterior (PA) view, especially if correctly centred films are not obtainable because of immobility of an elderly patient. The correct interpretation of any abnormal shadows seen on a PA view requires a lateral projection and it is best that this is taken together with the PA view.

A single haemoptysis at the time of an acute respiratory infection and with a normal chest radiograph may require no further investigation. Repeated haemoptysis or a radiological abnormality may demand difficult decisions if the patient is old or infirm. The decision as to whether to investigate further and how to do so rests on the benefits to the patient and the community of reaching a specific diagnosis.

The further investigation of an abnormality seen on the radiograph will be guided by the type of abnormality (a mass, atelectasis of a lobe or segment, patchy shadowing etc) and by the clinical situation. The commonest conditions which cause haemoptysis in the elderly and which are usually apparent on the chest radiograph are carcinoma, tuberculosis, pulmonary infarction and bronchiectasis. Haemoptysis in a patient with radiological evidence of previous tuberculosis may be the first sign of relapse of the infection and every effort must be made to collect sputum for bacteriological examination. An opacity in an area of previous tuberculosis may represent a fungus ball (mycetoma) due to colonisation of diseased lung with aspergillus fumigatus. Haemoptysis is frequent and may be severe or even fatal. Precipitins against the fungus are detectable at high titre in the serum of all such patients.

The chest radiograph of a patient who has had haemoptysis may be normal. Blood streaking may occur in the purulent sputum of exacerbations of chronic bronchitis, but such patients having smoked heavily are at risk of bronchial carcinoma and this cannot be excluded without bronchoscopy. Haemoptysis due to pulmonary thrombo-embolism is usually but not always associated with other symptoms such as breathlessness or pleuritic chest pain, but the chest radiograph may be normal in the absence of infarction or of pulmonary hypertension from previous episodes. If the clinical situation suggests the possibility of pulmonary embolism, as when an elderly person has been in bed or chair bound with swollen legs, an isotope perfusion lung scan is of value. Normal appearances in this relatively undemanding investigation virtually excludes embolism if carried out soon after the haemoptysis; but abnormal results are much more difficult to interpret. Any forms of airflow obstruction will result in abnormalities of lung perfusion and a small proximal tumour may cause surprising impairment of perfusion. In these situations a scan of ventilation is often of value, but does require more co-operation from the patient and is less widely available.

If thrombo-embolism is thought unlikely or has not been demonstrated on isotope scans the possibility of a proximal tumour arises. Such a tumour may remain invisible radiographically until it has reached considerable size or has blocked a bronchus. If a satisfactory specimen of sputum can be collected, malignant cells can be recognised by an experienced cytologist in about 80% of patients with proximal carcinomas, the highest yield being found if a blood stained specimen is examined (Oswald et al, 1971). Bronchoscopy with the fibre optic bronchoscope is now a relatively simple and undemanding procedure carried out under local analgesia which also enables biopsies to be obtained. It can be carried out on an outpatient, as a day case procedure or even at the bedside.

Chest pain

The causes of chest pain in the elderly are little different from those in other age groups but an accurate history may be more difficult to obtain. The features of cardiac, oesophageal and spinal pain are well recognised and will not be further discussed.

The cause of localised chest pain can usually be discovered by careful history and clinical examination. A diagnosis of pleurisy should not be made lightly because of the implications of severe underlying disease. An infective cause of acute pleurisy is rare unless associated with pneumonia, in which case the features of the pneumonia will usually be evident. Thrombo-embolism is an important cause of pleuritic pain but the implications for prognosis and management are such that further investigations to confirm this diagnosis are necesarry (see haemoptysis). Acute pleuritic pain is not a common initial manifestation of cancer or tuberculosis in the elderly.

Pain from ribs or from soft tissues of the chest wall can closely mimic pleurisy. Both may be worse on inspiration and movement but marked local tenderness suggests a chest wall rather than pleural source, and pain from the chest wall can usually be reproduced exactly by firm pressure over one spot on the chest, either over a rib or a costosternal joint. The severe burning pain which precedes the eruption of zoster may cause temporary diagnostic difficulty but there may be hyperaesthesia of the area and the diagnosis soon becomes apparent with the appearance of vesicles.

The pain of malignant deposits in the ribs or of direct involvement of the chest wall by tumour is more persistent and constant and local swelling or tenderness may be found.

The abnormal chest radiograph

With the increasing availability and use of chest radiology it is not uncommon to find abnormalities on a 'routine' film in a patient with or without pulmonary symptoms. An abnormality of this sort is likely in up to one third of

patients over the age of 60. Often investigations of the abnormality shown on the radiograph will provide the answer to the patient's symptoms. Some of the more common radiographic abnormalities are discussed below. In all cases differential diagnosis will depend not only on the radiographic appearances but on the clinical history, the abnormalities on previous films and the results of other investigations.

Localised pulmonary shadows

A single solitary mass is likely to represent malignancy in more than two thirds of cases in this age group. In the majority this will be a primary bronchogenic carcinoma but other causes that should be considered include metastases, tuberculosis, an abscess, a rheumatoid nodule and rarely an arteriovenus malformation or developmental cyst. Every effort should be made to find any previous chest films since these may reveal the chronic nature of such a benign shadow and save the patient undue anxiety and investigation. Single or multiple opacities may be due to infarcts in which case they will diminish in size on later films. Depending on the age, general health and condition of the patient investigation of well circumscribed pulmonary nodules should in the first instance be aimed at excluding malignant disease. To this end if examination of the sputum for malignant cells is negative, consideration should be given to percutaneous needle biopsy which has a very high yield and troubles the patient little. Alternatively bronchoscopy can be performed which is well tolerated by the elderly although the yield for peripheral well defined masses is less than for needle biopsy.

Atelectasis

Collapse of a lobe or segment of a lobe is due to the occlusion of a bronchus. Again the common cause in this age group is carcinoma and the relevant investigation, assuming the diagnosis has not been made by sputum cytology, is bronchoscopy to define the pathology of the lesion and its extent. Our preference is for a fibre optic bronchoscopy rather than a rigid bronchoscopy in the elderly since it does not involve a general anaesthetic nor extension of the neck which may be hazardous in the presence of severe cervical spondylosis. Segmental collapse may represent malignancy but occasionally may be due to retained secretions in an ill or immobile patient.

Pleural effusion

The most common cause of a pleural effusion at this age is an underlying malignancy. This may be suggested by the history or by finding other evidence of spread such as enlarged liver or lymph nodes. A large pleural effusion without the expected shift of the mediastinum to the opposite side suggests co-existent collapse of the underlying lung, a combination which is almost diagnostic of bronchial carcinoma. Aspirated fluid is often blood stained and may contain malignant cells. Bilateral pleural effusions commonly occur in congestive heart failure but may also develop in the diseases characterised by generalised oedema such as hypoalbuminaemia from cirrhosis or the nephrotic syndrome. They may also result from bilateral malignancy or rarely a collagen disorder and can occasionally occur as part of the post myocardial infarction syndrome. The pleural effusion which accompanies a bacterial pneumonia usually resolves as the infection is treated, but every post-pneumonic effusion is a potential empyema and in this setting a pleural aspiration is essential to determine if pus is present. Pleural effusion may result from a pulmonary infarct secondary to an embolus in which case there has usually been pleuritic pain and dyspnoea and the aspirated fluid is commonly blood stained.

Tuberculosis is an uncommon but important cause of pleural effusion in the elderly. The radiograph may show no other signs of tuberculous disease. The radiographic appearances of long standing 'pleural thickening' following inadequately treated tuberculosis many years previously may in fact be due to a chronic tuberculous empyema and any change in such shadowing should be investigated further with this possibility in mind.

Pleural effusion as a complication of rheumatoid arthritis is commoner in males than females and very occasionally may develop without severe joint disease. It is usually unilateral and may resolve spontaneously. The glucose content of aspirated pleural fluid is characteristically lower than plasma levels.

Finally it must be remembered that a pleural effusion may result from disease under the diaphragm, such as a subphrenic abscess, and in such circumstances investigation of the abdominal problem is the first priority.

Unfortunately examination of pleural fluid does not always lead to a diagnosis and pleural biopsy is more likely to confirm malignancy or tuberculosis (Abrams, 1958). For this reason we believe that pleural biopsy should be performed routinely whenever the chest is aspirated unless the fluid is purulent. Biopsy with an Abram's needle does not involve an additional procedure or any hazard. If fluid repeatedly reaccumulates after aspiration and rational treatment can be given only with a definite diagnosis, thorocoscopy under general anaesthetic may be useful but, as with all invasive procedures in the elderly, the risks and discomforts can be justified only if useful treatment is likely to follow.

Diffuse pulmonary shadowing

This will not be discussed in depth here since the causes in the elderly are not generally different from those in younger patients. Pulmonary oedema is unlikely to cause diffuse shadowing without characteristic clinical findings, and the patient is usually very breathless with other evidence of heart disease or hypertension. Miliary tuberculosis should always be borne in mind as although it

is very uncommon it still occurs and without treatment is invariably fatal.

Other causes of diffuse shadowing include malignancy, sarcoidosis, pneumoconiosis or aspiration of oesophageal contents. Fibrosing alveolitis and extrinsic allergic alveolitis may also occur in this age group. Unfortunately non-invasive techniques often fail to reveal the cause of widespread lung shadowing.

Mediastinal masses

Anterior mediastinal masses are less common in the elderly than the younger age groups but the possibility of an aortic aneurysm must be borne in mind. Bronchogenic carcinoma is by far the most likely cause of a mass in the middle mediastinum in this age group. Neurogenic and oesophageal lesions, as well as aortic aneurysms are the commonest cause of posterior mediastinal masses in the elderly.

SOME PROBLEMS OF MANAGEMENT

Tuberculosis

Although the incidence of tuberculosis is declining in developed countries it remains fairly constant in the elderly (Heffernan et al, 1975). The risk of acquiring new infection is now small but there remains a group of elderly people who acquired tuberculosis in early life and whose disease was either not recognised or became quiescent. It is in this group that viable tubercle bacilli may persist and reactivate after many years either spontaneously or as a result of an illness or therapy that suppresses their immunity. The symptoms of such reactivated tuberculosis may be slight with a low grade pyrexia, general malaise, some cough and sputum, symptoms that may well be ignored or attributed to 'bronchitis'; often there are no symptoms at all. There may be delay in diagnosis because of reluctance to arrange a radiograph in an elderly person with mild or non-specific symptoms but the diagnosis is usually made more rapidly if haemoptysis occurs since this symptom is generally taken seriously by patients and doctors alike.

On the radiograph the possibility of tuberculosis is usually suggested by the presence of upper zone shadowing, often with loss of volume and calcification reflecting the long previous history, but on occasions pneumonic spread to other areas may not immediately suggest tuberculosis. It must be emphasised that activity and infectivity of tuberculosis cannot be assessed from radiographic appearances and that patients with suggestive symptoms and radiograph should always have sputum examined and cultured. The chest film is almost invariably abnormal in patients with active pulmonary tuberculosis and a normal radiograph makes the diagnosis unlikely though not impossible. In patients with symptoms and radiographic shadowing that may represent active pulmonary tuberculosis but who cannot produce sputum, bronchoscopy is valuable with aspiration of secretions for microscopy and culture and if desired biopsy of lung tissue. These techniques have superceded laryngeal swabs or gastric aspiration in the search for tubercle bacilli.

Occasionally elderly patients with disseminated tuberculosis complain only of vague symptoms of loss of appetite and weight maybe with mild fever, and are found to have anaemia and abnormalities of liver and bone marrow function (Proudfoot, 1971). The chest radiograph may be normal and no acid-fast bacilli may be detectable in their sputum, in which case the possibility of tuberculosis may not be considered. Bone marrow aspirates and liver biopsy material should always be cultured for acid-fast bacilli but sometimes the diagnosis is made only on the basis of a clinical response to anti-tuberculous therapy choosing drugs which do not have a wide antibacterial spectrum.

Treatment of tuberculosis is now highly effective and is the same in the elderly as in other age groups. Rifampicin and isoniazid, with pyrazinamide or ethambutol are used in combination. Once appropriate chemotherapy has started the patient rapidly becomes non-infective, even if still coughing up demonstrable bacteria. Treatment can usually be given at home under careful supervision and bed rest and other 'traditional' measures can now happily be ignored. Nine months of therapy is sufficient and the main reason for failure of treatment is poor compliance with drug therapy (Ross & Horne, 1983). Close contacts of the patients with open (i.e. smear positive) tuberculosis must be traced and screened for tuberculosis.

Bronchial carcinoma

There has been a considerable increase in the incidence of bronchial carcinoma in the elderly in the last few decades; the peak mortality of the disease is in this age group and three quarters of all cases are first detected over the age of 60 (Belcher, 1975). The diagnosis is often delayed in the elderly because symptoms are ascribed to old age rather than medical illness. Cough and shortness of breath may be uncritically attributed to bronchitis or heart failure; pain and haemoptysis lead to earlier diagnosis. Occasionally an audible wheeze localised to one side may be heard in those complaining of shortness of breath suggesting occlusion of a major airway by tumour, or there is evidence of metastatic disease such as lymphadenopathy or hepatomegaly. Frequently however there are no helpful clinical signs and the presence of a tumour is revealed only by radiography.

An elderly person presenting with new and persisting symptoms should have a chest radiograph with a lateral view. Those with symptoms from a bronchial carcinoma will usually have abnormalities on these two views although a normal chest film does not exclude a small central tumour. To confirm the diagnosis sputum cytology has the attraction of simplicity and malignant cells can be then identified in 80% of cases in expert hands, although

the yield is much less for small peripheral tumours. At least four or five specimens must be examined if these figures are to be reached.

If the clinical and radiographic findings suggest a tumour but malignant cells are not found in the sputum a decision must be made about further investigation. Fibre-optic bronchoscopy is a relatively safe procedure in the elderly which does not require general anaesthetic; it may therefore be preferred to rigid bronchoscopy. Percutaneous needle biopsy is a useful method of obtaining tissue for cytology from peripheral lesions and again it does not require general anaesthetic and is painless in expert hands. It can yield diagnostic material in up to 85% of malignant tumours biopsied. A small pneumothorax develops after 15% of biopsies but less than 5% have significant haemorrhage. There is an understandable tendency to stop short of obtaining pathological proof of lung cancer in the elderly when the diagnosis seems likely. However management of a patient with a probable but unproven carcinoma may be difficult as subsequent symptoms develop, and it is our belief that the well tolerated procedures of fibre optic bronchoscopy and/or needle biopsy are often fully justified. The ability to provide a prognosis and to treat symptoms may make the patient's life easier even if it is not prolonged.

Surgery is still the treatment of choice for bronchial carcinoma, except in the case of an oat cell tumour. The risk of surgery does increase with age and pneumonectomy carries a mortality of 30% over the age of 70, and lobectomy a mortality of 15% (Bates, 1970). Most elderly patients will prove to be unsuitable for surgery as half will have disease which is too extensive locally and another quarter will be found to have distant spread or to be unfit for operation. It is difficult to predict whether the patient with chronic bronchitis is likely to become intolerably short of breath after lung resection. The decision to operate or not must also take account of general health, state of mind and home and family circumstances; no firm guidelines can be given. Radiotherapy may relieve symptoms of superior vena caval obstruction or haemoptysis and is effective in the treatment of pain from the primary tumour or from skeletal deposits. Occasionally radiotherapy will allow the re-expansion of a previously collapsed lobe or lung. Oral dexamethasone may produce dramatic if temporary relief from symptoms due to cerebral metastases.

In selected patients, particularly those with disseminated small cell carcinoma, chemotherapy may be considered. In expert hands relief of symptoms outweighs the risk of side-effects but life is rarely prolonged by more than a few months. Corticosteroids, such as prednisolone (30 mg daily) may provide relief from the malaise, lassitude and anorexia of malignant disease and suppresses raised levels of calcium in those with hypercalcemia. In patients with recurrent malignant pleural effusion in whom shortness of breath is a problem the introduction of tetracycline or a cytotoxic agent into the pleural space after removal of all fluid may limit the reaccumulation of fluid and relieve symptoms. Above all however, skilful and humane use of analgesic drugs, as well as care of the well-being of the patient, remain all-important.

Pneumonia

Pneumonia is especially common in the elderly and frail and is encouraged by the presence of oedema fluid and accumulation of secretions in areas of dependent lung. Aspiration of pharyngeal contents into the lung is probably not uncommon in the elderly and is, of course, a major problem in those with disorders of swallowing, as from a pseudobulbar palsy. In these so called 'secondary pneumonias' bacterial infection may be less important than stasis of secretions and antibacterial therapy is disappointing in the absence of effective expectoration. 'Primary pneumonia' in those who are normally in good health is most commonly due to *Streptococcus pneumoniae* but *Staphylococcus aureus* becomes important during epidemics of influenza. Less commonly, a gram negative organism such as *Klebsiella pneumoniae* or *Pseudomonas aeruginosa* is responsible, especially for pneumonia developing in hospital. Uncontaminated sputum samples are difficult to obtain from the elderly and ill and are often disappointing in defining a bacteriological cause. Gram negative organisms may have entered the specimen from the pharynx rather than the lung and often reflect no more than upper respiratory contamination, especially if the patient has received antibiotic treatment. Blood cultures are helpful and will be positive in many patients with untreated primary pneumonia.

The treatment of pneumonia in the elderly must include attention to the state of hydration and adequate oxygenation; the patient should be encouraged to cough to clear the secretions. It is open to question whether bed rest is of any benefit and the patient who is not extremely ill should remain mobile to avoid further stasis of secretions and the tendency to deep vein thrombosis. These aspects of management must not be overlooked and the prescribing of an antibiotic does not make them any less important. A wide spectrum antibiotic such as ampicillin is usually chosen but during an outbreak of influenza when staphylococcal pneumonia is common flucloxacillin should be used in addition. Failure to respond to the first antibiotic is an indication for a radiograph to exclude a complication such as a pleural effusion, empyema or abscess. Tuberculosis must be considered especially in upper lobe pneumonia and loss of volume of the affected part raises the possibility of occluding bronchial tumour. It is unusual for a patient with uncomplicated pneumonia to respond to a second drug having failed to respond to the first, and these possibilities should be carefully considered before embarking on a further course of antibiotics. A sudden deterioration after an initial improvement should suggest the possibility of a pulmonary embolus although this is often difficult to prove.

Chronic bronchitis and emphysema

Many patients who have 'simple' bronchitis with clear sputum and no breathlessness do not seek medical advice. Simple tests of lung function are normal, as is the chest radiograph. Persistent or recurrent purulent sputum is usually associated with *Haemophilus influenzae* or *Streptococcus pnemoniae* infection. Most but not all of such patients have effort dyspnoea related to airflow obstruction.

Two characteristic patterns of clinical features can be distinguished in patients with progressive chronic bronchitis and emphysema. The 'blue bloater' is often relatively free of breathlessness at rest and has prominent cough and sputum. On examination he is cyanosed and oedematous and the chest radiograph may reveal a rather large heart with little or no evidence or emphysema. Arterial blood gas analysis shows hypoxaemia and hypercapnia and secondary polycythaemia is common. The 'pink puffer' is breathless at rest, often breathing through pursed lips and has little sputum. He is usually thin without cyanosis or oedema and the arterial gases are well maintained until the late stages. The blue bloater may survive repeated episodes of cardiac failure usually precipitated by infection whereas the pink puffer who seems to have fewer infections, may succumb in his first bout of cardiac or respiratory failure.

All patients should be advised to stop smoking and, if obese, to lose weight. Regular bronchodilators such as the beta adrenergic agents salbutamol or terbutaline will usually produce a small improvement and are best given by inhalation since the effective dose is less than with oral preparations and side effects such as tremor are less of a problem. Some elderly patients find the technique of using pressurised aerosols difficult and for them inhaled powders administered by newer devices may be easier to use. Antibiotics are of value only when sputum is purulent on naked eye examination. Few now believe in the value of long term antibiotic therapy.

Acute exacerbations with worsening breathlessness and purulent sputum should be treated with physiotherapy and encouragement to cough. These may be more important than any other treatment but short courses of a wide spectrum antibiotic effective against *Haemophilus* and *Streptococcus pneumoniae* such as ampicillin, amoxycillin or co-trimoxazole are usually prescribed: tetracycline is best avoided because of the tendency to cause renal failure in the elderly. Bronchodilator therapy can be increased and if the patient is in hospital this may be given in a larger dose by nebuliser. Oxygen at low concentration can be safely given to most patients through the ventimask (24%) but higher concentrations carry the risk of exacerbating respiratory failure. Diuretic therapy may be required to reduce peripheral oedema in patients with cor pulmonale.

In the long-term, activity and exercise should be encouraged and good results have been obtained from schemes of graded exercise to increase exercise tolerance. Long-term oxygen give for at least 15 hours per day has been shown to improve the life expectancy of selected groups of patients with severe chronic airways obstruction but such patients need careful selection in a hospital laboratory before embarking on such a burdensome and expensive treatment.

Asthma

It is uncommon to identify any avoidable extrinsic cause for asthma in the elderly but the effort should be made to do so. Enquiries should be made about exposure to animals, chemicals or organic dusts, and it is important to ensure that the patient is not taking drugs such as beta adrenergic agents or possibly analgesics that may cause or increase airflow obstruction.

For treatment beta adrenergic and bronchodilators should always be tried first, preferably by inhalation.

Despite many ingenious devices for the delivery of aerosols or powders this may still prove difficult in the elderly. If, as if often the case, little improvement can be obtained from bronchodilator drugs alone corticosteriods should be prescribed. In the presence of severe airflow obstruction it is necessary to start with oral corticosteroids at high dosage (e.g. prednisolone 30 mg daily), but having obtained improvement the dosage can be slowly reduced. The introduction of inhaled corticosteroids has enabled many elderly asthmatics to control their symptoms on a lower dose of oral corticosteroids than otherwise or without the need for regular oral therapy. If oral corticosteroids prove necessary for the long term management of asthma an equivalent dose given on alternate days is effective and is less likely to cause side effects. Acute exacerbations of airflow obstruction should be treated with a short, sharp course of oral corticosteroids at high dosage. Unfortunately it is still insufficiently recognised that antibiotics are rarely of benefit in this context.

REFERENCES

Abrams L D 1958 A Pleural biopsy punch. Lancet 1: 30
Bates M 1970 Results of surgery for bronchial carcinoma in patients aged 70 and over. Thorax 25: 77–78
Belcher J R 1975 The changing pattern of bronchial carcinoma. British Journal of Diseases of the Chest 69: 247–258
Edge J R, Millard F J C, Reid L, Simon G 1964 The radiographic appearances of the chest in persons of advanced age. British Journal of Radiology 37: 769–774
Heffernan J F, Nunn A J, Peto J, Fox W 1975 Pulmonary tuberculosis in Scotland: a national sample survey and follow-up (1968–70) Tubercle 56: 253–267
Hendrick D J, Faux J A, Marshall R 178 Budgerigar-fanciers lung: the commonest variety of allergic alveolitis in Britain. British Medical Journal 2: 81–84
Lee H Y, Stretton T B 1972 Asthma in the elderly. British Medical Journal 4: 93–95
Oswald N C, Hinson K F W, Canti G, Miller A B 1971 The diagnosis of primary lung cancer with special reference to sputum cytology. Thorax 26: 623–631
Proudfoot A T 1971 Cryptic disseminated tuberculosis. British Journal of Hospital Medicine 773–780
Ross J D, Horne N W (Eds) 1983 Modern Drug Treatment in Tuberculosis. Chest, Heart and Stroke Association, London

28

Immunoprophylaxis

R. Austrian

INTRODUCTION

Since the development of medical specialties, immunoprophylaxis has become largely the province of pediatricians. Other than providing vaccines to travellers destined for areas where infections seldom encountered in highly developed nations pose a hazard, most physicians caring for adults have had limited involvement with this facet of preventive medicine. These circumstances notwithstanding, it is evident that certain illnesses of infectious origin causing significant morbidity and mortality in the elderly are amenable to prevention in varying degree, and that when simple means exist to reduce the likelihood of such illnesses they should be made available to those at risk.

Among the infectious disorders of importance in later life are those classified under the rubric 'pneumonia and influenza'. Illnesses in this category rank fourth among all causes of death among those over 65 years of age (Kovar, 1977). Although pneumonia is a clinical syndrome of diverse causes and one which, because of its complex pathogenesis, cannot be eliminated readily from any population, prevention of infection by some respiratory pathogens may lessen the total burden of such disorders and provide an initial step in the reduction of the total deaths resulting from respiratory infection. In addition, elderly persons not immune to tetanus, diphtheria and certain of the preventable diseases of childhood may be subject to serious or fatal illness of these kinds; the physicians caring for such individuals should be cognisant of and correct identifiable vulnerabilities when they exist.

It has been recognised for many years that both the morbidity and mortality of certain infections increase with advancing age (Gardner, 1980) and that the clinical patterns of some diseases, such as pneumonia, may be atypical in the elderly (Austrian, 1981a). The reasons for these phenomena are manifold and all are not fully understood. Both humoral and cellular immunity undergo changes throughout life. Alterations in cellular immunity, manifested by a decline in delayed cutaneous hypersensitivity, are accompanied by an increase in the incidence of reactivated tuberculosis and of malignancies;

among those over 80 years of age a complete loss of delayed cutaneous hypersensitivity may be associated with an early demise (Roberts-Thomson et al, 1974).

Changes in humoral immunity with advancing age were identified by Thomsen & Kettel (1929), who described the steady decline in the titer of the A, B, O blood group isoagglutinins. Since then, it has been recognised that levels of antibodies to the virus of influenza A (Howells et al, 1975) and to tetanus toxoid (Kishimoto et al, 1980) achieved following immunisation with their respective vaccines are lower in the elderly than they are in young adults. In addition, the mitogenic responsiveness of peripherial blood leucocytes to stimulation with tetanus toxoid declines in parallel fashion. Despite the fact that total levels of immunoglobulins in the elderly do not differ strikingly from those of their younger counterparts (Radl et al, 1975), it would appear that a smaller amount of specific antibody is formed in response to an antigenic sitmulus in older persons. Both a decline in helper T cell activity and a less well sustained production of specific antibody by B lymphocytes may contribute to the observed findings. Although the results summarised might suggest the inutility of immunoprophylaxis in the elderly, there are several epidemiologic observations which suggest that, although levels of specific antibodies may be reduced in those in later life, the reductions are not so great as to preclude protection against infection. For example recurrent infections with measles and rubella viruses are virtually unknown, and recurrent infection with the same pneumococcal type, in the absence of dysgamma-globulinemia, is very uncommon. In analogous fashion, although isoagglutinins of the major blood group antigens in the aged are strikingly reduced from their values in the prime of life, cross-matching of blood is still required for its transfusion into the elderly. The sharply higher incidence of tetanus in that segment of the population too old to have taken part in the programmes for universal immunisation against this disease suggest that lack of vaccination with tetanus toxoid, rather than inability to respond to it, is responsible for what the late Geoffry Edsall (1976) termed 'the inexcusable disease.'

Changes in the structure and functional capacity of the

lower respiratory tract would appear also to play a role in the increasing incidence of pneumonia with advancing age. Musculoskeletal alterations affect vital capacity and the forcefulness of cough; changes in neuromuscular function affect the cough reflex and glottal closure, increasing the likelihood of aspiration; and edema of the alveoli resulting from cardiac failure predisposes to impaired pulmonary clearance of bacteria and as a consequence thereof to pneumonia (Dher et al, 1976). It has been demonstrated also by roentgenographic studies that ingestion of food or liquids in the supine position by debilitated patients is followed frequently by their aspiration (Gardner, 1958). It is evident, therefore, that a multiplicity of factors may play a role in increasing the vulnerability of the elderly to respiratory infection and its consequences.

It is not the purpose of this report to deal at length with the topics either of influenza or of pneumococcal pneumonia but rather to consider the relevant features of these infections in the elderly and the measures available for their prevention.

PREVENTION OF INFLUENZA

Among the Orthomyxoviridae, the viruses of influenza A and B are the principal pathogens of man. Although an occasional outbreak of infection with influenza B virus may be associated with marked excess mortality in the community, the latter phenomenon is associated more often with epidemics of influenza A. The Centers for Disease Control estimate that outbreaks of influenza were associated with more than 200 000 excess deaths in the United States of America between 1968 and 1981 (Recommendations of the Immunization Practices Advisory Committee, 1982). The economic burden of influenza is high. The direct costs alone of the epidemic of the Hong Kong (H_3N_2) strain of influenza A virus in the United States in 1968 are estimated to have been 737 million dollars of which two-thirds were incurred by that segment of the population characterised as being 'at high risk' (Fedson, 1977).

Analysis of excess mortality following the epidemics of Asian influenza between 1957 and 1960 revealed that certain members of the population infected with this strain of the virus were at greater than average risk of death (Eickhoff et al, 1961). Among persons in this category were those over 65 years of age and those of lesser age with one or more of a variety of chronic illnesses including cardiovascular disease, bronchopulmonary disease, diabetes mellitus, hepatic cirrhosis and chronic renal disease. A more recent study of influenza epidemics involving members of a prepaid health plan in an American community has confirmed the earlier findings (Barker & Mullooly, 1980b & 1982). Among those in this population

between 15 and 44 years of age, there were no deaths, even of those with high risk conditions. In older otherwise healthy individuals, the death rate among those 65 years of age and older was 9 per 100 000 persons, more than 4 times that observed in those between 45 and 64 years of age. The presence of one underlying chronic illness increased the death rate in those 45 years of age and older 5 to 20 fold; and, in those with two or more so-called high risk conditions, the death rate per 100 000 individuals was 377 in those between 45 and 64 years of age and 797 in those over 65. These findings leave little doubt that the population in greatest need of prophylaxis against influenza can be identified with a considerable degree of accuracy. Several studies have shown moreover, that influenza viral infection remains endemic in many communities in interepidemic periods. Glezen and his associates (1982) reported that outbreaks have occurred annually in Houston, Texas, during the late autumn, winter or early spring months to be followed within two weeks by a peak in the deaths attributed to pneumonia and influenza. It is these deaths that give rise annually to the higher seasonal death rate in the colder months of the year and that contribute to the sinuous shape of the mortality curve used to establish the base line for deaths in the community. Their exclusion from calculations of excess mortality observed in more widespread epidemics leads to an underestimation of the true impact of influenza viral infection on the death rate.

In discussing the immunoprophylaxis of influenza, it is relevant to consider certain features of the viruses that cause it. Influenza viruses have multi-segmented genomes of ribonucleic acid (RNA), and genetic recombination between two viral strains can occur within the doubly infected cell. Two viral surface antigens, haemagglutinin (H antigen) and neuraminidase (N antigen) play a major role in infection, and influenza viruses of a given type are designated by the formula, HxNy. Antibodies to the H antigen prevent viral attachment to the cells of the host and, as a result, infection. Antibodies to the neuraminidase block release of virus from infected cells, and although they do not prevent infection, they limit its spread within the body. Both major and minor changes in the H and N antigens occur through mutation. Major changes in the H antigen tend to occur at intervals of 10 to 12 years and are accompanied often by major epidemics. Minor changes in the H antigen may result in reinfection with a virus bearing an altered H antigen of the same major group. Antibody tends to be highest to the H antigen to which the subject was first exposed, and it is possible, through serologic surveys, to determine retrospectively the time at which various H antigens (H_{sw}, H_0, H_1 etc) circulated in the community. It is evident also that an influenza vaccine, to be protective, must contain the H antigen of the strain of virus to which the recipient of vaccine will be exposed. To permit the proper selection of viral strains for the production of vaccine therefore, surveillance of influenzal infection is maintained continuously under the aegis of the World Health Organisation in sentinel laboratories throughout the world. Rapid production of a suitable vaccine is facilitated by the use of recombinant genetic techniques to obtain a viral variant growing rapidly in eggs and by modern methods of purification, including zonal centrifugation, which eliminates the preponderance of contaminating substances. Killed viral vaccines currently in use are standardised by their content of viral haemagglutinin and may include one or more strains of influenza A and B viruses. Because antigenic drift requires frequent changes in the composition of the vaccine and because the duration of protection following vaccination has not been elucidated fully, annual immunisation of those at high risk of serious or fatal illness is recommended.

Studies of the efficacy of vaccine in the prevention of influenza have given varying results. This finding is not altogether surprising when such factors as the diverse modes of preparing vaccines and the concordance, or lack thereof, of the strains included in them with those prevailing in the community at times proximal to immunisation are taken into account. The ability of the appropriate influenza A vaccine to protect the elderly is supported strongly by a retrospective analysis of two epidemic periods in the same population in which determinants of increased risk of fatal illness were examined by Barker & Mullooly (1980a). In both outbreaks of influenza A infection, an excess of pneumonic and influenzal illness and deaths was demonstrable in the population over 65 years of age. The first epidemic, in 1968–69 was caused by the A/Hong Kong 68 virus (H_3N_2). The vaccine administered to the population that year contained the type A antigen, A/Japan/62 (H_2N_2), and it failed to protect those at risk. In a second epidemic occurring in the same population and in which both the type A influenza strain A/England/72 causing infection, and the strain included in the vaccine employed that year A/Hong Kong/68, were of the similar major antigenic type H_3N_2, hospitalisations among vaccinees at high risk were reduced by 72%. There were no deaths among vaccinees in this age group in contrast to 13 fatalities among the unvaccinated, a death rate in the latter of 35 per 10 000 subjects at risk. These findings, as well as those of other studies, indicate that the appropriately formulated influenza vaccine can confer significant protection against infection with and death from influenza A viral infection. Comparable data on the efficacy of vaccine against influenza B viral infection are not available.

Reactions to influenza vaccine are usually mild, about a third of recipients developing discomfort, redness and induration at the site of injection lasting one to three days. Fever and myalgia lasting one to two days occur occasionally, more often in children than in adults. Because the vaccine is made from virus grown in eggs, it should not be given to anyone with a history of hypersensitivity to eggs or to egg products.

Widespread immunisation of Americans in 1976 with a vaccine containing the virus A/New Jersey/76 ($H_{sw}N_1$) was followed by reports of the development of the Guillain-Barré syndrome in approximately 13 per million recipients of the vaccine, an incidence four to five times that observed among those not given vaccine (Marks & Halpin, 1980) and one leading to the discontinuance of its use. The epidemiological association of the swine influenza vaccine with Guillain-Barré syndrome resulted in the establishment of continuing surveillance of this neurological disorder and of its possible relation to influenza viral vaccines. In the years 1979–80 and 1980–81, no evidence suggesting an increase in the risk of developing Guillain-Barré syndrome following immunisation with influenza vaccine was observed in either year (Kaplan et al, 1982). In light of this evidence, the events surrounding the vaccine used in 1976 ought not be viewed as a deterrent to the acceptance of influenza vaccine by those who should benefit most from prophylaxis.

A major problem in the control of influenza results from the limited administration of vaccine to those at highest risk of serious or fatal infection. Even prior to the association of the swine influenza vaccine and Guillain-Barré syndrome, there was marked underutilisation of vaccine (Kavet, 1976), so pronounced in fact that only enough vaccine was produced annually to immunise half those categorised as being at high risk. The reasons for failure of those in the target population to be immunised have been investigated and found to result either from ignorance of the vaccine or from the perception by potential recipients that it is not needed. Failure of physicians to advise patients regarding the potential seriousness of influenza and its complications doubtless plays a role also in the failure of elderly adults to be vaccinated.

Several strategies have been suggested to encourage annual immunisation with influenza vaccine. One such strategem is for the physician to send a postcard each autumn to those patients under his care who fall into the category of those at high risk of serious or fatal infection. Another approach is that proposed by Fedson (1977), who found that a high proportion of patients dying of disease categorised as 'influenza/pneumonia' had been hospitalised within the preceeding year. He has suggested that all individuals hospitalised for disorders placing them at high risk of death from respiratory infections and their sequelae be given influenza vaccine immediately prior to discharge from hospital. As noted by Barker & Mullooly (1982), although only approximately one fourth of those in 'high-risk categories' enrolled in their clinic had received influenza vaccine, nearly all had had contact with the clinic during the preceeding year. In view of the potential benefit to be derived from a potent influenza vaccine composed of the appropriate viral strains, it is evident that physicians and those for whom they care will have to achieve a higher level of awareness of its potential usefulness if the latter are to receive the optimal benefits of immunoprophylaxis as advocated by public health agencies.

For those who have not been immunised prior to the outbreak of influenza in the community or who have been given a vaccine lacking the antigens of the virus causing infection, chemoprophylaxis offers an alternative mode of protection. The drugs amantadine and rimantadine (Dolin et al, 1982), are effective both in preventing and in ameliorating infections caused by the viruses of influenza A but not by those of influenza B. Either drug in doses of 100 mg orally twice a day has been shown to reduce the incidence of infection approximately 90% and, if given early in the course of illness, to hasten defervescence and recovery. Both drugs are usually tolerated well although either may give rise to side-effects characterised by difficulty in concentrating, anxiety and insomnia. Individuals experiencing any untoward symptoms of cerebral or neural origin should not engage in potentially hazardous activities or drive a motor vehicle while taking the drug. If tolerated, amantadine or rimantadine should be taken throughout the course of the outbreak of influenza. In addition, in absence of sensitivity to eggs, unvaccinated persons should be immunised promptly.

PREVENTION OF PNEUMOCOCCAL INFECTION

Bacterial pneumonia in man is usually the sequel of viral, chemical or physical injury to the lungs and may follow viral infection, aspiration or contusion. It may be acquired outside or inside the hospital and its bacterial incitants may vary with the setting in which it arises. The pneumococcus *Streptococcus pneumoniae*, is still the most common cause of bacterial pneumonia acquired in the community and, as noted by Stuart-Harris & Schild (1976), pneumococcal infection is the most common bacterial complication of viral influenza. Among the pneumonias acquired by hospitalised patients, the pneumococcus plays a less prominent role, in part because many such individuals are receiving, for one reason or another, antimicrobial drugs which inhibit the pneumococcus.

The increased incidence and mortality from pneumococcal pneumonia and its not infrequently atypical presentation in the elderly have long been recognised (Austrian, 1981a). Both the former aspects of lobar pneumonia were well documented by Heffron (1939) in his recently republished classic monograph on this disease, and the insidious nature of the illness has been described in the last century as well as in this one (Hourmann & Dechambre, 1836).

Although the advent of antimicrobial drugs has brought about a significant reduction in the mortality of pneumococcal infections, there is no convincing evidence that the decline in their death rate has been accompanied by a reduction in their incidence. Unfortunately for a variety of reasons, accurate epidemiologic data regarding the incidence of pneumococcal pneumonia are fragmentary. Over-optimism regarding the efficacy of antibiotic drugs leading to removal of pneumococcal pneumonia from the list of reportable diseases, alterations of bacteriologic techniques in diagnostic laboratories, including abandonment of pneumococcal capsular typing, and failure to obtain appropriate materials for bacteriologic culture prior to institution of antimicrobial therapy have all contributed to the lack of knowledge. Such data as are available suggest that the attack rate of pneumococcal pneumonia in the United States is between 2 and 5 per 1000 persons per annum. A retrospective study of pneumococcal bacteremia which, for reasons set forth above, provides minimal attack rates, indicated the overall attack rate to be 8.5 per 100 000 persons per annum, with a rate of 21 per 100 000 persons 60 years of age and older per annum (Filice et al, 1980). It is not unlikely that the true attack rate of pneumococcal bacteremia in the elderly is two to four times this value.

Several studies of bacteremic pneumococcal pneumonia treated with antimicrobial drugs have shown it still to be a frequently fatal disease (Austrian & Gold, 1964; Mufson et al, 1974). The high mortality as shown by Mufson et al (1982), is not limited to populations served by municipal hospitals in inner cities but is observed also in small communities served by voluntary hospitals. It has been noted (Fig. 28.1) that there has been a proportionately smaller reduction in the mortality of bacteremic pneumococcal pneumonia treated with penicillin in those over 50 years of age than in their younger counterparts, and in the former age group, mortality from this infection still exceeds 25% (Austrian & Gold, 1964). In addition, it is apparent that a comparable mortality rate occurs from bacteremic pneumococcal pneumonia in those of any age with a variety of chronic illnesses which may affect cardiopulmonary function or the host's various defensive mechanisms against infection (Fig. 28.2). Further analysis of such illnesses shows that, for those destined at the onset of illness to die within five days (Fig. 28.3), antipneumococcal therapy has little if any influence on the outcome of the infection. Individuals included in this category are those who sustain very early in the course of illness irreversible physiologic injury, the nature of which is not understood and which is not affected by antibacterial drugs. Until the physiologic derangements of pneumococcal illness are defined and means devised to correct them, prophylaxis offers the only available alternative for those at high risk of serious or of fatal infection.

A second circumstance giving impetus to the availability of pneumococcal vaccine has been the slow but continuing

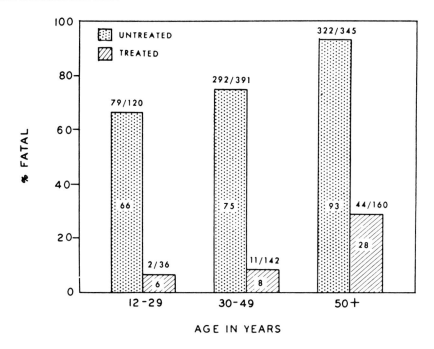

Fig. 28.1 Age adjusted fatality in untreated and penicillin treated pneumococcal bacteremia. The denominator of the fraction above the bar indicates the number of cases. The number within the bar indicates the percentage of fatal cases. Data for untreated cases include those of Tilghman & Finland (1937) and Bullowa (1937). (With the permission of the Association of American Physicians.)

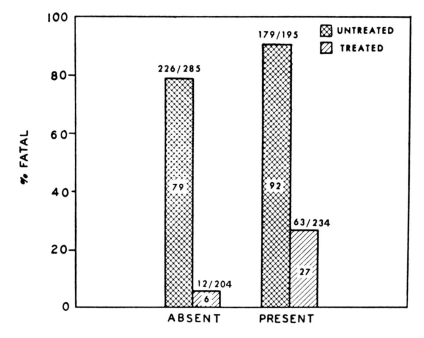

Fig. 28.2 The effect of complicating illness on fatality in untreated and treated pneumococcal bactermia, (For significance of fractions above and numbers within bars see Fig. 28.1: With the permission of the Association of American Physicians.)

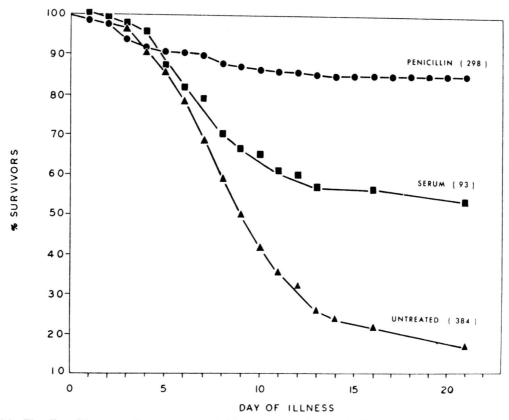

Fig. 28.3   The effect of therapy on the percentage survival in pneumococcal bacteremia. The numbers within parentheses indicate the size of each group of patients. Data for untreated and serum-treated patients (types 1 & 2 only) from Tilghman & Finland (1937). (With the permission of the Association of American Physicians.)

emergence of pneumococcal strains resistant to one or to multiple antimicrobial drugs which have been isolated from infected humans or from carriers living in Australia, Africa, Europe or North America (Ward, 1981). In some areas, the incidence of strains resistant to more than 0.1 μg/ml of penicillin and isolated from blood cultures now exceeds 5%. Because of therapeutic failures in the treatment of extrapulmonary infection caused by drug-resistant pneumococci with conventional doses of antimicrobial drugs, testing of the sensitivity of pneumococci isolated from such bodily sites to the therapeutic agent to be employed should be performed routinely.

Attempts to prevent pneumococcal pneumonia by immunisation with vaccines of intact heat-killed pneumococci were undertaken as long ago as 1911 but with equivocal results (Wright et al, 1914). Demonstration of the immunogenicity of pneumococcal capsular polysaccharides in man by Francis & Tillett (1930) was followed fifteen years later by the convincing demonstration in a military population that type specific protection against pneumococcal infection could be stimulated by injecting 30–60 μg of corresponding purified pneumococcal capsular polysaccharide (MacLeod et al, 1945). Similar studies,

performed in the last decade with a vaccine containing twelve rather than four capsular polysaccharides, have confirmed fully the results of the earlier investigations (Austrian et al, 1976).

Among the 83 capsular serotypes of the pneumococcus now recognised, all are not equally invasive. Although their rank order of frequency may vary with age, time and geography, there is, with a few exceptions, a remarkable constancy of those types accounting for the majority of illnesses. The presently licensed pneumococcal vaccine is required by regulatory authorities to contain the polysaccharides of those pneumococcal types or groups which are responsible for 80% or more of bacteremic pneumococcal infections. It is composed of the purified capsular polysaccharides of pneumococcal types 1,2,3,4,5, 6B,7F,8,9N,9V,10A,11A,12F,14,15B,17F,18C,19F,19A, 20,22F,23F and 33F dissolved in physiological salt solution in a concentration of 50 μg per millilitre with 0.5% phenol as a preservative. The dose of vaccine is 0.5 ml administered subcutaneously or intramuscularly. In adults 80–95% per cent of the anticipated serologic responses are observed. The higher the antibody level is prior to immunisation, the smaller is the fold increase likely to be found after vaccination. The magnitude of the rises in levels of antibodies to pneumococcal polysaccharides has been determined in more than 100 subjects over 50 years of age; in general, the increases have been comparable to those seen in younger subjects (Hilleman et al, 1981) although the levels of antibody to pneumococcus type 3 were somewhat lower and less well sustained with time in one study (Ammann et al, 1980). Pneumococcal polysaccharides appear not to be significantly biodegradable by mammalian enzymes, and antibodies to them persist for years following either recovery from infection or prophylactic immunisation. In adults, levels of antibodies five to eight years after vaccination remain at a third to a half their peak values immediately following administration of vaccine, and reimmunisation stimulates only a transitory rise in their titre. For these reasons and because some direct correlation has been observed between the aggregate level of antibodies to the antigens in the vaccine and the occurrence of local and febrile reactions to the vaccine, reinjection of pneumococcal vaccine is not presently advised (Carlson et al, 1979). Further data both on persistence of antibodies in the elderly and on the duration of protection against infection in persons in this age group are needed before more definitive recommendations regarding reimmunisation can be made.

Although the target populations for influenza vaccine and for pneumococcal vaccine are strikingly similar, it may be noted readily that the epidemiologic and immunologic features of influenzal and pneumococcal infection differ significantly. For these reasons, a combined influenza and pneumococcal vaccine appears unsuitable. In addition the additive effect of untoward reactions to each agent may produce ones of undesirable severity. The two vaccines may be given simultaneously if injected at separate sites and from separate syringes should circumstances dictate, but sequential administration on separate occasions is preferred (Carlson et al, 1979; Mufson et al, 1980). Unlike influenza vaccine and because of the long-lived immunologic response it engenders, pneumococcal vaccine may be given at any time of the year at the convenience of the physician and patient.

In assessing the efficacy of pneumococcal vaccine, it should be remembered that the currently licensed formulation is, in fact, a combination of 23 independent vaccines. If one elects to define a failure of pneumococcal vaccine as a failure of any one of its components, then one must anticipate a higher failure rate than one would expect if a vaccine were composed of a single antigen. In effect, according to the definition of failure set forth above, and assuming exposure to all the types represented in it, efficacy of the vaccine will be determined by the product of the efficacies of its 23 components. If each polysaccharide were 99% effective in preventing, in a homogenous population, disease caused by the homologous pneumococcal type and a failure of the vaccine were to be defined as a failure of a single component, then the

maximum achievable efficacy would be 0.99[23] or 79%, a protective value comparable to that of pertussis vaccine.

Trials of polyvalent pneumococcal vaccine in young adults have shown it to be 85% effective over periods up to two years in preventing bacteremic pneumococcal infection (Austrian et al, 1976). Trials in elderly subjects were conducted first by Kaufman (1947) between 1937 and 1943 and involved more than 10 000 subjects 50 years of age and older, approximately half of whom received bivalent or trivalent vaccines including the capsular polysaccharides of pneumococcal types 1, 2 and 3. Analysis of the collected data showed a 90% reduction both in putative pneumococcal pneumonia associated with the types in the vaccine and in proved bacteremic infection caused by the same types. The interpretation of these results, consistent with those of other trials of pneumococcal vaccine, has been clouded somewhat by the fact that the incidence of proved and putative pneumococcal infection associated with capsular types not included in the vaccine was less in the vaccinated than in the control population, raising some question regarding the comparability of two groups. A more recent trial involving 13 000 members 45 years of age and older, of a prepaid health plan in California, approximately half of whom received a dodecavalent pneumococcal vaccine, has also been indicative of the efficacy of the vaccine, but again does not resolve fully the issue of efficacy (Austrian, 1981b). In this trial, there was an 80% reduction in the incidence of infection associated with the pneumococcal types in the vaccine in vaccinees when contrasted with that in the control population, the diference having a p value of 0.0023 by the chi square test. The problems in evaluating this trial are related to the necessity of relying on seroconversion to confirm the diagnosis of pneumococcal infection in nonbacteremic pneumonia because of the low rate of bacteremic illness. The lack of definitive knowledge regarding the serologic behaviour of a vaccinee contracting infection with a pneumococcal type, the capsular antigen of which is included in the vaccine, renders the interpretation of such immunologic data debatable. Definitive data permitting such interpretation cannot be obtained without resort to transtracheal or lung puncture, the routine use of which could not be justified on ethical grounds. These problems notwithstanding, all the available data on pneumococcal vaccine in the older segment of the population are consistent with the view that it is immunogenic in older persons and reduces the incidence of type specific pneumococcal infection in its recipients.

An alternative epidemiologic approach suggested by Broome and her associates (1980) gives promise of defining further the efficacy of pneumococcal vaccine in various segments of the population without the need for controlled trials. The analytic method is based upon a comparison of the ratio of bacteremic disease caused by pneumococcal types in the vaccine in vaccinees and in unimmunised subjects with the ratio of infection caused by types excluded from the vaccine in the same two groups. The most recently published analysis by this method of efficacy of the vaccine in individuals over 10 years of age gives a value of 66% with a 95% confidence interval of 23–85% (Broome, 1981). Overall efficacy of the tetradecavalent pneumoccocal vaccine (14 antigens) is compatible with an average efficacy of its individual components in excess of 90% if exposure to four or more types represented in it is assumed. A similar assessment of the vaccine's efficacy has been derived from a case control study by Shapiro & Clemens (1983).

Vaccines both of whole pneumococci and of pneumococcal capsular polysaccharides are safe, and no deaths or permanent untoward sequelae have been associated with either. Among more than 6500 recipients 45 years of age and older of a dodecavalent vaccine (Austrian et al, 1976), 60% reported no untoward reaction whatever. Among the remainder, local discomfort, erythema and induration were noted, lasting 24 to 48 hours. Elevations of temperature of 1–2° F lasting 24 to 48 hours were recorded in 3% of vaccinees and 1% of those receiving a placebo. In general, reactions are comparable to those associated with other widely used vaccines and, with infrequent exceptions, less severe than those following parenteral administration of typhoid vaccine. Occasionally significant swelling and erythema will develop at the site of inoculation and persist for several days, most often in those with a high aggregate level of antibodies to the antigens in the vaccine prior to its administration (Carlson et al, 1979). Contraindications to giving pneumococcal vaccine are few and include febrile illness and pregnancy. Neither contraindication precludes immunisation at a later date. Two reports of reactivation of angioimmunoblastic lymphadenopathy following administration of pneumococcal vaccine (Schulman et al, 1979) suggest caution in its use in patients with this syndrome.

Problems surrounding the acceptance of pneumococcal vaccine are very similar, in many respects, to those related to the use of influenza vaccine, although the need to re-administer pneumococcal vaccine infrequently, if at all, should lessen difficulties concerning its administration. In the United States it is estimated that no more than 20% of those at greatest risk of serious or fatal pneumococcal infection have received the vaccine in the five years since it has been available, a figure comparable to that for the acceptance of influenza vaccine. In view of the observation that a mortality rate in excess of 25% from treated bacteremic pneumococcal infection in persons over 50 years of age has been confirmed repeatedly and in view of the fact that the incidence of such infection significantly exceeds that of tetanus, a disease for which universal prophylactic administration of toxoid is recommended, it would appear highly desirable that greater efforts be made to immunise more of the elderly. The observation of Sabin and his associates (1947) that primary immunisation with a viral vaccine was less effective in stimulating an antibody response in the elderly than in their younger counterparts, whereas secondary antibody responses were manifested by both groups, suggests the desirability of administering the first dose of pneumococcal vaccine by age 55 if feasible. Further data are needed to clarify this issue. Recently Fedson & Baldwin (1982) have carried out a study of pneumonia similar to Fedson's earlier investigation of influenza and have found that approximately half those over the age of 45 dying of pneumonia in hospitals had been hospitalised within the previous five years. On the basis of these findings, they have suggested that all persons 45 years of age and older hospitalised because of chronic illness be given pneumococcal vaccine prior to discharge if they have not been immunised previously.

Much lip service has been paid to preventive medicine in recent years, but lack of prophylactic vaccination of adults who could benefit significantly from it belies the seriousness of some who make such utterances. Education of the public and greater effort by those physicians who care for the elderly could significantly reduce the risk of influenza, pneumococcal infection and tetanus among this vulnerable segment of the population.

REFERENCES

Ammann A J, Schiffman G, Austrian R 1980 The antibody responses to pneumococcal capsular polysaccharides in aged individuals. Proceedings of the Society for Experimental Biology and Medicine 164: 312–316

Austrian R 1963 The current status of bacteremic pneumococcal pneumonia. Re-evaluation of an underemphasized clinical problem. Transactions of the Association of American Physicians 76: 117–124

Austrian R 1981a Pneumonia in the later years. Journal of the American Geriatrics Society 29: 481–489

Austrian R 1981b Some observations on the pneumococcus and on the current status of pneumococcal disease and its prevention. Reviews of Infectious Diseases Supplement: S1–S17

Austrian R, Gold J 1964 Pneumococcal bacteremia with especial reference to bacteremic pneumococcal pneumonia. Annals of Internal Medicine 60: 759–776

Austrian R, Douglas R M, Schiffman G, Coetzee A M, Koornhof H J, Hayden-Smith S, Reid R D W 1976 Prevention of pneumococcal pneumonia by vaccination. Transactions of the Association of American Physicians 89: 184–194

Barker W H, Mullooly J P 1980a Influenza vaccination of elderly persons. Reduction in pneumonia and influenza hospitalizations and deaths. Journal of the American Medical Association 244: 2547–2549

Barker W H, Mullooly J P 1980b Impact of epidemic type A influenza in a defined adult population. American Journal of Epidemiology 112: 798–813

Barker W H, Mullooly J P 1982 Pneumonia and influenza deaths during epidemics. Archives of Internal Medicine 142: 85–89

Broome C V 1981 Efficacy of pneumococcal polysaccharide vaccines. Reviews of Infectious Diseases Supplement: S82–S88

Broome C V, Facklam R R, Fraser D W 1980 Pneumococcal disease after pneumococcal vaccination. An alternative method to estimate the efficacy of pneumococcal vaccine. New England Journal of Medicine 303: 549–552

Bullowa J G M 1937 The management of the pneumonias. Oxford University Press, New York p 71

Carlson A J, Davidson W L, McLean A A , Vella P P, Weibel R F, Woodhour A F, Hilleman M R 1979 Pneumococcal vaccine: dose, revaccination and coadministration with influenza vaccine. Proceedings of the Society for Experimental Biology and Medicine 161: 558–563

Dhar S, Subramaniam R S, Lenora R A K 1976 Aging and the respiratory system. Medical Clinics of North America 60: 1121–1139

Dolin R, Reichman R C, Madore H P, Maynard R, Linton P N, Weber-Jones J 1982 A controlled trail of amantadine and rimantadine in the prophylaxis of influenza A infection. New England Journal of Medicine 307: 580–584

Edsall G 1976 The inexcusable disease (editorial). Journal of the American Medical Association 235: 62–63

Eickhoff T C, Sherman I L, Serfling R E 1961 Observations on excess mortality associated with epidemic influenza. Journal of the American Medical Association 176: 776–782

Fedson D S 1977 Influenza. The continuing need and justification for immunization. Primary Care 4: 761–779

Fedson D S, Baldwin J A 1982 Previous hospital care as a risk factor for pneumonia. Implications for immunization with pneumococcal vaccine. Journal of the American Medical Association 248: 1989–1995

Filice G A, Darby C P, Fraser D W 1980 Pneumococcal bacteremia in Charleston County, South Carolina. American Journal of Epidemiology 112: 828–835

Francis T J Jr, Tillett W S 1930 Cutaneous reactions in pneumonia. The development of antibodies following the intradermal injection of type-specific polysaccharide. Journal of Experimental Medicine 52: 573–585

Gardner A M N 1958 Aspiration of food and vomit. Quarterly Journal of Medicine 27: 227–242

Gardner I D 1980 The effect of aging on susceptibility to infection. Reviews of Infectious Diseases 2: 801–810

Glezen W P, Payne A A, Snyder D N, Downs T D 1982 Mortality and influenza. Journal of Infectious Diseases 146: 313–321

Heffron R 1939 Pneumonia with special reference to pneumococcus lobar pneumonia. Commonwealth Fund, New York

Hilleman M R, Carlson A J Jr, McLean A A, Vella P P, Weibel R E, Woodhour A F 1981 Streptococcus pneumoniae polysacharide vaccine: age and dose responses, safety, persistence of antibody, revaccination and simultaneous administration of pneumococcal and influenza vaccines. Reviews of Infectious Diseases Supplement: S31–S42

Hourmann, Dechambre 1836 Pneumonie des vieillards. – IIᵉ Partie – Etiologie et symptomatologie. Archives générales de Médicine, Journal Complémentaire des Sciénce Medicales. IIᵉ Serie 12: 27–51

Howells C H L, Vesselinova-Jenkins C K, Evans A D, James J 1975 Influenza vaccination and mortality from bronchopneumonia in the elderly. Lancet 1: 381–383

Kaplan J E, Katona P, Hurwitz E S, Schonberger L B 1982 Guillain-Barré syndrome in the United States 1979–1980 and 1980–1981 Lack of an association with influenza vaccination. Journal of the American Medical Association 248: 698–701

Kaufman P 1947 Pneumonia in old age. Active immunization against pneumonia with pneumococcus polysaccharide; results of a six year study. Archives of Internal Medicine 79: 518–531

Kavet J 1976 Vaccine utilization: trends in implementation of public policy in the USA. In: Selby P (ed) Influenza: Virus, Vaccines, and Strategy. Academic Press, New York, p 297–308

Kishimoto S, Tomino S, Mitsuya H, Fujiwara H, Tsuda H 1980 Age-related decline in the in vitro and in vivo syntheses of antitetanus toxoid antibody in humans. Journal of Immunology 125: 2347–2352

Kovar M G 1977 Health of the elderly and use of health services. Public Health Reports 92: 9–19

MacLeod C M, Hodges R G, Heidelberger M and Bernhard W G 1945 Prevention of pneumococcal pneumonia by immunization with specific capsular polysaccharides. Journal of Experimental Medicine 82: 445–465

Marks J S, Halpin T J 1980 Guillain-Barré syndrome in recipients of A/New Jersey influenza vaccine. Journal of the American Medical Association 243: 2490–2494

Mufson M A, Kruss D M, Wasil R E, Metzger W I 1974 Capsular types and outcome of bacteremic pneumococcal disease in the antibiotic era. Archives of Internal Medicine 134: 505–510

Mufson M A, Krause H E, Tarrant C J, Schiffman G, Cano F R 1980 Polyvalent pneumococcal vaccine given alone and in combination with bivalent influenza virus vaccine. Proceedings of the Society for Experimental Biology and Medicine 163: 498–505

Mufson M A, Oley G, Hughey D 1982 Pneumococcal disease in a medium-sized community in the United States. Journal of the American Medical Associaton 248: 1486–1489

Radl J, Sepers J M, Skvaril F, Morell A, Hijmans W 1975 Immunoglobulin patterns in humans over 95 years of age. Clinical and Experimental Immunology 22: 84–90

Recommendations of the Immunization Practices Advisory Committee (ACIP) 1982. Influenza Vaccines 1982–1983. Centers for Disease Control Morbidity and Mortality Weekly Report 31: 349–353

Roberts-Thomson I C, Whittingham S, Youngchaiyud U, MacKay I R 1974 Ageing, immune response, and mortality. Lancet 2: 368–370

Sabin A B, Ginder D R, Matumoto M, Schlesinger R W 1947 Serological response of Japanese children and old people to Japanese B encephalitis mouse brain vaccine. Proceedings of the Society for Experimental Biology and Medicine 65: 135–140

Schulman P, Budman D R, Vinciguerra V P, Degnan T J 1979 B-cell activation in angioimmunoblastic lymphadenopathy after immunization with multivalent pneumococcal vaccine. Lancet 2: 1141

Shapiro E D, Clemens J D 1983 Pneumococcal vaccine efficacy against serious pneumococcal infections in patients with vaccine indications. Clinical Research 31: 237 (abstract)

Stuart-Harris C H, Schild G C 1976 Influenza. The Viruses and the Disease. Publishing Sciences Group Inc, Littleton, Massachusetts, p 115

Thomsen O, Kettel K 1929 Die Stärke der menschlichen Isoagglutinine und entsprechenden Blutkörperchenreceptoren in verschiedenen Lebensaltern. Zeitschrift für Immunitätsforschung und experimentelle Therapie 63: 67–93

Tilghman R C, Finland M 1937 Clinical significance of bacteremia in pneumococcal pneumonia. Archives of Internal Medicine 52: 602–619

Ward J Antibiotic-resistant Streptococcus pneumoniae. Reviews of Infectious Diseases 3: 254–266

Wright A E, Parry Morgan W, Colebrook L V, Dodgson R W 1914 Observations on prophylactic inoculation against pneumococcus infections, and on the results which have been achieved by it. Lancet 1: 1–10, 87–95

29

Mouth and dentition

G. M. Ritchie

INTRODUCTION

A primary objective of geriatric medicine is to maintain the elderly person's independence within the community for as long as possible. The emphasis is on the quality of life in old age rather than the maximumisation of the life span. In order to achieve an optimum state of health, treatment is geared to the whole person rather than to a series of clinical pathologies. Attention is devoted to the provision of spectacles and hearing aids, improving mobility by physiotherapy and chiropody services with various facilities and services to improve their morale. It is therefore suprising that dental problems and needs are overlooked or at best accorded a low priority in health care programmes for the elderly.

Socio-economic factors

It is commonly assumed that the majority of elderly people are edentulous but surveys in various parts of the world have shown that 20% or more may have some of their natural teeth remaining. The retention of teeth is closely related to socio-economic factors and these are complicated by racial and regional differences, diet, availability and cost of dental services and attitudes, all of which are closely inter-related.

Generally people in the higher socio-economic categories have a better standard of dental health and care. A greater proportion will have natural teeth present in the mouth and these will probably be in a reasonably healthy condition. Similarly these people are more likely to have and wear dentures of fairly recent construction, if these are required. In addition these prostheses will probably be clean, hygienic and in a good state of repair.

Attitudes to dental treatment

The elderly as a group exhibit a variable degree of deprivation relative to the norm for the community in which they live. Their need for dental services has been shown by many surveys to be large, but their demands are small. The result is that most suffer from the effects of neglect (Ritchie et al, 1979).

There are a number of inter-related reasons for their reticence in seeking dental treatment. The most obvious are their fear of loosing the remaining teeth and the cost of treatment. However there are other equally important although less clearly expressed reasons such as not wishing to inconvenience a friend or relative, on whom they may already be heavily dependent, to arrange and accompany them on a visit to the dentist; a feeling that at their age, with perhaps little time to live, it is wasteful of the dentist's time and skills to seek treatment. An erroneous belief prevails that discomfort, disability or even pain is a function of old age and should be tolerated. Finally there is an apathy explicit in not wanting to be bothered, either because the effort required is too great or would become an unacceptable intrusion into an habituated life style.

It may be that some people may belong to a group identified in medicine who tend not to seek help from their medical practitioner, who is frequently ignorant of their current medical problems. Most of these elderly people live alone, often isolated by mobility problems. Dental treatment for the aged is not simply the provision of routine treatment for elderly people, it often requires special skills and techniques and above all an understanding of the biological and disease processes which contribute to senescence if appropriate and successful service is to be rendered.

Facial appearance

One of the first and most obvious signs of advancing years is the changes which take place to the facial appearance. Creasing of the facial skin, accentuation of the nasio-labial and inferior labial folds, the cheeks sag, fall inwards and may exhibit pouching. The lips may fall inwards or the lower lip may droop and become pendulous.

These topographical changes are the result of a depletion in replacement cell turnover, causing a reduction in the thickness of the skin and mucosa together with a loss of muscle bulk and tonus. There is an accompanying reduction is subcutaneous fat and tissue fluid. One other important factor is the loss or partial loss of teeth and their supporting alveolar bone, which greatly diminishes the support of the facial tissues.

SOFT TISSUE CHANGES AND THEIR EFFECTS

Oral mucosa

The physiological changes which take place with aging result in the oral mucosa becoming thinner, less resilient and more easily damaged by minor trauma. The tissues are less resistent to infection and slower to heal after damage. Most of the changes which are observed are the result of an interaction between degenerative changes resulting in atrophy, pathology and trauma and it is not easy to differentiate which of these is the predominating influence.

In the senescent oral mucosa, there is an inbalance between cell proliferation and cell death so that there is a reduction in the thickness of the cell layers and a decrease in the elasticity of the tissues. This is mainly due to diminution of capillary blood supply causing a deficit of oxygenation and nutrients. In addition there is a shift in the water balance reducing the cushioning effect in the tissues. The result is that both the oral mucosa and the gingivae become more friable and easily abraded.

Salivary glands

These are also affected by the atrophic processes so that the mouth becomes dryer. This is a frequent complaint amongst the elderly, and the reason why so many of them take to sucking boiled sweets in an attempt to moisten the mouth.

Xerostoma

Dry mouth is often a symptom of systemic disease, it is frequently seen in senile diabetes, uraemia and achlorhydria, and it is also an early sign in Sjögren's syndrome. Long standing chronic illness, dehydration and previous radiotherapy to the head or neck are further reasons for this problem (Kashima et al, 1965). Xerostoma may also be a side effect of a number of drugs that are frequently prescribed for the elderly, such as the antidepressants especially the phenothiazines, anti-hypertensive drugs, anticholinergic and relaxant drugs.

Salivary gland tumours

An additional cause of reduced salivary flow may be a salivary tumour which is more likely to affect the parotid gland than the others. These tumours may be adenocystic, mucoepidermoid or squamous cell carcinomas and are rarely painful unless they involve a branch of the facial or seventh cranial nerve. Due to their bulk in the cheek the patient may have difficulty in opening the mouth and initially this may be mistaken for a temporo-mandibular joint problem. These tumours rarely ulcerate externally and with treatment the prognosis is good although even when surgery is combined with radiotherapy a number of recurrences have been reported.

Parotitis

As a consequence of decreased salivary flow the glands, especially the parotids may become infected. The patient presents with pyrexia, an acute painful swelling of the gland and with gentle finger pressure pus can usually be expressed from the ducts of the gland.

Dental effect of Xerostoma

With dry mouth there is reduced salivary clearance resulting in an increased collection of food and epithelial debris in the mouth. This may initiate dental caries attack around the necks of the teeth just above the gum and also peridontal disease. Furring of the tongue occurs and the collection of epithelial debris may provide a suitable substrate for bacterial and fungal growth. Denture retention will be adversely affected and due to the loss of the lubricant effect, the tissues are more easily damaged during mastication. In addition there may be an increasing difficulty in bolus formation and deglutition. For this reason some patients may alter their food preference to dishes which are semi solids such as stews. In atrophic conditions and when the glands have been irreparably damaged by disease or radiotherapy, sialogues will be of no value and it may be necessaary to prescribe a saliva substitute to lubricate the tissues.

Taste aberrations

Reduced salivary secretion frequently results in the complaint that taste has been adversely affected; a bad taste in the mouth may be experienced and an aversion to bitter flavours sometimes develops. These manifestations may not only be a result of salivary insufficiency but may be related to atrophic changes in the taste buds arising from arteriosclerosis, hormonal changes or vitamin deficiencies. Alternatively they may be associated with disease in the oral cavity, bacterial plaque or even poor denture hygiene.

Hallitosis

Bad breath odour is associated with heavy smoking of tobacco, dry mouth or intra-oral disease but in most cases it is due to bacterial colonisation of oral or denture plaque. In the latter, attention should be directed to achieving good oral and denture hygiene, the prescription of mouth washes and the frequent intake of oral fluids.

DENTURE INDUCED LESIONS

Hyperaemic alveolar ridge

This is almost invariably the result of excessive loading from a denture which has an occlusal height which is too great. The inflamed area may be diffuse or patchy depending on whether the occlusal dimension of the whole denture is at fault or there is an error in the centric occlusal position so that certain teeth make contact prematurely. If the mucosa covering the alveolar ridge is atrophic then pressure ulcers may develop on the crest of the ridge. However it is more likely that the patient will discontinue wearing the dentures or just the lower denture since this is the one more likely to cause discomfort due to its smaller coverage of tissue, hence the load is greater relative to the unit tissue coverage. Referral to a prosthodontist is required to correct this defect which will almost certainly be related to new dentures.

Denture ulcers

These occur at the borders of the denture in the reflection of the sulci and are due to over extension of the denture flanges impinging on the movable investing tissues during function. Similar ulcers or hyperaemic abrasion areas may occur on the sides of the ridges due to instability of the denture during function movements such as grinding in mastication.

The length and depth of these ulcers, which are painful, will depend on the extent of the denture border causing the trauma. When these occur due to over extension of the posterior border of the upper denture onto the movable soft palate, long and very deep crater-like ulcers, which are frequently not painful, may be caused. Because of their apparent severity these lesions may be mistaken for a more serious condition.

These errors in the dentures can be easily rectified by the prosthodontist and seldom require medication.

Large chronic denture ulcers occurring in the floor of the mouth are occasionally mistaken for carcinomatous ulcers so it is wise to seek a dental opinion before disclosing the preliminary diagnosis to the patient or embarking on a biopsy. Inflamed mucosa or ulcers may also occur where dentures cover bony exostoses due to pressure on the thin covering of mucoperiosteum.

Denture hyperplasias

These may present in two forms, the denture hyperplasia or 'fibroma' and as granular or papillary hyperplasia. The former presents as a sausage-like fold of soft tissue at or in the reflection of the sulcus. The appearance is that of normal mucosa. A shallow fold in the tumour accommodates the border of the denture if still worn. The lesion results from a fibrous hyperplastic response to persistent irritation from an over extended denture border following the healing of a chronic ulcer. Often the tumour will regress and sometimes disappear if the border of the denture is reduced. The tumour is harmless but is sometimes removed surgically to facilitate construction of a new denture.

Papillary hyperplasia occurs on the palate, more commonly, but not exclusively in the rugae area. It appears as granular elevations of mucosa which may exhibit varying degrees of inflammation and is generally a response to irritation from antero-posterior or lateral rocking of the

upper denture in function. Generally no treatment other than prosthodontic service is required unless the papillae shelter bacterial growth, in which case removal by cryosurgery is indicated.

Fibrous or flabby ridge: hyperplastic maxillary tuberosities

Both of the above conditions are denture induced, the first by excessive load in function on the front of a complete upper denture causing bone resorption and the consequent antero-posterior rocking of the denture effecting a fibrous hyperplastic replacement of the lost tissue. This rocking of the denture in well fitting dentures may create a suction over the maxillary tuberosity and result in a fibrous hyperplasia of the covering mucosa. Although of no pathological significance, surgical reduction may be required in a healthy patient to facilitate the construction of new stable dentures.

Hyperkeratosis

This may arise anywhere in the mouth in response to chronic irritation; for example betel leaf and areca nut chewing on the cheeks and buccal pouches or heavy tobacco smoking on the anterior part of the hard palate. Spices and alcohol have also been implicated as possible initiating factors. In addition to these, chronic irritation may occasionally cause a small area of hyperkeratosis on the alveolar ridge. Since this is considered to be a pre-malignant lesion careful watch must be kept on the area after removal of the suspected irritant.

Suction disc lesion

Although suction discs are very rarely used now to assist in the retention of an upper denture, there are many elderly folk who are wearing dentures that are 20 even 30 years old when the use of this device was occasionally employed.

The lesion presents as a circular depression of variable depth corresponding to the suction cup, with raised rolled borders and a hyperaemic base. Rare cases have been reported in the past of perforation into the floor of the nose due to pressure atrophy of the mucosae and bone caused by the retaining stud of the disc. Due to their appearance these have sometimes been mistaken for malignant or gummatous lesions if the denture has been discarded.

Denture stomatitis

The incidence of denture stomatitis in the elderly who wear dentures was found to be high in the surveys of both Ritchie (1973) and Ettinger & Manderson (1973).

This lesion occurs almost exclusively under the fitting surface of an upper denture and is usually confined to the palate. It has been classified according to a visual assessment of its severity, ranging from patchy hyperaemia to a disquamating stomatitis sometimes with papillary hyperplasia of the palatal mucosa (Newton, 1962, Budtz-

Jorgensen, 1974). The lesion may occasionally extend beyond the posterior border of the denture to involve the palatal mucous glands posterior to the border of the hard and soft palate. Many aetiological factors have been cited but it is now generally believed that trauma from ill fitting dentures worn continuously is a predisposing factor, especially when the dentures are covered with plaque (Davenport, 1971). The plaque on the mucosa and on the denture becomes colonised by candida albicans and it is believed that exotoxins formed during the reproductive germ tube phase may be responsible for the mucosal inflammatory reaction. Invasion of the tissues rarely occurs and the lesions on the soft palate are due to hyphae blocking the openings of the large mucous gland causing a retention syndrome.

Debilitated people especially those suffering from a malignant lesion are prone to this condition, as are diabetics, patients with a folic acid or iron deficiency anaemia (Rose, 1968) and chronic bronchitics maintained for long periods on tetracyclins (McKendrick, 1968; Ritchie et al, 1969). In the latter it is probably because sputum containing candida albicans in its pathogenic stage is coughed up into the mouth and that this seeps under the ill fitting base of the upper denture.

Sometimes this lesion is misdiagnosed as an allergy to the denture base material but this occurs extremely rarely with polymethyl methacrylate, although a hypersensitivity reaction may occur to new dentures containing free unpolymerised resin. Allergy may manifest to metal based dentures constructed from alloys containing nickel or chromium, especially in patients who have been sensitised following a hip replacement with a prosthesis containing these metals.

Angular cheilitis, cheilosis or perleche
Thinning of the cell layers of the facial skin may result in the epidermal layer being only three cells thick in the skin folds, predisposing the inferior labial folds to angular lesions. A majority of patients with chronic persistent lesions at the corners of the mouth, known as angular cheilitis or cheilosis, may also be found to be suffering from denture stomatitis or oral candidosis (Ritchie & Fletcher, 1973). These lesions at the commisures of the mouth may extend for a considerable distance down the inferior labial fold especially when the lips and cheeks at the corners of the mouth are not adequately supported by teeth or dentures. This results in the tissues falling inwards and saliva flowing into the fold carrying a mixed bacterial flora including candida albicans.

In severe cases of chronic angular cheilitis there may be fairly considerable maceration of tissue and the lesion may also present in the intra-oral mucosa at the angles of the mouth. These cases invariably present with oral candidosis.

Although these lesions are not serious both denture stomatitis and angular cheilitis can be distressing and could become a focus for more serious infection elsewhere. The dentures should be thoroughly cleansed and disinfected (Olssen, 1971) and the patient instructed not to wear the dentures at night. Oral plaque should be removed with a mouth brush or by chewing bubble gum if the mucosa is very sensitive. Antimycotic drugs may be required; a gynaecological antimycotic cream applied to the fitting surface of the denture is a satisfactory form of medication. The patient should be referred for prosthodontic treatment. Angular cheilitis in the elderly frequently requires treatment with antimycotics combined with a broad spectrum antibiotic, however these lesions will recur unless the intra-oral condition is resolved.

MUCOSAL WHITE PATCHES

Thrush or chronic oral candidosis
This does not occur so frequently as in the past probably because more mouths now receive a better standard of oral and denture hygiene. When seen this condition almost invariably occurs in a severely debilitated person. The appearance varies according to the severity of the infection but may be differentiated from hyperkeratoses and leukoplakia by the fact that these often thick white filamentous plaques may be scraped away with a spatula.

Exfoliative cytology smears from underneath candida albicans lesions have occasionally shown the presence of 'tadpole cells' which are also seen in smears from carcinomatous ulcers but it is believed that in both cases these distorted cells arise from candida exotoxins and should not be considered as predictors of malignant or premalignant tissue changes (Ritchie et al, 1969).

Lichen planus
This distressing condition, which usually commences at an earlier age and continues in old age, appearing as white filaments or irregular raised white patches which may show atrophic changes. The usual presenting sites are the mandibular sulcus, buccal reflection and alveolar ridge but lesions are not confined to those sites. Lesions may also occur around the sexual organs and anus. In the differential diagnosis this condition is characterised by being painful, the lesions heal with scaring only to break out again at another site.

Hyperkeratosis
Mentioned earlier these patches which may occur at any intra-oral site, are generally considered to be caused by some form of chronic irritation although there is evidence that in certain cases deficiencies of vitamins A and B may have an aetiological significance. These white patches cannot be rubbed off but often disappear when the irritant factors are removed. Biopsy is a wise precaution especially if there is evidence of epithelial thinning around the lesion since this may be indicative of an early leukoplakia.

Leukoplakia

This condition usually presents as multiple lesions in the cheek especially near the occlusal line, and on the lips at the corners of the mouth. Chemical irritation has been implicated in the aetiology of this condition citing the same irritants as those initiating hyperkeratoses (Cummer, 1946). It is claimed that 30% of all leukoplakias become malignant and that those occurring in the floor of the mouth and on the tongue are particularly prone to neoplastic change.

These lesions which should certainly be regarded as pre-malignant, may present in a variety of forms which seem to bear some relation to the site of origin (Pindborg et al, 1968; Mehta et al, 1969). Smooth white patches with characteristic criss-cross markings relating to areas of atrophy tend to occur more commonly on the posterior park of the cheek, retromolar pad and tonsillar fossa regions. Raised plaques with irregular borders occur at the angles of the mouth, cheeks around the occlusal line and the floor of the mouth. The raised confluent type which may be papillomatous may cover the whole tongue but may occur at other sites also. These various types of presentation however can occur at any intra-oral site. Because of the high incidence of malignant change, biopsy should be considered mandatory (Pindborg, 1980).

Bowen's disease

This is a very rare condition that can occur at any site on the oral mucosa. It is considered a pre-malignancy and it occurs almost exclusively in elderly people. Presenting as a red velvety patch it may exhibit some white keratotic areas. Generally regarded as a precancerous dyskeratosis, some consider it to be a superficially spreading epidermoid carcinoma (Gorlin, 1950).

ORAL MALIGNANCIES OF SOFT TISSUES

The frequency with which certain areas of the mouth become sites of carcinomatous lesions seems to be related to a number of factors such as race, geography and habits; notable amongst the latter are the chewing of betal leaf and areca nut, and heavy smoking of tobacco. These factors are probably of some significance in the development of the premalignant lesions previously described. Although oral cancer is not a common disease the incidence of malignancy is greater amongst the elderly. In a survey of oral cancer cases Pogrel (1974) reported that a number of these patients had been recently examined by their dentist who had failed to detect or recognise the lesion. This serves to emphasise how vigilance is necessary when examining the mouth of an elderly person.

Lips

Nearly one third of all oral carcinomas are squamous cell carcinomas of the lips and the vast majority of these are on the lower lip. The subject is almost exclusively male and in excess of 55 years old. The papillary type of tumour before it proliferates and ulcerates may be mistaken for a wart. The nodular type, although raised, penetrates the submucosa early causing fixation; when initially it ulcerates it may be crusted or non-crusted, it then forms a deep crater with firm raised, pearly edges. It does not metastasise early but when it does so it is usually to the submaxillary or sublingual lymph nodes depending on the site and size of the lesion. With early treatment the prognosis is good.

Tongue

Squamous cell carcinoma of the tongue is also more prevalent in men than women and more commonly affects the tip, border and anterior two thirds of the dorsum. After the lip it is the second most frequent site of oral carcinoma. Presenting as a painless smooth white plaque or as a nodular or papillary growth, the latter progresses to become an extremely painful red nodule. As these tumours advance they become progressively more indurated and painful exhibiting first a shallow erosion and then the typical ulcer with a granular base and thick raised rolled borders. Dysphagia may result from restricted movement of the tongue. Metastases tend to occur early usually to the lymph nodes in the digastric triangle and the prognosis for these tumours is not good.

Floor of mouth

Carcinoma of the floor of the mouth presents in a similar manner to that of the tongue. Showing extensive induration it may restrict the movements of the floor of the mouth and tongue. The tumour may invade the ventral or underside of the tongue and accorrding to Cade (1949) metastases occur in 70% of cases.

Buccal sulcus and alveolar mucosa

Similar propensities for metastases occur when these neoplasms present in the buccal sulcus. They may appear as wart-like papillated tumours, ulcers or fissures. The fissured type more often presents in the distal part of the sulcus towards the retromolar pad area. Locally invasive, they may invade the adjacent muscle with subsequent fixation, which may be the first intimation the patient has of their presence. These tumours also mestastasise in about 40% of cases Cade, 1949). Carcinoma of the alveolar mucosa presents in a similar manner.

Gingivae

Although this is seldom seen because fewer old people have teeth remaining, the irritant effect of old, ill-fitting dentures, poor oral hygiene or opposing sharp traumatic teeth may play some initiating part in the aetiology of tumours at this site. The tumour may be smooth, papillated or fungating and frequently invades the underlying alveolar bone (Cady & Catlin, 1969).

Palate — hard and soft

These tumours may be papillated covering a wide area or present as a shallow ulcer with the typical firm, raised rolled edges. The 'verrucous' type of lesion is said to have a better prognosis as it metastaises less frequently. When occurring on the soft palate these may be extensions from, or recurrences of previously excised nasopharyngeal tumours. Carcinomas of the hard palate tend to infiltrate into the paranasal sinuses. Cade (1949) stated that 60% of carcinomas of the soft palate show metastases, which are often bilateral, whereas only half this number do so for hard palate lesions.

Distinction must be drawn between these carcinomas and pleomorphic adenomas or mixed salivary tumours which may also present on these sites in the older age group. These are red or reddish grey in colour, firm but freely movable. Slow growing, locally invasive they rarely metastasise (Crocker et al, 1970).

Nasopharynx

Nearly two thirds of these tumours are epidermoid or transitional cell carcinomas. From the dental aspect they may be the cause of asymmetric movement of the soft palate or a neuralgia of the second division of the fifth cranial nerve, which may be mistaken for some problem with the upper posterior teeth.

Basal cell carcimona

This is relatively common in the elderly usually presenting on the upper third of the face but it rarely occurs in the mouth. When it does, it commences as a small hard reddish-purple lump which later breaks down and ulcerates spreading slowly with the typical appearance of the rodent ulcer. With treatment the prognosis is good.

Transitional cell carcinoma or lympho-epithelioma

This is a variant of the epidermoid carcinoma which is rare in the mouth but much more likely to occur in the elderly than in younger patients. It presents as a soft polypoid mass usually on the tongue or base of the tonsillar fossa. A rapidly growing anaplastic tumour, it metastasises early and the prognosis is not good, (Vickers et al, 1963).

Malignant melanoma

This is a rare tumour in the mouth but more likely to occur in the fifth or sixth decade than earlier. It may be either pigmented or non-pigmented with a nodular surface which bleeds very easily. The site of predilection is the hard or soft palate. Lymph nodes are involved early and blood borne metastases occur, usually in the lungs. The prognosis is bad (Duckworth, 1962; Buckley & Russel, 1969; Trodahl & Sprague, 1970).

Adenocarcinoma

This is another neoplasm which is exceedingly rare in the mouth, but when it does occur, it is usually an intra-bony tumour metastasis from either the breast, thyroid, prostate or kidney (Basco, 1958). These metastatic neoplasms may cause expansion of bone and eventually ulcerate into the mouth. As these tumours normally metastasise late they may appear several years after the apparent successful removal of the primary tumour and when the patient has reached old age.

MUSCULAR CHANGES AND THEIR EFFECTS

Muscular ischaemia

In the absence of occlusion stress habits, the possibility of muscular ischaemia due to temporal arteritis should not be overlooked or mistaken for a temporo-mandibular joint dysfunction. A temporal arteritis may not only cause extreme pain and stiffness in the muscles but also decreased power and activity.

Physiological and neuromuscular changes

There are however physiological reasons why muscular power and activity may be diminished, such as reduced androgen secretion, potassium deficiency or failure to utilize sugars. In old age there is a general decline in neuromuscular status due to a reduction in muscle fibres and the motor end plates. These changes in addition to reducing masticatory chewing ability also affect the posture and result in the drooping of the facial musculature. When constructing dentures, difficulty may be encountered in recording a reproducible centric jaw recording which will make it difficult to construct dentures with a definitive occlusion. The result of this will be unstable dentures which the patient may be unable to control and these will cause discomfort and perhaps pain. This problem is often encountered in patients suffering from Parkinson's disease.

Stroke may also be the cause of neuromuscular weakness so that there is an imbalance between the oral musculature resulting in instability of a previously well controlled prosthesis. Because of defective control the tongue may become an active force dislodging the lower denture and there is the additional problem of the tongue and cheek being repeatedly bitten. The corner of the mouth on the affected side may fold inwards, loosing its competency to achieve an oral seal so that food and drink may escape from the mouth. Saliva may be seen dribbling from the corner of the mouth into the inferior labial skin fold and this may initiate an angular cheilitis.

In rehabilitative speech therapy the lower denture may initially become an impediment and is probably better removed until reasonable compensatory control of the tongue is achieved. Once this has been established the denture, if stable, should contribute to re-establishing a clear speech pattern.

An oral manifestation of senile chorea is the repeated flicking in and out of the tongue in snake-like fashion. This will also have a distinct destabilising effect on a lower denture. Any brain stem lesion may result in abnormal tongue movement and restricted mobility may be due to a malignancy in the floor of the mouth.

Alcoholism may exhibit a coarse tremor of the tongue and this may be confused with Parkinsonism, but can be differentiated by the fact that in the latter the movement is a slow rhythmic tremor which stops on voluntary extension of the tongue.

CONDITIONS OF THE TONGUE

The tongue is sometimes regarded as an indicator of general health and a number of systemic conditions show manifestations in the tongue. Malignant disease and abnormal movements of the tongue have already been dealt with, together with white patch lesions. The tongue is also affected by atrophic processes so that the neuromuscular control is reduced, the muscularity diminished and the dorsum exhibits degenerative changes which may result in alterations in the appreciation of taste and tactile sensations, both of which are intimately related.

Taste aberrations

Apart from degeneration of the taste buds as part of the general atrophy of the body tissues there are other factors to be considered, among these are glossitis, dehydration and xerostoma, candida plaques, hyperkeratotic lesions and neuroses. The causes of glossitis may range from pernicious anaemia and avitaminoses to chemical glossitis from mouthwashes.

Glossodynia

This is a frequent complaint amongst the elderly especially women. Often it is related to oestrogen deficiency but it may be a symptom of glossitis, arteriosclerosis, nasopharyngeal tumour or a neurosis. It has also been claimed that this may be a symptom of overclosure within the temporo-mandibular joint although there is little evidence to support this relation. Systemic causes can be diabetes, pernicious anaemia or it may be part of the Plummer-Vinson syndrome. In addition it may be related to some nutritional deficiency or even local irritation.

Varicosities

Surveys by Bhaskar (1968) and Ettinger & Manderson (1973) have shown that varicosities on the ventral side of the tongue are a frequent occurrence (Bean, 1955). These are of little clinical significance although they may be an indicator of the vascular system generally. Elsewhere it is mentioned that ossification sometimes takes place in the tendinous attachment of the genioglossus muscle to the genial tubercles on the mandible. These exostoses occasionally fracture off in function in grossly resorbed mandibles and if there are extensive varicosities in the floor of the mouth and tongue, trauma from these fragments may cause very large haematomas which may restrict tongue movement, cause pain and even difficulty in breathing, by impairing the airway (Carroll, 1983).

Pigmented tongue

Black hairy tongue is probably the most frequently seen of these pigmentations but other colourations also occur. These are due to the colonisation of dense epithelial plaques by bacteria, or staining by foodstuffs, drinks or smoking. Treatment is simply by removing the plaque and instituting a good standard of oral hygiene.

Fissured tongue

This is a fairly common condition which according to Colby et al (1971) shows progressive prevalence in each decade of adult life'. Although there is some suggestion that this may be linked with vitamin B deficiency it is of little significance except that in people with poor oral hygiene the fissures may become sites for the accumulation of debris and subsequent infection.

Atrophic luetic glossitis

A relatively common manifestation of tertiary syphilis, this form of glossitis is characterised by patches of leukoplakia and smooth shiny depapillated areas on the dorsum of the tongue. This is due to extensive syphilitic infiltration resulting in obliterative endarteritis and fibrous replacement.

Geographic tongue

This a harmless and usually symptomless form of glossitis of unknown aetiology, characterised by apparent migration of its depapillated patches. It may cause concern to the relative of an elderly person seeing the lesion for the first time.

Glossitis

Inflammatory lesions of the tongue may arise from a number of conditions which commonly occur among the elderly.

Sjögren's syndrome

The tongue is smooth with flattening of the filiform papillae and in addition the mouth is dry, smooth and shiny. Angular cheilitis may also be present.

Pernicious anaemia

This is a common complaint in the elderly especially among women and is due to vitamin B12 deficiency. The tongue is smooth with atrophy of the filiform papillae and the taste buds. The palate is usually a pale yellow colour and there may be brown pigmentation of the mucosa. Complaint is made of a sore burning mouth and abnormal taste sensations; angular cheilitis may also be present.

Vitamin B complex deficiency

It is unusual for one component only of the B complex vitamins to be deficient but these do seem to be of considerable significance with respect to oral lesions. Riboflavin deficiency results in a painful fissured glossitis in which the tongue appears glazed and magenta in colour. The lips crack, there may be angular cheilitis and the nasiolabial fold appears red and shiny. Deficiency of nicotinic acid causes glossodynia and a desquamating stomatitis which includes the tongue and is accompanied by swelling. The lower lip may also be affected.

Vitamin C deficiency

When severe this results in the typical scurvy, which is rarely seen now except occasionally in economically deprived elderly people living in cold northern climates. The tongue and mucosae become swollen, spongy and dark red or maroon in colour. The tissues bruise and bleed easily and because of dekeratinisation the alveolar mucosa abrades easily.

OTHER SOFT TISSUE LESIONS

Papilloma

These are relatively common tumours in the elderly and present as papillary or cauliflower-like lesions. They may be soft and red, or firm and white depending on the degree of keratinization. Occurring at any site in the mouth these tumours are considered benign but it is wiser to remove them, especially if they may be subject to traumatic irritation.

Traumatic ulcers

These more commonly occur on the margins of the tongue, cheek and lip. The causes may be accidental biting, abrasion from a sharp broken tooth, incorrect positioning of teeth on a denture or habitual chewing of the part; in addition neuromuscular disturbance may lead to frequent tongue or cheek biting.

Chronic traumatic ulcers of the tongue can easily be mistaken for a carcinomatous lesion because of the similarity in their appearance.

Other ulcers

There are other ulcerative conditions that may present in the elderly such as small lesions on the ventral surface of the tongue from thiamin deficiency, herpetic lesions and radionecrotic ulcers. The remote possibility of tertiary syphilitic lesions should not be overlooked.

Bruising

This may occur easily in an elderly debilitated or alcoholic person due to the fragility of the tissues. Scurvy has also been mentioned and if the haemorrhages are petechial, purpura is a possible cause, especially if the patient has received gold injections for an arthritic condition.

CHANGES IN BONE AND THEIR EFFECTS

Bone loss

Tallgren (1972) showed that although the majority of bone loss from the jaws occurs during the first seven years after the extraction of teeth, this loss of bone is a continuing process, certainly for at least 25 years. Further bone loss may result from denture trauma or physiological changes or from a combination of both these factors. There is however considerable individual variation in the rate and extent of loss of bone which seems to be related to a more generalised osteoporosis and pattern of skeletal bone resorption (Exton-Smith & Stewart, 1972).

Surveys of elderly populations in Britain (Ritchie, 1970) and in Australia (Ettinger, 1973), comment on the extensive mandibular bone resorption observed in a number of people. Negative mandibular alveolar ridge heights were recorded in 13% and 19% of these survey samples respectively. A majority of those exhibiting this gross resorption were women. Smaller mean mandibular ridge heights were also recorded in women by Heath (1973).

These findings may well relate to the high incidence of skeletal osteoporosity found in women by Exton-Smith & Stewart (1972). Anderson (1971) stated that osteomalacia occurs not infrequently in the elderly, especially in home-bound females. He attributed this mainly to vitamin D deficiency which due to the vagueness of the symptoms is misdiagnosed as hysteria or escapes diagnosis entirely. Although this may account for those cases where massive alveolar bone loss occurs rapidly in the elderly, in those where the loss has occurred more slowly it is probable that this commenced as part of a generalised post-menopausal osteoporosis.

In a majority of elderly edentulous people the integrity of the occlusal compact bone of the alveolar ridge is maintained, although the size of the medullary spaces in both the mandible and maxilla increases with age. Thinning of the cortical bone and an increase in the number of Haversian canals with resorption surfaces is exhibited so that the picture is one of decreasing mineralised bone mass (Atkinson & Woodhead, 1968). It has been suggested that radiographic assessment of skeletal bone loss can be accurately measured from the thickness of the mandibular angular cortex at the gonium (Bras et al, 1982).

The lamina dura is not normally lost from around the roots of the teeth providing these are periodontally healthy. In osteoporotic conditions, extensive rapid bone resorption may occur around peridontally involved teeth resulting in them becoming loose and inevitably their loss. An important aspect of the loss of bone from the jaws is the significant difference that results to the facial appearance, unless this can be adequately compensated for by well constructed dentures. Unfortunately where gross resorption has taken place, especially in the mandible, it is difficult to construct a well retained stable denture. Also the occlusal load-bearing properties are not conducive to comfort during mastication. In some cases the resorption of the body of the mandible may be so extensive that the posterior attachment of the mylohyoid muscle, the mylohyoid ridge, may project above the resting floor of the mouth and where formerly the alveolar ridge was present, there is a gutter bordered by the outer and inner plates of compact bone of the mandible. The roof of the mental nerve canal may be resorbed leaving the nerve exposed in a shallow trough.

In the mid-line of the mandible in the lingual sulcus, the genial tubercles may present as an elevated plateau which is considered due to a calcification or ossification around the tendonous attachment of the genioglossus muscle. A lower denture made for such cases will not only be unretentive and unstable but will elicit compression symptoms from the soft tissues covering the bony contours and from the mental nerve if this has become exposed.

Resorption may progress so far that little more than the lower border of compact bone remains so that mandibular fracture may occur from light trauma, even occasionally from masticatory load. Although extensive loss of maxillary bone may occur this rarely approaches the magnitude of mandibular bone loss. The maxilla generally maintains the integrity of the bony floor of the maxillary sinuses although excessive pressures from isolated mandibular teeth unopposed by a denture, may lead to the destruction of this thin layer of bone in a severely debilitated patient exhibiting generalised skeletal bone loss.

Intra-bony pathology

Radiographic surveys have shown that the increase of intra-bony pathology in the elderly is small and consists mainly of relatively unimportant dental pathology such as retained roots of teeth, unerupted teeth and residual cysts (Bhaskar, 1968; Ritchie, 1973; Ettinger & Manderson, 1973). Serious conditions such as tumours are rarely seen in the aged person, presumably because most of these generally manifest at an earlier age. When jaw tumours are detected in the elderly, these are more likely to be metastatic tumours and occur in the mandible rather than in the maxilla.

Bone expansion

Expansive bone-lesions seldom originate in the elderly patient but have commenced unobserved at an earlier age. Osteitis deformans or Paget's disease generally begins about the middle of the life span, however its progress may be so slow that it may not become apparent until the patient is well into the sixth decade. The facial bones, especially the maxilla, are frequently the first and sometimes the only bones to be affected by a slow irregular expansion caused by the deposition of coarse bone over areas of previous lacunar resorption. Radiographically the bones show a fluffy outline and the skull appearance is described as resembling cotton wool. The teeth may exhibit a bulbosity of the roots due to hypercementosis or show evidence of resorptions. The condition is generally but not always bilaterally symmetrical. An edentulous patient may complain that previously well-fitting dentures now seem too small for the jaws, which on examination is found to be the case.

Exostoses and osteomas

When these benign tumours are present they have rarely developed in old age with perhaps the exception of exostoses associated with the genial tubercles, which have been mentioned earlier. A palatal torus is present to some extent in the vast majority of adult populations of all ethnic groups and may be considered within the norm in spite of the fact that some of these may be quite large. Mandibular tori occurring on the lingual aspect of the mandible in the premolar region are far less common but occur quite frequently in mongoloid races.

Although these exostoses may be an impediment to the comfortable wearing of dentures they are otherwise of little significance. Enostosis and endosteal osteoma are rare but the latter may be the cause of neuralgia if it impinges on the inferior dental nerve.

Malignant tumours

Bone expansion may result from the growth of a central epidermoid carcinoma of the jaws. This may later erode the bone and perforate into the oral cavity, maxillary sinus or floor of the nose presenting an ulcer with the typical depressed base and everted margins. This tumour is extremely rare and should be differentiated from metastatic neoplasms having their probable origin in the prostate, breast, bronchus, thyroid or kidney (Meyer & Shklar, 1965).

These metastatic tumours often remain undetected as they are rarely symptomatic unless they cause pressure on a nerve, extensive bone expansion or ulcerate. Although more common in the mandible than the maxilla, the jaws are not common sites for the spread of metastases. Carcinomas of the lip, floor of mouth and maxillary sinuses may however infiltrate the bone of the jaws.

DEGENERATIVE JOINT DISEASES

Oral and dental health

These diseases are common among the elderly and the handicap may be so great that mobility is very severely restricted, precluding the possibility of the patient attending a practitioner for dental services. Those afflicted with arthritis of the fingers, hands, elbow or shoulder may have a considerable problem in maintaining good oral hygiene due to the difficulty of gripping a tooth brush or the physical restriction of getting the brush to the mouth and manipulating it once there. Similar difficulties may be encountered in trying to brush dentures to cleanse them. Various simple brush modifications may be made to help these handicapped people but for some, assistance is required to keep the mouth healthy and the dentures clean.

Attention should be given to the components of the diet to encourage low residual intra-oral food debris, especially highly refined carbohydrates and finishing a meal with a detergent food. For those who cannot manage fibrous foods a drink of water or preferably a mouthwash is helpful in removing food debris. Other caries and peridontal disease control measures are referred to later. Although these problems may seem insignificant in relation to the other problems caused by arthritic disease; failure to prescribe these simple measures will only serve to compound the patient's problems and discomfort.

TEMPORO-MANDIBULAR JOINT DYSFUNCTION

Arthritis

Prior to the studies of Carlsson et al (1967) it was commonly assumed that arthritic disease of the tempero-mandibular joint occurred only rarely because few complaints of pain or dysfunction were recorded in the elderly. Although a primary arthritis of this joint appears to be rare in the absence of arthritic disease in other joints, it is much more frequently present in the company of lesions elsewhere than previously thought. Presumably attention was focussed on those joints which exhibited the greater and more obvious functional limitations and pain; in addition medication probably has the effect of masking the temporo-mandibular joint symptoms.

Manifestations of rheumatic disease are likely to occur at a somewhat earlier age than osteo-arthritic changes. The lesions can be differentiated by the radiographic appearances of the joint although in the case of rheumatoid disease these may not be very obvious until the lesion is well established.

Occlusion problems

Although periarticular pain associated with the so-called muscles of mastication generally relate to occlusion problems with the teeth in younger patients, this may also occur in the partly dentate elderly person who has developed stress habits such as teeth clenching, bruxism or mandibular posturing.

THE DENTAL TISSUES

Teeth

The changes which take place in the teeth are not obvious becoming darker in hue as a result of thinning of the enamel in function and mineral deposits in the underlying dentine. These deposits occur mostly in the tubules of the dentine so that the tissue becomes less sensitive to stimuli. The reduction in sensitivity is further increased by degeneration of the pulp which becomes fibrotic, the blood supply is reduced and the odontoblast layer dies so that protective secondary dentine is no longer formed. Ultimately the whole pulp and root canal may become obliterated by calcified deposits. The cementum remains vital and in the absence of periodontal disease the attachment of the periodontal fibres to both cementum and bone remains intact. However in a majority of elderly people passive eruption occurs, this is a progressive apical proliferation of the epithelial attachment which results in an apparent elongation of the teeth. In spite of these changes the teeth still function perfectly effectively, but recession of the interdental papilla results in a space between the teeth in which food debris may lodge and initiate caries attack or periodontal disease.

A gradual attrition of the enamel of the incisal tips and occlusal surfaces of the teeth results in a small loss of height, but once the dentine which is softer is reached the rate of attrition is accelerated. This causes not only considerable loss of teeth height, perhaps even to gum level, but occlusal height so that the lower third of the face becomes shortened, which has an aging effect.

By abuse or the excessive intake of acid fruit juices, erosion of the teeth may occur either over the whole tooth surface or more extensively over those surfaces more exposed to the chelating substance. Another manifestation is cervical erosion, which is the smooth saucerised loss of tooth substance at the necks of the teeth, and this may be the result of toothbrush trauma.

Attrition, erosion and abrasion are slow processes so that it is only the manifestation of these that become apparent with age. Teeth abused in this fashion are saveable with modern restorative techniques and extractions need not be carried out. If the loss of enamel has occurred rapidly and the pulp is still vital and the dentine tubules not obliterated, these teeth will be painful to hot, cold, sweet and salty stimuli. Generally this is not the case as the loss of the protective enamel has occurred slowly over a considerable period of time.

Cervical abrasion may however, particularly in dry mouth sufferers where the salivary clearance of food debris is deficient, provide a protected site for caries attack and this is commonly seen in the elderly person. In fact it is the most likely area for caries attack at this age and may affect the whole neck of a tooth, causing a ring-like lesion. As the caries progresses, occlusal function may eventually cause the tooth to break at the neck, leaving only the root present at gum level. The dentist may decide to leave the root and not extract it if it is healthy; with suitable preparation these are useful and prevent the bone resorption that is a sequel to their removal.

Abrasion may not only result in disfigurement and sensitivity but the loss of occlusal height results in mandibular overclosure which may cause a temporo-mandibular joint dysfunction. This does not frequently occur because usually the loss occurs slowly and there is a gradual muscular and joint accommodation to the changed occlusal position.

Periodontal tissues

The incidence of periodontal disease increases with age as does its severity and it seems to be worse in men than in women probably because the latter generally attempt to maintain a better standard of oral hygiene. The factors associated with this disease are the accumulation of plaque, calculus and food debris, therefore people with defective salivary clearance and those who do not or cannot, due to physical handicap, keep their mouth clean will be in jeopardy.

There is debate regarding whether periodontal disease is a pathology or a senescent condition when it occurs in the elderly person and it would seem probable that it is both. Although the periodontal health may be maintained into old age, arteriosclerotic changes result in decreased vascularity of the gingivae which suffer a reduction in cellular composition. The gingivae loose their stippled appearance and become smooth, glazed and darker in colour. There is an increase in connective tissue and a reduction of tissue fluid so that the resilience of the gingivae is diminished and because the cell layers are thinner the gums are more easily abraded and less able to respond to local irritants. In addition the tissues repair is delayed. Further the inflamed tissues are conducive to the formation of dental plaque and denuded tissue to the omission of tooth brushing.

In such cases the avoidance of hard and abrasive foods is to be encouraged and the intake of fluids increased. The use of mouthwashes, (some authorities advocate the use of chlorhexidine) when the mouth is too sore to tolerate the use of a toothbrush also chewing gum or bubble gum have been found useful, but often the mouth needs to be moistened first to prevent the gum from adhering to the tissues.

DISEASES OF THE NERVOUS SYSTEM

Previous mention has been made of the diminishing neuromuscular status which results in reduced muscular power and co-ordination in the elderly. Nerve compression symptoms are also more common due to the reduced soft tissue protection offered. There is some sensory deprivation and nerve trauma seems to cause less pain but more disability than in a younger patient; as might be expected recovery is slower.

Neuralgic pain also occurs more commonly in elderly people, especially trigeminal neuralgia. This is usually related to the maxillary division of the trigeminal nerve, and the pain may be felt in the upper posterior teeth and gum, the check, the upper lip or the side of the nose. Commencing with occasional sharp electric-like pains, in time these bouts become more frequent and excruciating in character. Trigger-zones are a feature of this disease where the lightest touch triggers off an attack. Although recovery is rare, surgical section should be avoided as treatment with carbamazine usually provides a satisfactory alternative. When these characteristic pains are manifest in the base of the tongue, retromylohyoid fossa or ear, these sites may be indicative of a glossopharyngeal neuralgia or tumour. The same drug as above is valuable in treatment.

In both of these entities the pain which is reflex rarely disturbs sleep and this is a valuable diagnostic aid to distinguish this neuropathy from the migrainous type which may also affect the trigeminal region. Occurring in intermittent bouts of severe pain there are long periods free from pain. Characteristically the pain tends to occur at night disturbing sleep. Subcutaneous injection of ergotamine tartrate is the treatment of choice.

An acoustic nerve tumour may also give neuralgic pain which may initially be mistaken for a diseased upper molar tooth. The so-called typical facial neuralgia is very similar to the trigeminal variety except that there are no trigger zones. This condition however normally affects younger patients.

Other causes of severe facial pain may be an aneurism or a tumour causing pressure on a sensory nerve. In addition herpes, usually along the course of the mandibular nerve is another possible factor. A local source of severe pain, other than that caused by dental disease, may be a traumatic or amputation neuroma, which may be related to a site of previous physical or surgical trauma.

The causes of muscular weakness have already been mentioned except for the condition known as Bell's palsy. This may be temporary or permanent and is usually associated with trauma, compression or ischaemia of the facial nerve around the area of the stylomastoid foramen.

Psychiatric problems

Brain regression occurs early in life and may be accelerated by a series of mishaps such as minor traumatic injuries and infections. The active use of the brain in learning and training is important in both the development and maintainance of brain function. There is evidence to suggest that people of the higher developed intellects tend to suffer a slower rate of mental decline especially if they continue to exercise their mental faculties. The old adage of not being able to teach an old dog new tricks is not true but the learning process may be very much slower; much will depend on the individual's personality and motivation, as so often the old person will give up due to impatience with his slow rate of progress. This impatience may be misconstrued as a lack of interest. In addition self-critical ability and facility for solving problems becomes impaired as does short-term memory.

These changes have important implications with regard to dentistry, particularly the adaptability to new dentures and especially complete dentures. Alterations to the dimensions of new appliance relative to previous dentures may not be well tolerated even though these may improve the fit, function and appearance. It is for this reason that many prosthodontists prefer to modify an old existing denture than risk the rejection of a new appliance. In cases where substantial alterations are essential, denture copy techniques have been advocated with subsequent serial alteration made over a span of time with a period of habituation before commencing the next stage (Fish, 1969; Scher & Ritchie, 1978). This allows a variable period of adaptive learning and establishes an increasing tolerance to change and usually ensures success. However in certain conditions visual spatial perception is impaired and these people will not only experience great difficulty in adapting to new dentures, they may even reject appliances to which they had previously been well habituated (Joseph, 1982) and the dentures may be seen in the mouth in bizarre relation to each other and to the denture bearing tissues. There is evidence that certain combinations of drugs used in psychiatric treatment may produce this visual spatial impairment with subsequent rejection of dentures.

These problems are not confined to the wearing of dentures but also produce difficulties in maintaining or establishing oral hygiene regimens. Whilst the burnt out schizophrenics provide no difficulties with respect to treatment the presenile and senile dementias may be unresponsive to treatment and present a variable degree of difficulty or rejection due to emotional and behavioural problems; this may also be the case with people suffering from arteriosclerotic psychoses. Those with affective psychoses may lack interest or be excessively exacting and neurotic about their appliances and when in the demented state, untreatable. People suffering from late paraphenia, of which there are likely to be far more women than men, may cause difficulties due to their arrogant, quarrelsome and threatening attitude and may make unpleasant accusations against those attempting treatment. In the early stages of senile dementia patients may be treated with success if their unresponsiveness can be pierced, but once they enter the psychotic state they are better left alone.

As psychiatric patients and particularly the elderly tend to be isolated from the community, restorative dental treatment is not accorded a high priority which is why little is known about the techniques which may promote success when treatment is available. It may well be that further study might evince predictors of certain psychiatric states in those members of the public who present with irrational and unfounded complaints about their dentures.

Diet and mastication

The caloric intake of food should be reduced because the majority of elderly people undertake a smaller amount of physical work but the dietary intake should not be lowered as this is necessary for the normal reparative processes of the tissues. Managing the previously accustomed variety of food intake may become progressively more difficult due to problems with mastication. This may be due to a deficiency of teeth, painful teeth and gums or defective dentures and may lead to some dietary selection. The majority of people seem to manage extremely well even without dentures (Neill & Phillips, 1970, 1972; Heath, 1973), although many regret the restrictions placed upon them by decreased masticatory ability and complain of the monotony of a soft diet. In spite of this there is little evidence that restriction from this cause leads to malnutrition. Where nutritional deficiencies occur these are more likely to be related to financial limitations, mobility problems in obtaining food, difficulty in its preparation or perhaps due to apathy. Anderson (1971) has shown that undiagnosed potassium deficiency may lead to apathy, depression, mental confusion and muscular weakness thereby compounding the problem. Perhaps the more important aspect is that some are deprived of one of the prime enjoyments of life, the ability to enjoy a good meal of their choice.

The absence of dentures is frequently blamed for indigestion but research has shown no evidence of a cause and effect relationship, however it is possible that if a person strongly believes that one is the cause of the other, psychosomatically there may be some substance in this and certainly the provision of prostheses will be of benefit to the person, providing his expectations are not set unrealistically high.

DENTAL SERVICE CONSIDERATIONS

Indications from surveys of the elderly are that many people who have teeth remaining, due to neglect, often require extensive treatment including the extraction of badly diseased teeth. Many teeth are little more than decaying roots and periodontal disease is rife.

Clearly if teeth can be retained in later life with proper care and an effective oral hygiene regimen, there is no reason why the dental structures should not be maintained into old age. This however requires active participation on the part of the elderly person with organised services to help maintain a healthy mouth. This will be particularly required for the restricted mobility people and those who are handicapped. Perhaps most important of all is the education of people in the value of keeping the natural teeth as long as possible and keeping these in a healthy state.

It was mentioned earlier that the retention of teeth in a healthy state, promotes the maintainance and the quality of bone of the mandibule and maxilla. In turn the teeth and bone will help to retain the contour of the face, mitigating the aging process. Oral functions can be better carried out by the natural teeth than by prosthetic restorations and enables a wider range of foods to be managed in comfort. This together with the knowledge that natural teeth are still present has a beneficial psychological effect on an individual. Loss of teeth should not be considered any more inevitable than the previously mentioned attitude that 'pain and discomfort are functions of old age'.

Unfortunately many elderly edentulous people either have no dentures or have old, unhygienic or inadequate dentures that often cause damage, pain or promote disease to the wearer's oral tissues. Because of these problems the prostheses are discarded or worn only occasionally. This has given rise to the erronious impression that the elderly do not want to be bothered with dentures. There is a high degree of tolerance of infirmity and low expectation coupled with an apathy of age, which has resulted in a low level of demand on all medical services including dentistry. Whilst a sound case can be made for the maintenance of dental health in the dentate or partly dentate on the grounds of general health care, the benefits of prosthodontic service seem less clear. The provision and maintenance of partial dentures will help to maintain the health of the remaining teeth if the prostheses are well designed and constructed.

Complete dentures however may be considered unnecessary since a soft nourishing diet can be managed without prostheses. The value of dentures for the edentulous is that a greater variety of diet can be managed with comfort, they effect an aesthetic improvement and assist in the production of clear speech. These benefits, apart from conferring a psychological benefit, help to enable a person to remain with confidence in society and avoid, through embarrassment, isolation with the possible dementing effect to which this may eventually lead. Some of the senescent changes which make rendering prosthodontic service difficult have been covered but with modern techniques many of these problems can be at least partially overcome.

Although oral malignant disease is not common because a lot of elderly people have not visited a dentist for many years, the oral tissues should be carefully scrutinised for the presence of pathological lesions, remembering that the elderly are especially prone to most of the conditions that have been briefly covered earlier. When in doubt about any intra-oral lesion it is always wise to seek early consultation with a clinical oral pathologist since early dignosis may be crucial in effecting a speedy cure.

When patients are referred for dental treatment it is important that the dentist should be fully briefed on the patient's medical status in clear terms, together with any medication that has been prescribed. A great deal of modern dentistry is carried out with the patient in the prone position so it is important that postural problems are included in the information provided.

Little is known at present about overcoming problems with psychogeriatric patients and research needs to be carried out in this area, since it is possible that in some conditions successful dental treatment could be provided.

Although the tenor has been on reparative treatment, hopefully in the future the emphasis will be placed on preventive measures since tooth loss does not have to be an inevitable part of the aging process. The process of dental health education should be conducted throughout life and reinforced at pre-retirement age. This is where the medical profession can be helpful in bringing this to the notice of the potential 'geriatric' person, and the advisability of seeking a dental assessment. If an individual reaches old age with a good oral and dental status it should be relatively simple to maintain an optimum state of oral health for the remaining life span.

The team approach to geriatric care should include a dentist, not just to provide treatment where appropriate, but to provide input in the assessment and formulation of the care program for the aged person (Ritchie, 1978). Because the elderly are often under economic pressure and the size of the problem tends to be masked by mobility problems and lack of demand for dental treatment, government intervention is required to bring effective services to this deprived section of the community.

REFERENCES

Anderson W F 1971 Inter-relationships between physical and mental disease in the elderly In: Kay D W K, Walk A (eds) Recent Developments in Psychogeriatrics. Headley, Ashford p 19–24

Atkinson P J, Woodhead C 1968 Changes in human mandibular structure with age. Archives of Oral Biology 13: 1453–63

Bosco H F 1958 Metastatic adenocarcinoma of the mandible Oral Surgery 11: 86–88

Bean W D 1955 Caviar lesions of the tongue. In: Wolstenholme G E W, Cameron M P (eds) Colloquia on Ageing 1 Little Brown, Boston p 84–86

Bhaskar S N 1968 Oral lesions in the aged population Geriatrics 23: 137–149

Budtz-Jorgensen E 1974 The significance of Candida albicans in denture stomatitis. Scandinavian Journal of Dental Research 82: 151–90

Buckley D B, Russell J G 1969 Intra-oral blue naevus. British Dental Journal 127: 288

Bras J, Van Ooij C P, Abraham-Inpijn L, Wilmink J M, Kusen G J 1982 Radiographic interpretation of the mandibular angular cortex: a diagnostic tool in metabolic bone loss. Oral Surgery 53: 647–50

Cade S 1949 Maligant disease of the mouth annals of the Royal College of Surgeons 4: 381–391

Cady B, Catlin D 1969 Epidermoid carcinoma of the gum; a 20 years survey. Cancer 23: 551–69

Carlsson G E, Öberg T, Berman F, Fajers C M, 1967 Morphological changes in the mandibular joint disc in temporomandibular joint pain dysfunction syndrome. Acta Odontologica Scandinavica 25: 163–81

Carrol M J 1983 Spontaneous fracture of the genial tubercles. British Dental Journal 154: 47–48

Colby R A, Kerr D A, Robinson H B G 1971 Colour Atlas of Oral Pathology. Lippincott, Philadelphia

Crocker D J, Cavalaris C J, Finch R 1970 Intra-oral minor salivary gland tumours. Oral Surgery 29: 60–68

Cummer C L 1946 Leukoplakia (leukokeratosis) of the palate, papular forms; its relation to the use of tobacco. Journal American Medical Assocation 132: 493–498

Davenport J C 1970 The oral distribution of candida in denture stomatitis. British Dental Journal 129: 151–156

Duckworth R 1962 Malignant melanoma of the oral mucosa British Dental Journal 113: 73–82

Ettinger R L 1973 Diet, nutrition and masticatory ability in a group of elderly edentulous patients. Australian Dental Journal 18: 12–19

Ettinger R L, Manderson R D 1973 An investigation of the dental status and needs of the institutional elderly population of Edinburgh. Report of the Scottish Home and Health Department.

Exton-Smith A N, Stewart R J C 1972 Bone resorption in old age. Proceedings of the Royal Society of Medicine 65: 674

Fish S F 1969 Adaptation and habituation to full dentures. British Dental Journal 127: 19–26

Gorlin R J 1950 Bowen's disease of the mucous membrane of the mouth. Oral Surgery 3: 35–51

Heath M R 1973 Dental state and bone loss in the elderly. Proceedings of the Royal Society of Medicine 66: 590–594

Joseph E L 1982 Personal communication.

Kashima H K, Kirkham W R, Andrews J R 1965 Post-irradiation sialadenitis: a study of the clinical features, histopathologic changes and serum enzyme variations following irradiation of human salivary glands. American Journal of Roentgenology 94: 271–291

McKendrick A J W 1968 Denture stomatitis and angular cheilitis in patients receiving long-term tetracycline therapy. British Dental Journal 124: 412–417

Mehta F S, Pindbory J J, Gupta P C, Daftary D K 1969 Epidemiologic and histologic study of oral cancer and leukoplakia among 50 915 villagers in India. Cancer 24: 832–849

Meyer I, Shklar G 1965 Malignant tumours metastatic to mouth and jaws. Oral Surgery 20: 350–362

Neill D J, Phillips H I 1970 The masticatory performance, dental state and dietary intake of a group of elderly army pensioners. British Dental Journal 128: 581–585

Neill D J, Phillips H I 1972 The masticatory performance and dietary intake of elderly edentulous patients. Dental Practitioner and Dental Record 22: 384–389

Newton A V 1962 Denture sore mouth: a possible aetiology. British Dental Journal 112: 357–360

Olsson K A, Bergman B 1971 A comparison of two prosthetic methods for the treatment of denture stomatitis. Acta Odontologica Scandinavica 29: 745–753

Pindborg J J 1980 Oral cancer and precancer. Wright, Bristol.

Pindborg J J, Renstrup G, Jølst O, Roed-Peterson B 1968 Studies in oral leukoplakia. Preliminary report on the period prevalance of malignant transformation in leukoplakia based on a follow-up study of 248 patients. Journal American Dental Association 76: 767–771

Pogrel M A 1974 The dentist and oral cancer in the North-east of Scotland. British Dental Journal 137: 15–20

Ritchie G M 1970 A survey of the Oral and Dental State of Geriatric patients with particular reference to prosthetic problems. MDS Thesis. London University.

Ritchie G M, 1973 A report of dental findings in a survey of geriatric patients. Journal of Dentistry 1: 106–112

Ritchie G M 1978 The dental care of geriatric patients; a community responsibility. Quintessence International 9: 83–88

Ritchie G M, Fletcher A M, Main D M G, Prophet A S 1969 The aetiology, exfoliative cytology and treatment of denture stomatitis. Journal of Prosthetic Dentistry 22: 185–200

Ritchie G M, Fletcher A M 1973 Angular inflammation. Oral Surgery 36: 358–366

Ritchie G M, Turner C H, Fletcher A M 1979 An assessment of dental requirements of elderly people. Quintessence International 10: 81–88

Rose J A 1968 Aetiology of angular cheilitis. Iron metabolism. British Dental Journal 125: 67–72

Scher E A, Ritchie G M, 1978 Prosthodontic treatment of the elderly by incremental modifications to old dentures. Quintessence International 9: 47–53

Tallgren A 1972 The continuing reduction of the residual ridges in complete denture wearers. A mixed longitudinal study covering 25 years. Journal of Prosthetic Dentistry 26: 120–32

Trodahl J N, Sprague W G 1970 Benign and malignant melanocytic lesions of the oral mucosa. Cancer 25: 812–823

Vickers R A, Gorlin R J, Smart E A 1963 Lympho-epithelial lesions of the oral cavity: report of four cases. Oral Surgery 16: 1214–1222

30

Oesophagus and stomach

K. Arnold

SYMPTOMATOLOGY AND DIFFERENTIAL DIAGNOSIS

Anorexia, nausea and vomiting

The causes of these symptoms in the elderly are legion and may relate to disease in almost any system. Anorexia is frequently due to depression or fairly advanced dementia. Depressive anorexia is occasionally very severe and chronic, leading to profound weight loss, weakness and sometimes development of pressure sores. Before making the diagnosis, search should be made for other features of depressive illness and pointers to an organic cause of anorexia. These patients usually improve dramatically with treatment of the underlying depression, whether by alleviation of social isolation, drug therapy or electroconvulsive therapy (ECT). When weight loss and weakness are advanced, care must be taken to distinguish depressive illness from malaise, with apathy and anorexia, due to organic disease. Malignancy, tuberculosis and malabsorption should be borne in mind particularly.

Anorexia occurs fairly early in faecal impaction. Nausea, vomiting and the characteristic picture of intestinal obstruction may follow. These symptoms may also relate to medication. Drugs may act directly on the vomiting centre, cause gastric irritation, constipation or occasionally metabolic disturbances. Common offenders are digoxin, L-dopa, non-steroidal anti-inflammatory drugs, sulphonamides and opiates, including codeine and dextropropoxyphene (in Distalgesic). Excessive sedation causes anorexia.

Neurological disorders are easily forgotten as causes of vomiting. When due to raised intracranial pressure, vomiting is often projectile, particularly with cerebellar tumours, when it may be induced by changes in posture. Vertigo and nystagmus may be absent.

Vomiting may be one of the few presenting symptoms in an elderly patient with an acute abdominal emergency, since pain and muscle rigidity may be absent. Vomiting may also cause secondary problems. Dehydration and electrolyte disturbances occur when vomiting is prolonged or associated with diarrhoea. Aspiration is likely when the state of consciousness is reduced. A Mallory Weiss tear may cause haemorrhage, sometimes massive, and even perforation.

Dysphagia

Dysphagia is a common symptom in the elderly and a question about swallowing difficulties should form part of complete history taking. Dysphagia means the retardation of easy passage of food and fluid from pharynx to stomach. It should not be confused with other symptoms which occur frequently, but not necessarily, in association with it. These include difficulties in mastication, regurgitation, nasopharyngeal reflux, tracheal aspiration, painful swallowing and a sensation of a lump in the throat. The latter is not always psychogenic in origin, so that 'globus hystericus' may be a misnomer (Watson & Sullivan, 1974). Dysphagia may be due to extrinsic or intrinsic obstruction, neuromuscular disorders or failure of the mouth to deliver a suitably small and lubricated bolus of food to the pharynx. Enquiry should thus be made regarding chewing problems, with reference to teeth and dentures particularly. Dryness of the mouth (xerostomia) may be due to drugs, dehydration, fever, mouth breathing, infections of the salivary glands and Sjögren's and Mikulicz's syndromes.

The patient who has far more difficulty with solids than with liquids is less likely to have dysphagia of neuromuscular origin. Aspiration on the other hand occurs most often with liquids. The sensible patient can normally localise accurately the level at which food sticks, although sometimes in oesophageal obstruction it seems somewhat higher than the true level of the lesion. Painful low dysphagia is usually due to oesophagitis with stricture formation. High (oropharyngeal) dysphagia is most often of neuromuscular origin, but webs, vertebral osteophytes, pharyngeal diverticula and tumours are occasionally responsible. Likewise, although nasopharyngeal reflux and tracheal aspiration may be associated with dysphagia of any cause, they are most often seen with neuromuscular dysphagia. Reflux into the nose occurs readily when there is paralysis of the palate and pharyngeal constrictors, so that the nasopharynx cannot be sealed off during swallowing and regurgitation.

Bouts of coughing occurring only after eating and

drinking indicate tracheal aspiration. This is sometimes a manifestation of dysfunction of the upper oesophageal sphincter; in health the vagus sends excitatory impulses continuously to the cricopharyngeus muscle and these are inhibited only briefly to allow relaxation of the muscle at precisely the correct phase of deglutition. If the sphincter tone is always reduced, perhaps through damage to the vagus or nucleus ambiguus, upward oesophago-pharyngeal reflux will occur, sometimes against a closed mid-pharynx, so forcing the contents into the larynx. When infrequently, this is an isolated neuromuscular lesion, these features will be observed in the absence of dysphagia.

Gerhardt et al (1980) found a very high incidence of aspiration pneumonitis in subjects with oesophago-pharyngeal reflux and cricopharyngeal hypotension. Lung disease is especially frequent and severe, often fatal, when gastro-oesophageal and oesophago-pharyngeal reflux co-exist, because of the corrosive effect of gastric juice and bile. Cricopharyngeal myotomy is thus contraindicated in the presence of gastro-oesophageal reflux.

Cricopharyngeal hypertension, also called cricopharyngeal achalasia or spasm, as a cause of dysphagia is more controversial. There is little double that it occurs when a large object such as an endoscope, is rammed ineptly into the lower pharynx. The presence of acid in the oesophagus may also increase sphincter tone. Nevertheless the common finding of a radiographically prominent cricopharyngeal indentation is not usually associated with increased sphincter tone as measured by manometry (Daniel & Benacerraf, 1978). There is some evidence however, that the sphincter may not relax sufficiently during swallowing in several of the neuromuscular disorders associated with dysphagia. In this situation the food bolus may be redirected into the nasopharynx or larynx. Myotomy may be helpful.

Dysphagia requires specialist management. Its severity, the state of nutrition and evidence of aspiration into the airways should determine whether this is provided on an in or out-patient basis. Its management must include general examination, inspection of the mouth, examination of the nervous system and cranial nerves in particular. It is sometimes useful to observe the patient during the act of swallowing liquids and solids.

Dysphagia is one of the few situations where radiology with cinematographic or video screening is better than endoscopy, since pharyngo-oesophageal motility may be observed closely during the act of deglutition. It is sometimes useful to mix barium with solid food. Nevertheless, endoscopy may be required subsequently when an anatomical obstruction is demonstrated. It is sometimes necessary to proceed to other studies, including manometry, laryngeal inspection and electromyography of the buccal and pharyngeal muscles.

Unless or until specific treatment becomes effective, it is often helpful to give a diet of porridgy consistency to a patient with neuromuscular dysphagia. The semi-fluid bolus will pass easily but without too great a risk of aspiration. Others will require enteral feeding via a fine bore nasograstric tube. These are much better tolerated than tubes of standard bore and are less often dislodged by the confused patient. There is also greater risk of gastro-oesophageal reflux and airways aspiration with standard bore tubes. Several well balanced liquid enteral feed preparations are now available. With complete oesophageal obstruction, short term parenteral feeding may be required prior to surgery. Patients with a tendency to aspirate should be nursed sitting up. Drugs with sedative action should be avoided.

Otherwise, the treatment of dysphagia depends on the cause. A decision to proceed to cricopharyngeal myotomy should be weighed carefully, since aspiration is often provoked. In particular, gastro-oesophageal reflux must first be excluded. Hurwitz & Duranceau (1978) have indicated by collating studies, that myotomy in approprairte subjects is usually beneficial. However myotomy should be delayed if there is any possiblity of spontaneous improvement, as in dysphagia due to recent stroke disease. Fibre optic endoscopy now allows non-surgical dilatation of peptic oesophageal stricture and even insertion of intra-luminal by-pass tubes in oesophageal carcinoma (Mee et al, 1981).

Commoner causes of dysphagia are listed in Table 30.1. The fibrotic degeneration in systemic sclerosis chiefly

Table 30.1   Some common causes of dysphagia

Neuromuscular	Intrinsic obstruction	Extrinsic obstruction
Brain stem lesions	Carcinoma of	Cardiac enlargement
Pseudo-bulbar palsy	pharynx	Unfolded aorta
Multiple sclerosis	oesophagus	Aortic aneurysm
Motor neuron disease	stomach	Goitre
Parkinsonism	Web	Retropharyngeal
		abscess
Syringobulbia	Peptic stricture	Carcinoma of
		bronchus
Myasthenia gravis	Pouch	larynx
Myositides	Foreign body	thyroid
Systemic sclerosis		Lymphadenopathy
Presbyoesophagus		Spondylotic
		osteophyte

affects the oesophageal smooth muscle and thus its predominant effects are neuromuscular. Achalasia of the cardia rarely presents in the very elderly. By contrast presbyoesophagus is present in most people over 85 years of age. In this condition, peristaltic contractions are to varying degrees replaced by static or inco-ordinated contractions. Very few are symptomatic however. Pharyngeal diverticula occasionally cause dysphagia when they become distended with food, but oesophageal diverticular rarely cause such problems.

The neuromuscular control of deglutition and aetiology

of oropharyngeal dysphagia have recently been thoroughly reviewed by Hellemans et al (1982).

Oesophageal pain

This is usually due to gastro-oesophageal reflux (see later) and appears to be due to continued exposure of the mucosa to gastric acid, even in the absence of frank oesophagitis. Although normally a retrosternal burning sensation, it may mimic cardiac pain in its character, distribution and radiation. Furthermore, it may be relieved by organic nitrates and nitrites, possibly because of reduced gastric peristalsis. Thus it is important to obtain a full history of precipitating and relieving factors and of other symptoms which help to distinguish cardiac and oesophageal disease. Investigations should include cardiac enzymes and electrocardiography after exercise when appropriate, proceeding to barium swallow and endoscopy if these are satisfactory. Since both ischaemic heart disease and reflux are common in the elderly, the two conditions may co-exist.

Abdominal pain

Visceral pain is sometimes diminished in old age and this is possibly related to the frequency of autonomic dysfunction. An acute surgical abdominal emergency may present with little or no pain and rigidity of the abdominal musculature. Pyrexia and leucocytosis may also be absent. As recommended by Coleman & Denham (1980), there should be a high index of suspicion and, when intra-abdominal pathology is suspected, repeated X-rays may be necessary to reveal pneumo-peritoneum. Although steroids are not now thought to contribute significantly in the aetiology of peptic ulceration, except possibly in very high doses (Conn et al, 1976), patients receiving them are particularly prone to 'silent' presentation of an acute abdomen.

Otherwise, patterns of abdominal pain are similar to those found in younger patients and the differential diagnosis is described in standard textbooks of medicine and surgery. The affected system can sometimes be identified from precipitating factors in the history, e.g. relationships to meals, to defaecation, to micturition or to movements of the trunk. Diagnoses which are easily missed include acute pancreatitis, radicular pain, herpes zoster and leaky or dissecting aortic aneurysm. Appendicitis is less common in the elderly but it is not a rarity, so that the possibility of it should not be dismissed out of hand.

Haematemesis and melaena

Mortality rates from upper gastro-intestinal haemorrhage are high in the elderly. There are several reasons for this. Arteriosclerotic vessels will not retract well so that prolonged bleeding and rebleeding are more likely. Pre-existing diseases, particularly myocardial pump failure, coronary and cerebral atheroma reduce tolerance to shock states. Post-operative mortality is high, although surgery is frequently of necessity the treatment of choice. Of no small importance is the delay in hospital admission so often apparent in this age group, for a variety of medical and social reasons. The greatest hope of improving mortality lies in prevention, particularly by judicious prescribing of aspirin and non-steroidal anti-inflammatory drugs, with follow-up of patients receiving them. In an unpublished survey by the writer, of 106 elderly patients endoscoped at a district general hospital following acute gastro-intestinal bleeding, 55% had been taking these drugs. Excellent symptom control might be achieved with paracetamol alone in many such patients.

There should rarely be diagnostic difficulties. Haematemesis may occasionally result from swallowed blood, but the source is usually obvious. When the patient is a poor historian, it is not always possible to distinguish haematemesis from haemoptysis. The odour of melaena is characteristic; its presence renders faecal occult blood testing unnecessary, even when the stools are black from oral iron therapy.

The patient should be dispatched to hospital with the minimum delay. If facilities are available, an intravenous line should be inserted while the ambulance is awaited, samples for haemoglobin, cross-match and electrolytes being taken at insertion. Unless features of shock are already apparent, isotonic saline need be run in only slowly to keep the line open. Otherwise, these measures should be undertaken on arrival in hospital, before a full history and examination are completed.

Shock should, of course, be corrected swiftly by the normal means, bearing in mind the danger of overcorrection and fluid overload. A central venous pressure (CVP) line is invaluable but its insertion and subsequent reading should be undertaken by experienced personnel. Due regard must be given to the total state of the patient since CVP readings are occasionally artefactual. The elderly are likely to require more transfused blood than younger patients. Opiates should be used for severe pain only. When sedatives are required to allay anxiety or prior to endoscopy, initial doses should be very small, particularly in the frail and very elderly. The surgical team should be informed about the patient as soon as possible, even when surgery would appear to be unnecessary.

Endoscopy is the investigation of choice, this being the best method of identifying the underlying lesion and of observing continued bleeding. There is a high risk of rebleeding when blood clot is found in ulcer craters (Foster et al, 1978). With widespread use of endoscopy, it is now appreciated that massive bleeding from oesophagitis and Mallory-Weiss tears is not uncommon.

Those patients with massive, prolonged or recurrent bleeding will require surgery; new drugs and techniques such as endoscopic laser photocoagulation, have done little so far to change this. The mortality rate is about 20% following operation for upper gastro-intestinal bleeding in the elderly, being lower for the younger elderly and very much higher over 80 years. It is particularly high when the bleeding lesions are gastric carcinoma or oesophageal varices.

Iron deficiency anaemia

This is usually due to occult gastro-intestinal bleeding (Croker & Beynon, 1981). The bleeding site is sometimes elusive, escaping detection by barium studies and endoscopy alone. A very few isolated demented or depressed patients may develop anaemia purely from dietary deficiency. Such patients will usually have features of generalised malnutrition. Iron deficiency anaemia is discussed at greater length in chapter 34.

COMMON DISORDERS

Gastro-oesophageal reflux

Gastro-oesophageal reflux is due to incompetence of the lower oesophageal sphincter, rather than hiatus hernia per se. Whilst it is true that sliding hiatus herniae are often associated with lack of sphincter tone and reflux, the latter may occur without demonstrable herniation. Furthermore, the vast majority of hiatus herniae are asymptomatic, mainly because sphincter function is normal or only slightly impaired (Cohen & Harris, 1971).

It is by no means certain what causes sphincteric incompetence. Rarely, contractility is lost through a process such as systemic sclerosis or malignant infiltration. There is some evidence that vagal damage may play a part (Angorn et al, 1977). Vagotomy and diabetic autonomic neuropathy may be associated with reflux

Occasional reflux is physiological and usually painless. It may be that gastric acid sensitises the mucosa so that frequent copious reflex causes oesophageal pain. Many patients with painful reflex do not have frank oesophagitis but only a hyperplasia of the oesophageal epithelium, which looks normal macroscopically. Pain occurs when posture encourages reflux under gravity and when intra-abdominal pressure is raised. There may be an associated acid taste in the mouth. This is useful diagnostically.

When frank oesophagitis results, painful swallowing, iron deficiency anaemia and even massive haemorrhage may occur. Widespread use of endoscopy has revealed that significant bleeding from oesophagitis is much more common than was once thought. It may occur in the absence of oesophageal pain.

Associated ulceration may cause fibrosis and stricture formation, with dysphagia which may be painful. Occasionally dysphagia is caused by non-propulsive contractions which are common in reflux. They frequently delay oesophageal emptying, thus exacerbating the oesophagitis, but are not normally sufficiently sustained to cause dysphagia. Atkinson (1980) has reviewed their importance.

Sometimes oesophageal ulcers heal by extension of the gastric columnar epithelium. There is frequently residual ulceration with stricture formation (Barrett, 1950). These patients should receive regular endoscopy because malignant change in the columnar epithelium is not uncommon.

Initially the diagnosis of reflux is best confirmed by barium swallow, since the procedure of endoscopy may provoke reflux, even in the normal subject. Subsequent endoscopy will show the extent of oesophagitis or biopsy may reveal the histological changes associated with reflux. Biopsy and cytology help to confirm that a stricture is benign.

In treatment, general measures are as important as drug therapy. The patient should avoid bending at the waist. The head of the bed should be raised; this is better than the use of extra pillows, since flexion of the trunk will increase intra-abdominal pressure. A high fibre diet will reduce colonic loading and straining at stool; it should be formulated as a low calorie diet for the obese. Smoking should be avoided, since nicotine causes relaxation of the sphincter.

With these measures and antacids, adequate symptom control is usually achieved. Alginate antacids have the theoretical advantage of forming a protective coating on the mucosa. Cimetidine also helps symptoms but may not accelerate the healing of oesophagitis (Behar et al, 1978). Metoclopramide increases sphincter tone, but extrapyramidal side effects are not uncommon and it should only be used when the above measures have failed. In a preparation such as Pyrogastrone, carbenoxolone sodium acts locally and need not be given in large doses. Nevertheless electrolytes should be monitored regularly in elderly patients receiving it. Strictures can normally be dilated endoscopically by the Eder-Puestow method (Royston et al, 1976). Surgery is occasionally required for persistent severe reflux.

Gastric ulcer

The prevalence of these in the elderly is difficult to ascertain accurately because of ulcer-associated deaths and pre-mortem stress ulceration in autopsy series, and because many ulcers are 'silent'. There is no doubt that they are common however, with an approximately equal sex incidence and much higher mortality than in the young. Some gastric ulcers in the elderly are very large, occupying a substantial proportion of the stomach wall. These giant ulcers are benign and often superficial, although bleeding and perforation may occur.

The aetiology remains obscure. Associated factors include liver disease, renal failure, hyperparathyroidism, family history, ingestion of aspirin and non-steroidal anti-inflammatory drugs.

It is impossible to distinguish reliably between gastric ulcer, duodenal ulcer, gastric carcinoma and several other afflictions on history alone. Thus night pain occurs in about one third of patients with symptomatic gastric ulceration (Horrocks & de Dombal, 1978). However food rarely causes pain, unlike duodenal ulceration. Some patients present with acute or chronic bleeding and occasionally perforation with little or no prior dyspepsia. Thus a high index of suspicion is required and dyspeptic symptoms should be taken seriously. It is particularly important to forewarn and arrange follow-up for patients starting anti-inflammatory drugs. Diagnosis is best made by endoscopy when benignity may be assessed, macroscopically, by biopsy and cytology.

There is some evidence that ulcers heal more rapidly after cessation of smoking. Causative drugs should be stopped. Bed rest will provoke more problems in the elderly than it will cure. Antacids and H_2 receptor antagonists undoubtedly help symptoms, but the evidence concerning promotion of ulcer healing is conflicting, in contrast to the proven value of cimetidine in duodenal ulceration. Controlled trials have been reviewed by Baron et al (1980). A more recent study suggests that tripotassium dicitrato bismuthate is effective (Sutton, 1982). Older patients achieve high serum levels of carbenoxolone sodium (Hayes et al, 1978), but it remains to be demonstrated whether smaller doses would be safe and effective in the elderly.

When cimetidine in full dosage is abruptly withdrawn, there is a high relapse rate. The value of low-dose maintenance cimetidine in preventing recurrence has not yet been established. The H_2 receptor antagonist ranitidine promises to be even safer than cimetidine, but it is a comparatively new drug.

Endoscopy should be repeated in about six weeks to ensure healing. A few of those ulcers which fail to heal will prove to be malignant. Surgery is usually indicated for persistent or recurrent ulceration, perforation and acute bleeding in the elderly.

Pyloric stenosis

Whereas the commonest cause of pyloric stenosis in the young is duodenal ulceration, in the elderly it is infiltrating gastric carcinoma. Copious vomitus of offensive odour, succussion splash and visible gastric peristalsis are found. The elderly will succumb readily to the effects of fluid and electrolyte loss and these must be corrected prior to surgery. Gastric aspiration is also essential. With these measures, oedema around the pylorus will occasionally clear sufficiently to allow elective investigation and treatment. Nevertheless the surgical team should always be consulted at an early stage.

Complications of gastric surgery

About 10% of patients develop long term symptomatic complications and, after partial gastrectomy, a much higher proportion develop anaemia.

The dumping syndrome occurs when the pylorus is rendered non-functioning, that is its ability to regulate outflow of gastric contents is lost. Symptoms occur after meals and include sweating, flushing, faintness, epigastric fullness, nausea and occasionally vomiting. It is uncommon after proximal gastric vagotomy and thus its frequency in the UK should decrease. Generally, symptoms can be controlled by taking small meals with water and by avoidance of foodstuffs found to be troublesome. Surgical revision is rarely required and may be unsuccessful.

Vomiting of bile propably occurs because of copious biliary reflux into the stomach. This is sometimes due to the afferent loop syndrome.

Stomal ulcers occur mostly after surgery for duodenal ulceration. They occasionally cause colonic fistulae. Diagnosis is technically more difficult than for other peptic ulcers, but is best made by endoscopy. Treatment is usually surgical.

Diarrhoea is common after vagotomy but is usually mild. Steatorrhoea and malabsorption occur occasionally from the blind loop syndrome. Anaemia is much more common, however. It is usually due to iron deficiency, mostly because of reduced absorption, infrequently because of chronic bleeding from a stomal ulcer. Vitamin B_{12} and rarely folate deficiency are also seen.

REFERENCES

Angorn I B, Dimopoulos G, Hegarty M M, Moshal M G 1977 The effect of vagotomy on the lower oesophageal sphincter — a manometric study. British Journal of Surgery 64: 466–469

Atkinson M 1980 The oesophagus. In: Bouchier I A D (ed) Recent Advances in Gastroenterology — 4. Churchill Livingstone, Edinburgh, p 7

Baron J H, Langman M J S, Wastell C 1980 Stomach and duodenum. In: Bouchier I A D (ed) Recent Advances in Gastroenterology — 4. Churchill Livingstone, Edinburgh, p 52

Barrett N R 1950 Chronic peptic ulcer of the oesophagus and oesophagitis. British Journal of Surgery 38: 175–182

Behar J et al 1978 Cimetidine in the treatment of symptomatic gastro-oesophageal reflux — a double blind controlled trial. Gastroenterology 74: 441–448

Cohen S, Harris L D 1971 Does hiatal hernia affect competence of the gastro-oesophageal sphincter? New England Journal of Medicine 284: 1053–1056

Coleman J A, Denham M J 1980 Perforation of peptic ulceration in the elderly. Age and Ageing 9: 257–261

Conn H O, Blitzer B L 1976 Non-association of adrenocorticosteroid therapy and peptic ulcer. New England Journal of Medicine 294: 473–479

Croker J R, Beynon G 1981 Gastro-intestinal bleeding — a major cause of iron deficiency in the elderly. Age and Ageing 10: 40–43

Daniel B, Benacerraf R 1978 La dysphagie par dyskinésie de la bouche oesophagienne. Journal de Radiologie, d'Electrologie et de Médecine Nucléaire 59: 731–734

Foster D N, Miloszewski K J A, Losowsky M S 1978 Stigmata of recent haemorrhage in diagnosis and prognisis of upper gastroinestinal bleeding. British Medical Journal i: 1173–1177

Gerhardt D C, Castell D O, Winship D H, Shuck J J 1980 Esophageal dysfunction in esophagopharyngeal regurgitation. Gastroenterology 78: 893–897

Hayes M J, Sprackling M, Langman M J S 1978 Changes in the plasma clearance and protein binding of carbenoxolone with age and their possible relationship with adverse drug effects. Gut 18: 1054–1058

Hellemans J, Vantrappen G, Pelemans W 1982 Oesophageal disorders in old people. In: Isaacs B (ed) Recent Advances in Geriatric Medicine — 2. Churchill Livingstone, Edinburgh, p 91–110

Horrocks J C, de Dombal F T 1978 Clinical presentation of patients with dyspepsia. Gut 19: 19–26

Hurwitz A L, Duranceau A 1978 Upper esophageal sphincter dysfunction. Pathogenesis and treatment. American Journal of Digestive Diseases 23: 275–281

Mee A S, Jaiswal M, Croker J R, Cotton P B 1981 Non-surgical palliation of malignant oesophageal obstruction in the elderly. Age and Ageing 10: 123–126

Royston C N, Dowling B L, Gear M J 1975 Oesophageal dilatation using Eder Puestow dilators. Gut 16: 411

Sutton D R 1982 Gastric ulcer healing with tripotassium dicitrato bismuthate and subsequent relapse. Gut 23: 621–624

Watson W C, Sullivan S N 1974 Hypertonicity of the cricopharyngeal sphincter: a cause of globus sensation. Lancet ii: 1417–1418

31

Small bowel and pancreas

S. G. P. Webster

It is very difficult to be precise about the incidence of malabsorption in the elderly. Its frequency is likely to be underestimated as it is not often regarded as a common diagnosis. When deficiency states are identified in the elderly they are in many instances assumed to be due to dietary defects. However this is too simplistic and frequently cannot be substantiated. In fact when dietary intake in old age is measured it is seen that the majority eat adequately (Exton-Smith, 1979). For example, osteomalacia when first described in geriatric patients was thought to have a dietary cause (Dent & Smith, 1969), but closer observation has forced investigators to consider alternative mechanisms (Webster et al, 1976). It is easily shown in many osteomalacic subjects that their daily intake of vitamin D is no worse than that of their contemporaries or even that of fit young controls.

Results of attempts to find the frequency of malabsorption in old age are surprising. Pelz et al (1968) reported an incidence of 7% in elderly residents of a home who were losing weight but were otherwise in a stable condition. Montgomery et al (1978) found in a survey to investigate malabsorption in old age that they detected such abnormalities in 12% of their small control group. Findings such as these may indicate malabsorption in old age is often silent and much more frequent than previously anticipated. Alternatively the high incidence of abnormal results may signify the tests used were inappropriate. It is of course possible that a combination of both explanations is responsible.

The investigation of frail elderly patients is always difficult. There are considerable practical problems with many tests of absorption. Many patients find it difficult to take the essential loading dose — for example the high fat intake for faecal fat estimations. Specimen collections are fraught with problems due to forgetfulness and incontinence. Physiological changes associated with aging also complicate many desirable investigations. Impairment of renal function invalidates tests based on the measurement of urinary excretion of test substances. Delayed bowel emptying and prolonged transit times interfere with whole body counting techniques in oral isotope tests.

Great care is therefore needed in both the selection of tests for the investigation of malabsorption in old age and in the interpretation of the results. Unfortunately it is not always possible to be as precise and exhaustive as one would wish.

CLUES TO DEFECTIVE FUNCTION

Symptoms

The most striking feature about symptoms in old age is their silence or absence. This is as true of gastro-intestinal disease as of disorders in any other system. Even conditions with dramatic symptomatology in the young may arise without warning in the elderly. Acute pancreatitis is an excellent example. So called silent pancreatitis is more common in the very old (Norris et al, 1961). Victims may suddenly collapse without obvious clues — without pain and without abdominal signs. The true diagnosis may only become apparent at examination after death. However pain is more closely associated with pancreatic disease than with small bowel disorders. Both acute and chronic pancreatitis may present with abdominal pain, sometimes also radiating into the back. Unfortunately the pain is not always clearly defined and may be difficult to differentiate from the pain of peptic ulceration and gallstones. A past history of the latter but with variation of the type of pain can be a good arouser of the suspicion of pancreatitis.

Small bowel disease is unlikely to present with pain — unless the patient has Crohn's disease — where colic may occur. Mesenteric ischaemia is also likely to be painful. The pain of the latter is usually aching in nature and the patient may be able to liken it to that of angina of effort or claudication which he may have previously experienced. In old age mesenteric ischaemia is unlikely to arise without similar vascular changes in other systems. The post prandial nature of the pain may lead to confusion with peptic ulceration.

Diarrhoea is generally another disappointingly rare symptom in gut disease in the elderly. Even where severe steatorrhoea can be recorded the patient may not be aware of any significant change in bowel habit (Ryder, 1963).

When steatorrhoea is observed it is more likely to be due to pancreatic disease than secondary to pathology in the small bowel. Abnormal bacterial colonisation of the small bowel is the most likely duodenal or jejunal cause of diarrhoea. Post-infective enzyme deficiency — especially alactasia — can also lead to prolonged episodes of loose motions. In fact milky food and drinks taken to build up the convalescent patient may prolong and aggravate the symptoms.

'Failure to thrive' is the most common symptomatic pattern to be associated with malabsorption. This may consist of weight loss associated with the symptoms due to anaemia and vague aches and pains due to bone disease. Unfortunately the causes of such vague complaints are legion and can be found in most systems. They can therefore do little more than alert the physicians to the possibility of underlying impairment of bowel and pancreatic function.

Signs

Unfortunately clinical examination of an elderly patient with pancreatic disease or malabsorption is unlikely to reveal any pathognomonic signs. General features such as wasting and cachexia may be apparent. Physical signs of anaemia and vitamin deficiencies may be observed. Pallor, atrophic changes of the skin and mucous membranes are the usual findings while pigmentation of the skin may occur in more severe cases. Finger clubbing can be manifest in severe cases of inflammatory bowel disease and chronic diarrhoea. Neurological damage due to vitamin B12 and folic acid deficiency will only rarely be found. Evidence of widespread vascular disease should be sought in suspected cases of mesenteric ischaemia. Both absent peripheral pulses and the presence of abdominal bruits and the cardiac murmurs of aortic sclerosis are all helpful signs if detected.

Examination of the abdomen generally reveals little of significance. Observation may bring to light evidence of previous surgery to the gallbladder or stomach. The former can be significant in suspected cases of pancreatitis and the latter in patients with malabsorption. Only when a carcinoma of the pancreas has spread to cause liver enlargement due to metastases is an abnormal finding likely to reward palpation of the abdomen.

ROUTINE LABORATORY TESTS

Simple laboratory tests such as the haemoglobin and peripheral blood film, urea, electrolytes and liver function tests are as routine as the extraction of the fullest possible history and a thorough physical examination. All three approaches are essential in the assessment of any elderly person presenting with an alteration of health status. Abnormalities in the laboratory tests may provide the first evidence of the possibility of underlying gastro-intestinal disease. The results may be the only early clues in the detection of the pathological mechanisms. Further tests will be necessary for the complete solution to be obtained. Much care will be required in the interpretation of all the laboratory tests, for demonstrated abnormalities may have many potential causes which may be located in any system.

Haematinic deficiencies due to malabsorption will lead to anaemia. Estimation of the haemoglobin level must be accompanied by the measurement of the red cell indices. The most commonly detected abnormality will be that of a microcytic hypochromic anaemia. Overall occult bleeding will be the most likely responsible cause but impaired absorption of iron should be considered, especially if examination of the stools for occult blood proves to be negative. Substantiation of the nature of the disorder by the measurement of the serum iron and total iron binding capacity can also be helpful.

The reporting of a macrocytic anaemia with hyperchromia is generally a more valuable finding when malabsorption is being considered. Other causes of macrocytosis, such as myxoedema, liver disease and haemolysis need to be excluded, but gut disease is the most likely underlying pathology. Further confirmation may be obtained by performing a bone marrow examination; not only may megaloblastosis be seen on the slides but an estimation can also be made about the available iron stores. Whether the megaloblastic marrow picture is due to either vitamin B12 or folic acid deficiency can only be decided by direct measurement of each substance.

In patients with macrocytic anaemia it is most common to find reduced B12 levels. The majority of these patients will be suffering from pernicious anaemia and the primary pathological fault will lie in their gastric mucosa. In only a few will a terminal ileal defect be responsible. Differentiation between the two groups will usually be made by isotope tests (see below).

Folic acid deficiency is much more common — in about 20% of elderly patients (Webster & Leeming, 1979) — but the majority of these people are not anaemic. Although dietary insufficiency is often blamed for the high incidence of folate deficiency the evidence is not very convincing. In many instances impaired small bowel function will also be contributing (Webster & Leeming, 1979).

Standard liver function tests are also useful in revealing potential causes of malabsorption and pancreatic disease. Low albumin levels are not uncommon in ill elderly patients (Hodkinson, 1977). The finding is very non-specific as it may represent malnutrition, excess loss in the urine, reduced protein metabolism by the liver or gastro-intestinal protein loss secondary to inflammatory and malignant disease as well as protein malabsorption.

A raised alkaline phosphatase level may suggest several underlying pathologies. If the enzyme can be shown, by electrophoretic techniques, to be of liver origin then metastatic disease and bile duct obstruction should be considered. Carcinoma of the pancreas would be the most likely condition amongst those discussed in this chapter. Where the elevation can be shown to be due to bone disease then osteomalacia becomes a possibility, in which case all those causes of fat malabsorption and maldigestion need to be considered — including pancreatitis, carcinoma of the pancreas, abnormal bacterial colonisation and small bowel mucosal defects. The raised alkaline phosphatase of osteomalacia may be accompanied by low calcium and phosphate levels, but this is not mandatory and should not always be expected.

Biochemical evidence of obstructive jaundice can be associated with primary carcinoma of the pancreas but other causes (metastatic disease, drug cholestasis and gallstones) need to be actively excluded.

DIFFERENTIATION BETWEEN PANCREATIC AND SMALL BOWEL DISEASE

Acute pancreatitis is a relatively easy diagnosis to make and confirm. Exceptions are those silent cases which can occur in old age. Although silent they are usually dramatic with sudden collapse of the patient and rapid deterioration. In such circumstances acute pancreatitis must be considered, along with other disasters such as perforation of a viscus, massive bleeding and myocardial infarction. The recording of a raised serum amylase level will confirm the diagnosis. Artificial elevation can be caused in patients with uraemia but the high levels which can be anticipated in genuine cases will rarely lead to confusion.

Abdominal pain, weight loss and steatorrhoea but without anaemia are a combination of findings which would suggest chronic pancreatic disease.

Steatorrhoea is still used as the first marker of bowel dysfunction. The measurement of faecal fats is difficult, tiresome and unpleasant for all concerned. However it remains the most tried and tested of the early laboratory tests. Special difficulties are likely to be encountered in geriatric patients. There may be problems in persuading the patient to take an adequate fat load in their diet of 60–100 g. Constipation (even with steatorrhoea) may mean that the faecal collection period may have to be prolonged. Memory impairment may prevent the complete and accurate collection of all specimens. When these practical complications are not applicable it remains as a useful test and one which can be very helpful in making an initial differentiation between pancreatic and small bowel disease. Pancreatic disease is likely to be responsible in over 50% of cases where any abnormality is detected, and especially so if marked steatorrhoea is recorded (Price et al, 1977).

Patients with marked steatorrhoea but a normal result to an absorption test — such as xylose absorption — will almost certainly have pancreatic disease and not a small bowel condition.

FURTHER INVESTIGATION OF THE PANCREAS

As described above the diagnosis of acute pancreatitis is relatively simple. However considerable problems are associated with the identification and differentiation of chronic and progressive pancreatic disorders. Since we have no methods of reversing chronic pancreatitis or malignant disease it is essential that such diagnoses are made early in order that the pathology may be halted or removed. By the time that gross steatorrhoea can be demonstrated on fat balance studies or jaundice due to obstruction has arisen, it will be too late for little but symptomatic intervention.

Special tests for pancreatic disease

Tests of function:
1. Serum amylase for acute pancreatitis
2. Faecal fats
3. Lundh test
4. Secretion tests

Structural examination:
1. Straight X-ray abdomen — ? calcification
2. Barium meal — may exclude gastric lesion. Duodenal loop abnormalities may be seen in pancreatic disease.
3. Ultrasound of pancreas or CAT
4. ERCP and cytology

The search continues for tubeless tests of pancreatic function. Stool examinations for fat globules, undigested meat fibres and enzyme levels can do little more than add support to a diagnostic suspicion. The glucose tolerance test is usually abnormal in young patients with pancreatic disease — but this test loses its value in the elderly because of the high frequency of altered carbohydrate metabolism with aging.

Alternatives to faecal fat balance:
1. Fluorescein test
2. Triolein breath test.

The fluorescein dilurate test may prove itself to be useful (Barry et al, 1982). The urinary excretion of fluorescein is compared after esterified and non-esterified oral doses. Renal and small bowel disturbances should not influence the results as the patient is acting as his own control, but ten hour urinary collections are needed on two separate days.

A triolein breath test (Newcome et al, 1979) is available for the study of fat absorption. However it is expensive to perform and the accuracy of the results is variable (especially in patients with respiratory disorders). Essentially 5 μCi of glyceryl C14 triolein are given with a 20 g liquid fat meal and the percentage of labelled carbon dioxide is measured in the expired air for six hours after ingestion. Steatorrhoea is suggested if less than 6% is recorded.

The most valuable tests for the functional assessment of the pancreas require intubation. There is therefore a natural reluctance to undertake them because of the inconvenience and unpleasantness for patient and investigator. However the early detection of abnormalities can only be achieved by the direct measurement of the excretions of the pancreas and their varying response to stimuli.

The Lundh test (Lundh, 1962) is the most frequently used and measures the pancreatic response to a test meal consisting of 18 g of corn or soya bean oil, 15 g of Casilan and 40 g of glucose all made up in 300 ml of water. The tryptic activity of duodenal juice obtained for two hours after ingestion of the test meal is used as a measure of pancreatic efficiency. Reduced levels of less than 10 international units or 150 μg of trypsin per ml are compatible with pancreatic disease but false positives can occur in other non-pancreatic causes of steatorrhoea. The lower the level of trypsin activity the more severe is the pancreatic disease but the results cannot differentiate between chronic pancreatitis and malignant disease (although the lowest results generally occur in the former).

Attempts can be made to try to differentiate between chronic pancreatitis and carcinoma on the basis of response to the intravenous injection of secretin (Moeller et al, 1972). In this test one unit of secretin per kg body weight is given. The duodenal aspirate is collected during the 60 minutes after the injection. A reduced volume of aspirate but with a normal bicarbonate level is suggestive of obstruction due to a carcinoma but a normal value with reduced bicarbonate suggests chronic pancreatitis. However carcinoma of the tail may give misleading results as obstruction is not a prominent feature.

In general, tests of pancreatic function do not provide sufficient information for an accurate diagnosis of the nature of any pancreatic pathology. They must be combined with attempts to visualise structural changes in the organ if a complete diagnosis is to be achieved.

In recent years there have been great developments in our ability to visualise the pancreas. Its deep-seated position had previously made the examination of its structure a difficult task. Radiology provided the first techniques for studying the anatomy of the organ (Broadbent & Kerman, 1951). Unfortunately only gross abnormalities were likely to be demonstrated, e.g. calcification in cases of chronic pancreatitis and expansion of the duodenal loop on barium meal studies by malignant growths of the pancreas. On occasions an eroding pancreatic neoplasm could be seen roughening the duodenal mucosa in contrast studies. Hypertonic duodenography has extended the value of these X-ray techniques. When allied to endoscopic retrograde cholangio-pancreatography (ERCP) the X-ray department can obtain information from the interior of the gland as the ducts and any distortions or blockages can be demonstrated. Aspiration of pancreatic excretions can be made at the same time and the fluid can be examined both biochemically and cytologically.

Although ERCP is a fruitful procedure it requires much skill and practice on the part of the operator. The patient also has to be willing and able to withstand the endoscopy. There are also potential complications, especially aggravation of pancreatitis if contrast is instilled in great volumes and under pressure. Non-invasive methods of investigation are therefore preferable if information of equally high quality can be guaranteed (Mackie et al, 1979). Isotope screening with radioactive selenium was tried but the results were disappointing and the method has fallen into disuse.

Fortunately the newer techniques of imaging are proving to be of great value in the investigation of pancreatic disease. Computer assisted tomography (Fawcitt et al, 1978) and ultrasoundography (Lees et al, 1979) appear to be equally successful in the study of structural changes in the pancreas. The latter is more freely available and is a very suitable method of examination in geriatric patients (Coles et al, 1982). Either mode of investigation can differentiate between malignant, inflammatory and fibrotic changes. They are both of value in monitoring progress in benign conditions, e.g. the follow up of cystic areas or inflammatory masses after an episode of acute pancreatitis.

It is hoped that the use of these new methods of investigation of the pancreas will lead to the early detection of treatable lesions and prevent unnecessary laparotomies and other operations in cases where the opportunity of worthwhile intervention has been lost.

INVESTIGATION OF THE SMALL BOWEL

The small bowel has several inter-related functions. Within its lumen digestion takes place, the results then need to passively or actively traverse the gut wall and finally the products need to be distributed around the body. Although these activities do not occur in isolation it is helpful to discuss individually their investigation.

Digestion is the main lumenal function and depends on the presence of adequate amounts of exocrine secretions. The pancreas is the main source and the investigation of the function of this organ has been discussed above. Consideration of enzymes released from the small bowel mucosa will be dealt with later.

Special tests for bacterial overgrowth
  1. Aspiration and culture
  2. Urinary indicans
  3. Bile salt breath test

The bacteriology of the bowel lumen is of great importance and can significantly alter the effectiveness of its function. The main concern is with changes in the normal flora and in particular with colonisation by excessive and abnormal organisms. The direct approach is to intubate, aspirate and culture. However this is an unpleasant procedure for the patient (who must be fasted overnight and must not be receiving antibiotics). Culture for anaerobic as well as aerobic organisms may be beyond the scope of a routine laboratory. Bacterial overgrowth is judged to be evident when bacteroids or E coli are found in concentrations greater than 10^5/ml (King & Toskes, 1979).

More convenient indirect methods of investigation are also available. The most convenient is the examination of the urine for indicans. An increase will be caused by bacterial overgrowth in the small bowel — levels above 80 mg per 24 hours are significant. There are problems in the elderly, especially that of ensuring that the 24 hour urine collection is complete. It has been suggested that false high levels may occur in the elderly but there appears to be no substantiating evidence for this claim (Kirkland et al, 1982).

An alternative non-invasive test is that of the C14 breath test. The procedure consists of giving (by mouth) 5 μCi of C14 labelled glycine glycocholic acid to a fasting patient. Bacteria present in the gut will then deconjugate the bile salt thus releasing the C14 which can be measured as radioactivity in expired carbondioxide — raised levels indicating increased bacterial activity. Breath collection can be difficult in elderly subjects and those with chronic respiratory disease and obesity may give false negative results (James et al, 1973).

Unfortunately both these non-invasive techniques fail to give clear-cut results in many instances.

Radiological examination by barium meal with follow through is of value in suspected cases. The demonstration of a potential site for bacterial overgrowth is an important step in making the diagnosis. Patients with small bowel diverticular disease, previous surgery (especially postgastrectomy patients with a blind loop) and patients with strictures and slow gut motility are worthy of further investigation, along the lines described above.

Special tests for small bowel disease
1. Combined oral and intravenous xylose tests
2. Dicopac to measure B12 absorption in presence of low B12
3. Small bowel biopsy

Unfortunately there is no single simple test of function for the small bowel mucosa. The xylose tolerance test has been used for the longest period of time and in spite of its drawbacks probably remains the best screening test. There are particular problems related to its use in the elderly. The greatest difficulty is the concomitant renal deterioration associated with aging. This change invalidates the usual test of oral administration linked with estimation of renal excretion of the test substance. However the renal complications can be circumvented by the combination of an intravenous test together with the more usual oral technique (Webster & Leeming, 1975b). In this method the renal impairment, which may be associated with the patient's age, will affect both tests to an equal extent. However the tests become very time consuming, needing to be separated by several days and requiring the patient to be fasted overnight on each occasion. Then either an oral dose of xylose (25 g) or an intravenous dose (5 g) is given and urine collection completed for the next 5 hours. The result must be expressed as a ratio of the excretion of the oral dose divided by the amount recovered after the intravenous test. A result greater than 1.8 represents normal function.

In the elderly the most satisfactory estimation of B12 absorption is made by using the Dicopac variation of the Schilling test (Bell et al, 1965). In this method two isotopes are needed (Cobalt 57 and Cobalt 58) to label either 'free' or 'bound' (i.e. with intrinsic factor) vitamin B12. The ratio between the two isotopes is then measured in a urine sample. Normally the result will be 1 but will depart from this if the free B12 is not properly absorbed, as in pernicious anaemia. Terminal ileum defects causing B12 deficiency will still give a result of 1. If a 24 hour urine specimen can be collected the total absorption of the test substance can be estimated but renal complications tend to invalidate this procedure in old age. B12 deficiency due to bacterial overgrowth will also give potentially misleading results.

There are also problems in the interpretation of small bowel biopsies taken from elderly patients. On dissecting microscope examination there is an increase in leaf-shaped villi. Even broader forms may also be seen but the changes of total or subtotal/villous atrophy have the same significance as in the young. Measurements of villi taken from elderly patients will also show a reduction in height of villi (Webster & Leeming, 1975a).

The technique to obtain a small bowel biopsy is unchanged in old age — tolerance to the procedure seems to be high in old subjects as their tendency to gag on swallowing the biopsy capsule appears to be reduced. It has been suggested that the investigation may be more dangerous in the elderly but this has been based on a very small number of examinations. Nevertheless extra care should be taken and careful observation should be made after the biopsy has been obtained as perforation may occur late and relatively silently (Linaker & Calam, 1978).

Biopsies may also be examined by histochemical methods in order to demonstrate any alteration in enzyme content. Polypeptide hormones may be similarly identified in special centres and valuable information about gut function and dysfunction in old age may become available from such investigations.

A damaged or inflamed small bowel mucosa may not only act as an obstacle for absorption but may also provide a site for nutrient loss. Protein loss is perhaps the most frequent and obvious problem. Confirmation of this event is very difficult. Studies with radioactive iodine labelled protein are complicated as the iodine is usually absorbed and recirculated once it has been separated from the albumin when in the gut. Chromic chloride 51 when injected intravenously attaches itself mainly to the albumin — if it then enters the gut lumen it remains unabsorbed. Estimation of the stool concentration of radioactive chromium therefore gives an indication of protein loss. Five day collections of stools are required and this makes it a difficult test to use in geriatric practice (Kerr et al, 1967).

Barium studies may demonstrate structural abnormalities, for example in Crohn's disease, but most gut wall pathologies will not be revealed on X-ray examination. If non-flocculating barium is used then the non-specific sign of clumping of the barium may be seen in the presence of steatorrhoea, whatever its cause.

Arteriography and lymphangiography are the only available methods of studying the vessels serving the gut wall. These procedures can be performed in the elderly but are rarely carried out. Such investigations can only be justified if there is the possibility of finding and locating a single well demarcated lesion. Vascular disease in old age is usually widespread and therefore not amenable to surgical intervention. Under such circumstances the majority of patients should be spared from these expensive and inconvenient investigations (Table 31.1).

Table 31.1 Interpretation of special tests for the investigation of pancreatic and small bowel disorders

	Pancreatic disease	Small bowel disease	Bacterial overgrowth
Steatorrhoea	+++	+	++
Deficient fat soluble units	+++	+	++
RCF	N	↓	N or ↑
B$_{12}$	N or ↓	↓↓	↓

+ mild increase, + + moderate increase, + + + marked increase, N normal, ↓ mild reduction, ↓↓ moderate reduction, ↑ raised.

THE MANAGEMENT OF PANCREATIC DISEASE

The management of pancreatic disease can be subdivided into patterns of measures needed during acute episodes or those required to supplement a patient with chronic pancreatic failure. These categories do tend to merge, for although acute pancreatitis may occur as an isolated incident it is more likely to be part of a relapsing picture which may proceed to a state of chronic failure.

In acute episodes the main task will be to deal with pain and to support vital functions. The pain in acute attacks may be very severe and analgesics of maximum potency may therefore be required. Pethidine is the most frequently used preparation as it is less likely than the opiates to cause nausea or vomiting or sphincter spasm. In cases of relapsing pancreatitis it may not be necessary to use such

potent preparations, although at all times it is essential that a drug is used which is sufficient to control the symptoms.

Many of these acute patients will be severely shocked and intensive supportive action will be needed. Attention will have to be paid to fluid and electrolyte correction, temperature control and respiration. Careful checking of vital signs and fluid balance will be required. Clearly many such patients will be most conveniently cared for in an intensive care unit.

It is difficult to know how much can be done to protect and encourage pancreatic function during and after these acute episodes. There is general agreement that the organ should be rested, i.e. no oral fluids should be given and the stomach and below should be kept empty by regular gastric aspiration via a nasogastric tube. Broad spectrum antibiotics are also given in many cases, the intravenous route being the most convenient as a drip is usually available. Several other interventions have been recommended but without conclusive evidence of effectiveness. The multiplicity of suggestion tends to emphasise the lack of clear-cut benefit. The use of apaprotein, glucagon and cimetidine and steroids have all been advocated and all are used, but caution is required if only on the basis of the expense of some of these preparations.

The patient's progress may be monitored by the regular checking of serum amylase levels. Structural changes can be conveniently reviewed by repeat ultrasoundography, especially in the suspected presence of pseudocyst formation. After recovery a search should be started in order to identify the underlying cause. The majority will be secondary to gallstones or alcoholism. Corrective treatment will then be required. This is much more easily achieved in the former if the patient is willing and fit enough to undergo surgery. In cases of alcohol abuse it may be possible to demonstrate to the patient a connection between binges and pain and this may be helpful in persuading the patient to regulate his lifestyle. Rarer causes of pancreatitis, such as hypercalcaemia and hyperlipidaemia should also be sought.

The correction of steatorrhoea will be the main aim in the management of patients with chronic pancreatitis. Some benefit can be gained by reducing the fat content of their diet. The alternative approach is to give oral pancreatic supplements but large amounts may be needed and thus interfere with the patient's enjoyment of his food. Up to 10 g daily may be needed in divided doses taken before meals. The precise requirements for each patient can only be calculated by titrating the effect of treatment against the patient's symptoms (steatorrhoea). In patients with gross destruction of their pancreas there may also be the problem of secondary diabetes mellitus. This should be managed in the usual ways available — depending on the severity of the condition and the patient's expected prognosis.

The place of surgery in pancreatic disease is currently

very limited. The value of cholecystectomy is clear in patients with recurrent pancreatitis due to gallstones. Pancreatectomy may be required in patients with severe pain due to chronic pancreatitis. Operations to relieve obstruction to the bile ducts would be justified in some patients with carcinoma of the pancreas. In most cases with malignant pancreatic disease the diagnosis is made at such a late stage that the possiblity of a surgical cure is very remote. When operations are attempted they are of major dimensions e.g. Whipples resection, and can only be sustained by otherwise fit patients.

All patients with steatorrhoea should be regularly reviewed with particular attention to the possibility of the development of deficiency diseases due to impaired fat absorption. Osteomalacia and a prolonged bleeding time are both worth seeking as they will respond to supplements of either vitamin D or K.

THE CAUSES AND MANAGEMENT OF SMALL BOWEL DISEASE

Advanced age does not offer protection from the familiar causes of small bowel disorders. All conditions reported in younger subjects can be encountered in geriatric practice. However the silence of the symptoms and the frailty of the patient with multiple pathology may prohibit the desired investigation and subsequent management. In very frail patients it may be impossible or inhumane to do more than identify and correct any deficiency states.

Coeliac disease
Although usually considered a condition of the young, it may be diagnosed for the first time at the end of life. Badenoch (1970) reported cases where presentation occurred after the age of 60. To confirm the diagnosis it would be necessary to show impaired xylose absorption (using an oral plus an intravenous test) in conjunction with the typical small bowel mucosal appearance on dissecting microscope examination. Ideally the small bowel biopsy should be performed initially when the patient is on a normal diet and then repeated after the exclusion of gluten from his food. A return to a normal structure after dietary adjustment adds significant strength to the diagnosis. If the patient is expected to keep to a gluten free diet it is important that the diagnosis has been confirmed beyond doubt. Initially correction of deficiency states will be required but they should not recur if the patient can be established on the gluten free diet.

Bacterial overgrowth
The lesions which encourage bacterial overgrowth are more frequently found in the elderly than in any other group. Blind loops associated with partial gastrectomies are predominantly found in patients who had troublesome

peptic ulceration in the 1940s and 1950s when they were themselves middle aged (Mellstrom & Rundgren, 1982). Small bowel diverticular disease becomes increasingly frequent with increasing age, reaching 20% of patients undergoing barium meals in a department of geriatric medicine (Pearce, 1980). Gut transit times become prolonged in old age (McEvoy et al, 1982) even without the presence of strictures or scleroderma. All these structural changes are best demonstrated by barium studies. The presence and nature of bacterial changes can be shown by the direct and indirect methods described previously. Changes in ability to absorb can be revealed by peforming tests of function before and after treatment. A course of broad spectrum antibiotic, usually tetracycline, is employed to reverse the bacterial changes. Repeat courses of treatment may be required as recolonisation can always occur while structural lesions persist. If necessary they may be removed surgically.

Mesenteric ischaemia
Acute mesenteric ischaemia is dramatic in presentation in the form of abdominal pain followed by the symptoms and signs of ileus and peritonitis. Such serious cases require urgent surgical intervention to remove the gangrenous length of small bowel. Some minor cases may be managed by resting the bowel and supporting the patient. The underlying embolic cause, such as subacute bacterial endocarditis, cardiac arrhythmia, valve disorders or myocardial infarction, should be sought and treated appropriately. Chronic mesenteric ischaemia is a less serious, but in many ways a more troublesome disorder. The pain may be difficult to differentiate from other causes; although intermittent it will be unrelenting. Deficiency states can arise because of impaired small bowel function. Steatorrhoea may be confirmed and impaired absorption of xylose demonstrated. Arteriography will rarely be justified as the patient's vascular disease is usually advanced and widespread.

Management will consist of a correction of identified nutritional deficiencies. The patient's pains may be relieved by advising small and frequent meals in order to avoid excessive functional stressing of the gut.

Inflammatory bowel disease
Crohn's disease may affect any part of the gastro-intestinal tract. It can be one of the few pathological changes that affect the terminal ileum, in which case an isolated B12 deficiency can arise. This is best differentiated from the more common pernicious anaemia by use of the double isotope Schilling test (Dycopac test). In pernicious anaemia unequal amounts of both isotopes will be found in urinary estimations; this will not be so in disorders of the terminal ileum. The diagnosis usually has to be made on the basis of radiological examinations. Intermittent areas of narrowing (string sign) with crypt formation and cobblestone

appearance of the mucosa are all highly suggestive of Crohn's disease.

Crohn's disease responds best to oral steroids — the dose being decided by the patient's symptom and response. Because of the risk of steroid side effects the total dose must be kept as low as possible. Sulphasalazine may also have a role to play in the long term management of this condition. Surgical intervention will be required in the presence of obstructive complications or significant fistula formation.

Protein-losing gastroenteropathy
This is always a difficult diagnosis to prove, especially in the elderly. However it is in this age group that causes are more frequent. The best documented cases are due to lesions in the upper gastro-intestinal tract, especially atrophic gastritis and carcinoma of the stomach. In addition it may accompany small bowel causes of malabsorption and also inflammatory disease of the duodenum, jejunum and ileum. Amyloidosis is another reported cause; although rare it is more likely to be found in the elderly where a generalised increase in amyloid tissue is sometimes reported as part of the aging process. Encouragement to take a high protein diet is clearly going to be an important part in the management of these patients, especially where the underlying disease has no specific treatment.

Gastro-intestinal infections
The majority of these are viral in nature and will resolve spontaneously but during this period the patient may need expertly supervised management of fluid and electrolyte replacement. Bacterial infections will also be treated conservatively in most instances, unless evidence can be shown of widespread dispersion of the organism (e.g. positive blood cultures). Specific antibiotic treatment will then be required. It should also be remembered that gastro-intestinal TB still occurs and especially in the elderly where ileal disease may still be encountered.

Miscellaneous
Malabsorption can occur as a complication of several systemic diseases or their treatment. The association between skin and gut disorders should not be forgotten. Patients with dermatitis herpetiformis and psoriasis seem most at risk. Vascular disorders, such as arteritis and slow flow diseases (e.g. polycythaemia) may also have gut symptoms and signs. Malignant disease and rheumatoid disease may also influence the efficiency of the small bowel. Patients receiving neomycin, alcohol, biguanides and cholestyramine are all at risk from developing mild malabsorption.

REFERENCES

Badenoch J 1960 Steatorrhoea in the adult. British Medical Journal 2: 879–887

Barry R E, Barry R, Erie M D, Parker G 1982 Fluorescein dilaurate — tubeless test for pancreatic exocrine failure. Lancet 2: 742–744

Bell T K, Bridges J M, Nelson M G 1965 Simultaneous free and bound radioactive vitamin B12 urinary excretion test. Journal of Clinical Pathology 18: 611–613

Broadbent T R, Kerman H D 1951 100 cases of carcinoma of the pancreas — a clinical and roentgenological analysis. Gastroenterology 17: 163–177

Coles J A, Beynon G P J, Lees W R 1982 The use of ultrasoundography in Geriatric Medicine. Age and Ageing 11: 145–152

Dent C E, Smith R 1969 Nutritional osteomalacia. Quarterly Journal of Medicine 38: 195–209

Exton-Smith A N 1979 Nutrition and Health in Old Age. DHSS Report on Health and Social Subjects. HMSO, London

Fawcitt R A, Forbes W A C, Isherwood I, Braganza J M, Howat H T 1978 Computed tomography in pancreatic disease. British Journal of Radiology 51: 1–4

Hodkinson H M 1977 Biochemical diagnosis of the elderly. Chapman and Hall, London

James O F W, Agnew J E, Bouchier I A D 1973 Assessment of the C14 glycocholic acid breath test. British Medical Journal 3: 191–195

Kerr R M, Dubois J J, Holt P R 1967 Use of I and Cr labelled albumin for the measurement of gastrointestinal and total albumin catabolism. Journal of Clinical Investigation 46: 2064–2082

King C E, Toskes C P 1979 Small intestinal bacterial overgrowth. Gastroenterology 76: 1035–1055

Kirkland J L, Vargar E, Brocklehurst J 1982 Indican excretion in healthy young and old control subjects and chronically ill elderly patients. British Geriatrics Society 27

Lees W R, Vallon A G, Denyer M E, Vahl S P, Cotton P B 1979 Prospective study of ultrasoundography in chronic pancreatic disease. British Medical Journal 1: 162–164

Linaker B D, Calam J 1978 Jejunal biopsy with the Watson capsule and perforation in the elderly. Gastroenterology 75: 723–725

Lundh G 1962 Pancreatic exocrine function in neoplastic and inflammatory disease — a simple and reliable new test. Gastroenterology 42: 275–280

McEvoy A W, Fenwick J D, Boddy K, James O F W 1982 Vitamin B12 absorption from the gut does not decline with age in normal elderly humans. Age and Ageing 11: 180–183

Mackie C B, Cooper M J, Lewis M H, Moosa A R 1979 Non-operative differentiation between pancreatic cancer and chronic pancreatitis. Annals of Surgery 189: 480–487

Mellström D, Rundgren A 1982 Long-term effects after partial gastrectomy in elderly men. Scandinavian Journal of Gastroenterology 17: 433–439

Moeller D D, Dunn G D, Klotz A P 1972 Comparison of the pancreozymin-secretion test and the Lundh test meal. American Journal of Digestive Disease 17: 799–805

Montgomery R D, Haeney M R, Ross I N, Sammons H G, Barford A V, Balakrishnan S, Meyer P P, Culank L S, Field J, Gosling P 1978 The ageing gut: a study of intestinal absorption in relation to nutrition in the elderly. Quarterly Journal of Medicine 186: 197–211

Newcomer A D, Hofmann A F, Dimagnio E P, Thomas P J, Carlson G L 1979 Triolein breath test — A sensitive and specific test for fat malabsorption. Gastroenterology 76: 6–13

Norris T St M, Good C J 1961 Pancreatitis: a retrospective review of 92 cases. Postgraduate Medical Journal 37: 792–797

Pearce V R 1980 The importance of duodenal diverticular in the elderly. Postgraduate Medical Journal 56: 777–780

Pelz K S, Gottfried S P, Soos E 1968 Intestinal absorption studies in the aged. Geriatrics 23: 149–153

Price H L, Gaszard B G, Dawson A M 1977 Steatorrhoea in the elderly. British Medical Journal 1: 1582–1584

Rubini M E, Sheahy T W 1961 Exudative enteropathy. A comparative study of $^{51}CrCl_3$ and $^{131}IPVP$. Journal of Laboratory and Clinical Medicine 58: 892–901

Ryder J B 1963 Steatorrhoea in the elderly. Gerontologia Clinica 5: 30–37

Webster S G P 1973 Small bowel function and structure in the elderly. M.D. Thesis. London University

Webster S G P, Leeming J T 1975a The appearance of the small bowel mucosa in old age. Age and Ageing 4: 168–174

Webster S G P, Leeming J T 1975b Assessment of small bowel function in the elderly using a modified xylose tolerance test. Gut 16: 109–113

Webster S G P, Leeming J T, Wilkinson E M 1976 The causes of osteomalacia in the elderly. Age and Ageing 5: 119–122

Webster S G P, Leeming J T 1979 Erythrocyte folate levels in young and old. Journal of the American Geriatrics Society 27: 451–454

32

Disorders of the lower bowel

J. C. Brocklehurst

Disorders of the lower bowel in old age can be divided into three main categories — those which are common at any age, those which become increasingly more prevalent with advancing age and constipation. Since the first two groups are well dealt with in textbooks of general medicine and surgery, less emphasis will be laid upon them here. Constipation and its complication, faecal incontinence, are major geriatric problems and will be dealt with in more detail.

CONSTIPATION

Constipation means a frequency of defaecation which is diminished below the subject's normal habit, a difficulty in passing stools because of their hardness or a combination of both of these things. The range of normal bowel habit described by Connell and his associates (1965) lies between three stools a week and three stools a day. This frequency did not change in the over 65s. They found however that the over 65s are greater consumers of laxatives, and, while it might be argued that this is evidence of a tendency to constipation, it is also arguable that this is a cohort effect stemming from the first two decades of this century when the theory of auto-intoxication from the colon was rife and laxative taking became an almost universal habit. Constipation however is a very real problem with the immobile and this includes that group of old people who are extremely disabled, many of them living in institutions.

There are probably two reasons why immobile people become constipated. The first is because the gastrocolic reflex (the production of mass peristalsis of the colon as a result of food entering the stomach and duodenum) is unlikely to occur in association with total immobility. In these people therefore the call to stool may not develop and constipation ensues. The other reason is that if the gastrocolic reflex is present, the disabled person may be unable to respond to it without the help of a nurse or other attendant, and if help is not forthcoming at the appropriate time, the need for defaecation is suppressed and may not be recalled at will later. The constipated old person gradually develops the 'terminal reservoir syndrome' — the gradual build up of faeces in the sigmoid and rectum and eventually more proximally to the colon. If it persists, the extraction of water may lead to hard scybalous masses which in turn produce faecal impaction.

Constipation of course may be a symptom of intrinsic disease of the lower bowel, of some generalised diseases such as hypothyroidism and depression or may be the effect of drugs including codeine and the anticholinergics. If there is uncertainty from the history and clinical examination as to whether or not constipation is present, it may usually be confirmed by straight X-ray of the abdomen or by a measurement of intestinal transit time. The simplest method of undertaking the transit time is for the patient to swallow one or more capsules containing 20 or 25 tiny radio-opaque markers and for the abdomen to be X-rayed three and six days later. Normally 80% of the markers should have been passed by the third day. If they persist, then their disposition in the rectum and lower sigmoid will be indicated.

The prevention of constipation requires exercise and the ingestion of a reasonable quantity of fibre. In all but the very immobile, 20 g a day of unprocessed bran is usually effective.

Once constipation has developed it may be successfully dealt with by laxatives, but if the terminal reservoir syndrome is present it will almost certainly require treatment from below — by enemas and/or suppositories. The 130 ml phosphate enema (Fletchers, Fleet) is usually effective but two in succession may be required and a long nozzle may be necessary to get above the impacting mass at the anus. This is best done by adding a piece of rubber tubing to the nozzle. Care must be taken with the plastic nozzle since necrosis of the bowel wall has been reported as a result of injury during insertion followed by the necrotic effect of the hypertonic solution. A 5 ml enema (Micralax) is sometimes effective. Bisocodil or glycerol suppositories may be used as alternatives. If a good result follows this treatment then the procedure should be repeated every day until no more faecal matter is passed. This may require 7–10 days of treatment.

In order to overcome this prolonged treatment and obtain a complete evacuation at one time, two other methods have been proposed. One is whole gut irrigation by normal saline run through an intragastric tube at the rate of 2.5 1 per hour. In a patient prepared by intravenous frusemide and metoclopramide, an average of 8 1 over three hours is required for complete emptying (Smith et al, 1978). The other approach is by the use of mannitol 10% solution, cooled and flavoured with fruit. One litre followed by up to 2 1 of normal saline (or other clear fluid) should be drunk over 1–2 hours.

Once the severe constipation has been cleared, its recurrence must be prevented in patients who remain immobile. A high fibre diet and phosphate enemas once or twice a week is probably the best preventative treatment.

There are two important complications of severe constipation in the elderly — idiopathic megacolon and faecal incontinence. The former may be further complicated by volvulus of the sigmoid colon or by diarrhoea due to bacterial overgrowth, requiring treatment with metronidazole.

FAECAL INCONTINENCE

Faecal incontinence is one of the most unpleasant and degrading conditions that can afflict an old person. It is extremely common in long-stay wards — prevalence rates of up to 50% have been reported. Very largely it is preventable. An understanding of the causes of this important condition requires first a consideration of the mechanisms which normally maintain anal continence. There are at least three of these. The first is the ano-rectal angle maintained by the puborectalis muscle which acts as a sling (Fig. 32.1). This angle provides an effective valve but if it is increased above 115° incontinence will follow. The

second is the flutter valve formed by the slit-like anal canal, which maintains closure without the need for great external force above that of the atmospheric pressure. The third is the constant contraction of the internal and external anal sphincters.

The normal process of defaecation follows the entry of faeces into the rectum as the result of a gastrocolic reflex. This is immediately followed by an increase in intrarectal pressure, a relaxation of the internal sphincter and a sensation of distension and desire to defaecate. This may be followed by relaxation of the levator ani, obliterating the anorectal angle and allowing the bolus to impinge on the upper end of the anal canal where there are nerve sensors which can discriminate between faeces, fluid and flatus. If time and place are appropriate defaecation may follow, but if not, the person with an intact nervous system is able to resist the urge to defaecate, the bolus returns to the rectum and the anorectal angle is restored. Contraction reappears in the internal sphincter and the faeces may indeed pass back to the sigmoid.

These mechanisms may be impaired in various ways. In the chronically constipated person the faecal mass will obliterate the anorectal angle (Fig. 32.2). The sphincter may have diminished contractility and semi-solid faeces may seep through the anus, producing a fairly continuous faecal incontinence. Recent work by Percy and colleagues (1982) suggests a partial denervation of the muscles of the external sphincter, the puborectalis and the levator ani, possibly as a result of aging or following a trauma at childbirth or in other ways. This is accompanied by impairment of sensation, loss of sphincter tone leading to a patulous anus and loss of the anorectal angle. All of these changes may predispose to incontinence, not only in the presence of constipation but also in diarrhoeal states. In

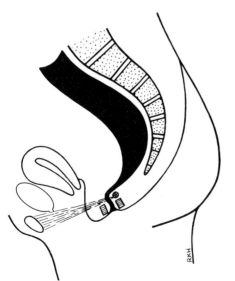

Fig. 32.1 The ano-rectal angle maintained by the pubo-rectalis muscle

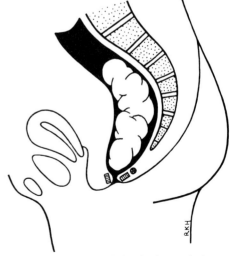

Fig. 32.2 The ano-rectal angle lost in the terminal reservoir syndrome

these conditions the sampling of the bolus may be less critical and it may be interpreted as flatus rather than fluid. The other continence mechanisms are also impaired.

Another cause of faecal incontinence in the elderly is loss of the power to resist voluntarily the rectal distension reflex and so an uninhibited defaecation occurs. This is most commonly the case in patients with multiple cerebrovascular disease or severe Alzheimer's disease in whom a formed stool may be passed once or twice a day in association with the mass peristalsis of the gastrocolic reflex.

A classification of faecal incontinence is shown in Table 32.1. Its treatment requires first a diagnosis of the cause and the treatment of that condition. If it is neurogenic

Table 32.1 Classification of faecal incontinence

Constipation	— Retention with overflow
Neurogenic	
Cortical	— Loss of inhibition
Spinal	— Reflex
Muscle atrophy	— 'Stress' incontinence
Diarrhoeal states	— Local causes

incontinence due to cerebral cortical disease, control may be achieved by a regime alternating a laxative such as Senokot at night and a constipating mixture such as codeine phosphate or chalk and opium in the morning. Alternatively, attempts at re-education in this condition and in loss of function in motor units (stress incontinence) may be by the use of biofeedback mechanisms together with pelvic floor exercises (MacLeod, 1979).

DIVERTICULAR DISEASE

In Western countries the development of colonic diverticula is an age-associated phenomenon and a great deal of evidence suggests that it is secondary to a life-long low fibre diet. The diverticula develop first in the sigmoid and then may spread in a cephalic direction throughout the whole colon. They are associated with high pressures, generated within the haustra of the colon, and these in turn are due to an overactivity of the segmental motility (sometimes described as shuttling motility since it moves the colonic bolus backwards and forwards). It is thought that this segmental motility at the sigmorectal junction has the effect of a functional sphincter — preventing the onward movement of colonic contents into the rectum. The lower the residue of these contents, the harder this mechanism has to work and the higher pressures are generated. The diverticula themselves develop in the pathway of the perforating branch of the marginal artery (Fig. 32.3) and so the developed diverticulum has this artery in its wall. This is the reason why bleeding is a common complication of diverticular disease (Meyers et al, 1976).

Pain is the most common presenting symptom of

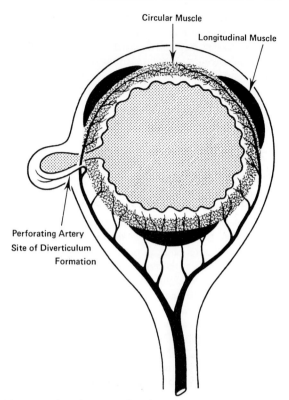

Fig. 32.3 Site of development of colonic diverticulum — showing intimate relationship with perforating artery (Brocklehurst & Hanley, 1982: With the permission of Churchill-Livingstone)

diverticular disease, characteristically in the left iliac fossa. It is a colicky pain due to contraction of the circular muscle. In the presence of diverticulitis the character of the pain is different and is due to peritoneal irritation. Alteration in bowel habit is another important symptom, constipation being more common than diarrhoea. Both may be present. Rectal bleeding occurs in about 30% and urinary symptoms in about half that number due either to an inflamed diverticulum in contact with the bladder or, rarely, to a colovesical fistula. In the latter case, gas may be passed after micturition and there may be faecal matter in the urine. Nausea and vomiting are also common symptoms of diverticular disease.

Tenderness and a mass are often palpable in the left iliac fossa. In the presence of diverticulitis there may be constitutional signs of infection and all the signs of peritoneal irritation.

A number of conditions are associated with diverticular disease which probably have a common aetiology in low fibre intake over a long period of time. These include haemorrhoids, varicose veins, hiatus hernia, abdominal hernia and gallstones (Brodribb & Humphreys, 1976).

A high fibre diet (containing 20 g of unrefined bran) or two or more sachets of ispaghula (fibogel) or other bulking agent such as methyl cellulose will remove pain due to colic and correct associated constipation. An antispasmodic such as propantheline may also be used. Haemorrhage from a diverticulum requires blood transfusion in the first instance and in most cases surgery is not necessary. Diverticulitis requires antibiotics; abscess or fistula need surgical intervention.

ISCHAEMIC COLITIS

Since atherosclerosis is so commonly the cause of disease in most organs of the body, it is surprising that vascular disorders of the alimentary tract are not more common. The colon has a particularly rich anastomotic circulation through a marginal artery which distributes blood from the superior and inferior mesenteric arteries. The most vulnerable point is at the splenic flexure 'Griffith's point'. In fact quite considerable arteriosclerotic change in the long colic arteries (from the marginal artery to the gut wall) has been demonstrated (Bins & Isaacson, 1978).

In addition to impairment of blood vessels, drop in blood pressure is an equally important factor and commonly precipitates the attack of ischaemic colitis. This may be due to dehydration, congestive cardiac failure or haemorrhage. Other associated conditions are polycythaemia, arteritis and the use of digitalis.

Ischaemic colitis is probably under-diagnosed because it is a transient ischaemic condition. It presents most commonly with left-sided abdominal pain and loose and blood stained stools. Abdominal tenderness, abdominal distension, pyrexia and loss of intestinal sounds may all be present. The diagnosis is confirmed by findings on barium enema, which are mostly due to mucosal oedema. These include the thumb-print sign, the saw-tooth sign and sometimes an appearance of pseudopolyps.

Treatment should be conservative with fluids, antibiotics and low molecular weight dextran. If the condition progresses to gangrene, colectomy will be required and the prognosis is poor.

ULCERATIVE COLITIS

Ulcerative colitis may present for the first time in old age and probably about a quarter of all cases occur in the elderly. The most common presenting symptom is diarrhoea which may be associated with faecal incontinence. This may be associated with lower abdominal pain, tenesmus and urgency of micturition. Haemorrhage is less common than in younger patients. Perforation with acute peritonitis may be a difficult diagnosis to make in old age because of the absence of pain. The patient may present with acute brain failure and the appearances of a toxic state.

In about a quarter of patients ulcerative colitis is confined to the rectum and in some cases there is a mild granular proctitis without ulceration. The diagnosis depends on sigmoidoscopy and biopsy and the treatment is the same as in younger patients. Either sulphasalazine (0.5 g twice daily, which may be increased to a total of 2 g daily) or else prednisolone (20 mg daily) are required. If this is unsuccessful then panproctocolectomy with the formation of an ileostomy may be necessary. In acute fulminating cases dilatation of the colon may present as an acute surgical emergency.

CROHN'S DISEASE

Around 15% of cases of Crohn's disease present in old age. It is then more common in females and more likely to affect the left side of the colon and rectum. Histologically the disease differs from ulcerative colitis in affecting the whole thickness of the bowel wall and also in being discontinuous. Anal lesions and fistulae between the lower rectum and the skin are not uncommon in this disease. The presenting symptoms are similar to those of ulcerative colitis but the above features are characteristic of Crohn's disease. Medical treatment of the condition is similar to that for ulcerative colitis — sulphasalazine and corticosteroids being the first line of approach. If this fails, or in the presence of abscess and fistula, surgical treatment may be necessary.

CARCINOMA OF THE COLON AND RECTUM

Lower bowel cancer is the commonest form of malignant disease in old age. Carcinoma of the rectum occurs twice as often in males as in females but in the colon the sex incidence is similar. Lower bowel cancer has considerable geographical variations, being relatively rare in Africa and Asia, and differences in dietary habits may account for this variation. High fibre diet may be protective by increasing the bulk of the stool and also increasing the rate of its passage. This may dilute the effect of any carcinogenic material contained in the faeces. One suggestion is that unsaturated bile acids provide this carcinogenic factor.

Cancers in the lower bowel develop from adenomas and occasionally more than one carcinoma may be present. The importance of early diagnosis is stressed by the good results of radical surgery — around 70% five year survival. There is some variation according to whether or not treatment is carried out at a specialist centre.

Since this disease is common and since early treatment provides optimistic results the possibility of a screening procedure to provide early diagnosis has been considered by many workers. However no cost effective programme has yet been forthcoming.

ANGIODYSPLASIA OF THE COLON

It is suggested that the commonest cause of colonic bleeding and so one of the main causes of iron deficiency anaemia is the recently described condition of colonic angiodysplasia. These angiomas or vascular ectasias develop particularly in the ascending colon and it is suggested that they are age-associated phenomena, similar in that respect to diverticula. Indeed one theory is that circular muscle contraction throughout a life time may obstruct the small venules returning from the colonic villi and so cause submucous varicosities — the ectasias. It is only recently that they have been described since they cannot be recognised at operation nor at autopsy. They can be diagnosed only by colonoscopy or on arteriography and one or other of these methods must be employed in their treatment — which is either by endoscopic coagulation or by surgical resection (Leading article, 1981).

REFERENCES

Bins J C, Isaacson P 1978 Age related changes in the colonic blood supply: their relevance to ischaemic colitis. Gut 19: 384–390

Brocklehurst J C, Hanley T 1982 Geriatric Medicine for Students, 2nd edn. Churchill-Livingstone, Edinburgh

Brodribb A J M, Humphreys D M 1976 Diverticular disease — three studies. British Medical Journal 1: 424–429

Connell A M, Hilton C, Irving G, Lennard-Jones J E, Misiewicz J J 1965 Variations of bowel habit in two population samples. British Medical Journal 2: 1095–1099

Leading article 1981 Angiodysplasia. Lancet 2: 1086–1087

MacLeod J H 1979 Biofeedback in the management of partial anal incontinence. Diseases of Colon and Rectum 22: 169–171

Meyers M A 1976 Griffith's point — critical anastomosis at the splenic flexure. American Journal of Roentology 126: 77–94

Percy J P, Neill M E, Kandiah T K, Swash M 1982 A neurogenic factor in faecal incontinence in the elderly. Age and Ageing 11: 175–179

Smith R G, Curry A E J, Walls A D F 1978 Whole gut irrigation, new treatment for constipation British Medical Journal 3: 396–397

33

Liver and gallbladder disease

O.F.W. James

INTRODUCTION

In normal man the liver accounts for about 2.5% body weight at the age of 50 and subsequently becomes gradually both relatively and absolutely smaller so that by the age of 90 it represents only c.1.6% body weight. Liver blood flow decreases in parallel with declining liver volume and falls from maximum c.1400 ml/min to 1000 ml/min age 65 and 800 ml/min age 75.

LIVER FUNCTION

Conventional liver function tests — serum bilirubin, alkaline phosphatase and transaminases (LFTs) — do not alter with increasing age in normal man. There may be a slight mean fall in serum albumin but results stay within what may be regarded as the normal range for all adults (James, 1983).

The effect of increased age upon the metabolic activities of the liver is very variable. Broadly speaking microsomal enzyme activity (oxidation, hydroxylation, demethylation) is mildly or moderately impaired whereas conjugation reactions (sulphation or glucuronidation for example) do not apear to decline markedly. Other extraneous factors like changes in nutrition, alcohol and cigarette consumption may also play an important part in determining changes in hepatic function in the elderly. Drug extraction from the portal blood (first pass effect) may be substantially reduced so that the systemic bioavailability and hence activity may be substantially enhanced. To summarise, it appears that hepatic function declines slowly with age, probably roughly in proportion to its decreasing size and declining blood flow. Such a deterioration does not affect the normal static conventional measurements of liver function but the interaction between increased age and stress due to one or more diseases may lead to a marked decline in such dynamic functions as protein synthesis or the clearance of foreign or toxic material and this may become of considerable clinical importance.

INVESTIGATION OF HEPATOBILIARY DISEASE

The object of investigation of hepatobiliary disease in an elderly individual is to arrive at a diagnosis as quickly and with as little discomfort or danger to the patient as possible. The flow charts (Fig. 33.1) summarise diagnostic strategies.

Basic blood tests

All elderly patients with suspected liver disease should have a complete set of blood tests (McIntyre, 1982).

Basic blood tests
Liver function tests (LFTs)
Blood count, film, clotting
Serum Proteins
HBV markers
Autoantibody screen
 + immunoglobulins

'Secondary blood tests'
Alphafaetoprotein
Ferritin
α-l-antitrypsin
Gamma G T
Blood ethanol (outpatient)

1. Liver function tests: Bilirubin, Alkaline Phosphatase, Transaminase (AST)
If serum AST is elevated to a markedly greater extent than alkaline phosphatase then LFTs may be considered 'hepatitic'. If the abnormality is roughly equivalent then LFTs may be considered equivocal. If alkaline phosphatase is markedly more elevated then LFTs may be considered cholestatic (obstructive). Serum gamma glutamyl-transpeptidase (γGT) is a useful enzyme to confirm cholestasis i.e. that an elevated alkaline phosphate is due to hepatobiliary disease, not to bone disease.

2. Blood count and film: (Mean corpuscular volume (MCV), Platelet count, Reticulocytes)
The MCV is often elevated in alcoholic liver disease, even in the presence of normal serum folate and B12. If alcoholic

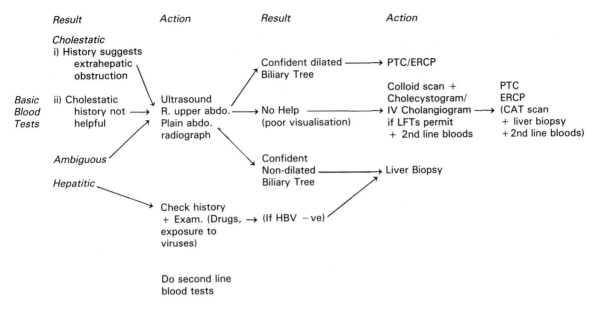

Fig. 33.1 Diagnostic strategies in hepatobiliary disease in the elderly

liver disease is suspect a random blood ethanol in clinic may be useful (Chanarin, 1979).

3. Serum proteins:

4. Hepatitis B virus (HBV) markers: HBsAg (Australia antigen), Anti HBs, Anti HBc
If HBsAg +ve then e antigen/antibody; HBsAg should be checked immediately on all patients with suspected liver disease. The e antigen is part of the HB virus core. Its presence in the serum indicates continuing active replication of whole virus in the liver thus high infectivity. Antibody to e (anti HBe) implies little or no active replication of whole virus in the liver. Antibody to the core of the HBV – anti HBc is the most sensitive serum marker of previous HBV infection. It appears shortly after the outset of an HBV infection and remains present in the serum for many years, often for life. HBsAg –ve anti HBc +ve patients are not infectious.

5. Autoantibody screen: Antimitochondrial antibody (AMA), Antismoothmuscle antibody (SMA) Antinuclear factor (ANA)
While low titre (1 in 10) of AMA, SMA or ANA are regarded as non specific findings not only in a variety of liver diseases but occasionally in apparently normal individuals, higher titres of these antibodies are of great significance. A positive AMA ≥ 1/40 together with any elevation of alkaline phosphatase is highly suggestive of primary biliary cirrhosis (PBC) (James et al, 1981); similarly positive SMA ≥ 1/40 suggests chronic active hepatitis; ANA may also be elevated in this group of diseases (Sherlock, 1981).

Non-invasive hepatobiliary imaging

Ultrasound
The great advantages of ultrasound are that it is painless, safe and rapid. Despite major advances in recent technology the great disadvantages of ultrasound examination of the hepatobiliary system are:
1. It is highly operator dependent.
2. A proportion of patients are poor sonar subjects because of gas in the upper abdomen or obesity (Okuda, 1981).
For these reasons published reports of the diagnostic efficacy and accuracy of ultrasound appear overoptimistic to many who obtain a routine ultrasound service from busy radiological departments. With the above caveat ultrasound should now be regarded as the first investigation (together with plain abdominal radiograph) of possible hepatobiliary disease after history taking, clinical examination and initial laboratory tests. It is claimed that in good hands ultrasonography is capable of distinguishing the nature of a case of jaundice with over 95% accuracy; that is to say that it can distinguish extrahepatic obstruction versus parenchymal liver disease, and can indicate the site of obstruction i.e. above or below the gallbladder. It is far less reliable at distinguishing the exact nature of such obstruction and it is unwise to rely on ultrasound to distinguish the cause of obstruction at the lower end of the common bile duct (Frommhold & Wolf, 1983). If ultrasound examination confidently shows a non-dilated biliary tree then, assuming clotting and platelets are satisfactory, needle biopsy of the liver is safe and may well be the next investigation (Fig. 33.1). Ultrasound may be less reliable in the diagnosis of intrahepatic lesions apart from those filled with fluid since the sonar interface between a tumour and surrounding liver may be ill-defined.

Radio-isotope imaging

Injection of a labelled colloid (usually ^{99m}Tc colloid) leads to uptake by the reticuloendothelial system, notably the Kuppfer cells within the liver. This procedure is again safe and simple for the patient. Whereas ultrasound is best for possible extrahepatic disease colloid scanning is most useful for intrahepatic disease. The scan can detect space occupying lesions (SOL) of greater than c.3 cm within the liver since tumours, cysts, abscesses etc do not contain Kuppfer cells and thus do not take up colloid. The second use of isotope scan is in the evaluation of chronic liver disease since patchy uptake of colloid and 'spill-over' into an enlarged spleen is suggestive of chronic liver disease although it does not exclude infiltration of the liver (Mountford, 1982). In a second form of hepatobiliary isotope scanning derivatives of iminodiacetic acid (IDA) are injected intravenously. IDA compounds are taken up by the hepatocytes and excreted into the bile; the gallbladder is usually outlined within an hour. Concentration of labelled IDA in a large gallbladder on scan indicates low biliary obstruction. In patients with cholecystitis there is little or no uptake of the IDA compound into the gallbladder, often because of cystic duct obstruction. This is therefore an attractive method of confirming a diagnosis of cholecystitis in patients with abnormal LFTs in whom oral cholecystography would not be successful. As with all imaging techniques it should be stressed that experience in use and interpretation is vital. Occasional recourse to such investigations will lead to misleading results or poor interpretation (Taylor et al, 1980).

Computed tomography (CT)

CT scanning has comparable sensitivity in the investigation of the extrahepatic biliary tree and adjacent organs to that of a real-time ultrasound examination by an experienced operator. Since CT is painless and safe it is an attractive imaging method but 1. it is time consuming, 2. extremely expensive and 3. by no means universally available (Frommhold & Wolf, 1983). At present therefore, CT scanning cannot be said to have a place in the 'routine' investigation of hepatobiliary disease in the elderly. In cases where other diagnostic methods have provided conflicting results or in the careful consideration of the operability of tumours it has an invaluable place if available (Levitt et al, 1977).

Biliary radiology

Cholecystography and intravenous cholangiography

With the advent of other non-invasive hepatobiliary imaging techniques on the one hand and of ERCP and PTC (see below) on the other the indications for oral cholecystography and intravenous cholangiography are much reduced (Berk et al, 1981). In patients with suspected gallbladder disease and with normal LFTs a clear ultrasound view of stones in the gallbladder and a normal CBD probably obviates the necessity for cholecystography. Poor ultrasound examination or inadequate facilities mean that oral cholecystography may still be usefully carried out in many centres however. Similarly in patients without marked cholestasis in whom an inadequate visualisation of the biliary tree has been obtained by other means and in whom common bile duct stones or obstruction are suspected, an infusion intravenous cholangiogram, preferably with tomograms, is a reasonable investigation, particularly in circumstances where ERCP is impossible to obtain.

ERCP and PTC

After ultrasound scan direct visualisation of the biliary tree either by percutaneous transhepatic cholangiography (PTC) or by endoscopic retrograde cholangiography (ERCP) is the method of choice in providing precise information as to the presence or absence of biliary obstruction and pathology and its possible site. The advantages and drawbacks of each technique are shown in Table 33.1. In very experienced hands ERCP probably has the edge in diagnostic and therapeutic yield but not only is

Table 33.1 The advantages and disadvantages of ERCP and PTC in the investigation of hepatobiliary disease in the elderly.

	Advantages	Disadvantages
ERCP	1. Visualisation of ampulla + of stomach + duodenum	1. Technically difficult + needs sophisticated interaction of staff + equipment
	2. Additional information from pancreatogram likely.	2. Success rate in showing biliary tree c.60% in most hands (85% in super centres)
	3. Possibility of therapeutic procedures (mostly stones) a) endoscopic papillotomy b) insertion of biliary drain or prosthesis	3. Sepsis + cholangitis, pancreatitis are complications
	4. Easier than PTC for undilated ducts	4. Impossible after some gastric surgery
PTC	1. Relatively simple to learn; no sophisticated equipment needed	1. Less successful in non-dilated biliary tree (Depends on number of passes into liver) – average c.70%
	2. Almost always successful in patients with dilated biliary tree (over 95%) 3. Possibility of therapeutic procedures (mostly tumour); insertion of prostheses through tumours in biliary tree.	2. Complications of cholangitis/Septicaemia + biliary leak

it technically more difficult but hospital stay and complications after ERCP, particularly after sphincter-otomy, are perhaps greater than sometimes realised (Sloof et al, 1980). In less experienced centres PTC, particularly if dilated ducts have been demonstrated by ultrasound, is probably the investigation of choice (Cotton, 1983). In either instance elderly patients should a) be receiving intravenous fluids for at least 12 hours after the procedure to guard against dehydration; b) receive a dose of intravenous antibiotic – usually an aminoglycoside – just prior to the examination and c) receive 200 ml 10% mannitol IV just after the procedure if biliary obstruction is confirmed.

Liver biopsy
Percutaneous needle biopsy of the liver is the cornerstone of diagnosis in parenchymal liver disease (Burroughs & Scheuer, 1982).

It is well tolerated by the elderly and is safe. The management of liver disease rests upon reliable interpretation of hepatic histology. Routine stains should include haematoxylin and eosin, an iron stain and a stain for connective tissue. Other special stains may be necessary (Scheuer, 1980).

PARENCHYMAL LIVER DISEASE

The spectrum of liver disease seen in the elderly is as wide as that seen in younger patients but diagnostic expectations may be different. Whereas few patients presenting with jaundice aged 20 have extrahepatic obstruction due to pancreatic cancer the reverse is true in those aged 80. Estimates of the relative frequency of malignant disease, gallstones or parenchymal disease as a cause of jaundice in the elderly vary substantially. Some authors find that over 80% elderly patients presenting with jaundice have cancer or gallstones, in other series these diagnoses account for less than 50% patients (Croker, 1982).

Acute hepatitis
The clinical features of acute viral hepatitis are similar in elderly and younger patients. In developed countries type A hepatitis is becoming commoner in patients over the age of 50 as sanitation improves and the proportion of the population with immunity to the HA virus acquired in childhood decreases. It is now worthwhile testing HAV IgM in an elderly patient with an acute hepatitic illness, Serum IgM antibody to HAV indicates a recent infection. Studies by Goodson et al (1982) have suggested that the clinical course of presumed non-A non-B (NANB) acute hepatitis is similar in patients over age 60 to younger ones, the vast majority making a clinical recovery within six months although a proportion still have mild abnormalities of LFTs and hepatic histology indicating chronic persistent

hepatitis. By contrast the prognosis for acute type B hepatitis (HBV) is probably worse in the elderly, a greater proportion of patients proceeding to fulminant hepatic failure (Fenster, 1965). If severe hepatic necrosis occurs in the elderly, whether virally induced or caused by paracetamol (acetaminophen) overdose, mortality is higher in the elderly (Sherlock, 1981). Since immunisation against the HBV is now becoming available the finding that older individuals are less reliable in their production of antibodies in response to the HB vaccine than younger subjects may be important; clarification of the ability of the elderly to develop immunity to the HBV following vaccination is needed (Maupas et al, 1981).

Drug induced liver disease
Since they consume a disproportionate quantity of drugs it is hardly surprising that adverse effects of such drugs upon the liver are commonly seen in the elderly. Adverse reactions in the liver may be classified as direct – usually related to the production of a toxic metabolite of a drug or as 'unpredictable' – usually due to an immunological reaction to the drug. It is extremely hard to be certain whether alterations in hepatic metabolism or the aging immune system render the elderly patient more susceptible to adverse drug reactions. It seems likely however, that severe drug related damage whether metabolite related as in paracetamol (acetaminophen) overdose, or possibly immunologically mediated as with halothane associated hepatitis or nitrofurantoin induced chronic active hepatitis, is worse in elderly subjects (Inman & Mushin, 1978; James, 1983). Recently severe cholestatic liver disease associated with the non-steroidal anti-inflammatory drug benoxaprofen has been detected almost exclusively in elderly patients (Taggart & Alderdice, 1982).

Chronic liver disease
Alcoholic
Alcoholic liver disease often presenting with jaundice or the complications of portal hypertension is increasingly apparent in the elderly. In France over 20% patients with alcoholic cirrhosis have been found to be over the age of 70 (Aron et al, 1979) and while the clinical course of the disease appeared similar to younger patients, those elderly subjects with evidence of malnutrition were said to have a considerably worse prognosis than their younger counterparts. In the United States the peak decade for alcoholic cirrhosis in a survey of whites was found to be the seventh (Garagliano et al, 1979). Particular attention should be paid to nutrition in elderly patients with alcoholic liver disease.

Immunological
No major differences in the clinical features or prognosis of the immunological diseases chronic active hepatitis (CAH) and primary biliary cirrhosis (PBC) occur in the elderly

compared with young subjects. In CAH it is suggested that although treatment with prednisolone ± azothiaprine is effective in aggressive disease, it is unnecessary to treat elderly patients with these drugs unless symptoms become troublesome or LFTs decline (Knodell & Farleigh, 1981). Nevertheless since autoimmune CAH responds so well to immunosuppressant treatment it is important to make the diagnosis. The combination of raised SMA or ANF and suggestive hepatic histology is usually sufficient to confirm the diagnosis.

PBC frequently presents in patients over the age of 65 (35 of 121 in our own series). The clinical spectrum of the disease is unchanged in the older age group except more patients may be asymptomatic of liver disease at the time of diagnosis. PBC should be suspected when raised AMA titre is detected on an autoimmune screen, or in females with raised serum alkaline phosphatase of hepatic type and with no evidence of biliary disease (James et al, 1981). After exhoneration of the biliary tree, liver biopsy should be carried out to confirm the diagnosis. Since patients with PBC – particularly postmenopausal women – may be susceptible to osteoporosis and osteomalacia, routine monthly injections of vitamin D together with oral calcium supplements are recommended.

Miscellaneous cirrhosis

As diagnostic accuracy improves, the proportion of patients with cryptogenic cirrhosis has declined. One possible clue to the cause of the occasional cases of inactive cirrhosis encountered in old people or found by chance at post mortem has been the description of elderly cirrhotic patients with the histological features of a-1 antitrypsin deficiency, these have been both heterozygous MZ and homozygous ZZ individuals (Battle et al, 1982).

Treatment of cirrhosis

Bleeding varices

Bleeding from oesophageal varices is rare in elderly patients and the principles of treatment are similar to those in younger individuals. Roberts et al (1983) have compared the outcome of treatment using fibre optic oesophageal sclerotherapy for bleeding varices in over 65 year olds against that in younger patients. The mortality and morbidity in the two groups over a limited (around six months) follow-up was similar. The results of the treatment suggest that this is probably the best way to manage such patients.

Ascites

More common than bleeding varices is the occurrence of ascites in the elderly cirrhotic; this may be accompanied by hypokalaemia, malnutrition and incipient impairment of renal function. A suggested plan of management for such patients is outlined in Fig. 33.2. The importance of a high protein diet with vitamin supplements is stressed. If patients are anorexic a fine bore soft nasogastric tube may be passed and a liquid feed may be added. Parenteral nutrition is seldom if ever indicated. Intravenous infusions of amino acid solutions are of no proven benefit.

Encephalopathy

Again the treatment of portosystemic encephalopathy is the same for young and old alike. It is vital to avoid constipation in the elderly cirrhotic. Regular lactulose – usually 20 ml b.i.d. – is helpful but occasionally patients develop gaseous abdominal distention after treatment. A faecal softener and suppository treatment may also be useful. Long-term neomycin treatment is not recommended in the elderly since they appear more susceptible to nerve deafness.

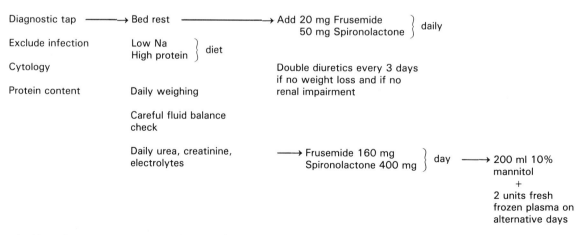

n.b. Aim to lose no more than c. 500 g/day. If encephalopathy occurs stop therapy. If creatinine rises progressively over more than 3 days, cut back on treatment.

Fig. 33.2 The management of elderly cirrhotic patients with ascites (progressive treatment until control is achieved)

In summary, the management of the elderly cirrhotic consists of:
1. Treatment of complications (infection, bleeding, ascites etc).
2. Nutritious diet, mineral and vitamin supplements – notably thiamine, pyridoxine, vitamins A, C, D, K, folic acid, check Mg, Zn.
3. Rest then rehabilitation.
4. Have patience, and avoid unnecessary intravenous intervention.

BILIARY TRACT DISEASE

By the age of 70 about 30% of women and 15% of men in Europe and the US will have developed gallstones although in many instances these may be asymptomatic and only discovered at post-mortem (Bateson & Bouchier, 1975). Gallstone disease will be considered in three catagories and the management of each group will be discussed.

1. Asymptomatic stones in gallbladder alone

These may be detected on plain abdominal radiographs or as a result of abdominal ultrasound examination for an unrelated condition. It has been suggested that up to 50% of patients with asymptomatic gallstones will develop symptoms and complications in the elderly and that obstructive jaundice, pancreatitis or cholangitis may lead to subsequent mortality as high as 15% (Wenkert & Robertson, 1966). More recently Gracie & Ransohoff (1982) suggested that the cumulative probability of developing biliary pain from truly asymptomatic gallstones is as low as 15%, mortality being very low. Furthermore although cancer of the gall-bladder is associated with stones in almost all instances, the risk of cancer developing in a gallbladder with stones is c.1%. Surgeons urge that elective cholecystectomy with its mortality of c.1% in patients over the age of 60 should be carried out in these patients (Stubbs et al, 1983). However modern operative mortality for elective cholecystectomy in those over 70 rises to over 3% (Chigot, 1981). Therefore in truly asymptomatic stones in the very elderly, prophylactic cholecystectomy is probably not indicated (Bouchier, 1983).

For this reason medical treatment of gallstones using oral bile acid therapy with either ursodeoxycholic acid (usually 600 mg taken at night) or chenodeoxycholic acid (usually 750 mg to 1 g) may be recommended in patients with asymptomatic small radiolucent stones in a functioning gallbladder (Dowling, 1983). In patients with doubtful or minimum symptoms the decision, surgery versus medical treatment versus no treatment, is difficult and must depend upon the wishes of individual patients and the other conditions which may complicate their management.

2. Symptomatic stones in gallbladder alone

Acute cholecystitis
Acute cholecystitis, usually caused by obstruction to the cystic duct by a stone and accompanied by bacterial infection is a serious emergency. Symptoms are of severe persistent pain in the right upper abdomen accompanied by nausea and vomiting. Fever, raised white cell count and abnormal liver function tests follow the onset of pain (Fenyo, 1982). The clinical diagnosis is confirmed by ultrasound or scan as outlined in Figure 33.1. Not all elderly patients have the classical presentation. Up to 40% do not have a very elevated temperature and peritoneal signs may not be prominent; toxic confusion may be an important sign in the presence of markedly abnormal LFTs (Morrow et al, 1978). Although conservative management of acute cholecystitis in the elderly has been recommended using antibiotic treatment (IV ampicillin, metronidazole and aminoglycoside) together with intravenous fluids and analgesia, it now seems clear that early surgery even in the acute phase of the inflammation carries a better prognosis. Glenn (1981) summarises this view: 'the elderly patient with acute cholecystitis requires meticulous management, pre-operative preparation and undelayed surgery'.

Chronic cholecystitis
The symptoms of chronic gallbladder inflammation almost always associated with gallstones, are very variable and often non-specific. Pain either intermittent and colicky or a more continuous ache, sometimes in the epigastrium is usually a prominent finding, but intermittent pyrexia, sometimes with non-specific abnormality of LFTs or a toxic confusional state are frequent presenting complaints; septicaemia is not infrequent. Diagnosis is as suggested in Figure 33.1 and in the earlier diagnostic section. Cholecystectomy should be accompanied by antibiotic cover, a single dose of IV cephalosporin being effective. All elderly patients undergoing cholecystectomy should have a per-operative cholangiogram to exclude common duct stones (Stubbs et al, 1983). Chronic gallbladder disease in the elderly may lead to such complications as mucocoele, empyema, subphrenic abscess or biliary-enteric fistula. Frequently these complications are only realised at operation and they contribute to the mortality of biliary tract disease in the elderly.

3. Stones in the biliary tree

Stones in bile ducts alone
Bile duct stones with none in the gallbladder (or following cholecystectomy) typically present either with obstructive jaundice or without jaundice but with symptoms or signs of infection together with abnormal LFTs. They must also be suspected in elderly patients presenting with far more non-specific complaints attributable to general decline in health in whom abnormal LFTs, particularly elevated alkaline

phosphatase are found (Cobden et al, 1984; Jones et al, 1982). Although stones in the biliary tree are usually associated with cholestatic LFTs the transaminase level may occasionally be very high, mimicking LFTs seen in acute hepatitis. The diagnostic decisions are made as already described. Acute cholangitis requires similar urgent antibiotic treatment and intravenous fluid support to that described for acute cholecystitis.

If stones are found in the bile duct alone (or in patients with previous cholecystectomy) then the treatment of choice in experienced hands is endoscopic sphincterotomy (Kozareck & Sanowski, 1981). The management of stones in the biliary tree is outlined in Figure 33.1. Mortality associated with exploration of the biliary tree in patients over the age of 70 may be as high as 28% whereas it is under 1% in experienced hands following endoscopic sphincterotomy. Over 80% of patients will have the biliary tree cleared of stones following this procedure (Cotton, 1980).

Stones in gallbladder and bile ducts
If stones are found in both the biliary tree and the gallbladder treatment is controversial. If this diagnosis is made during ERCP then a sphincterotomy with full supportive treatment is probablay the treatment of choice, allowing subsequent elective cholecystectomy to be carried out; occasionally endoscopic sphincterotomy is followed by disappearance of gallbladder stones as well as those in the CBD. In other circumstances cholecystectomy with exploration of the CBD is satisfactory; the supraduodenal rather than the transduodenal approach for the removal of stones in the CBD has a lower mortality.

OBSTRUCTIVE JAUNDICE IN THE ELDERLY

Probably the commonest single problem associated with hepatobiliary disease in the elderly is that of obstructive jaundice. The diagnostic choices are described above and in Figure 33.1; the differential diagnosis, listed in approximate order of likelihood is as follows:

Stones in biliary tree
Pancreatic carcinoma/Ampullary carcinoma
Bile duct carcinoma (cholangiocarcinoma)
Carcinoma of gallbladder
Metastatic carcinoma (within liver or in obstructing biliary tree) or Primary liver cell cancer
Sclerosing cholangitis
Cholestasis – not obstruction
i.e. Drugs
   PBC/CAH
   Cholestatic hepatitis
   Heart failure

Biliary stones have been discussed and pancreatic carcinoma appears elsewhere. Bile duct carcinoma and in particular carcinoma of the gallbladder are predominantly diseases of the elderly. Bile duct carcinoma almost always presents with jaundice, sometimes fluctuating; pain is often not a prominent feature. Features of cholangitis are usually absent. The diagnosis is confirmed at PTC or ERCP. Laparotomy is the treatment of choice since tumours at the lower end of the CBD may be resected; tumours in the hilum of the liver cannot often be fully resected but insertion of a prosthesis may be carried out; mean survival of all tumours is about one year (Tomkins et al, 1981). Recent developments in the transhepatic percutaneous insertion of prostheses or even endoscopic insertion of biliary prostheses may enable elderly frail patients to obtain relief of jaundice and accompanying pruritus for periods of months. These are highly skilled techniques to be undertaken only in special centres (Hagenmuller & Soehendra, 1983). Carcinoma of the gallbladder presents with abdominal pain in almost all patients, obstructive jaundice is frequent. The diagnosis is often not made until laparotomy or post-mortem. In patients presenting with biliary obstruction the prognosis is very bad, paliative relief of jaundice by hepaticojejunostomy or insertion of a prosthesis should be carried out (Shieh et al, 1981). Occasionally a small carcinoma of gallbladder may be found by chance at cholecystectomy for gallstones. Such tumours have a much better prognosis, possibly 65% with a five year survival (Liguory & Canard, 1983). Primary sclerosing cholangitis is associated with inflammatory bowel disease in about 50% of patients. Unlike other mechanical causes of obstructive jaundice it is not commoner with advancing age; clinical features and management are reviewed by Chapman et al (1980).

Carcinoma in the liver
Metastatic disease
Metastatic cancer within the liver may present either with symptoms and signs of liver disease – jaundice, upper abdominal pain, pruritus – or as a more non-specific general deterioration in health with anorexia, weight loss and weakness. In the first instance examination often reveals an enlarged liver, sometimes with an adjacent abdominal mass indicating a primary site nearby; investigation is then as for any cause of obstructive jaundice. In the more occult presentation examination also often reveals a firm enlargement of the liver, investigation shows raised alkaline phosphatase; colloid scan, ultrasound or computed tomography scan will reveal a space occupying lesion or lesions within the liver. Guided percutaneous liver biopsy is then performed. Treatment of multiple metastases within the liver is usually paliative at best but single hepatic metastases, particularly from colonic primary tumours may be removed with a reasonable prognosis (Sherlock, 1981).

Primary hepatocellular cancer

In western countries this is often a disease of advanced years. The majority of such tumours are associated with previous exposure to the Hepatitis B virus – usually many years previously. Alcoholic cirrhosis, haemochromatosis and alpha-1-antitrypsin deficiency also predispose to its development (Kew, 1982). Primary liver cancer usually presents late and may be clinically indistinguishable from metastatic disease, pancreatic or biliary carcinoma. The underlying liver is usually cirrhotic thus patients frequently also have features of hepatocellular failure. Serum alphafoetoprotein is markedly elevated in about 70% of patients and if over 1000 iu/1 (upper limit of normal about 10) in an elderly patient with liver disease is diagnostic of primary hepatocellular carcinoma. Occasionally early or limited tumours may be resected, chemotherapy with adriamycin is beneficial in about one third of patients. Mean prognosis is about six months (Johnson et al, 1978).

The liver in other diseases in the elderly

Although it is very difficult to classify and enumerate the many disorders in which an abnormality – usually not very severe – of LFTs is encountered in the elderly, it is nonetheless important to be aware of the commoner circumstances in which this occurs and to deal with any such abnormality intelligently, or to know when further investigation is probably not necessary. Table 33.2 lists these major 'secondary' causes of abnormal LFTs in geriatric patients.

The investigation and management of a non-specific abnormality of LFT in a 'typical' geriatric patient (using multiple diagnosis and medications) is as follows:

1. Check that LFT abnormality is persistent, not very transient (i.e. only present in very acute stage of illness).

2. If alkaline phosphatase elevated alone check Gamma GT or alkaline phosphatase isoenzymes (is it really hepatic alkaline phosphatase?).

3. Check HBV markers auto-antibodies, alcohol history, MCV. Order hepatobiliary ultrasound.

4. If LFTs still abnormal, no explanation from above investigations then:

a) examine medications – could any be responsible for abnormal LFTs?

b) examine clinical course of patient. Are they improving generally (i.e. from heart failure or pneumonia) while LFTs remain abnormal/worse?

5. If any medication could well be responsible (i.e. phenothiazine) – stop and wait. If patient remains ill with e.g. severe heart failure or systemic infection then treat this, do not worry too much about liver.

6. If LFTs remain significantly abnormal despite marked improvement in 'systemic' condition – then suspect two diagnoses i.e. 'systemic' condition + hepatobiliary disease.

Table 33.2 'Secondary' causes of abnormal LFTs in geriatric patients.

Diagnosis	Abnormality
1. *Heart failure*	*Variable: Chronic heart failure* → ↑ Bili, A.P. Acute heart failure → ↑ Transaminase Recover as heart failure improves
2. *Systemic infections* i.e. T.B. Abdominal sepsis	Variable: usually mild elevation of Bili., A.P., less in transaminase Recover on treatment of infections
Severe urinary infections + septicaemia n.b. 'old' syphilis hydatid disease	
3. *Rheumatoid arthritis/* other rheumatoid disorders (not osteoarthritis)	Variable: usually ↑ A.P.
4. *Collagen diseases*	Variable: usually ↑ A.P.
5. *Pneumonia* (noteably pneumococcal)	Variable: usually ↑ Bilirubin
6. *Drug related*	Variable
7. *Metabolic/nutritional*	Alkaline phosphatase (rarely hepatic fibrosis)
Myxoedema Amyloid (very rare) Arsenic ingestion (old R̠ for syphilis + skin disorders)	Non-specific

In these circumstances follow diagnostic path shown in Figure 33.1. Suspect:

1. Occult biliary disease
2. Alcohol
3. Occult neoplasm (pancreas common)
4. Drugs

These abnormalities of LFT may occur either in the context of the severely ill old person, often with multiple pathologies in whom the investigation of abnormal LFTs must take second place to the management of life threatening disease; or abnormal LFTs may be found as part of a general assessment in an elderly person with less immediately severe or obvious illness.

CONCLUSION

The investigation and management of hepatobiliary disease in an old person is both interesting to the physician and potentially rewarding for the patient. Our realisation that occult disease may severely affect the general health of old persons, and recent advances in both non-invasive and invasive investigation and treatment have radically altered the outlook for our patients with such diseases.

REFERENCES

Aron E, Dupin M, Jobard P 1979 Les cirrhoses du troisieme age. Annals Gastroenterologie Hepatologie 15: 558–563

Bateson M C, Bouchier I A D 1975 Prevalence of gallstones in Dundee: a necropsy study. British Medical Journal 4: 427–430

Battle W M, Matarazzo A, Selhat G F, Catalano E 1982 Alpha-l-antitrypsin deficiency – A cause of cryptogenic liver disease in the elderly. Journal of Clinical Gastroenterology 4: 269–273

Bert R N, Ferrucci J T, Fordtran J S et al 1981 The radiological diagnosis of gallbladder disease. Radiology 141: 49–56

Bouchier I A D 1983 Brides of quietness: silent gallstones. British Medical Journal i: 415–416

Burroughs A K, Scheuer P J 1982 Liver biopsy: indications and procedure. Medicine 16: 718–719

Chanarin I 1979 Alcohol, liver disease and the blood. In: Chanarin I The Megaloblastic Anaemias, 2nd edn. Blackwell, Oxford p 504–515

Chapman R W G, Marborgh B A, Rhodes J M et al 1980 Primary sclerosing cholangitis. Gut 21: 870–877

Chigot J P 1981 Le risque operatoire dans la lithiase biliare. Semains Hopital (Paris) 57: 1311–1319

Cobden I, Lendrum R, Venables C W, James O F W 1984 Biliary tract disease as a cause of unexplained deterioration in health in the elderly. Lancet i 1062–1064

Cotton P B 1980 Non-operative removal of bile duct stones by duodenoscopic sphincterotomy. British Journal of Surgery 67:

Cotton P B 1983 Direct choledochography. Clinics of Gastroenterology 12: 101–107

Croker J R 1982 Gallstone disease in the elderly. In: Evans J G, Caird F I (eds) Advanced Geriatric Medicine 2. Pitman, London

Dowling R H 1983 Management of stones in the biliary tree. Gut 24: 599–608

Fenster L F 1965 Viral hepatitis in the elderly. Gastroenterology 49: 262–271

Fenyo G 1982 Acute abdominal disease in the elderly. American Journal of Surgery 143: 751–754

Frommhold W, Wolf F 1983 Radiological and radionucleide methods for the diagnosis of biliary disorders. Clinics in Gastroenterology 12: 65–100

Garagliano C F, Lilenfeld A M, Mendelhoff A I 1979 Incidence rates of liver cirrhosis and related diseases in Baltimore and selected areas of the United States. Journal of Chronic Diseases 32: 543–544

Glenn F 1981 Surgical management of acute cholecystitis in patients 65 years of age and older. Annals of Surgery 193: 56–59

Goodson J D, Taylor P, Campion E W et al 1982 The clinical course of acute hepatitis in the elderly patient. Archives of Internal Medicine 142: 1485–1488

Gracie W A, Ransohoff D F 1982 The natural history of silent gallstones. The innocent gallstone is not a myth. New England Journal of Medicine 307: 798–800

Hagenmuller F, Soehendra N 1983 Non-surgical biliary drainage. Clinics in Gastroenterology 12: 297–316

Inman W H W, Mushin W W 1978 Jaundice after repeated exposure to halothane. British Medical Journal ii: 1455–1456

James O F W 1983 Gastrointestinal and liver function in old age. Clinics in Gastroenterology 12: 671–691

James O F W, Macklon A F, Watson A J 1981 Primary biliary cirrhosis – a revised clinical spectrum. Lancet i: 1281–1284

Johnson P J, Williams R, Thomas H et al 1978 Induction of remission of hepatocellular carcinoma with doxoribicin. Lancet i: 1006–1008

Jones S N, Askew C M, Beynon G P, Croker J R 1982 Isolated elevation of serum alkaline phosphatase and biliary disease in the elderly. Postgraduate Medical Journal 58: 85–86

Kew M C 1982 Tumours of the liver. In: Zakim, Boyer (eds) Hepatology New York, Saunders p 1048–1079

Knodell R G, Farleigh R M 1981 Chronic active hepatitis: A plea for conservative management. Geriatrics 36: 111–115

Kozarek R A, Sanowski R A 1981 Endoscopic papillotomy in the geriatric patient with complicated biliary tract disease. Journal of American Geriatrics Society 29: 70–73

Levitt R G, Sagel S, Stanley R J, Jost R G 1977 Accuracy of computed tomography of the liver and biliary tract. Radiology 124: 123–128

Liguory C, Canard J M 1983 Tumours of the biliary system. Clinics of Gastroenterology 12: 269–295

McIntyre N 1982 Testing liver function. Medicine 16: 711–713

Maupas P, Goudeau A, Dubois et al 1981 Potency and efficacy of HB vaccine applied to a high risk population, a five year study. In: Maupas P, Guesny P (eds) Hepatitis B Vaccine INSERM Symposium 18. Elsevier North-Holland, Amsterdam p 177–231

Morrow D J, Thompson J, Wilson S E 1978 Acute cholecystitis in the elderly. Archives of Surgery 113: 1149–1152

Mountford D 1982 Imaging the liver. Medicine 16: 720–722

Okuda K 1981 Advances in hepatobiliary ultrasonography. Hepatology 1: 662–672

Roberts C M, Casey B, Foizallah R, Walker R J, Krasner N, Morris A I, Marcus S N 1983 Injection sclerotherapy for oesophageal varices in the elderly. Age and Ageing 12: 139–143

Scheuer P J 1980 Liver Biopsy Interpretation. 3rd edn. Balliere Tindall London

Sherlock S 1981 Diseases of the Liver and Biliary System. 6th edn. Blackwell, Oxford

Shieh C J, Dunn E, Standard J E 1981 Primary carcinoma of the gallbladder. Cancer 47: 996–1004

Sloof M, Baker R, Lavelle M I, Lendrum R, Venables C W 1980 What is involved in endoscopic sphincterotomy for gallstones? British Journal of Surgery 67: 18–21

Stubbs R S, McCloy R F, Blumgart L H 1983 Surgery in cholelithiasis and cholecystitis. Clinics in Gastroenterology 12: 179–201

Taggart H McA, Alderdice J M 1982 Fatal cholestatic jaundice in elderly patients taking benoxaprofen. British Medical Journal ii: 372

Taylor T V, Summerling M D, Carter D C et al 1980 An evaluation of ^{99m}Tc-labelled HIDA in hepatobiliary scanning. British Journal of Surgery 67: 325–328

Tomkins R K, Thomas D, Wile A, Longmire W P 1981 Prognostic factors in bile duct carcinoma. Annals of Surgery 194: 447–455

Vellacott K D, Powell P H 1979 Exploration of the common bile duct, a comparative study. British Journal of Surgery 66: 389–391

Wenkert A, Robertson B 1966 The natural cause of gallstone disease. Eleven year review of 781 non-operative cases. Gastroenterology 50: 376–381

34

Anaemia

D.A. Lipschitz

INTRODUCTION

Little information is available on the effects of age on haematopoiesis. Most evidence indicates that changes are minor and that only minimal reductions in circulating formed blood elements occur with aging. Animal studies have shown that haematopoietic stem cell depletion does not occur as they age. There is however, increasing evidence that the responsiveness of haematopoietic stem cells becomes impaired with age. Thus, the erythropoietic response of the marrow following stimulation is reduced. In addition, the ability to mount a granulocyte response to infection is decreased. This chapter deals with the problem of anaemia in the elderly. The disorder is very prevalent in older subjects and the complex inter-relationship among age, nutrition, disease and drugs used in treatment, all of which may affect haematopoiesis, makes the diagnosis and management of anaemia difficult.

PREVALENCE

The consensus of many studies is that anaemia in the elderly should not be considered a normal part of aging (Lewis, 1976). The incidence of anaemia is greater in the institutionalised and hospitalised than among the healthy elderly (Evans et al, 1968). The definition of anaemia is arbitrary and a wide overlap in haemoglobin values occurs between subjects subsequently proven to be anaemic and those in whom the haemoglobin value is merely low. Thus the best method of expressing incidence of anaemia is to determine the fraction of the group at low, moderate or high risk of being anaemic (US Department of Health, Education and Welfare, 1968–1980; Nutrition Canada, 1973). Males are at low risk of anaemia if the haemoglobin level is greater than 14 g/dl. Females are at low risk if the haemoglobin level is greater than 12 g/dl. Moderate risk of anaemia is defined as a value between 12 and 14 g/dl for males and between 10 and 12 g/dl for females. High risk of anaemia is indicated by a value below 12 g/dl for males and

10 g/dl for females. Large epidemiological as well as community and clinical studies have analysed the prevalence of anaemia in the elderly (US Department of Health, Education and Welfare, 1968–1980; Nutrition Canada, 1973). From these investigations the following generalities seem appropriate. Approximately 6–10% of females above the age of 60 are at moderate risk of anaemia which is very similar to the risk found in middle-aged females. In men above the age of 60 approximately 15% are at moderate risk of anaemia which is much higher than that found in younger males. Only a small fraction (1–2%) of males and females above the age of 60 are at high risk of anaemia. Small community studies are important because they have examined larger numbers of subjects in the eighth and ninth decades (Hill, 1967; Myers et al, 1968; McLennan et al, 1973). In both males and females the incidence of anaemia in the eighth decade is significantly higher than in the seventh with an even higher incidence in subjects aged over 80. These observations indicate that the prevalence of anaemia does indeed increase with advancing age. In any age group and in both sexes the incidence of anaemia is higher in blacks than in whites and irrespective of race the prevalence is invariably higher in subjects from low income compared to high income groups (US Department of Health, Education and Welfare, 1968–1980; Nutrition Canada, 1973). The actual incidence of anaemia in hospitalised patients is difficult to determine and depends upon the group studied. For example, on the Geriatric Evaluation Unit located at the Little Rock VA Hospital, 48% of all admissions to this acute care facility had haemoglobin levels below the commonly recognised lower limit of normal. The prevalence of anaemia in chronic institutionalised patients or in those attending out-patient clinics tends to be substantially less than that in acutely ill subjects but greater than the incidence in the general community. Because of the complexities of diseases presenting in the elderly in general and in the hospitalised patient in particular, clinical judgment is essential in deciding how extensive a workup for anaemia should be. This especially applies to those subjects with only a modest reduction in haemoglobin values.

Signs and symptoms

The subtle signs and symptoms of anaemia are harder to detect in the elderly than in young adults. Anaemia itself is frequently a symptom of an underlying disease such as tumour, ulcer, infection etc which usually determines the clinical presentation. Oxygen delivery to tissue depends not only on red cell mass but also on cardiopulmonary function which is frequently compromised in the elderly. As a result the symptoms of anaemia generally occur more frequently in older persons with the disorder. Dyspnoea, weakness and excessive sweating with exertion occur when the haemoglobin concentration decreases by about 30%. However, the rate of decrease in haemoglobin and the degree of physical activity are important in determining when anaemia becomes symptomatic. Anaemia may produce local symptoms such as intermittent claudication, angina, disorientation or behavioural disorders when there is localised vascular insufficiency. Syncope may occur and anorexia and abdominal discomfort after large meals may result from decreased tissue perfusion of the gut.

There are few clues on physical examination of anaemia. Pallor of conjuctivae and mucous membranes may suggest a low haemoglobin concentration. Findings related to the specific etiology of anaemia are relatively infrequent. Glossitis suggests a deficiency of iron, folate or vitamin B_{12}. Jaundice, splenomegaly, lymphadenopathy, evidence of neoplasia, or an active inflammatory disease will aid greatly in delineating the cause of anaemia.

DIFFERENTIAL DIAGNOSIS OF ANAEMIA

In general the causes of anaemia in the elderly are very similar to those in younger subjects. Anaemias may be classified as hypoproliferative (decreased red cell production), ineffective and haemolytic types (Hillman & Finch, 1974). These are summarised in Table 34.1. The vast majority of anaemia in patients of all ages is hypoproliferative but haemolytic anaemia and maturation abnormalities resulting in ineffective erythropoiesis must also be considered. The most efficient approach to the diagnosis of hypoproliferative anaemia is to exclude haemolysis by the absence of significant reticulocytosis (see below) and ineffective erythropoiesis by the absence of macrocytosis, red cell fragmentation with a normal indirect bilirubin and LDH level.

THE HYPOPROLIFERATIVE ANAEMIAS

The differential diagnosis of hypoproliferative anaemia includes inadequate supply of iron for haemoglobin synthesis, an intrinsic lesion of the marrow affecting erythroid stem cells and a decreased marrow stimulation by

Table 34.1 Classification of anaemia

Hypoproliferative	Ineffective	Haemolytic
1. Iron deficient erythropoiesis	1. Megaloblastic	1. Immunologic
a. Blood loss anaemia	a. B_{12}	a. Idiopathic
b. Inflammation	b. Folate	b. Secondary to drug, tumour, or disease
c. Protein calorie malnutrition	c. Refractory	
2. Erythropoietin lack	2. Microcytic	2. Intrinsic
a. Renal failure	a. Thalassaemia	a. Metabolic
b. Myxoedema	b. Sideroblstic anaemia	b. Abnormal haemoglobin
		c. Membrane defect
3. Marrow failure	3. Normocytic	3. Extrinsic
a. Hypolastic anaemia	a. Stromal disese	a. Mechanical
b. tumour	b. Dimorphic	b. Lytic substance
c. Fibrosis		

erythropoietin. A rational approach to the diagnosis of the hypoproliferative anaemias is shown in Figure 34.1.

Inadequate iron supply is the most frequent cause of hypoproliferative anaemia and results either from blood loss (true iron deficiency) or from a wide variety of acute and chronic diseases that are associated with a decreased ability of the reticuloendothelial system to utilise iron from senescent red cells. Diseases associated with 'the anaemia of chronic disease' include acute or chronic infections, collagen vascular disease and cancer. Inadequate iron supply is also often found in protein calorie malnutrition which is frequent in hospitalised elderly patients. In all the above disorders iron deficient erythropoiesis can be diagnosed by the presence of microcytosis (mean corpuscular volume (MCV) less than 84 fl), a transferrin saturation less than 20%, a red blood cell protoporphyin/heme ratio greater than 30 μmol/mol and absent sideroblasts on histologic examination of the bone marrow (Hillman & Finch, 1974). In general, the abnormalities in laboratory tests occurring in chronic disease and malnutrition are usually less severe than in blood loss anaemia which is the likely diagnosis when the MCV is less than 75 fl or the transferrin saturation less than 16%.

Anaemia from blood loss occurs only after tissue iron stores are totally depleted. Serum ferritin reflects iron stores and is usually less than 12 ng/ml when iron stores are absent (Lipschitz et al, 1974). In such situations, histologic examination of the marrow will reveal no stainable reticuloendothelial iron. In contrast, a decreased ability to

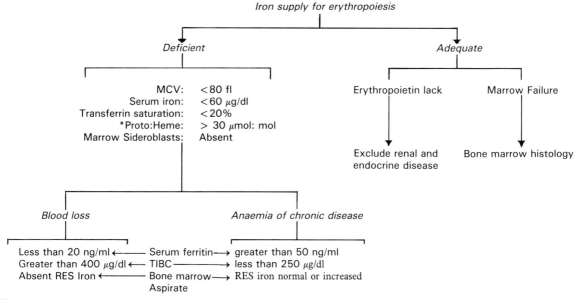

Fig. 34.1 The approach to the diagnosis of hypoproliferative anaemia

release iron from the reticuloendothelial system is the initial abnormality in chronic disease and malnutrition and hence in these conditions iron deficient erythropoiesis develops in the presence of normal or increased tissue iron stores. The serum ferritin is usually greater than 50 ng/ml and bone marrow examination shows adequate to increased reticuloendothelial iron. The total iron binding capacity (TIBC) varies inversely with tissue iron stores and tends to be increased in blood loss anaemia and decreased in chronic disease (see Fig. 34.1). In all causes of iron deficient erythropoiesis, irrespective of the level of tissue iron stores, sideroblast number is reduced.

The characteristics of anaemias associated with chronic disease and that with protein calorie malnutrition in the elderly are very similar (Lipschitz, 1982). In the hospitalised elderly patient malnutrition is best diagnosed by hypo-albuminaemia (less than 3 g/dl), lymphocytopenia (less than 1.6×10^3 cells/μl) and anergy. In addition, neutropenia, marrow hypocellularity and decreased myeloid precursors are usual in malnutrition. When anaemia is associated with other chronic diseases (cancer, acute and chronic infections, collagen vascular disease) peripheral granulocytosis and increased marrow myeloid precursors are usually found.

Of particular concern in the evaluation of the hospitalised elderly patient is the presence of multiple disease which may directly or indirectly affect the haemoglobin level. When a hypoproliferative anaemia exists in this clinical setting peripheral blood measurements frequently fail to ascertain whether the anaemia is due to blood loss or to failure of the reticuloendothelial system to recircuit iron as

occurs in the 'anaemia of chronic disease'. When peripheral blood measurements fail to make the diagnosis of blood loss, histologic examination of the bone marrow is the best method of demonstrating absent iron stores. Alternatively in relatively healthy ambulatory elderly subjects a therapeutic trial of oral iron may be indicated (see below). It is extremely important that protein calorie malnutrition in the elderly be detected as a substantial improvement in haemotopoietic function has recently been shown when malnutrition is corrected (Lipschitz & Mitchell, 1982).

Once a diagnosis of blood loss anaemia, the anaemia of chronic disease or malnutrition has been made further investigation to establish the cause may be indicated. Pathologic blood loss, primarily from the gastro-intestinal tract is the commonest cause of iron deficiency anaemia in the elderly. Despite aggressive diagnostic studies to exclude gastro-intestinal disease the cause of blood loss anaemia in the elderly will frequently not be found. Nutritional iron deficiency is rare and older females have significantly higher tissue iron reserves than do those in the child bearing age. Although post-menopausal bleeding is common in elderly females, blood loss sufficient to cause anaemia is unusual. There is no good data available to determine how frequent anaemia is the initial manifestation of an underlying acute or chronic disease in the elderly.

The management of iron deficiency in older subjects is similar to that in younger individuals. Intolerance of oral iron is no more common in the elderly and a usual dose of about 70 mg of ferrous iron given 3 times a day, is adequate to return the haemoglobin to normal and replete tissue iron stores. In general a 2 gm% increase in circulating haemoglobin is seen after a three week trial of oral iron. Once the haemoglobin has returned to normal iron therapy should be continued for a further six months to allow the replenishment of tissue iron stores. Intolerance to oral iron or poor patient compliance are the main indications for parenteral iron therapy. Iron dextran is the preparation of choice. After testing for hypersensitivity, 5–10 ml of undiluted iron dextran may be administered intravenously over a period of 5 minutes. Injections may be repeated daily until the required dose is given. Alternatively multiple intramuscular injections may be given. The details of calculating the dose and the side effects of iron dextran have been reported extensively elsewhere (Hillman & Finch, 1974). Generally when a chronic disease co-exists with iron deficiency anaemia significant increase in the haemoglobin will occur following iron therapy even though the chronic disease is not improved. In contrast when the anaemia of chronic disease or malnutrition is the prime diagnosis a response to oral iron will not be detected. A rise in haemoglobin occurs when protein calorie malnutrition is corrected. Like malnourished young children however, the haemoglobin is the last nutritional parameter to return to normal with subtle increases that only become apparent after six weeks of nutritional repletion.

Marrow failure

An intrinsic marrow failure due to drug toxicity, tumour or fibrosis is more frequent in older than young subjects. The classic examples of drug that cause aplastic anaemia are chloramphenicol and phenylbutazone. The list of agents associated with the hypoplastic anaemia is very large. For this reason a standard text should always be referred to when drug induced marrow failure is suspected (Wintrobe, 1981a). The diagnosis will usually be made by the associated presence of neutropenia and thrombocytopenia. The true prevalence of mild marrow failure in the elderly remains to be determined. A recent survey has shown that the mild anaemia in apparently healthy elderly subjects is frequently not due to iron deficiency, chronic disease or malnutrition (Lipschitz et al, 1981). In these anaemic subjects neutrophil and platelet counts are significantly lower than non-anaemic subjects and a recent study of their bone marrow has demonstrated a reduction in all haematopoietic cell lines (Lipschitz et al, 1984). These findings suggest that mild marrow failure may be frequent in the elderly. The etiology of this disorder, its relation to the aging process and its clinical significance remain to be determined.

MATURATION ABNORMALITIES IN THE ELDERLY

The mechanism of anaemia in this group of disorders includes cytoplasmic abnormalities resulting in reduction in haemoglobin formation and nuclear maturation abnormalities producing megaloblastic changes in the marrow and peripheral blood (Hillman & Finch, 1974). Cytoplasmic disorders are generally associated with microcytosis whereas the nuclear disorders classically have macrocytosis. With the exception of iron deficiency anaemia the remaining disorders all present clinically with varying degrees of ineffective erythropoiesis.

Cytoplasmic abnormalities

The cytoplasmic abnormalities resulting in decreased haemoglobin synthesis include iron deficiency anaemia, defective production of haemoglobin chains as occurs in thalassaemia syndromes, and disorders of porphyrin metabolism which include the entire spectrum of the sideroblastic anaemias. A uniform feature of these diseases in the presence of microcytosis which is frequently below 75 fl. Iron deficiency can usually be distinguished from thalassaemia or sideroblastic anaemia by the presence or absence of iron deficient erythropoiesis. In the latter disorders ineffective erythropoiesis is present and as a result indirect hyperbilirubinaemia or an elevated LDH are usually found. Thalassaemia minor and alpha thalassaemia are very prevalent amongst various ethnic groups and may remain undetected until late in life. They should therefore always be included in the differential diagnosis of mild microcytic anaemia in elderly subjects.

Sideroblastic anaemia is a disease of later life and must be suspected in an elderly subject with microcytic anaemia not due to iron deficiency. The etiology of the disease in the elderly is frequently of the acquired type with the idiopathic variety predominating over those secondary to alcohol, drugs or a variety of chronic diseases. Disorders associated with sideroblastic anaemia include neoplasia (particularly gastro-intestinal, renal and lymphoma) inflammatory diseases (rheumatoid arthritis, systemic lupus erythematosus) and chronic infections. The diagnosis is usually made by finding increased serum iron and serum ferritin levels with significant numbers of ringed sideroblasts on histologic examination of the bone marrow. Iron absorption is increased and if transfusions are required excessive accumulation of iron stores occurs. Secondary haemochormatosis may develop which results in cardiomyopathy, hepatocellular disease, diabetes and a variety of endocrine syndromes. In general in the elderly there is no satisfactory therapy for this condition. Most recent evidence suggests that the idiopathic variety is a relatively benign disease and rarely limits life. Subjects who have a large transfusion requirement generally have a poorer prognosis. Like younger subjects, a fraction of elderly individuals will show a significant elevation in the haemoglobin level when pharmacologic doses of pyridoxine or pyridoxal phosphate are administered. For this reason a trial of one or other of these agents is usually indicated.

The megaloblastic anaemias

The cardinal features of this disease is the presence of macrocytosis and hypersegmented granulocytes in the peripheral blood smear. The MCV is frequently greater than 110 fl, indirect hyperbilirubinaemia is usual and the mean corpuscular haemoglobin concentration (MCHC) is normal. Examination of the bone marrow reveals megaloblastic erythroid precursors and giant metamyelocytes and band forms in the granulocytic series. In the elderly the differential diagnosis centres around folate or B_{12} deficiency. Although a careful clinical examination may assist in distinguishing the two deficiencies, the correct diagnosis requires the measurement of vitamin levels in the peripheral blood.

Numerous surveys have shown a modest reduction in folate levels in the elderly, thought to be due to inadequate dietry intake of folate (US Department of Health, Education and Welfare, 1968–1980; Nutrition Canada, 1973; Girdwood et al, 1969). A folate value low enough to be associated with anaemia is however, exceptionally rare. If a diagnosis of folate deficient megaloblastic anaemia is made, other conditions associated with deficiency of this vitamin must be considered. Of these the most important is chronic alcoholism which is not uncommon in the elderly. Megaloblastic anaemia due to folate deficiency has been observed in as many of 20% of patients with alcoholic cirrhosis (Krasnow, 1957). The mechanism of the deficiency relates not only to inadequate dietary intake but also to disordered folate metabolism. A variety of anti-convulsant drugs is associated with folate deficiency (Reynolds et al, 1966). These include diphenylhydantoin, primidone and phenobarbitol used either alone or in combination. Although a frank megaloblastic anaemia is unusual evidence of folate deficiency and mild haematologic changes are relatively common. The mechanism of the abnormality is unclear. A reduction in folate absorption has been reported as has an alteration in folate metabolism. The modest reduction in folate stores in older people makes this side effect of anti-convulsant drugs more likely.

Although vitamin B_{12} deficiency is a relatively rare disorder, its prevalence increases with each advancing decade. The commonest cause of vitamin B_{12} deficiency in the elderly is pernicious anaemia. This systemic disease has been described extensively and will not be reviewed in great detail here (Wintrobe, 1981). However some points bear special mention. The disorder is primarily a disease of old age, the peak incidence being the age of 60. In the seventh and eighth decade the frequency may be as much as 0.1–0.2% of the population. The disease is more frequent in northern countries and is more prevalent in woman. It is not uncommon for the initial manifestation of this disease to be a severe anaemia which is frequently asymptomatic. Occasionally other systemic symptoms of pernicious anaemia may precede the haematologic manifestions. An alteration in mental status and neurologic changes are most important. The incidence of carcinoma of the stomach is also higher in subjects with pernicious anaemia. The differential diagnosis of vitamin B_{12} in the elderly is wider than in younger subjects. A reduction in intrinsic factor due to primary atrophic gastritis must be considered. Of particular importance is small bowel bacterial overgrowth due to blind loops or diverticuli. Malabsorption of the vitamin due to ileal malfunction associated with myxoedema and diabetes has also been described. Finally megaloblastic anaemia due to vitamin B_{12} deficiency is a rare side effect of a variety of drugs including para-aminosalicylic acid (PAS), neomycin, ethanol and potassium chloride.

As indicated above the peripheral blood and bone marrow findings of megaloblastic anaemia due to folate and vitamin B_{12} deficiency are identical. When either deficiency is suspected appropriate measurements of the vitamins in the peripheral blood should be undertaken. A diagnosis of vitamin B_{12} deficiency can be made if the serum value is less than 120 ng/ml. Values between 120 and 180 ng/ml are in a 'grey zone' that is neither clearly normal nor clearly abnormal. In contrast to vitamin B_{12}, serum folate is labile and sensitive to short-term changes in folate balance. The measurement of erythrocyte folate provides a more accurate reflection of folate stores. The erythrocyte level is established during formation of the red cell and persists throughout its life span. Thus it may take 3–4 months of folate deprivation before low values are obtained.

DiGuiglielmo's disease

In the elderly the erythropoietic anaemias due to an intrinsic acquired nuclear maturation abnormalities of the marrow must be included in the differential diagnosis. This group of conditions is generally referred to as DiGuiglielmo's anaemia and are classically associated with the presence of pancytopenia, megaloblastic erythriod precursors and significant increases in myeloblasts. Prognosis of this disease can vary from relatively mild to severe; the rate limiting factors being the development of pancytopenia or acute leukaemia. The diagnosis is usually made by examination of the bone marrow.

THE HEMOLYTIC ANAEMIAS

The cardinal diagnostic feature of haemolytic anaemia is the presence of a significant reticulocytosis. Reticulocytes are young cells containing ribonucleic acid (RNA) strands which take up a super vital stain that allows their detection on peripheral smears. The value is usually reported as a percentage of the number of erythrocytes in the sample evaluted. The percentage can increase either because the absolute number of reticulocytes increase or because the number of adult erythrocytes decrease as occurs in anaemia. Furthermore in response to a lower haemoglobin concentration erythrocyte production increases and red cells that are more immature (shift cells) enter the circulation. The prolonged maturation time of these shift cells results in an apparently higher reticulocyte count. In diagnosing haemolytic anaemia the number of circulating reticulocytes must be absolutely increased. This can be determined by calculating the reticulocyte production index (RPI) that corrects the reticulocyte count for the lower erythrocyte concentration and for the longer maturation time (Hillman & Finch, 1974). The calculation used is as follows:

$$RPI = \frac{Reticulocytes}{maturation\ time} + \frac{Observed\ haemotocrit\ (\%)}{45}$$

Where:

1) 45% is used as a normal haematocrit.

2) Maturation time = 1 day at a haematocrit of 45%, 1.5 days at a haematocrit of 35%, 2 days at a haematocrit of 25% and 2.5 days at a haematocrit of 15% etc.

If the RPI is greater than 3 a diagnosis of haemolytic anaemia is extremely likely. If the RPI is less than 2.5 haemolytic anaemia is unusual.

The differential diagnosis of the haemolytic anaemias is extremely large (see Table 34.1). In general the distribution of etiologies of haemolytic anaemia in the elderly is different from that found in young subjects. An occasional patient with a congenital haemolytic anaemia may present for the first time in old age. A classic example is congenital spherocytosis which has been reported to present with worsening anaemia and/or cholycystitis in the elderly. Far more frequently however, the haemolytic anaemia is of the acquired type with auto-immune disease being the most frequent. The diagnosis is made by the presence of a positive Coomb's test and the disorder may be primary or secondary to a wide variety of underlying diseases. These tend to predominate in the elderly the more frequent being lymphoma, chronic lymphatic leukaemia, collagen vascular disease, and polymyalga rheumatica. Drug induced auto-immune haemolytic anaemia is common in the elderly. The list is extensive and has been reported in detail elsewhere (Williams et al, 1977).

In the secondary auto-immune haemolytic anaemia treatment should be directed at the underlying disease. The presence of auto-immune disease is an absolute indication to treat lymphoma or chronic lymphatic leukaemia. Steroids constitute the initial treatment of choice for the remaining auto-immune diseases there being no evidence that the elderly respond less well to the drug than do young individuals. The use of long term steroids in older subjects however, is particularly hazardous and for this reason early splenectomy or the use of cytotoxic agents is often indicated in the more severely ill individual.

CONCLUSIONS

From the above discussion it is clear that anaemia is a common disorder in the elderly and provides a difficult challenge for the clinician. The chances that the etiology of anaemia is multifactorial is higher in the elderly than in young subjects and therefore a rational approach to evaluation is particularly important. Based upon current state of knowledge it is not appropriate to consider reductions in haemoglobin and haematocrit values a normal consequence of the aging process. However, the high prevalence of modest reductions in haemoglobin and haematocrit levels in the elderly make clinical judgment important in deciding how extensive a diagnostic workup of anaemia should be. In general when an individual is at high risk of anaemia (haemoglobin < 12 gm/dl for males and < 10 gm/dl for females) a greater effort to determine the cause is warranted. Future studies will be required to determine how frequently anaemia is the initial manifestation of a serious underlying disease in the elderly.

REFERENCES

Evans D M D, Pathy M S, Sanerkin M C et al 1968 Anaemia in geriatric patients. Gerontologia Clinica 10: 228–241

Girdwood R H, Thompson A D, Williamson J 1969 Folate status in the elderly. British Medical Journal 1: 670–671

Hill R D 1967 The prevalence of anaemia in the over-65s in a rural practice. Practitioner 217: 936–967

Hillman R S, Finch C A 1974 Red Cell Manual. F A Davis, Philadelphia

Krasnow S E 1957 Megaloblastic anaemia in 'alcoholic cirrhosis'. Archives of Internal Medicine 100: 870–872

Lewis R 1976 Anaemia – a common but never a normal concomitant of aging. Geriatrics 31: 53–61

Lipschitz D A 1982 Protein calorie malnutrition in the hospitalized elderly patient. Primary Care 9: 531–538

Lipschitz D A, Mitchell C O 1982 The correctability of the nutrition, immune and hematopoietic manifestations of protein calorie malnutrition in the elderly. Journal of American College Nutrition 1: 17–25

Lipschitz D A, Cook J D, Finch C A 1974 The clinical evaluation of serum ferritin as an index of iron stores. New England Journal of Medicine 290: 1213–1216

Lipschitz D A, Milton K Y, Thompson C Effect of age on hematopoiesis in man. Blood. In press

Lipschitz D A, Mitchell C O, Thompson C 1981 The anaemia of senescence. American Journal of Hematology 11: 47–54

McLennan W J, Andrews G R, Macleod C, Caird F I 1973 Anaemia in the elderly. Quarterly Journal of Medicine 52: 1–13

Myers M A, Saunders C R G, Chalmers D G 1968 The hemoglobin level of fit elderly people. Lancet 2: 261–263

Nutrition Canada 1973 Natural Survey. Information Canada. Ottowa

Reynolds J H, Milner G, Mathew D M, Chanarin I 1966 Anticonvulsant therapy, megaloblastic haemopoiesis and folic acid metabolism. Quarterly Journal of Medicine 35: 521–534

U.S. Department of Health, Education and Welfare 1968–1980 Ten-State Nutrition Survey

Williams W J, Beutler E, Erslew A S, Rundles R W (eds) 1977 Drug reactions involving antibodies reacting with erythrocytes. In: Hematology. McGraw Hill, New York, p 605–610

Wintrobe M M (ed) 1981a Pancytopenia, aplastic anaemia and pure red cell aplasia. In: Clinical Hematology. Lea and Febiger, Philadelphia, p 698–733

Wintrobe M M (ed) 1981b Megaloblastic and non-megaloblastic macrocytic anemias. In: Clinical Hematology. Lea and Febiger, Philadelphia, p 559–604

35

Coagulation and bleeding problems

B. B. Weksler

INTRODUCTION

Blood clotting involves interactions among platelets, plasma coagulation factors and the blood vessel wall. When injury to a blood vessel occurs, platelets are rapidly activated, adhere to the site of injury and aggregate (clump) forming a platelet plug (primary haemostasis). During this activation process the platelet membrane becomes a catalytic surface upon which blood coagulation takes place. At the same time vasoactive mediators released by the activated platelets further augment their aggregation and constrict the injured vessel. Platelet plug formation halts bleeding from small vessels within one to five minutes. This primary phase of haemostasis is measured by the bleeding time.

Tissue injury also initiates the activation cascade of plasma procoagulant factors. These factors interact sequentially to produce the enzyme thrombin, which cleaves soluble plasma fibrinogen, forming an insoluble fibrin clot (secondary haemostasis). Thrombin also activates platelets. In turn, thrombin generation is markedly accelerated in the presence of platelets and becomes much more efficient. The integrity of the activation cascade of plasma coagulation factors is measured by the prothrombin time (PT) and partial thromboplastin time (PTT). The prothrombin time measures the extrinsic pathway of coagulation starting with tissue thromboplastin (including factors VII, X and II), while the partial thromboplastin time measures the intrinsic pathway which generates blood thromboplastin (factors XII, XI, IX, VIII, X and II). Thus general screening for blood clotting capacity can be accomplished with a combination of bleeding time, PT, PTT and a platelet count.

The platelet count and the levels of plasma coagulation factors do not change with age. In the elderly, probably because vascular disease (atherosclerosis) is common, providing an abnormal surface for platelets to contact, the platelets may appear more active than in younger subjects (Hamilton et al, 1974b; Couch & Hassanein, 1976; Zahavi et al, 1980). Bleeding time may be slightly shorter in the elderly than in young adults, and plasma levels of released platelet products higher (Jorgensen et al, 1980; Sie et al, 1981). In the presence of atherosclerosis or chronic inflammatory diseases, the levels of certain coagulation factors may be increased, particularly factor VIII (antihaemophilic globulin – Von Willebrand's Factor) and fibrinogen (Hamilton et al, 1974a). Thus in the elderly, both platelet activation and plasma coagulation factors may be increased, indicating a potentially 'hypercoagulable' state.

Balancing the process of blood coagulation is the process of clot dissolution: fibrinolysis. The main plasma pro-enzyme involved in this process, plasminogen, does not change in amount or activity with age. Indeed tissue plasminogen activator released from the blood vessel wall to initiate the fibrinolytic cascade by cleaving plasminogen to its active form, plasmin, may be increased in the elderly (Hamilton et al, 1974b). Fibrinolytic capacity tends to be maintained with age. However, immobility and vascular stasis may reduce the release of plasminogen activator, resulting in an overall age-related decrease in fibrinolysis. Thus the enzyme systems involved in control of blood clotting may all change with increasing age in a prothrombotic direction. In contrast, bleeding tendencies in the elderly usually represent the effects of drugs or of specific diseases on platelets, plasma clotting factors or fibrinolysis.

Causes of a bleeding tendency in the elderly

New manifestations of a bleeding tendency in the elderly patient usually represent an acquired disorder. It is possible that a mild congenital bleeding diathesis such as mild haemophilia, Von Willebrand's disease or factor XI deficiency may be recognised for the first time in an elderly person, previously undiagnosed until a stress such as surgery is imposed. This is unusual. Common reasons for an acquired bleeding tendency manifested in the older age group, are listed in Table 35.1. First and most common, is an anatomical lesion in the gastro-intestinal (GI) or gastro-urinary (GU) tract such as diverticula, ulcers, polyps, hiatus hernia or carcinoma. Such lesions may present as occult anaemia or as overt, localised bleeding. The next most common reason for a bleeding tendency in the elderly is ingestion of drugs which may cause thrombocytopenia or abnormal platelet function. Aspirin-containing medications provide the leading cause of platelet dysfunction, whereas quinidine or thiazides most commonly cause thrombocytopenia. Hepatic or renal disease may also result in a bleeding tendency. Chronic liver disease, whether hepatitis or cirrhosis, especially if combined with alcoholism, is associated with reduced synthesis of clotting factors (II, VII, IX, X and in severe disease V and fibronogen). Liver disease also produces a chronic, mild, disseminated intravascular coagulation and thrombocytopenia. Thrombocytopenia often results from hypersplenism which can accompany liver disease with portal hypertension. Renal insufficiency may cause abnormal platelet function and a long bleeding time. Diseases of the bone marrow, such as chronic or acute leukaemias, myeloma and the myeloproliferative diseases may be accompanied by bleeding often related to thrombocytopenia or abnormal platelet function. Nutritional deficiencies such as pernicious anaemia or folic acid deficiency also manifest thrombocytopenia, and vitamin C deficiency can lead to abnormal platelet function. Bone marrow failure resulting in refractory sideroblastic anaemia or aplastic anaemia is also characterised by thrombocytopenia. Auto-immune diseases such as idiopathic thrombocytopenic purpura (ITP), auto-immune hemolytic anaemia with thrombocytopenia (Evan's syndrome) or systemic lupus erythematosus may also present as bleeding tendencies. Amyloidosis characteristically is accompanied by severe purpura. Acquired circulating anticoagulants directed against factor VIII or the prothrombin complex may also produce bleeding.

Table 35.1 Common reasons for an acquired bleeding tendency

Anatomic lesions	ulcer, tumor, diverticuli
	Telangectasis
	Gastritis
Drug ingestion	Aspirin
	Non-steroidal anti-inflammatory drugs
	Anticoagulants
	Quinidine
	Thiazides
	Gold
Liver disease	
Renal disease	
Hematologic malignancy	Leukaemia
	Myeloproliferative disease
	Aplastic anaemia
	Multiple myeloma
Immunologic disorder	Systemic lupus erythematosus
	Idiopathic thrombocytopenic purpura
	Circulating anticoagulant

Evaluation of a bleeding tendency

Evaluation of a bleeding tendency requires an accurate patient history, with particular attention to family and patient history of bleeding problems, prior anaemia or need for transfusion and bleeding at tooth extraction or at surgery. A careful enumeration of drugs being currently taken and those taken in the past is essential. Clinical clues to the presence of a bleeding tendency may relate to the site of bleeding: skin and mucosal membrane, joint and muscle bleeding or bleeding from the GI or GU tracts tend to have different mechanisms. Thrombocytopenia or platelet dysfunction characteristically present with bruising, petechiae, epistaxis or gum bleeding, whereas joint or muscle bleeding is associated with circulating anticoagulants, clotting factor deficiencies and amyloid. Epistaxis in the elderly more frequently relates to local factors such as nose-picking or drying of the nasal mucosa than to haemostatic defects. Chronic GI or GU tract bleeding is most commonly associated with discrete anatomic lesions such as diverticula, ulcer or carcinoma. Such bleeding can be exacerbated by platelet or coagulation factor defects or by drugs. Haematuria may signal a coagulation or platelet defect as well as anatomic lesions such as stone or tumor.

Clues from the physical examination include the presence of ecchymosis or purpura, especially petechiae or bruises on the trunk, face, conjunctiva or retina, and the presence of palpable ecchymoses. In contrast, small bruises on the lower legs or hands more often relate to local trauma than to haemostatic defects. Lymphadenopathy, hepatosplenomegaly and telangectasia should be sought. Laboratory screening should include (Table 35.2) a complete blood count with differential white cell count, a platelet count, prothrombin time and activated partial thromboplastin time and, if the platelet count is normal, a bleeding time. The peripheral blood smear should be examined for platelet and red cell morphology. Specific features sought should include thrombocytopenia, presence of giant platelets, spherocytes, schistocytes or immature leukocytes. A urinalysis with microscopic examination for red cells and examination of the stool for occult blood should be done. Liver function tests, serum protein examination and serum creatinine may also aid in defining underlying disorders affecting haemostasis.

Table 35.2 Laboratory screening for haemostatic disorders

Complete blood count
    Differential white cell count
    Platelet count
Prothrombin time
Activated partial thromboplastin time
Bleeding time
Urinalysis with microscopic examination
Stool for occult blood
Serum creatinine
Serum protein electrophoresis

COMMON BLEEDING DISORDERS IN THE ELDERLY ASSOCIATED WITH ABNORMAL PLATELET NUMBERS OR FUNCTION

Thrombocytopenia

A marked reduction in platelet number frequently leads to mucosal and superficial bleeding which may present as bruising, petechiae, epistaxis, GI bleeding and occasionally intracerebral bleeding. Platelet counts below 50 000 per μl are more frequently associated with bleeding. However if the thrombocytopenia is of gradual onset, patients with counts of as low as 10–20 000/μl may be relatively asymptomatic. At such low counts a bleeding time will always be prolonged and should not be done. Thrombocytopenia may be related to drug ingestion, auto-immunity, marrow failure, malignancy, infection, or disseminated intravascular coagulation. The key diagnostic test in evaluating thrombocytopenia is a bone marrow examination; an increased number of megakaryocytes is strongly suggestive of peripheral platelet destruction which may be autoimmune or drug related, whereas decreased or absent megakaryocytes signal marrow depression and a production defect. The most common drugs causing thrombocytopenia include thiazides, quinidine, digitalis, gold, penicillins, ethanol or estrogens (Hackett et al, 1982) – but many other drugs may be implicated. The platelets often are 'innocent bystanders' which become coated with drug-antidrug immune complexes and are secondarily removed from circulation by the spleen or liver. The key to management of a drug-induced immune purpura is to stop or change the drug. Recovery will occur in one to two weeks depending upon the rate of clearance of the offending drug from the circulation.

Auto-immune thrombocytopenic purpura (ITP) in the elderly may be associated with an underlying disease such as lymphoma, chronic lymphocytic leukaemia, auto-immune haemolytic anaemia or collagen vascular disease (Kaden et al, 1979). In ITP the bone marrow reveals increased megakaryocytes, while the peripheral platelet count may be profoundly depressed. Platelet associated IgG may be markedly increased and platelets on the peripheral smear tend to be large (i.e. young). Platelet survival is short and transfused platelets are destroyed as quickly as the patient's own. Management of ITP include steroid therapy (40–60 mg/d prednisone) which controls the purpura and corrects the thrombocytopenia in about 70% of the cases within two weeks. Transfusion of platelets is to be avoided except in central nervous system bleeding, because of the rapid destruction of all platelets. Patients who are refractory to steroids or heavily steroid-dependent may require splenectomy or the administration of immunosuppressive drugs such as vincristine or cytoxan. An experimental therapy temporarily useful in steroid-refractory patients is administration of high-dose gamma globulin intravenously. In contrast to the acute and self-limited course of ITP in children, in the adult ITP tends to be chronic. In many cases, the function of those platelets present is normal to enhanced, reflecting their large size and rapid turnover rate. In some cases, especially those associated with systemic lupus erythematosus, platelet function may be poor contributing further to bleeding phenomena. ITP in patients with chronic lymphocytic leukaemia or Hodgkin's disease may reflect activity of the underlying disease and may be responsive to treatment of the latter. Rarely, ITP may present in patients with disseminated carcinoma (Spivak et al, 1979; Schwartz et al, 1982).

Thrombocytopenia commonly develops in severe infections, disseminated intravascular coagulation (DIC), refractory anaemia or aplastic anaemia. These situations represent marrow failure of different degrees of severity. Bone marrow reserve may be depressed in the elderly person so that platelet as well as neutrophil production may be inadequate during stress states such as sepsis, especially when platelet consumption is augmented as in accompanying DIC. In refractory anaemia, which may represent a pre-leukaemic state and in bone marrow failure, whether idiopathic or related to drugs, radiation or chemotherapy, thrombocytopenia may herald worsening of marrow function. In refractory anaemia, the appearance of thrombocytopenia is a prognostic sign of leukaemic transformation. Bone marrow examination shows decreased megakaryocytes. The peripheral smear displays small platelets rather than the large ones which may be seen in ITP. Steroid treatment generally fails to correct the thrombocytopenia of bone marrow failure and platelet transfusion is the most useful modality to control bleeding if the underlying condition, especially infection, cannot be corrected.

Thrombocytosis

A marked increase in platelet count may be seen with chronic infection such as tuberculosis or chronic bowel disease, after splenectomy and in the myeloproliferative syndromes – polycythemia vera, chronic myelogenous leukaemia, myeloid metaplasia and essential thrombocythaemia. A raised platelet count may also be an early manifestation of visceral malignancy. Counts may be as high as several million in thrombocytosis secondary to infection or cancer; platelet size and function are usually normal and platelet count falls with correction of the underlying disease. In contrast, thrombocytosis in the myeloproliferative syndromes is characterised by bizarre, giant platelets, platelet mass increased out of proportion to the platelet count, abnormalities of platelet function and a combination of bleeding and thrombotic tendencies. The characteristic functional abnormality of myeloproliferative platelets is the absence of aggregation in response to epinephrine. The bleeding time may be abnormal (prolonged) in myeloproliferative syndromes despite the high platelet count, but does not correlate well with either bleeding or thrombotic complications. The platelet count may be controlled in the myeloproliferative syndromes by treatment with cytostatic drugs such as hydroxyurea or busulfan. These drugs must be administered with great care because of variable sensitivity and duration of response. Once the platelet count is normalised, the tendency towards bleeding or thrombosis may be lessened but the measurable abnormalities in platelet function are not corrected.

Drug induced changes in platelet function

One of the most common reasons for a bleeding tendency in the elderly is the depressive effect of commonly ingested drugs upon platelet function. Aspirin-containing medications and the non-steroidal, anti-inflammatory drugs (indomethacin, ibuprofen, fenamates etc) inhibit arachidonic acid metabolism in platelets, depressing the platelet release reaction and impairing platelet aggregation. These drugs specifically inhibit the platelet enzyme cyclooxygenase, which mediates production of thromboxane A_2, a substance which normally causes platelet aggregation and vasoconstriction. Thus these drugs prolong the bleeding time and exacerbate any underlying bleeding tendency. This is why aspirin-like drugs should be avoided in anticoagulated patients. It has recently been shown that ingestion of alcohol together with aspirin results in extreme prolongation of bleeding time and a further impairment of platelet function (Deykin et al, 1982). The inhibitory effect of a single dose of aspirin on platelet function may last as long as a week, the lifespan of platelets, because platelets cannot generate new cyclooxygenase after inhibition by aspirin. However, the effects on platelets of other non-steroidal anti-inflammatory agents are reversible and last less than 24 hours. Many other drugs impair platelet function including penicillin and cephalosporin type antibiotics when administered intravenously in high dosage.

Non-thrombocytopenic purpuras

If the platelet count and platelet function are normal, the presence of purpura suggests an abnormality in vascular factors contributing to haemostasis. Senile purpura, a common and benign condition, results from a gradual loss of sub-cutaneous fat and the degeneration of elastic and connective tissue fibres of the skin, particularly in sun-exposed areas. Because of the loss of the supporting tissue network around small skin vessels, minimal trauma can produce bruising. In addition, a decrease in the inflammatory response to resorb the extravasated blood, leads to persistence of the purpura. Senile purpura is harmless and requires no treatment. Similar changes in the skin leading to easy bruising are observed in Cushing's syndrome or, more frequently, after administration of corticosteroids.

More serious purpura can be caused by abnormal plasma proteins such as those present in the dysproteinaemias. In multiple myeloma, macroglobulinaemia and cryoglobulinaemia, circulating monoclonal immunoglobulins may interfere with platelet function or with coagulation. Monoclonal immunoglobulins can coat platelets and prevent their normal interaction, slow or inhibit the polymerisation of fibrin or prevent clot retraction. These plasma abnormalities may result in purpura or in a severe bleeding tendency, particularly at surgery. Cryoglobulinaemia may be accompanied by vasculitis which can also produce a thrombotic tendency in the affected vessels. In amyloidosis, either associated with multiple myeloma or secondary to other diseases, purpura is common and may be severe. Here the purpura is related to the increased fragility of small vessels infiltrated with deposits of friable amyloid, especially in loose or dependent tissues such as under the eyes. Rarely, vascular deposits of amyloid adsorb coagulation factor X leading to an acquired factor X deficiency with a severe bleeding tendency. Finally, benign hyperglobulinaemic purpura occurs in older women who have a diffuse polyclonal increase in plasma immunoglobulins, pruritic purpura of the legs and deposition of an antibody to IgG in the purpuric lesions. This condition appears to represent a cutaneous vasculitis.

Hereditary haemorrhagic telangiectasia (Osler-Weber-Rendu Disease) is a congenital bleeding disorder with a dominant inheritance which can become more severe in the elderly. The fragile telangiectasias appear on the skin and mucosal membranes and may cause severe and repeated epistaxis, GI or urinary bleeding. Patients may require life-long iron supplementation because of recurrent bleeding. In addition to the mucosal lesions, older patients (commonly 30%) develop pulmonary arteriovenous fistulae which may produce bleeding, hypoxaemia or thrombo-embolism.

COAGULATION DISORDERS IN THE ELDERLY

While lifespan in severe congenital coagulation disorders may be shortened, patients with mild haemophilia A or B (deficiency of factor VIII or IX respectively), Von Willebrand's disease or factor XI deficiency may enjoy a normal lifespan. Bleeding problems may be unrecognised or only appreciated when haemorrhage occurs at surgery or with trauma. The presence of a life-long coagulation defect does not appear to prevent the onset of atherosclerosis, and both coronary artery disease and cerebro-vascular disease may present in patients with mild haemophilia at appropriate ages. However acquired coagulation defects are a common cause for impaired haemostasis in the elderly.

The most common causes for acquired coagulation defects in the elderly include vitamin K deficiency, liver disease or the ingestion of anticoagulants. Since vitamin K is obtained from the diet plus synthesis by intestinal bacteria, vitamin K deficiency can be associated with poor nutrition, prolonged antibiotic ingestion or biliary obstruction. Alcoholism, which also impairs platelet production by the bone marrow and is frequently accompanied by poor nutrition, is a common associated factor in vitamin K deficiency. These conditions may result in decreased levels of the vitamin K – dependent coagulation factors which are synthesised in the liver; factors II (prothrombin), VII, IX, X. In severe liver disease factors V and fibrinogen, which are also produced in the liver but do not require vitamin K, may also be diminished. A decrease in the liver related factors leads to a prolongation of the PT and PTT. Severe liver disease is also accompanied by local intravascular coagulation and fibrinogen consumption. In such cases, both vitamin K replacement and plasma therapy may be needed to restore coagulation to normal. The combination of limited food intake plus antibiotic therapy post-operatively in patients undergoing bowel surgery for example, is a particular hazard for the development of vitamin K deficiency in the elderly.

Patients taking oral anticoagulants may unintentionally become over anti-coagulated because of drug interaction with other medications being taken. Moreover, surreptitious ingestion of anticoagulants must always be considered when a bleeding disorder is otherwise unexplained and the PT is markedly prolonged.

Circulating anticoagulants

Spontaneous appearance of inhibitors of the normal coagulation mechanism may occur in collagen vascular disease, multiple myeloma, with chlorpromazine therapy or in the absence of any disease. These circulating anticoagulants are antibodies usually directed against factor VIII or against the prothrombin complex. Inhibitors to Von Willebrand's factor are rare, occurring mainly in patients with lymphoma or chronic lymphocytic leukaemia. Inhibitors of Factor VIII: antihaemophilic factor can cause severe bleeding. The appearance of a 'lupus anticoagulant' directed against the prothrombin complex occurs in 10% of patients with systemic lupus erythematosus, but also in a large number of otherwise normal individuals. This anticoagulant is directed against phospholipid-containing molecules in cell membranes and is associated with a positive VDRL or ANA. It is detected by a prolonged PTT (less often, prolonged PT) which is not corrected by mixing with normal plasma. The lupus anticoagulant is not associated with a bleeding tendency unless a second lesion in the haemostatic pathway, such as thrombocytopenia or platelet dysfunction is also present. Indeed, the presence of a lupus anticoagulant may be associated with a thrombotic rather than a haemorrhagic tendency. When this anticoagulant occurs in the presence of clinical systemic lupus erythematosus, both bleeding and haemorrhagic episodes are observed with increased incidence.

Disseminated intravascular coagulation

Intravascular activation of the coagulation system, with consumption of platelets and coagulation factors, occurs in the elderly in three main clinical settings. The first is severe infection: classically gram-negative sepsis, but also severe gram-positive bacterial infections, viral infections or malaria. The second area is trauma and shock. Shock from any cause can produce a burst of DIC, including hypotension associated with severe infection, surgery, myocardial infarction or trauma. A third area in which DIC occurs commonly in the elderly – in a chronic rather than an acute form – is widespread visceral malignancy. Here DIC is associated with migratory thrombophlebitis (Trousseau's syndrome). Carcinoma of the colon, prostate, pancreas, lung, stomach or breast can cause this syndrome (Sack et al, 1977) as can promyelocytic leukaemia. The mechanism appears to be the release of procoagulant materials from tumour tissue: tissue thromboplastins or proteases. In acute promyelocytic leukaemia, release of granule thromboplastins from the leukaemic cells can also produce severe DIC. Rarer causes of DIC include haemolytic transfusion reactions, acute vasculitis, massive venous thrombosis, hepatic necrosis, heat stroke, snake bite and cardiac arrest.

In acute DIC, diagnostic clues can be obtained from peripheral blood smear and coagulation screening tests (Ockelford & Carter, 1983). Because of consumption of platelets and coagulation factors the platelet count is decreased, the PT and PTT are prolonged and fibrinogen and factor VIII levels are low. The peripheral smear reflects not only the thrombocytopenia but also shows schistocytes, fragmented red cells damaged by passage over intravascular fibrin strands. These reflect a micro-angiopathic haemolytic anaemia. Tests for the presence of fibrin split products, indicating secondary activation of the fibrinolytic system, are positive. In chronic DIC such as in malignancy, the laboratory signs may be much more subtle. The PT and PTT may be normal, or even short if there is an increased production of coagulation factors to meet the increased consumption. Fibrinogen and factor VIII levels may be normal to increased for the same reason. The platelet count is usually slightly decreased. The peripheral smear may continue to show schistocytes and the fibrin split products remain elevated.

The primary therapy of acute DIC is to treat the underlying cause: sepsis, malignancy etc. Supportive therapy may be necessary if the patient is actively bleeding and consists of cryoprecipitate (to supply fibrinogen), platelets and packed red blood cells. If clotting factors are low but there is no bleeding, such replacement is probably unnecessary, especially when the DIC is self-limited. If the clinical manifestations are thrombosis rather than bleeding, as frequently occurs in malignancy, therapy with full doses of heparin may be crucial. In Trousseau's syndrome, oral anticoagulants are not efficacious and chronic heparin therapy may be necessary. Heparin will also control DIC and bleeding in patients with acute promyelocytic leukaemia.

HYPERCOAGULABILITY AND THROMBOSIS

Certain conditions prevalent among the elderly result in a thrombotic tendency. These include immobility and venous stasis; atherosclerotic cardiovascular and cerebrovascular disease; malignancy; chronic inflammatory diseases; vasculitis and the myeloproliferative syndromes. In addition, acute inflammatory states, trauma and surgery can temporarily activate the coagulation mechanism and lead to thrombotic complications. Hypercoagulability is a difficult state to define. It is best considered a condition in which there is an increase in activated clotting factors either because of increased activation rates or decreased clearance of activated factors. Interaction of platelets with the abnormal surface of atherosclerotic blood vessels can result in platelet activation, so called spontaneous platelet aggregation, and can further promote thrombosis.

It is difficult to measure hypercoagulability in the laboratory. Plasma levels of coagulation factors are often raised in inflammatory states, in malignancy or after surgery or trauma. Such elevated levels do not necessarily indicate an increased tendency to thrombosis. Similarly in these conditions the PTT may be short, but a clinical correlation with thrombosis is not well established. High platelet counts also seen in these settings may be associated with thrombosis but also with bleeding. Thus while these conditions overall are clinically linked with increased venous or arterial thrombosis, no simple prognostic laboratory approach is presently available to guide prophylaxis or acute interventive therapy (Hirsh, 1981).

Prophylactic use of antithrombotic therapy

In general, prevention of venous thrombosis differs from the prevention of arterial thrombosis. In venous thrombosis, where stasis is a prominent factor and thrombi are 'red' i.e. composed mainly of fibrin and enmeshed red cells, anticoagulant therapy is preferred. In arterial thrombosis, where vascular injury and consequent platelet activation are prominent inciting factors, thrombi are 'white' i.e. composed of platelets and fibrin, and therapy directed against platelet activation is used. In patients who are haemostatically intact, recommendations for anticoagulant or antiplatelet therapy to prevent thrombo-embolism in the elderly are similar to those for younger individuals.

Prophylaxis against venous thrombosis and pulmonary embolism in the elderly depends upon the clinical setting. In patients undergoing elective abdominal or gynaecologic surgery, 'miniheparin' administered pre- and post-operatively has been shown to decrease the incidence of

post-operative venous thrombosis. The dosage recommended is 5000 units every 8–12 hours subcutaneously. This dose schedule does not prolong the PTT. Low-dose heparin may also reduce DVT in patients immobilised after completed stroke or myocardial infarction. However low dose heparin prophylaxis has not been beneficial in preventing DVT or pulmonary embolism in patients with hip fracture or those undergoing elective reconstructive hip surgery, where its use may result in increased wound haematomas and infections. Miniheparin acts mainly to prevent factor X activation. Since activated factor X (Xa) catalyses thrombin formation, a small dose of heparin can prevent the formation of large amounts of thrombin. Far higher (full) heparin dosage is needed to inhibit the action of thrombin already generated. Thus in conditions where thrombus formation has already begun – as in hip fracture or deep venous thrombosis; where large amounts of thrombin are being produced as in trauma associated with hip surgery, or in acute pulmonary embolism – full dose heparin is required to control thrombosis. In patients undergoing orthopaedic procedures, venous thrombosis near the operated area is very common. For elective hip or knee surgery, venograms show thrombosis on the operated side in 70–80% of patients and on the contralateral side in 50%. Antithrombotic drug use is directed against thrombus propagation and possible consequent pulmonary embolism. Aspirin pre and post-operatively or dextran infusion post-operatively both reduce the incidence of pulmonary embolism in patients undergoing elective hip surgery. In hip fracture by contrast, antiplatelet drugs such as aspirin are not efficacious prophylaxis against DVT (Morris & Mitchell, 1977). Post-operative full-dose heparin followed by oral anticoagulation is useful in preventing pulmonary emboli in hip fracture patients. Low-dose warfarin started 10 days pre-operatively (PT 3–5 seconds greater than control) followed by dose adjustment to keep PT 1.5 times control after hip or knee surgery has been another effective and safe method to prevent DVT and pulmonary embolism (Francis et al, 1983). An alternative means of protecting against post-operative DVT is the use of sequential leg compression boots, which have been especially useful in patients with intracranial disease as well as abdominal disease (Turpie et al, 1979).

When deep venous thrombosis is diagnosed, therapy should be started promptly after ascertaining the patient's baseline haemostatic status (PT, PTT, complete blood count and platelet count). Heparin at full dosage is given, 5000–10 000 units as a bolus injection intravenously followed by 1000 units/h by infusion to keep the activated PTT at 2–2.5 times the patient's baseline. Renal and hepatic disease diminish heparin clearance and require downward dose adjustment. After a week of heparin therapy, oral anticoagulation can be substituted. It should be started during heparin therapy at 15 mg coumadin the first day then 5–10 mg daily until the PT is 1.5–2 times control, when heparin is discontinued. For deep venous thrombosis in the legs, anticoagulation should be continued at least 2 months, while for pulmonary embolism it should be continued at least 3–4 months. Fresh thrombi (within 2–7 days) either pulmonary or in the extremities can also be treated with thrombolytic drugs such as streptokinase or urokinase if there has been no recent surgery, trauma, cerebrovascular process or bleeding (Sharma et al, 1982). Thrombolytic therapy can promptly relieve vascular obstruction (which heparin does not), but carries a much higher risk of bleeding than does anticoagulation.

Venous thrombosis occurring in malignancy offers several special cases. The superficial thrombophlebitis and DIC associated with visceral malignancy respond to chronic full-dose heparin therapy, but are poorly controlled by oral anticoagulants (Sack et al, 1977) or miniheparin. This may result in part from production by tumour cells of enzymes which directly activate factor X. These are better inhibited by heparin, which prevents factor X activation, than by coumarins. In women with breast carcinoma who are receiving adjuvant chemotherapy, an increased incidence of deep venous thrombosis has recently been observed. This complication may require not only acute heparin therapy for the thrombosis but long-term oral anticoagulation to prevent recurrent thrombosis while chemotherapy is continued. Thrombosis in the myeloproliferative syndromes responds best to control of the blood count: reduction of red cell mass and viscosity in polycythaemia vera, and reduction of thrombocytosis by cytostatic drugs (e.g. hydroxyurea) in other myeloproliferative diseases. Anticoagulation of such patients may be hazardous because of the paradoxical bleeding tendencies also found. Phlebotomy for polycythaemia vera is an effective means of lowering red cell mass but may lead to a 'rebound' thrombocytosis if carried out too vigorously.

Prophylaxis against arterial thrombo-embolism must also be tailored to the clinical setting. Prevention of cerebral or systemic embolism of cardiac origin in patients with valvular heart disease, left ventricular aneurysm or prosthetic heart valves requires chronic oral anticoagulation. In patients whose thrombotic tendency is resistant to anticoagulants alone, the addition of dipyridamole or sulfinpyrazone may help to limit recurrent thrombosis. Patients who respond to such combination therapy are those who have increased platelet activity or platelet consumption (Steele & Rainwater, 1980). While aspirin theoretically could inhibit platelet activation in such patients, the combination of aspirin with anticoagulants presents an unacceptably high risk of haemorrhage (Yett et al, 1978). Dipyridamole acts as an antiplatelet agent in this setting without increasing the risk of bleeding.

The use of anticoagulants or antiplatelet agents to prevent recurrence of myocardial infarction remains a controversial subject. Numerous trials of either therapy have produced statistically questionable benefit. However in one well-controlled clinical study of patients over the age of 65 who were anticoagulated following one myocardial infarction, long-term oral anticoagulation clearly improved outcome, reducing both the incidence of recurrent infarction and mortality (Sixty Plus Reinfarction Study Group, 1980). The complication rate was not greater than for younger patients although patients with prior bleeding tendency, congestive heart failure or renal disease were excluded from study. In other studies, the administration of beta-adrenergic blocking drugs have also prevented recurrent infarction or sudden death following infarction, in contrast to the lack of effect of antiplatelet agents.

In atherosclerotic cerebrovascular disease characterised by transient ischaemic attacks (TIA), the risk of stroke has been estimated at 5% per year (Genton et al, 1977). Aspirin therapy is recommended to prevent TIA, stroke or death in men (Canadian Cooperative Study, 1980). A recent multicentre trial suggests that women over 50 with TIA or prior stroke may also benefit from aspirin prophylaxis (Bousser et al, 1983). The dosage of aspirin is a matter of current controversy. Most studies used 1 g daily or higher dosage. However recent evidence suggests that the anti-platelet effects of aspirin are maximal at 80 mg daily and that higher doses of aspirin may concurrently inhibit vascular producton of the natural anti-platelet and vasodilator substance, prostacyclin (Weksler et al, 1983). Thus higher aspirin dosage may cancel out anti-platelet effects, cause gastric bleeding and depress renal function. Low aspirin dosage e.g. 80 mg/day will have an equivalent anti-platelet effect without other actions. Vasculitis, in particular temporal arteritis common in older persons, may also lead to vascular occlusion. Steroid therapy is the treatment of choice in vasculitis to prevent thrombo-embolic complications, such as blindness.

Hazards and complications of antithrombotic therapy in the elderly

The major risks associated with anticoagulant or antiplatelet therapy in the elderly include haemorrhage, thrombocytopenia and renal dysfunction (Kelton & Hirsh, 1980).

The main risks of heparin therapy are haemorrhage and thrombocytopenia. Elderly women have appeared to be at greater risk of bleeding during heparin therapy than were men or younger women when heparin was administered by bolus injection (Jick et al, 1968; Vieweg et al, 1970). Comparison of the efficacy and toxicities of heparin administered by bolus injection versus continuous infusion however, has shown that intermittent therapy required 25% more heparin and produced seven times more frequent bleeding complications than did continuous infusion. Infusion of heparin produced equal clinical benefit. No added risk related to age or sex was observed (Salzman et al, 1975). Thrombocytopenia may occur during heparin therapy, usually within the first week. The mechanism may be immunologic, with demonstration of a circulating platelet-aggregant factor in the patient's plasma. More commonly a component of the heparin itself may directly cause platelet clumping, leading to thrombocytopenia. Arterial thrombosis as well as haemorrhage may accompany heparin-induced thrombocytopenia. Some evidence exists that porcine intestinal heparin produces fewer instances of thrombocytopenia than bovine lung heparin; treatment of the thrombocytopenia requires discontinuation of heparin if the platelet count falls below 100 000 mm^3 or if bleeding occurs.

Bleeding due to oral anticoagulants is most often associated with poor control of therapy, interaction of the anticoagulant with other medications being taken, or the presence of a second haemostatic defect. There is an increased sensitivity to the effects of warfarin with increasing age, which is independent of body weight (Shepherd et al, 1977). The pharmacokinetics of warfarin do not change with age. The therapeutic range for oral anticoagulant therapy is better established than that for heparin therapy. The desired prolongation of the PT depends upon the type of test used: thus, bleeding complications can be minimised if the dose is adjusted to maintain the PT at 1.5 times control using rabbit brain thromboplastin, 2–3 times control using human brain thromboplastin or thrombotest 5–10%. In many studies, rates of haemorrhage correlate with increased PT beyond these ranges. In the Sixty Plus Reinfarction Study Group (1982), 75% of bleeding episodes in patients receiving coumarins occurred when the prothrombin time was prolonged 2.7–4.5 times control. Overall, the incidence of bleeding complications did not increase with increasing age in the 878 patients studied.

Bleeding from oral anticoagulant therapy occurs most commonly at sites of recent surgery or trauma, the GI tract or the urine. Intracranial bleeding is the most frequent fatal haemorrhagic complication of oral anticoagulant therapy; the risk is greatest in patients with hypertension or recent cerebral infarction. In the elderly, subdural haematoma is another important haemorrhagic complication, especially as clinical signs may be very subtle.

Ingestion of aspirin or other non-steroidal anti-inflammatory drugs, antibiotics or other drugs which displace coumarins from albumin binding sites and the presence of liver or kidney disease may all increase the biologic response to oral anticoagulants and may lead to bleeding. Treatment of such bleeding is based on the following principles: discontinue the oral anticoagulant; administer vitamin K_1 (5–10 mg) if the coagulation defect must be reversed within 6–12 hours; administer fresh frozen plasma if the defect must be reversed more quickly, or prothrombin complex concentrate if volume is a problem.

CONCLUSION

Elderly patients are susceptible to a variety of acquired bleeding disorders and, as a result of greater immobility and vascular disease, to increased incidence of thrombosis especially in association with the presence of other disease. While no specific tests are available to predict a prothrombotic tendency, simple prophylactic measures can be used and accessible tests employed to monitor coagulation problems. In employing antithrombotic therapy in the elderly, their altered pharmacokinetics related to age-associated changes in liver or renal function as well as drug interactions may require modifications of dosage schedules.

REFERENCES

Andersen L A, Gormsen J 1976 Platelet aggregation and fibrinolytic activity in transient cerebral ischemia. Acta Neurologica Scandanavica 55: 76–82

Bousser M G, Eschwege E, Haguenau M, Lefaucconnier J M, Thibult N, Touboul D, Touboul P 1983 'AICLA' Controlled trial of aspirin and Dipyridemole in the secondary prevention of athero-thrombotic cerebral ischemia. Stroke 14: 5–22

Browse N L, Gray L, Jarret P E, Morland M 1977 Blood and vein wall fibrinolytic activity in health and vascular disease. British Medical Journal 1: 478

Canadian Cooperative Study Group 1980 A randomized trial of aspirin and sulfinpyrazone in threatened stroke. New England Journal of Medicine 299: 53–57

Couth J R, Hassanein R S 1976 Platelet aggregation, stroke and transient ischemic attack in middle-aged elderly patients. Neurology 26: 888–895

Deykin D, Janson P, McMahon L 1982 Ethanol potentiation of aspirin-induced prolongation of the bleeding time. New England Journal of Medicine 306: 852–854

Ettinger M G, Kusonoki R, Fusishima H 1969 Blood coagulation studies. Geriatrics 24: 116–125

Francis C W, Marder V J, Evarts C M, Yaukoolbodi S 1983 Two step warfarin therapy. Prevention of postoperative venous thrombosis without excessive bleeding. Journal of the American Medical Association 249: 374

Gaston L, Brooks J, Blumenthal H, Miller C 1971 A study of blood coagulation following an acute stroke. Stroke 2: 81–87

Genton E, Barnett H J M, Fields W S, Gent M, Hoak J C 1977 XIV Cerebral ischemia: The role of thrombosis and of antithrombotic therapy. Stroke 8: 148–175

Hackett T, Kelton J, Powers P 1982 Drug-induced platelet destruction. Seminars in Thrombosis and Hemostasis 8: 116–137

Hamilton P J, Dawson A, Ogston D, Douglas A S 1974a The effect of age on the fibrinolytic system. Journal of Clinical Pathology 27: 326–329

Hamilton P J, Allardyce M, Ogston D, Dawson A, Douglas A S 1974b The effect of age upon the coagulation system. Journal of Clinical Pathology 27: 980–982

Hirsh J 1981 Blood tests for the diagnosis of venous and arterial thrombosis. Blood 57: 1–8

Hochman R, Clark J, Rolla A, Thomas S, Kaldany A, D'Elia J 1982 Bleeding in patients with infections: are antibodies helping or hurting? Archives of Internal Medicine 142: 1440–1442

Jick H, Slone D, Borda I T, Shapiro S 1968 Efficacy and toxicity of heparin in relation to age and sex. New England Journal of Medicine 279: 284–286

Jorgensen K, Dyerberg J, Olesen A, Stoffersen E 1980 Acetyl salicylic acid, bleeding time and age. Thrombosis Research 19: 799–805

Kaden G R, Rosse W F, Hauch T W 1979 Immune thrombocytopenia in lymphoproliferative diseases. Blood 53: 545–551

Kelton J G, Hirsh J 1980 Bleeding associated with antithrombotic therapy. Seminars in Hematology 17: 259–291

Morris G K, Mitchell J R A 1977 Preventing venous thrombo-embolism in elderly patients with hip fractures: studies of low-dose heparin, dipyridamole aspirin and flurbiprofen. British Medical Journal 1: 535–537

Ockelford P A, Carter C J 1983 Disseminated intravascular coagulation: the applicaton and utility of diagnostic tests. Seminars in Thrombosis and Hemostasis 8: 198–216

Sack G H Jr, Levin J, Bell W R 1977 Trousseau's syndrome and other manifestations of chronic disseminated coagulopathy in patients with neoplasms: clinical, pathophysiologie and therapeutic features. Medicine (Baltimore) 56: 1–37

Salzman E, Deykin K, Shapiro R, Rosenberg R 1975 Management of heparin therapy: controlled prospective trial. New England Journal of Medicine 1046–1050

Schwartz K, Slichter S, Harker L 1982 Immune-mediated platelet destruction and thrombocytopenia in patients with solid tumours. British Journal of Haematology 51: 17–24

Sharma G, Cella G, Parisi A, Sasahara A 1982 Thrombolytic therapy. New England Journal of Medicine 306: 1268–1276

Shepherd A M, Hewick D S, Moreland T A, Stevenson I H 1977 Age as a determinant of sensitivity to warfarin. British Journal of Clinical Pharmacology 4: 315–320

Sie P, Montagut J, Blanc M, Boneu B, Caranobe C, Cazard J, Bierme R 1981 Evaluation of some platelet parameters in a group of elderly people. Thrombosis and Haemostasis 45: 197–199

Sixty Plus Reinfarction Study Research Group 1980 A double-blind trial to assess long-term oral anticoagulant therapy in elderly patients after myocardial infarction. Lancet ii: 989–994

Sixty Plus Reinfarction Study Research Group 1982 Risks of long-term oral anticoagulant therapy in elderly patients after myocardial infarction. Lancet 1: 64–68

Spivak M, Brenner S, Markham M, Snyder E, Berkowitz D 1979 Presumed immune thrombocytopenia and carcinoma: report of 3 cases and review of the literature. American Journal of the Medical Sciences 278: 153–156

Steele P, Rainwater J 1980 Favourable effect of sulfinpyrazone on thromboembolism in patients with rheumatic heart disease. Circulation 62: 462–465

Telford A M, Wilson C 1981 Trial of heparin versus alenolol in prevention of myocardial infarction in intermediary coronary syndrome. Lancet 1: 1225–1228

Turpie A G, Delmore T, Hirsh J, Hull R, Genton E, Hiscoe C, Gent M 1979 Prevention of venous thrombosis by intermittent sequential calf compression in patients with intracranial disease. Thrombosis Research 15: 611–616

Vieweg W, Piscatelli R, Houser J, Proulx R 1970 Complications of intravenous administration of heparin in elderly women. Journal of the American Medical Association 213: 1303–1306

Weksler B, Pett S, Alonso D, Richter R Stelzer P, Subramanian V, Tack-Goldman K, Gay W A Jr. 1983 Differential inhibition by aspirin of vascular and platelet prostaglandin synthesis in atherosclerotic patients. New England Journal of Medicine 308: 800–805

Yett H, Skillman J, Salzman E W 1978 The hazards of aspirin plus heparin. New England Journal of Medicine 298: 1092

Zahavi J, Jones N, Leyton J, Dubiel M, Kakkar V 1980 Enhanced in vivo platelet 'release reactor' in old healthy individuals. Thrombosis Research 17: 329–336

36

Gonadal function and sexual potency in aging men

H. R. Nankin & S. M. Harman

INTRODUCTION

During the past two decades there has been a remarkable expansion and refinement of knowledge relating to the endocrinology of reproduction. A variety of technical advancements have given tools that could be applied to human and animal in vivo and in vitro studies, but the application of radioimmunoassay, originally described by S. Berson and R. Yalow, for the measurement of glycoprotein gonadotropins released by the pituitary, then to steroid hormones produced by the testis, and more recently to hypothalamic releasing factors which regulate the anterior pituitary, has probably had the greatest impact. It is beyond the scope of this chapter to give a detailed review of the hypothalamic-pituitary-gonadal relationship, and the readers are referred to standard textbooks (some are mentioned herein: *Endocrinology and Metabolism*, Felig, Baxter, Broadus, Frohman eds., McGraw Hill, 1981; *Textbook of Endocrinology*, Williams ed., W.B. Saunders, 1981; *Reproductive Endocrinology*, Yen and Jaffe eds., Saunders, 1978) or review books (for example, *Manual of Clinical Endocrinology and Metabolism*, J.E. Griffin, McGraw-Hill Pre Test Series, 1982). A short synopsis of feedback regulation and steroid hormone action will be presented to facilitate comprehension of portions of the present chapter. Table 36.1 depicts usual normal ranges for common reproductive tests in men.

Through the efforts of Schally and co-workers we have learned that the hypothalamus produces a decapeptide called gonadotropin releasing hormone (GnRH, LHRH, LRF) and the hypothalamic release of this peptide after sensing circulating feedback hormones regulates pituitary release of luteinizing hormone (LH) and follicle stimulating hormone (FSH). The two pituitary gonadotropins directly stimulate testis function. LH has specific receptors on Leydig cells in the small interstitial compartment and causes these cells to produce the biologically effective androgen, testosterone. The concentration of testosterone in the testis is about 50 times that of circulating levels, and local actions of androgens appear to be important in spermatogenesis. FSH has specific receptors on the Sertoli cells of the seminiferous tubules. The latter comprise about

85% of testis volume. The Sertoli cells have major roles in the entire process of germ cell maturation, from immature stem cells to mature spermatozoa. In response to FSH, a variety of Sertoli cell functions are stimulated, one of the most important being the production of androgen-binding protein (ABP). This protein binds testosterone and delivers this steroid to the milieu of the seminiferous tubules.

By way of draining lymphatics and venous effluent, Leydig cell products including testosterone and some biologically active precursor steroids (for example progesterone), as well as steroids which can be converted to androgens and oestrogens in peripheral tissues, and 5α reduced testosterone (dihydrotestosterone, which is the active androgen in certain sex organs) all are carried into the systemic circulation and appear to have feedback potential for both gonadotropins. In addition, Leydig and Sertoli cells can convert androgens to oestrogens which also may help regulate gonadotropins. Sertoli cells also produce and release the peptide hormone inhibin which appears to block the secretion of only FSH, probably at the pituitary level.

Testosterone and other androgens have biologic actions on virtually every tissue in the body. In utero testosterone directly causes wolffian duct differentiation and on end organ conversion to dihydrotestosterone, the external genitalia are masculinized. Linear growth, muscle development, nitrogen retention, maturation of the external genitalia and maturation of secondary sexual organs (penis, scrotum, prostate and seminal vesicles) are due to pubertal increases in testosterone production. Testosterone production increases to 5–10 mg per day in 20–50 year old normal men and also causes enlargement of the larynx and thickening of the vocal cords, male-pattern sexual hair, male-pattern genetically related balding, and increases libido and potency. In some tissues testosterone is biologically active, in other tissues that steroid is 5α reduced to dihydrotestosterone which is the active hormone, and in other tissues the androgen is aromatised to oestrogen (oestradiol) which may cause or modify the testosterone action. Only a small per cent of oestradiol is normally produced by the testis, the amount increases with increasing LH stimulation. Steroid hormones passively diffuse into cells, where directly or after conversion, they are bound to cytoplasmic high affinity receptors and the steroid/receptor complex induces final actions. Thus throughout the life of a male, the reproductive system has both androgenic and anabolic effects.

There is dramatic gonadal failure during the menopause in women occurring over a few years, however, reproductive senescence in men appears to be a gradual process. In fact it is still questionable whether or not true gonadal failure occurs at all as men age. Some men retain full reproductive function into extreme old age. There is however, considerable published data that males of various animal species, including man, do show reduced reproductive capacity with age. The subject of sexual function in older men arouses interest. This is because, in humans, sexual activity is not only associated with reproduction, but also serves deeply felt personal needs which reinforce the permanence of couples and the stability of families. The hormones which regulate reproductive function are the same ones which support and modulate sexual capacity and drive. Alterations in hormone secretion by aging or disease can produce deleterious effects on sexuality. These effects can be of concern to men of any age. There is substantial agreement that aging in men is accompanied by reduced sexual interest, activity and capacity. However several factors may result in reduced sexuality and these will be reviewed later.

GONADOTROPIC FUNCTION

Primary testis failure with advancing years should be

Table 36.1 Normal values for adult men

Serum testosterone	250–350* to 800–1100* ng/dl
Serum luteinizing hormone	5–20* mIU/ml
Serum follicle stimulating hormone	5–20* mIU/ml

* Check reference lab ranges, these values can vary with the methodology and standards used.

Bulbocavernosus latency time	32–44 ms

Penile systolic blood pressure in R & L dorsal and R & L cavernosal arteries — either within 40 mmHg of brachial, or ratio of penile to brachial ≥ .75 (normal), .60–.75 (indeterminant), <0.6 (reduced blood pressure)

Nocturnal tumescence — a) flat for three nights — no tumescence
b) 1 cm or less = partial tumescence
c) greater than 1 cm can be full or partial erection

Semen volume	1.5–5.0 ml
Sperm count	>20 000 000/ml of ejaculate
Sperm motility	>60% actively motile
Sperm cytology	>60% normal morphology
Testis size	4–6 cm in longest diameter or 15–25 ml using orchidometer

associated with increased gonadotropins. Increased excretion of urinary gonadotropins in aging men was first reported by Pedersen-Bjergaard & Jonnesen (1948) using bioassay methods. Albert (1956) and Christiansen (1972) both reported that although both LH and FSH were elevated in urine from aging men, the increase in FSH was more prominent. Using radioimmunoassay methods, recent studies have nearly all demonstrated increased circulating gonadotropin concentrations in men after the age of about 50 (Harman et al, 1982). Some aged subjects have LH and FSH concentrations as high as those found in post-menopausal women or castrated men. The clearance of LH from plasma appears to be unrelated to age (Kohler et al, 1968; Pepperell et al, 1975), so increased pituitary secretion appears to be the cause. The latter is thought to be due to a reduction in feedback inhibition of the hypothalamic-pituitary axis. The greater increase in FSH than LH may result from reduced inhibin, which becomes deficient as tubular function decreases with age (Baker et al, 1976). This hypothesis is consistent with experiments showing increased FSH but no increase in LH in healthy elderly men with unaltered (Sparrow, et al, 1980) or even moderately decreased (Zumoff et al, 1982) plasma testosterone concentrations. In healthy aged men, Harman et al (1982) found increases in both serum FSH and LH levels despite unchanged plasma sex steroid concentrations. They concluded that the increased LH might represent compensation for mild Leydig cell failure, reduction in feedback sensitivity of the hypothalamic-pituitary axis (as suggested by Dilman & Anasimov, 1979), or a combination of factors. Muta et al (1981) showed greater steroid dose requirements for inhibition of gonadotropin secretion in old men. Reduced aged human Leydig cell responses to hCG (gonadotropin-like LH) have been reported (Nankin et al, 1981). There is increased pituitary LH content with age (Ryan, 1962). As reviewed by Harman et al (1982), use of LHRH to test pituitary secretory reserve for LH and FSH has given various results. Although studies provide evidence for some impairment of pituitary response pituitary gonadotropic reserve was demonstrated. Clearly, elevated LH can sometimes result in normal testosterone (Harman & Tsitouras, 1980). Failure for full compensation in other studies may be due to a variety of factors.

SEMINIFEROUS TUBULAR FUNCTION

There is constant maturation of germ cells in adult men. The length of time required for mature spermatozoa to develop from spermatogonia does not appear to be influenced by age (Talbert, 1977), but is species specific. In humans the process typically requires about 10 weeks. On the other hand, a woman is born with her full supply of eggs. These eggs are therefore exposed to mutagens until ovulation. This sex difference may explain why paternal age appears to be a relatively less important factor in production of chromosomal aneuploidy in a fetus than does maternal age. However, there are data to suggest increased spontaneous translocations in aged mouse spermatogonia (Leonard & DeKnudt, 1970; Murumatsu, 1974) and an increased percentage of sperm bearing two Ys (aneuploidy) in sperm from older men (Bynum et al, 1982).

Semen quality has been correlated with aging. Blum (1936) reported that the per cent of semen samples containing spermatozoa decreased from 68.5% in the sixth to 48% in the eighth decade. MacLeod & Gold (1953) in a study of over 1500 men aged 20–50, reported reduced fertility from the age of 25 on. They also reported a decreased intercourse frequency in older men resulted in increased total sperm counts and ejaculate volumes, but reduced sperm motility. After correcting their data for the effects of continence, they still found increasing sperm concentrations up to the age of 50, with no apparent age effects on sperm morphology. Recently Nieschlag et al (1982) reported unchanged sperm number and morphology in healthy older men of proven fertility. Although motility was somewhat decreased in aged men, the ability of their sperm to penetrate ova in a heterologous ovum penetration test was unimpaired. This in vitro test gives a better estimate of sperm fertility potential than does motility or count.

Degenerative histologic changes of the seminiferous tubules in the testis have been reported to increase with aging. In order of increasing severity, these include: basement membrane thickening; reduced germ cells; peritubular fibrosis; germ cell arrest; only Sertoli cells remaining; and narrowing and obliteration of tubule lumens (Sniffen, 1950; Tillenger, 1957; Burgi & Hedinger, 1959; Sokal, 1964; Sasano & Ichigo, 1969; Suoranta, 1971; Kothari & Gupta, 1974). In addition, Schulze & Schulze (1981) have described an increase in the number of multinucleate germ cells in seminiferous tubules of aging men.

There is general agreement that focal regions showing degeneration of tubules are typically interspersed among areas with grossly normal morphology in older males. Engle (1952) reported that 50% of men aged 70 or over still had some regions of apparently normal spermatogenesis. Sasano and Ichigo (1969) found that the percentage of tubules containing spermatids fell with progressive aging. Fewer patent capillaries (Sasano & Ichigo, 1969; Suoranta, 1971), focal inflammation (Suoranta, 1971; Frick, 1969) and auto-immune disease (Fjallbrant, 1975) have all been suggested as age-related causes of testis deterioration.

Whether testis size and weight normally decrease with aging remains controversial and this may depend on patient selection. Apparent decreases in testis volume with age were reported by Longcope (1973), Stearns et al (1974) and Baker et al (1976), while Kothari & Gupta (1974) and Harman et al (1982) found no reductions when selected healthy men were examined.

LEYDIG CELL FUNCTION

Using bioassay, Pederson-Bjergaard & Jonnesen (1948) first demonstrated that urinary androgen progressively decreased after age 40, falling to very low levels by the eighth decade. Hollander & Hollander (1958) found similar changes in testosterone concentrations with aging in testicular vein blood obtained during surgery. In the past decade, a large number of investigations using radio-immunoassay techniques have shown varying decreases in plasma testosterone concentrations as men age. In general, a decline in mean serum testosterone seems to begin at about age 50 and progresses into the eighth or ninth decades. However, even in studies showing a decrease in mean plasma testosterone, individual concentrations are quite variable, so that although some men in their 70s to 90s have testosterone levels well below the lower limit of normal, other men of the same ages have even high normal testosterone concentrations. This was reviewed by Nankin et al (1981). Furthermore, two recent large studies of selected healthy American men have not demonstrated decreases in serum testosterone with age (Harman & Tsitouras, 1980; Sparrow et al, 1980). Nieschlag et al (1982) now also have data from healthy European young fathers and older grandfathers which reveals similar testosterone levels in both groups.

Testosterone (T), dihydrotestosterone (DHT) and oestradiol (E_2) circulate in plasma free and bound to proteins. All three are bound with high affinity to sex hormone binding globulin (SHBG) (in order of decreasing affinity — DHT > T > E_2) and with low affinity they are bound to albumin, only a small per cent of each being free or metabolically active, although albumin-bound appears to be readily available. A number of studies have suggested that SHBG capacity increases with age producing a decrease in the free testosterone fraction in plasma. This decrease of free testosterone appears more prominent than the decrease in total plasma testosterone in some studies (Hallberg, et al, 1976; Baker et al, 1976; Kley et al, 1974; Pirke & Doerr, 1973 & 1975; Rubens et al, 1974; Purifoy et al, 1981). The increase in SHBG might be secondary to an increase in plasma oestrogenic steroids, since it is known that oestrogens promote synthesis of SHBG by the liver. Increased plasma concentrations of unconjugated oestradiol and oestrone have indeed been demonstrated in older men in many of these same studies (Hallberg et al, 1976; Kley et al, 1974; Kley et al, 1975; Pirke & Doerr, 1975; Rubens et al, 1974).

In five separate reports other workers have not found altered basal plasma estrogen concentrations in older men. Harman & Tsitouras (1980) found only a slight increase in SHBG binding of testosterone in healthy older men, which was insufficient to produce a significant reduction in free testosterone with age. They also reported no alteration with age in serum oestrone or oestradiol concentrations. Similarly, Zumoff et al (1982) found no increase in SHBG binding fraction so that measurement of free testosterone added no independent information beyond that obtained from the total plasma testosterone. Furthermore total oestrogen excretion (conjugates and free) are not changed with age. Factors that could increase oestrogens in men of all ages include obesity, alcohol ingestion, hyperthyroidism and a failing testis.

Various studies have demonstrated lower, unchanged, or increased concentrations of dihydrotestosterone in aged men. About 80% of circulating DHT results from peripheral conversion of testosterone in target cells and subsequent release of this steroid into circulation. The remaining 20% of DHT is from direct testis secretion.

The reasons for the wide variety of results obtained for plasma sex steroids of aging men are not clear. It is possible that in some studies altered sex steroid levels may be due to the influence of chronic illness, medications, obesity, alcohol intake or environmental stress (all of which can affect plasma testosterone and/or oestradiol), rather than age per se. In normal 20–50 year old men circulating levels of testosterone have a diurnal rhythm, with highest values between 6 a.m. and 9 a.m., falling by an average of 20% to a late evening nadir. Superimposed on the diurnal rhythm are sporadic increases. Therefore studies based on single samples, or where sampling was done throughout the day may vary from other studies. Bremner & Prinz (1981) did find a loss of diurnal testosterone in elderly men, so that morning but not afternoon values appeared to decrease with age. In contrast Murono et al (1982a) have found a persistent diurnal rhythm of testosterone in their older healthy population of men. The diurnal effect would not account for the observation of unchanged plasma testosterone in morning samples by Sparrow et al (1980), Tsitouras et al (1982) and Nieschlag et al (1982). On the other hand, Zumoff et al (1982) found significantly reduced 24-hour mean integrated plasma testosterone in older men, whom they describe as healthy and ambulatory. The issue is not yet settled.

Human chorionic gonadotropin (hCG), an LH-like material, has been administered to aged men by several groups of investigators. Virtually all studies demonstrate reduced Leydig cell responses in older males (Nankin et al, 1981). Although some in vitro studies suggested altered biosynthesis because of reduced enzyme activity in old men, in vivo studies have not demonstrated precursor buildup in circulating plasma (Murono et al, 1982b). The data on testosterone degradation are also complicated and there are no consistent findings.

Sarjent & McDonald (1948) compared the number of Leydig cells per 100 seminiferous tubules and found a progressive reduction from the age of 20 on. Decreased Leydig cells have also been reported by Tillenger (1957) and Frick (1969). Harbitz (1973) and Kaler & Neaves (1978) using sophisticated morphometric techniques confirmed these findings. However Harbitz (1973), noted

that the greatest decrease in Leydig cell number was associated with prolonged illness. In contrast Sniffen (1950) and Sokal (1964) found no decrease in number of Leydig cells with age, while Kothari & Gupta (1974) reported total Leydig cell mass to be increased in testes from older men. It is unclear whether the reported decrease in Leydig cells is an effect of age, or whether it reflects debilitating diseases in some of the populations studied.

It may be that certain androgen target tissues have altered sensitivity with age. The findings by Muta et al (1981) that more testosterone is required to inhibit gonadotropin secretion in aged men and by Desleypere & Vermeulen (1981) that binding of DHT to androgen-responsive skin is reduced in older men, suggest that tissue responsiveness to androgens may be reduced with age.

Male accessory organs

The prostate, seminal vesicles and the epididymides are the main accessory organs. The human prostate gland develops secretory alveoli with a tall, columnar epithelium and contributes to the ejaculate numerous enzymes, citric acid and zinc. The tall columnar cells and surrounding stroma are progressively replaced by collagen after the age of 40 (Moore, 1952). There is nearly universal occurrence of benign prostatic nodular hyperplasia consisting of focal proliferations of stromal and glandular tissue. The earliest changes occur in the peri-urethral area (Harbitz & Raugen, 1972) and then spreads primarily to the lateral and medial lobes. The exact cause of prostate hyperplasia is not known but several hypotheses have been suggested (Baranowska et al, 1980; Ortega et al, 1979; Sarofi et al, 1980; Wilson, 1980; Trachtenberg et al, 1982; Ron et al, 1981).

The epididymis stores and capacitates spermatozoa. The latter process is essential for fertility. With aging the columnar epithelium becomes cuboidal and the epithelium demonstrates increasing pigment granules (Mainwaring & Brandes, 1974).

Alkaline seminal fluid containing fructose, prostaglandins, proteins including basic proteins, other carbohydrates, enzymes and potassium is added to the ejaculate during orgasm by the sacular shaped seminal vesicles. Older men have a sharp reduction in secretory surface and glands. Cholinergic nerves innervate this organ and may become abnormal with neurogenic disorders. The capacity of the organ reduces from about 5 ml at the age of 60, to 2.2 ml in 80-year old men. However there are relatively few studies of other aging changes.

SEXUAL POTENCY

Since the end of World War II, there has been a marked increase in our understanding of sexual behaviour, the problems causing impaired sexual activity and the ramifications of impaired sexual activity. However, most studies involve younger patients and there is little data about patients beyond the age of 60. Only recently has society begun to consider sexual desires and contacts between older people as normal and acceptable. The fact is of course, that sexuality is neither unusual nor immoral (Botwinick, 1978). There is no question that the human male's sexual responsiveness wanes as he 'ages'. This waning is gradual and drops almost linearly until the age of 60 (Botwinick, 1978). At the age of 60 most male subjects are still sexually active. Long-term longitudinal studies of people between 60 and 94 years of age have found that about 15% of older persons actually increased their sexual activity and interest as they aged (Butler & Lewis, 1977). Men between 50 and 75 years of age can make love for a more protracted time before coming to orgasm. Older men may experience a reduction in seminal fluid volume and a decrease in pressure to ejaculate. Orgasm is experienced as a shorter one-stage event as compared to two stages in earlier life — but it remains pleasurable. After the age of 50 there is a physiologically extended refractory period after orgasm (Masters & Johnson, 1966). Loss of sexuality can be due to a number of factors: boredom, fatigue, over-eating, excessive drinking, medical and psychiatric disabilities (impotence can be one of the first signs of depression) and fear of failure. A wide variety of drugs can interfere with sexual function. Horowitz & Goble (1979) report that impaired sexual function may take the form of reduced libido, impotence, failure of ejaculation or a combination of these. By far the most frequent symptom is impotence. Erectile difficulty may occur in the presence or absence of any significant change in libido. In 1948, Kinsey et al reported only occasional cases of impotence under the age of 45 years. The incidence rose sharply after this to 25% at 65 years and 50% at 75 years. Burger & Rose (1979) note that impotence rises from 1 per 1000 at the age of 20 to 75% of all males at the age of 75 and older. Impotence is almost certainly under-reported because of men's fears of exposing themselves to real and imagined ridicule. The incidence of transient episodes is far higher still. Impotent males are often urged to seek treatment by their spouses. This is emotionally threatening to men. Some aging males voluntarily withdraw from coital activity rather than face the ego-shattering experiences of repeated episodes of sexual inadequacy (Botwinick, 1978). Any physical disability, acute or chronic, may and usually does lower the sexual responsiveness of the involved male. There are anecdotal reports that anxiety arising out of sexual problems can precede and may contribute to a heart attack. Fears of sex may lead to abstinence. Currents of anxiety, depression and hostility can accompany these fears as sexuality is inhibited.

Physiology of erections and ejaculation

In simplified terms sexuality depends on four components — libido, erection, emission/orgasm, and ejaculation.

Libido can be altered by the mental state. Sedation, preoccupation with significant problems and fear of failure can reduce libido. Erection is a reflex phenomenon and dependent on psychogenic and/or reflex stimuli (Weiss, 1972). Auditory, visual, olfactory, gustatory, tactile and imaginative stimuli cause the psychogenic erection. Stimulation of the genital region produces a reflexogenic erection. Erections can be facilitated by autonomic events — interoceptive erections. The neurophysiology of erection is not completely known. Weiss (1972) reviewed the neurogenic input. The tactile afferent impulses are carried through the pudendal nerves. Sacral roots S_2, S_3 and S_4 carry the efferent parasympathetic fibres (nervi erigentes). Impotence is found with neurologic disease involving the limbic system, spinal cord and pelvic nerve lesions. The cerebral cortex and limbic system impulses eventually reach the sympathetic ganglia (thoracolumbar and hypogastric) and then the sacral parasympathetic nerves. In some 25% of patients with the entire pelvic region denervated (below T_{12}) erotic psychic stimuli still caused erection. More than 90% of men with complete cord transection well above the sacral area are able to have erections, but these erections occur only after reflex stimulation. Temporal lobe lesions in men are associated with decreased erections but normal libido. Why cerebral dysfunction causes impotence is not known. Horowitz & Goble (1979) note that cortical impulses on sexual arousal may include inhibition of reflex stimuli. Drugs which depress cortical centers, may, depending upon circumstances and dosage, either initiate or relieve sexual dysfunction.

Erection

The penile erectile tissues consists of two corpora cavernosa and a single corpus spongiosum. Increased delivery of blood, decreased venous outflow or a combination of these may be present during erection. Smooth muscles known as polsters, appear to usually limit entry of arterial blood to the corpora cavernosa and spongiosa and these muscles can be relaxed by both sympathetic and parasympathetic fibres (Horowitz & Goble, 1979). Erection normally occurs and is maintained when 20–50 ml of blood remains within the corpora. Only the corpora cavernosa are compressed against a thick fibrous outer covering, the tunical albuginea and attain rigidity. Littre's glands start to secrete with erection.

Orgasm/emission

Orgasm is identical with the emission phase. Emission is the discharge of the Cowper's glands, vasa deferentia, prostate, epididymides and seminal vesicles causing semen to be propelled into the bulbar urethra (Millar, 1979). This is thought to be a sympathetic reflex relayed from the lumbar sympathetic chain and superior hypogastric plexus.

Ejaculation

After emission there is contraction of the bulbocavernosus and the ischiocavernosus muscles resulting in the expulsion of seminal fluid. The bladder neck is tightly closed. This phase is thought to be under parasympathetic and sympathetic innervation. The corpus spongiosum forms a pressure chamber within the posterior urethra with semen discharged distally (Marberger, 1974). Ejaculation causes constriction of the vessels supplying blood to the erectile tissues and the penis becomes flaccid.

Impotence

Impotence can be defined as erectile failure in at least 25% of attempts (Shrom et al, 1979) and also as inability to maintain erection for penetration or an erection without sufficient rigidity for vaginal penetration (Wasserman et al, 1980).

Failure of ejaculation

Sympathetic neuropathy, drugs which interfere with the sympathetic nerves (chlordiazepoxide and tricyclic antidepressants) and surgery (lumbar sympathectomy, aortic aneurysm repair, rectal resection) could cause this.

Reduction or loss of libido

This could be due to reduced testosterone, increased oestrogen and increased prolactin, psychologic causes and drugs. Of these three complaints, impotence is by far the most common and most distressing sexual problem.

The causes of impotence

Aetiology can be divided into six primary areas: psychologic; hormonal; vascular; medications; neuropathy; and miscellaneous. Some patients will have combined problems. In one study of 27 consecutive men with erectile impotence of at least six months' duration, evaluated for neurologic, psychiatric and vascular abnormalities, 48% of the patients had combined disorders (Blaivas et al, 1980).

Psychogenic impotence has been reported as causing impotence in 35–90% of subjects, depending on the population studied. It tends to have an abrupt onset, to be episodic or selective, is associated with reduced libido and is more common in younger men. Sometimes it is difficult to differentiate psychogenic from organic causes of impotence. Wasserman et al (1980) reviewed the literature regarding nocturnal penile tumescence disturbances. About 20% of patients with probably psychogenic causes have impaired nocturnal penile tumescence. Cortical impulses on sexual arousal may include inhibition of reflex stimuli (Horowitz & Goble, 1979). Psychogenic causes tend to be associated with stressful events, marital difficulties and states such as depression. Some women cause psychogenic impotence in their partners. The impairment may be episodic or selective and may not affect masturbation or nocturnal penile tumescence. Desire is usually not impaired in organically impotent men but lowering of desire can occur in response to anxiety and frustration associated with repeated erectile failure.

It has been demonstrated that androgen deficiency is associated with reduced sexual function and that this is treatable with appropriate replacement therapy. Hypogonadal subjects were treated with testosterone or vehicle in double-blind fashion. The frequencies of erections, including nocturnal erections and coitus showed significant dose-related responses to androgen treatment (Davidson et al, 1979). Montague et al (1979) studied 165 impotent men and found that 13% of the patients had hypogonadism. Burger & Rose (1979) noted a variety of endocrine disturbances which can cause impotence. Spark et al (1980) reported endocrine abnormalities causing impotence in 37 of 105 men. Patients who use narcotics and chronic methadone users tend to have reduced testosterone levels (Mirin et al, 1980). Chronic digoxin therapy was associated with a lowered testosterone, a lowered circulating LH, elevated oestradiol and reduced sexuality (Neri et al, 1980). Unpublished data in 104 consecutive men seen for impotence in a Veterans' Administratioin Hospital outpatient clinic, reveal about 30% have low testosterone levels (Nankin et al, unpublished). Early results suggest that many of these androgen-deficient men can be helped with replacement therapy. Elevated prolactin is associated with decreased libido and impotence in men. The effects of prolactin on libido and potency are usually independent of endogenous gonadotropin and testosterone. Bromocriptine has improved libido and potency in most men who had increased pituitary production of prolactin and impotent patients with chronic renal failure have been successfully treated with bromocriptine (Gura et al, 1980). Morley & Melmid (1979) reviewed gonadal dysfunction with a wide variety of systemic disorders. Cirrhosis of the liver, haemochromatosis, sickle cell disease, myotonia dystrophica, hypo and hyperthyroidism, elevated blood glucose, Cushing's syndrome, renal failure, malnutrition and obesity have been linked with endocrine dysfunction and impotence.

Occlusive vascular disease, complications of Peyronie's disease, complications of priapism and occasional unusual problems all can result in vascular insufficiency. Montague et al (1979) report a vascular basis for 25% of impotent men, whereas Blaivas et al (1980) report vascular abnormalities in 67% of impotent men. Aorto-iliac bypass surgery and renal transplantation can result in vascular impotence (Morley & Melmid, 1979; Quayle, 1980).

Virtually all psychotropic drugs, most antihypertensive drugs (except furosemide, hydralazine and prazosin), most depressants, oestrogens, spironolactone, antineoplastic agents, narcotics, alpha blockers, anticholinergic drugs and alcohol all can reduce sexual function (Lipman, 1977).

Some of the neurologic causes for impotence were

mentioned above. Alcoholism, multiple sclerosis and diabetes mellitus are the more common causes of neuropathies. Surgery and trauma can also result in neuropathy. Montague et al (1979) reported the incidence between 10% and 20%; Blaivas et al (1980) found neurologic abnormalities in 41% of impotent men and Quayle (1980) reported neurogenic impotence after aorto-iliac surgical procedures. Ertekin & Reel (1976) found neuropathy in one quarter of impotent men.

Miscellaneous causes of impotence include renal failure, paraplegia and quadraplegia, sickle cell disease and myotonic dystrophy where the cause or causes are not definite.

Workup of impotence

Practically speaking, aged men should be able to perform sexually unless there are reasons why they are unable. Some men are too ill or too debilitated or have major physical limitations, and these can be considered in the evaluation and a decision made not to proceed with a workup. When such contra-indications are not present, the patient and his partner should be interviewed so that the presence of impotence can be confirmed and the impact on their relationship assessed. Some couples willingly accept impotence and seek alternative activities as acceptable substitutes for vaginal sex. Both partners should have reasonable aspirations.

After an initial screening interview both partners should have comprehensive physical examinations with special attention to the reproductive portions. For the male a varicocele should be looked for before he lies down. The testes, breasts, prostate and penis are carefully examined. Neurologic and peripheral vascular assessments are performed. Penile blood pressure is obtained as suggested by Goldstein et al (1982). A bulbocavernosus reflex is attempted and all patients are also sent for a bulbocavernosus latency time (Ertekin & Reel, 1976). A prolonged latency time suggests nerve damage. Both partners can take a Minnesota Multiphasic Personality Index and can be screened by a clinical psychologist. A wide variety of other suitable psychologic tests are available (LoPicollo & Steger, 1974; Locke & Wallace, 1959; Janda & O'Grady, 1980). Sex education and sex therapy may be helpful even if organic problems are detected (Schumacher & Lloyd, 1981).

For the male, standard laboratory screening studies are done and special tests include two to three separate (consecutive days) early morning (7–9 a.m.) blood samples for luteinizing hormone, testosterone and prolactin. Oestradiol and follicle stimulating hormone are not routinely obtained. Nocturnal tumescence monitoring is performed for three nights. If all three nights reveal no tumescence, then psychologic causes are unlikely but not excluded (Cunningham et al, 1982). If tumescence is less than 1 cm then erections are almost certainly partial. If tumescence increases 1 cm or more, then two techniques are available to quantitate the erections: direct observation and measurement of rigidity, or performing an artificial erection (Morales et al, 1982). These techniques allow differentiation between partial and full erections.

Treatment of impotence

Once impotence (no or partial erections) has been documented and evaluated, treatment would include sex education and switching or deleting medications if possible. Elimination of alcohol prior to attempted sex may also improve potency. Hyperprolactinaemia should be evaluated and treated. In our experience men with low or borderline low circulating levels of testosterone very commonly respond to intramuscular (im) testosterone (enanthate or cypionate). We prefer im testosterone to current oral preparations because the former has less hepatoxicity. We give im hormone every 14 days based on body weight (100 mg $\leqslant$ 125 lbs, 150 mg for 125–174 lbs, 200 mg $\geqslant$ 175 lbs) and give the medication for about two months as a trial. The beneficial effects may slowly appear. If this is successful, it can be maintained, although we examine the effects of withdrawal after six months of treatment. Prostate cancer is a contra-indication to this therapy. With persistent impotence and vascular or neurologic aetiologies, a penile implant may be considered (Beaser et al, 1982; Furlow, 1978). Sex therapy is helpful for psychologic impotence. At present we have no set scheme for men with major psychiatric disorders who are controlled by medications. Some of them do have stable partner relationships and if they remain impotent, if psychiatric clearance is obtained and if the man and woman are medically suited, we have tried testosterone therapy in appropriate individuals and referred a limited number of such men for implants. However the long-term results are not yet available.

In summary, in unusually healthy aged men circulating levels of testosterone should not decrease, but some Leydig cell failure occurs as circulating luteinizing hormone increases and old Leydig cells probably do not respond as well to injections of large doses of gonadotropin. Ejaculation and semen can remain reasonably unchanged. On the other hand a wide variety of systemic diseases, vascular disease, and probably auto-immune disease may deleteriously alter testis function and libido. Impotence becomes increasingly more common in men over the age of 50 and may have a variety of aetiologies. The approach to workup and treatment is outlined. How sexual dysfunction is perceived varies tremendously and those treating older individuals must carefully consider all ramifications. The return of potency in some individuals can dramatically enhance the quality of life and may mean more to them than medical care given to prolong survival.

REFERENCES

Albert A 1956 Human urinary gonadotropins. Recent Progress Hormone Research 12: 266–282

Baker H W G, Burger H G, DeKretser D M, Hudson E, O'Connor S, Wang C, Mirovics A, Court J, Dunlop M, Rennie G C 1976 Changes in the pituitary testicular system with age. Clinical Endocrinology 5: 349–372

Baranowska B, Zgliczynski S, Szymanski J 1980 Hormonal disturbances in men with prostatic adenoma. Journal of Urology 86: 551–558

Beaser R S, Van der Hoek C, Jacobson A M, Flood T M, Desautels R E 1982 Experience with penile prostheses in the treatment of impotence in diabetic men. Journal of the American Medical Association 248: 943–948

Blaivas J G, O'Donnell T F, Gottlieb P, Labib K B 1980 Comprehensive laboratory evaluation of impotent men. Journal of Urology 124: 201–204

Blum V 1936 Das Problem des mannlichen Klimakteriums. Wein Klin Wochnschr 2: 1133–1140

Botwinick J 1978 Aging and Behavior. 2nd edn, Spring Publishing, New York, p 38–58

Bremner W J, Prinz P N 1981 The diurnal rhythm in testosterone levels is lost with aging in normal men. Endocrine Society 63rd Annual Meeting. Abstract 480, p 202

Burger H, Rose M 1979 Sexual impotence. Medical Journal of Australia 2: 24–26

Butler R N, Lewis N I 1977 Aging and mental health. 2nd edn, C.V. Mosby Co, St Louis, p 112–117

Burgi Von H, Hedinger C 1959 Histologische hodenveranderung im hohen alter. Schweiz Med. Wochschr. 89: 1236–1239

Bynum G, Becker D, Schneider E 1982 (unpublished) Examination of the effect of Paternal aging on human meiotic chromosomal nondisjunction.

Christiansen P 1972 Urinary follicle stimulating hormone and luteinizing hormone in normal adult men. Acta Endocrinologica 71: 1–6

Cunningham G R, Karacan I, Catesby Ware J, Lantz G D, Thornby J I 1982 The relationship between serum testosterone and prolactin levels and nocturnal penile tumescence in impotent men. Journal of Andrology 3: 241–247

Davidson J M, Camargo C A, Smith E R 1979 Effects of androgen on sexual behavior in hypogonadal men. Journal of Clinical Endocrinology and Metabolism 48: 955–958

Desleypere J P, Vermeulen A 1981 Aging and tissue androgens. Journal of Clinical Endocrinology and Metabolism 53: 430–434

Dilman V M, Anisimov V N 1979 Hypothalamic mechanisms of aging and of specific age pathology I. On the sensitivity threshold of hypothalamic-pituitary complex to homeostatic stimuli in the reproductive system. Experimental Gerontology 14: 161–174

Engle E T 1952 The male reproductive system. In: Lansing A I (ed) Cowdry's Problems of Aging. 3rd edn, Williams and Wilkins, Baltimore, p 708–729

Ertekin C, Reel F 1976 Bulbocavernosus reflex in normal men and in patients with neurogenic bladder and/or impotence. Journal of Neurological Sciences 28: 1–15

Fjallbrant B 1975 Autoimmune human sperm antibodies and age in males. Journal of Reproduction and Fertility 43: 145–148

Frick J 1969 Darstellung eine Methode (competitive protein binding) zur bestimmung des testosteronspiegels im plasma und studie uber den testosteronmetabolismus beim mann uber 60 jahre. Urology International 24: 481–501

Furlow W L (ed) 1981 Male sexual dysfunction. The Urologic Clinics of North America 8: 79–194

Goldstein I, Siroky M B, Nath R L, McMillan T N, Menzoian J O, Krane R J 1982 Vasculogenic impotence: role of the pelvic steal test. Journal of Urology 128: 300–306

Gura V, Weizman A, Maoz B, Zevin D, Ben-David M 1980 Hyperprolactinemia — a possible cause of sexual impotence in male patients undergoing chronic hemodialysis. Nephron 26: 53–54

Hallberg M C, Wieland R G, Zoin E M, Furst B H, Wieland J M 1976 Impaired Leydig cell reserve and altered serum androgen in the aging male. Fertility and Sterility 27: 812–814

Harbitz T B 1973 Morphometric studies of the Leydig cells in elderly men with special reference to the histology of the prostate. Acta Pathologica Microbiologica Scandanavia 81A: 301–313

Harbitz T B, Haugen O A 1972 Histology of the prostate in elderly men. Acta Pathologica Microbiologica Scandanavia 80A: 756–768

Harman S M, Tsitouras P D 1980 Reproductive hormones in aging men I: Measurement of sex steroids, basal LH, and Leydig cell response to hCG. Journal of Clinical Endocrinology and Metabolism 51: 35–40

Harman S M, Tsitouras P D, Costa P T, Blackman M R 1982 Reproductive hormones in aging men II: Basal pituitary gonadotropins and gonadotropin response to luteinizing hormone releasing hormone. Journal of Clinical Endocrinology and Metabolism 54: 537–541

Horowitz J D, Goble A J 1979 Drugs and impaired male sexual function. Drugs 18: 206–217

Janda L H, O'Grady K E 1980 Development of a sex anxiety inventory. Journal of Consulting and Clinical Psychology 48: 169–175

Kaler L W, Neaves W B 1978 Attrition of the human Leydig cell population with advancing age. Anatomic Recordings 192: 513–518

Kinsey A C, Pomeroy W B, Martin C E 1948 Sexual behavior in the human male. W.B. Saunders, Philadelphia

Kley H K, Nieschlag E, Bidlingmaier F, Kruskemper H L 1974 Possible age dependent influence of estrogens on the binding of testosterone in plasma of adult men. Hormone and Metabolic Research 6: 213–215

Kley H K, Nieschlag E, Kruskemper H L 1975 Age dependence of plasma estrogen response to hCG and ACTH in men. Acta Endocrinologica 79: 95–101

Kohler P C, Ross G T, Odell W D 1968 Metabolic clearance and production rates of human luteinizing hormone in pre and postmenopausal women. Journal of Clinical Investigation 47: 38–47

Kothari K L, Gupta A S 1974 Effect of aging on the volume, structure, and total Leydig cell content of the human testis. International Journal of Fertility 19: 140–146

Hollander N, Hollander V P 1958 The microdetermination of testosterone in human spermatic vein blood. Journal of Clinical Endocrinology and Metabolism 38: 966–971

Leonard A, DeKnudt G 1970 Persistence of chromosome rearrangements induced in male mice by X-irradiation on premeiotic germ cells. Mutation Research 9: 127–133

Lipman A G 1977 Drugs associated with impotence. Modern Medicine 81–82

Locke H J, Wallace K M 1959 Short marital and prediction tests: their reliability and validity. Married Family Living 21: 251–255

Longcope C 1973 The effect of human chorionic gonadotropin on plasma steroid levels in young and old men. Steroids 21: 583–592

Lo Piccolo J, Steger J C 1974 The sexual interaction inventory: a new instrument for assessment of sexual dysfunction. Archives of Sexual Behavior 3: 585–595

MacLeod J, Gold R Z 1953 The male factor in fertility and infertility. VII. Semen quality in relation to age and sexual activity. Fertility and Sterility 4: 194–207

Mainwaring W I P, Brandes D 1974 Functional and structural changes in accessory sex organs during aging. In: Brandes D (ed) Male accessory Sex Organs, Academic Press, New York, p 469–500

Marberger H 1974 The mechanisms of ejaculation. In: Coutenho E M, Fuch F (eds) Basic life sciences, Physiology and Genetics of Reproduction

Masters W H, Johnson V E 1966 Human sexual response. Churchill, London

Millar J G B 1977 Drug-induced impotence. The Practitioner 223: 634–639

Mirin S M, Meyer R E, Mendelson J H, Ellingboe J 1980 Opiate use and sexual function. American Journal of Psychiatry 173: 909–915

Montague D K, James Jr R E, DeWolfe V G, Martin L N 1979 Diagnostic evaluation. Classification and treatment of men with sexual dysfunction. Urology XIV: 545–548

Moore R A 1952 Male secondary sexual organs. In: Lansing A I (ed) Cowdrey's Problems of Ageing. 3rd edn, Williams and Wilkins, Baltimore. p 686–707

Morales A, Surridge D H C, Marshall P G, Fenemore J 1982 Nonhormonal pharmacologic treatment of organic impotence. Journal of Urology 128: 45–47

Morley J E, Melmid S 1979 Gonadal dysfunction and systemic disorders. Metabolism 28: 1051–1073

Muramatsu S 1974 Frequency of spontaneous translocations in mouse spermatogonia. Mutation Research 24: 81–82

Murono E P, Nankin H R, Lin T, Osterman J 1982a The aging Leydig cell V. Diurnal rhythms in aged men. Acta Endocrinologica 99: 619–623

Murono E P, Nankin H R, Lin T, Osterman J 1982b The aging Leydig cell VI. Response of testosterone precursors to gonadotropin in men. Acta Endocrinologica 100: 455–461

Muta K, Kato K, Akamine Y, Ibayashi H 1981 Age-related changes in the feedback regulation of gonadotropin secretion by sex steroids in men. Acta Endocrinologica 96: 154–162

Nankin H R, Lin, T, Murono E P, Osterman J 1981 The aging Leydig cell III. Gonadotropin stimulation in men. Journal of Andrology 2: 181–189

Nankin H R, Lin T, Osterman J, Murono E P, Carnes J, Krzyzaniak K, Markuck D, Powell D Evaluation of impotent men referred to a Veterans' Administration Endocrine Clinic

Neri A, Aygen M, Zukerman Z, Bahary C 1980 Subjective assessment of sexual dysfunction of patients on long-term administration of digoxin. Archives of Sexual Behavior 9: 343–347

Nieschlag E, Lammers U, Freischem C W, Langer K, Wickings E J 1982 Reproductive function in young fathers and grandfathers. Journal of Clinical Endocrinology and Metabolism 55: 676–681

Ortega E, Ruiz E, Mendoza M C, Martin-Andres A, Osorio C 1979 Plasma steroid and protein hormone concentrations in patients with benign prostatic hypertrophy and in normal men. Experentia 35: 844–845

Pedersen-Bjergaard K, Jonneson M 1948 Sex hormones analysis: excretion of sexual hormones by normal males, impotent males, polyarthritics, and prostatics. Acta Medica Scandanavia 213: 284–291

Pepperell R J, deKretser D M, Burger H G 1975 Studies on the metabolic clearance rate and production rate of human luteinizing hormone and on the initial half-time of its subunits in man. Journal of Clinical Investigation 56: 118–126

Pirke K M, Doerr P 1973 Age-related changes and inter-relationships between plasma testosterone, estradiol, and testosterone binding globulin in normal adult males. Acta Endocrinologica 74: 792–800

Pirke K M, Doerr P 1975 Age-related changes in free plasma testosterone, dihydrotestosterone, and oestradiol. Acta Endocrinologica 80: 171–178

Quayle J B 1980 Sexual function after bilaterial lumbar sympathectomy and aorto-iliac bypass surgery. Journal of Cardiovascular Surgery 21: 215–218

Ron M, Fich A, Shapiro A, Caine M, Ben-David M 1981 Prolactin concentration in prostates with benign hypertrophy. Urology 17: 235–237

Rubens R, Dhont M, Vermeulen A 1974 Further studies on Leydig cell function in old age. Journal of Clinical Endocrinology and Metabolism 39: 40–45

Ryan R J 1962 The luteinizing hormone content of human pituitaries. I Variations with sex and age. Journal of Clinical Endocrinology and Metabolism 22: 300–303

Sarjent J W, McDonald J R 1984 A method for quantitative measurement of Leydig cells in the human testis. Mayo Clinic Proceedings 23: 249–254

Saroff J, Kirdani R Y, Chu T M, Wajsman Z, Murphy G P 1980 Measurements of prolactin and androgen in patients with prostatic diseases. Oncology 37: 46–52

Sasano N, Ichigo S 1969 Vascular patterns of the human testis with special reference to its senile changes. Tohuku Journal Experimental Medicine 99: 269–276

Schumacher S, Lloyd C W 1981 Physiological and psychological factors in impotence. Journal of Sex Research 17: 40–53

Shrom S H, Leif H I, Wein A J 1979 Clinical profile of experience with 130 consecutive cases of impotent men. Urology 13: 511–515

Sniffen R C 1950 The testis I The normal testis. Archives of Pathology 50: 259–284

Sokal Z 1964 Morphology of the human testes in various periods of life. Folia Morphologica 23: 102–111

Spark R F, White R A, Connolly P B 1980 Impotence is not always psychogenic. Newer insights into hypothalamic-pituitary-gonadal dysfunction. Journal of the American Medical Association 243: 750–755

Sparrow D, Bosse R, Rowe J W 1980 The influence of age, alcohol consumption, and body build on gonadal function in men. Journal of Clinical Endocrinology and Metabolism 51: 508–512

Stearns E L, MacDonald J A, Kauffman B J, Lucman T S, Winters J S, Faiman C 1974 Declining testis function with age: hormonal and clinical correlates. American Journal of Medicine 57: 761–766

Suoranta H 1971 Changes in the small blood vessels of the adult human testis in relation to age and some pathological conditions. Virchows Archives (Pathological, Anatomy and Histology) 352: 165–181

Tillenger K G 1975 Testicular morphology. Acta Endocrinologica 30: 28–39

Trachtenberg J, Bujnovszky P, Walsh P C 1982 Androgen receptor content of normal and hyperplastic human prostate. Journal of Clinical Endocrinology and Metabolism 54: 17–21

Tsitouras P D, Martin C E, Harman S M 1982 Relationship of serum testosterone to sexual activity in healthy elderly men. Journal of Gerontology 37: 288–293

Wasserman M D, Pollak C P, Spielman A J, Weitzman E D
   1980 The differential diagnosis of impotence. Journal of the
   American Medical Association 243: 2038–2042
Weiss H D 1972 The physiology of human penile erection.
   Annals of Internal Medicine 76: 793–799
Wilson J D 1980 The pathogenesis of benign prostatic

hyperplasia. American Journal of Medicine 68: 745–756
Zumoff B, Strain G W, Kream J, O'Connor J, Rosenfeld R S,
   Levin J, Fukushima D K 1982 Age variation of the 24-hour
   mean plasma concentration of androgens, estrogens, and
   gonadotropins in normal adult men. Journal of Clinical
   Endocrinology and Metabolism 54: 534–538

37

Thyroid disorders

C. I. Gryfe

Thyroid disease in old age tends to be under-diagnosed on clinical grounds, and over-diagnosed using laboratory criteria. These diagnostic traps make it difficult to assess the impact of thyroid disorders on the overall function of elderly patients, although the general importance of thyroid hormone in metabolic processes is obvious.

The hypothalamic-pituitary-thyroid axis regulates the availability of thyroid hormone (Larsen, 1982), but non-endocrinologic factors can influence the results of thyroid function tests. Among these many factors are the diseases found so commonly in old people. Because of the high prevalence of extra-thyroidal disease it is very difficult to find appropriate test subjects in whom normal thyroid function can be defined and then used as a standard for detecting and quantifying thyroid disease. With these limitations constantly in mind, it is still useful to review published studies and attempt to understand normal, age-related changes in thyroid function.

STRUCTURE, FUNCTION AND CHEMISTRY

Consistent with the general phenomenon of senescent involution and atrophy of organs, the normal thyroid gland does not enlarge with age. Follicular size decreases and connective tissue increases, and these apparently normal, age-related changes, together with an increased frequency of pathologic nodules give the appearance of thyroid enlargement (Stoffer et al, 1961). However, usually it may be concluded that a palpable thyroid gland in an elderly patient is abnormally enlarged, analogous to the palpable spleen.

Thyroid hormone action determines the total rate of oxygen consumption. Although thryoxine (T4) is not the direct effector of this process, it has been and remains the key to our understanding of thyroid function. Thyroxine is produced in the thyroid follicle cells by the coupling of the di-iodinated forms of the amino acids tyrosine or hydroxphenylpyruvic acid (Taurog & Nakashima, 1978). Once synthesised, thyroxine may be stored in the colloid content of the follicular lumen or released immediately to the general circulation. Stored hormone is bound to thyroglobulin, the protein matrix on which it is synthesised.

After release from the gland, the hormone is deiodinated to produce most importantly, tri-iodothyronine (T3) the agent directly acting on peripheral cells (Larsen, 1972a). Two primary senescent processes alter the rate but not the quality of this basic economy of thyroid hormone: declining renal glomerular capacity and diminishing total target cell mass.

The loss of nephrons in normal aging causes a decline in glomerular filtration rate and hence a decrease in iodide clearance (Oddie et al, 1966) and a rise in plasma iodide concentration. Some unknown intra-thyroidal regulatory mechanism neutralises this tendency to an increased plasma-gland gradient of iodide by allowing the establishment of relatively high intra-thyroidal iodide levels, and a decreased rate of iodide trapping (Gaffney et al, 1962). The net effect is a diminished absolute iodine uptake and a minor reduction in the rate of iodine uptake, as measured by the 24-hour 131 I-uptake test or RIU. (Perlmutter & Riggs, 1949).

These consequences of decreasing glomerular filtration of iodide set the stage for a reduction in the rate of thyroid hormone synthesis, but this is balanced by a diminished need for hormones, resulting from a smaller peripheral target cell mass. There is indeed a lower turnover rate of iodide and of thyroid hormone (Gregerman et al, 1962) but no defect in thyroid function.

The reduced rate of turnover is reflected in an age-related reduction in basal metabolic rate (BMR), but this is the direct result of declining lean body mass and is not caused by failing thyroid capacity (Shock et al 1963).

Despite the slower turnover of thyroid hormone serum T4 concentrations do not differ in healthy young and old people (Snyder & Utiger, 1972). Immediately after release from the gland into the blood, T4 is bound to specific carrier proteins, mostly thyroid-binding globulin (60–70%) but also thyroid-binding pre-albumin (20%) and thyroid-binding albumin (10%). The bonding force is greatest for thyroid-binding globulin (TBG), but is reversible in all cases, resulting in a small fraction (0.02–0.04%) of free hormone in a dynamic equilibrium and available for actual metabolic action. Healthy elderly subjects exhibit an increased binding of T4 by TBG but a decrease in binding by pre-albumin with the net result that hormone binding to serum protein does not account for age-related differences in thyroid hormone metabolism (Braverman et al, 1966). However binding is markedly influenced by a variety of acute and chronic illnesses and by some drugs commonly used in geriatric practice.

The small fraction of circulating T4 which is unbound is available for metabolic action but this is mostly effected through conversion to T3 (Schimmel & Utiger, 1977). Although low serum concentrations of T3 are frequently found in old age they are almost always due to disease both thyroidal and non-thyroidal, and not to normal aging (Olsen et al, 1978).

Peripheral conversion of T4 normally occurs through two alternative steps. The enzyme 5'-deiodinase indiscriminately and randomly removes an iodide molecule from either the 5' or 5 position, producing T3 or reverse tri-iodothyronine respectively (Chopra, 1976). The latter has virtually no metabolic effect (Pittman et al, 1962) and both T3 and reverse tri-iodothyronine (rT3) are further deiodinated to produce 3,3'-diiodothyronine (T2), also metabolically inert (Stasilli et al, 1959). Under normal circumstances the net yield of T3 and rT3 is almost equal (Schimmel & Utiger, 1977) but when there is decreased synthesis of T4, as in hypothyroidism, conversion to T3 occurs preferentially, and in effect compensates for diminished T4. In the presence of various systemic diseases, the alternative deiodination predominates (Chopra et al, 1975), producing more rT3, whose accumulation in preference to T3 is further enhanced by decreased conversion to T2. Many of the common diseases of old age can produce this increase in rT3.

Regulation of T4 synthesis and release is controlled by the pituitary hormone, thyrotropin or thyroid-stimulating hormone (TSH), which appears in peripheral blood at essentially the same concentration in healthy young and old, under basal conditions (Olsen et al, 1978). The normal negative-feedback effect of thyroid hormone on TSH prevails in old age, but stimulation of TSH by hypothalamic thyrotropin-releasing hormone (TRH) appears to be blunted in old men (Snyder & Utiger, 1972).

THE FREQUENCY OF THYROID DISEASE

An enlarged gland is the commonest clinical abnormality of the thyroid but usually of no importance. Many are impalpable because of the distortion of the lower neck by a kyphotic, osteoporotic cervico-thoracic spine or by changes in the rib cage from senescent lung expansion. The weight of an enlarged gland may cause it to descend into the upper mediastinum with consequent traction tracheomalacia. Thus, on rare occasions tracheal obstruction may occur. This common enlargement is the result of multiple nodules, usually of the colloid type and often with secondary degenerative changes.

Although people over 60 years of age comprise less than 15% of the population in most industrialised countries, they represent about 30% of the prevalence of discrete, solid, non-functioning thyroid nodules. Autonomously functioning solitary nodules appear with increasing frequency in advancing age causing clinical thyrotoxicosis in the elderly more often than does Graves' disease (Bartels, 1965).

Reports of the frequency of hypothyroidism after the age of 65 give widely varying figures. Some of this variation may be attributable to the difficulty in distinguishing the classic hypothyroid state from the common findings in old age which together resemble the clinical syndrome of myxoedema i.e. the general slowing of function, tendencies to hypothermia, atherosclerosis, hyperlipidaemias, elevated blood pressure and anaemia. The wide difference in reported prevalence is due to the selection of the study populations. It appears that in community-based subjects over 65 years old, about 2% are hypothyroid (Hodkinson & Denham, 1977), and the frequency increases with age, perhaps twofold within the average expected lifespan, and with the increasing proportion of women in advanced age groups (Taylor et al, 1974). In hospitalised old patients, the prevalence is also about 2–4% (Jefferys, 1972; Bahemuka & Hodkinson, 1975; Burrows et al, 1975; Atkinson et al, 1978), demonstrating that hypothyroidism is second only to diabetes as an endocrine disorder in old age.

Hyperthyroidism after 60 years of age comprises about one-third to one-half of all cases (Rønov-Jessen & Kirkegaard, 1973), with an annual incidence of 0.98 per 1000, seven times the frequency in the younger population. Unlike younger patients in whom Graves' disease is the commonest cause, toxic nodules and thyroiditis are the usual associated pathology.

Regardless of pathology or direction of aberrant function, thyroid disease is more frequent in women. In all types of thyroid disease, diagnosis in the elderly is difficult and requires a high index of suspicion.

THYROID TESTING

The purpose of each of the many available thyroid function tests should be clearly understood in order to make appropriate selection. They may be usefully classified as tests for: the evaluation of thyroid function; the detection of specific thyroid diseases; and the structural definition of the thyroid gland.

The position, size, shape and macroscopic homogeneity

of the gland can be defined by radio-isotope scintigraphy and ultrasound imaging, and focal abnormalities can then be assessed histologically after needle biopsy. Scintigraphy is useful in the detection, localisation and characterisation of nodules ('hot' vs 'cold'), but gives no real information regarding histopathology. Ultrasound differentiates between cystic and solid structure in nodules but definitive diagnosis requires biopsy which can be accomplished effectively using a fine-needle technique. While minimally traumatic, fine-needle biopsy requires interpretation by an experienced pathologist (Walfish et al, 1977).

Immunopathic disease such as Hashimoto's disease, subacute thyroiditis and Graves' disease can be detected by the use of appropriate antibody tests. Recurrent follicular carcinoma of the thyroid can be detected by serum thyroglobulin monitoring, and medullary carcinoma may be discovered by serum calcitonin assays.

Tests used to measure various parameters of thyroid function include the very commonly employed assays of serum hormone concentrations and their degree of protein-binding, but true evaluation of the functional status of the gland requires tests of thyroid iodine turnover, peripheral hormone effects or the integrity of the hypothalamic-pituitary-thyroid axis.

Measurement of total serum T4 is the key screening test for hypo or hyper-thyroidism, but a concurrent test of hormone protein-binding, such as a T3-resin uptake (T3U) is required to interpret abnormal or unexpected values. The increasing availability of total serum T3 radio-immunoassay has expanded the 'routine' thyroid function test battery, but confusion of T3U & T3 test results is still common and must be avoided. Direct tests of free T4 and T3 concentrations in serum are complex and expensive but similar information usually can be deduced by the calculation of the free hormone indices (T4 × T3U = FT4I; T3 × T3U = FT3I).

The most commonly used test of thyroid iodine turnover, the 24-hour RIU is obsolete for the diagnosis of hypothyroidism and of thyrotoxicosis, but remains useful for the detection and monitoring of subacute thyroiditis.

There are still no adequately precise or accurate measurements of peripheral hormonal effects, although some indication of thyroid hormone action may be seen in BMR, in serum concentrations of cholesterol (Kritchevsky, 1960), or creatinephosphokinase (CPK) (King & Zapf, 1972), or in Achilles reflex time (Gibson, 1959).

A wide variety of non-thyroidal illnesses can produce abnormal values in the common thyroid function tests. In younger patients these abnormalities usually are associated with severe illness, but less marked degrees of illness appear to perturb thyroid function in the elderly. Diagnostic and therapeutic agents used in connection with these diseases can also produce misleading results, such as the obfuscation of thyroid function tests for up to 3 weeks after oral cholecystography (Reiner et al, 1980).

Because disease states are more frequent in old age, the circumstances under which thyroid testing is undertaken are particularly important. In general it is better to defer thyroid function testing until the patient's condition has stabilised, unless there is good clinical evidence to support a suspicion of life-threatening thyroid disease.

HYPOTHYROIDISM

If hypothyroidism is suspected, routine laboratory tests should include serum T4 concentration and T3U or other test of protein-binding. If the test results are equivocal, high serum TSH values will confirm the diagnosis of hypothyroidism. However elevated serum TSH values without low serum T4 are found frequently in old age and their significance is controversial (Gryfe et al, 1978). Much of the evidence indicates this is a compensated state of diminished thyroid reserve but these patients are likely not functionally hypothyroid and require no replacement therapy. However the patient with an isolated elevation of serum TSH should have serum assay for thyroid antibodies, and if positive, repeat serum T4 at 6 to 12 month intervals is advisable.

When serum TSH is only slightly elevated and myxoedema is suspected, provocation of the hypothalamic pituitary-thyroid axis is indicated. The TRH stimulation test is preferred to the TSH stimulation test because it minimises the risk of activating a latent hyperthyroid state and is more convenient, without repeat visits or handling of radio-isotopes. The response standards established for younger patients are appropriate for testing aged subjects.

Except in the rare case of myxoedema coma, treatment of hypothyroidism is not urgent. Replacement therapy with pure l-thyroxine is standard and the usual maintenance dose is 0.15 or 0.2 mg per day. Because of the very common concurrence of ischaemic heart disease, therapy must be initiated at low doses and increased cautiously. Starting at 0.025 mg per day and incrementing by the same dose every 2 to 3 weeks is usually well tolerated, but the patient must be monitored regularly and frequently for angina, tachycardia and heart failure. Diabetes may be precipitated or aggravated by thyroid replacement therapy.

Effectiveness of treatment usually can be guaged by improvement in clinical symptoms and signs, but objective, quantitative evidence seems to satisfy the practitioner more. If serum CPK has been found elevated prior to treatment, its return to normal is a readily available and inexpensive indicator of response (King & Zapf, 1972), but is not very precise (McConahey, 1969). Normalisation of serum T4 or serum TSH does not reflect accurately the effectiveness of therapy at the cellular level, but the restoration of normal serum T3 is a reliable index of euthyroidism.

If angina limits dosage to suboptimal levels, increments

of 0.0125 mg every 3 weeks with concurrent propranolol therapy may be tried, but with great caution. The discovery of hypothyroidism within 6 months after acute myocardial infarction presents a particularly thorny dilemma for which there is no concensus for resolution.

When hypothyroidism is diagnosed in association with a chronic dementing syndrome, hope inevitably arises that adequate hormone replacement may reverse the brain failure. However in the author's experience, this is rarely if ever realised.

HYPERTHYROIDISM

The classical features of thyrotoxicosis are not easily recognisable as a constellation in old age, and the diagnosis also must be entertained under less typical circumstances such as heart failure, angina pectoris, supraventricular tachyarrhythmias (Davis & Davis, 1974), discomfort about the thyroid gland, and even psychomotor retardation (Thomas et al, 1970). Hormone excess is usually demonstrable in an elevated serum T4, but normal values may be found in 14% of cases (Caplan et al, 1978) and rarely, isolated T3-toxicosis is present, particularly in association with nodular goitre (Sterling et al, 1970). It should also be noted that T4 may be elevated without increased serum T3 (Caplan et al, 1978; Birkhauser et al, 1977). Therefore, laboratory confirmation requires measurement of serum T4, T3U and T3. If there is T4-T3 dissociation, the TRH stimulation test is indicated, to probe the pituitary-thyroid axis.

Marked decreases in the TSH response to TRH follow small increases in endogenous serum T4 and T3 concentrations (Snyder & Utiger, 1973). The TSH response to TRH is, accordingly, almost uniformly absent in patients with hyperthyroidism (Ormston et al, 1971). An absent TSH response to TRH in the patient suspected of having hyperthyroidism does not establish that clinically significant hyperthyroidism is present; it does however, strongly suggest that thyroid function is to some extent autonomous or both. A normal TSH response to TRH on the other hand conclusively excludes a diagnosis of hyperthyroidism (Utiger, 1978).

The size, texture and consistency of the thyroid gland during thyrotoxicosis are important considerations before undertaking treatment. If the gland is palpably enlarged, it is usually due to multinodular disease, or an isolated nodule may be responsible for the hyperthyroidism. Tenderness is an important clue to the presence of subacute thyroiditis as the cause of thyrotoxicosis, in which case thyroid ablative measures are not indicated.

Most elderly patients with toxic nodular goitre can be and should be treated with radio-iodine, except in the presence of a large, obstructing gland or when cancer is

suspected. Lifelong follow-up is required because of the virtually inevitable development of hypothyroidism.

THYROIDITIS

Non-suppurative, acute or subacute inflammation of the thyroid gland is being recognised with increasing frequency. Probably due to viral infection and affecting people with a particular genetic predisposition (Volpe, 1979), subacute or deQuervain's thyroiditis goes through a destructive phase during which excess release of hormone produces a mild thyrotoxic state. The inflammation characteristically produces thyroid pain of variable intensity, and the coincidence of neck or jaw pain plus tachycardia may lead the unwary physician primarily to a diagnosis of ischaemic myocardial disease. However the lack of typical, clinical features of hyperthyroidism must be kept in mind in geriatric practice, and subacute thyroiditis should be considered in any elderly woman with non-specific complaints, even in the absence of thyroid pain or tenderness (Gordon & Gryfe, 1981). Thyroid antibodies, if elevated, are usually so only transiently and do not reach the high levels seen in Hashimoto's auto-immune thyroiditis. Serum thyroid hormone concentrations are typical of hyperthyroidism early in the disease, and the cause of the elevation can be demonstrated by RIU or radio-isotope scan of the thyroid gland. Unlike Graves' disease or toxic nodular disease, where high uptake or 'hot' scans occur, subacute thyroiditis produces a diagnostic syndrome of low RIU and high serum T4 and T3. Later, with depletion of thyroid colloid, about one quarter of patients enter a typical hypothyroid phase, but eventual spontaneous recovery is the rule. Treatment should be expectant and supportive only, with analgesics for any pain and beta-adrenergic blockers for thyrotoxic symptoms. Corticosteroids have been strongly recommended for younger patients but do not appear to be necessary in the elderly.

NON-THYROIDAL DISEASE

Not infrequently suspicion of thyroid disease arises while patients are being investigated or treated for recognised non-thyroidal illness, many of which are common in the polypathology of old age. Acute febrile illnesses (Burger et al, 1976), chronic liver and renal disease (Chopra et al, 1975), chronic obstructive lung disease, malignant neoplasia (Carter et al, 1974), as well as non-specific stresses such as major surgery (Burr et al, 1975), treatment in intensive care units (Carter et al, 1974) and fasting in obese subjects (Spaulding et al, 1976) can alter the metabolism of thyroid hormone. Under these circumstances it is very difficult to substantiate a diagnosis of thyroid disease using the results of only two or three thyroid function tests.

The common clinical scenarios are either suspected hypothyroidism in a generally debilitated patient with chronic, multisystem disease, or possible thyrotoxicosis in association with hyperkinetic cardiac illness such as paroxysmal atrial fibrillation. In the first instance, there is the temptation to diagnose hypothyroidism if a low serum T4 is reported. Often serum T3 is also low but this cannot be taken as evidence of thyroid gland insufficiency. The associated FT4I is not usually depressed, thereby excluding hypothyroidism (Olsen et al, 1978) but if it is, TSH assay can usually distinguish between spurious and true primary hypothyroidism. However TSH elevation must be substantial to be diagnostic. Conversely, normal serum TSH excludes the diagnosis of primary hypothyroidism (Melmed et al, 1982). The less readily available tests for rT3 and direct free T4 can also help to make the distinction (Chopra et al, 1979).

When hyperthyroidism is suspected in association with non-thyroidal illness, elevated serum T4 may also be spurious (Britton et al, 1975; Burrows et al, 1975; Birkhauser et al, 1977). Total serum T3 values are unpredictable in the combined presence of thyrotoxicosis and severe non-thyroidal disease; rT3 assay or direct free T3 are usually not readily available under the circumstances. However the absence of a suppressed TSH response to a 400 μg intravenous dose of TRH effectively excludes hyperthyroidism.

EFFECTS OF DRUGS ON THYROID FUNCTION

The polypathology which characterises old age inevitably increases the use of medications, further confounding the diagnosis of thyroid disease, whether based on symptomatology or on interpretation of laboratory tests. Clinically overt side effects of drugs initially may resemble the presenting symptoms of thyroid disease and the results of thyroid function tests may also be perturbed by these drugs.

Oestrogens are widely used to control menopausal symptoms, metastatic carcinoma of the prostate or to prevent senescent osteoporosis, and their ability to influence thyroid hormone economy in several ways has important effects on thyroid function tests. The most prominent is an increase of serum T4 concentration, which may reach twice pre-treatment levels, and is mediated by an increased concentration of TBG.

At pharmacologic doses, corticosteroids also have wide effects on thyroid hormone economy, mostly through the inhibition of TSH secretion. As a consequence serum T4 values are reduced.

Greater sophistication in the diagnosis and treatment of behavioural disturbances in old age has led to increased recognition of depressive illness and its treatment with lithium carbonate, a potent inhibitor of thyroid hormone secretion. Most patients remain euthyroid but underlying auto-immune thyroiditis may be unmasked when low serum T4 values are discovered (Emerson et al, 1973).

Analine derivative compounds have demonstrated antithyroid properties but those derivatives which have been developed and adopted for clinical practice have not been found sufficiently potent to affect thyroid function. These agents include the sulphonamide antimicrobials, the sulphonylurea antidiabetic drugs and the benzothiadiazine diuretics. However para-aminosalicyclic acid, still used extensively in treating tuberculosis, has occasionally caused goitre.

Serum concentrations of T3 and T4 are reduced by 15–20% in patients using salicylates (Larsen, 1972b) or phenytoin (Hansen et al, 1974). High FT4I is frequently found in ill elderly women (Britton et al, 1975) and this appears often to be due to the drugs being used, particularly digitalis, cotrimoxazole, diuretics and levodopa (Baruch et al, 1976). Protein-binding of T4 is also influenced by diazepam (Schussler, 1971).

REFERENCES

Atkinson R L, Dahms W T, Fisher D A, Nichols A L 1978 Occult thyroid disease in an elderly hospitalized population. Journal of Gerontology 33: 372–376

Bahemuka M, Hodkinson H M 1975 Screening for hypothyroidism in elderly patients. British Medical Journal 2: 601–603

Bartels E C 1965 Hyperthyroidism in patients over 65. Geriatrics 20: 459–462

Baruch A L H, Davis C, Hodkinson H M 1976 Causes of high free-thyroxine-index values in sick euthyroid elderly patients. Age Ageing 5: 224–227

Birkhauser M, Busset R, Burer T, Burger A 1977 Diagnosis of hyperthyroidism when serum-thyroxine alone is raised. Lancet 2: 53–56

Braverman L E, Dawber N A A, Ingbar S H 1966 Observations concerning the binding of thyroid hormones in sera of normal subjects of varying ages. Journal of Clinical Investigation 45:1273–1279

Britton K E, Ellis S M, Miralles J M, Quinn V, Cayley A C D, Brown B L, Ekins R P 1975 Is 'T4 toxicosis' a normal biochemical finding in elderly women? Lancet 2: 141–142

Burger A, Suter P, Nocid P, Vallotton M B, Vagenakis A, Braverman L 1976 Reduced active thyroid hormone levels in acute illness. Lancet 1: 653–655

Burr W A, Black E G, Griffiths R S, Hoffenberg R, Meinhold H, Weinzel K W 1975 Serum triiodothyronine and reverse triiodothyronine concentrations after surgical operation. Lancet 2: 1277–1279

Burrows A W, Shakespear R A, Hesch R D, Cooper E, Aickin C M, Burke C W 1975 Thyroid hormones in the elderly sick: 'T4-euthyroidism'. British Medical Journal 4: 437–439

Caplan R H, Glasser J E, Davis K, Foster L, Wickus G 1978 Thyroid function tests in elderly hyperthyroid patients. Journal of the American Geriatrics Society 26: 116–120

Carter J N, Corcoran J M, Eastman C J, Lazarus L 1974 Effects of severe, chronic illness on thyroid function. Lancet 2: 971–974

Chopra I J 1976 An assessment of daily production and significance of thyroidal 3,3′,5′ triiodothyronine (reverse T3) in man. Journal of Clinical Investigation 58: 32–40

Chopra I J, Chopra U, Smith S R, Reza M, Solomon D H 1975 Reciprocal changes in serum concentrations of 3,3′5′-triiodothyronine (reverse T3) and 3,3′,5-triiodothyronine (T3) in systemic illnesses. Journal of Clinical Endocrinology and Metabolism 41: 1043–1049

Chopra I J, Solomon D H, Hepner G W, Morgenstein A A 1979 Misleadingly low free thyroxine index and usefulness of reverse triiodothyronine measurement in nonthyroidal illness. Annals of Internal Medicine 90: 905–912

Davis P J, Davis F B 1974 Hyperthyroidism in patients over the age of 60 years. Medicine 53: 151–181

Emerson C H, Dyson W L, Utiger R D 1973 Serum thyrotropin and thyroxine concentrations in patients receiving lithium carbonate. Journal of Clinical Endocrinology and Metabolism 36: 338–346

Gaffney G W, Gregerman R I, Shock N W 1962 The relationship of age to the thyroidal accumulation, renal excretion and distribution of radioiodide in euthyroid man. Journal of Clinical Endocrinology and Metabolism 22: 784–794

Gibson W E 1959 Achilles-reflex recording with a simple photomotograph. New England Journal of Medicine 260: 1027–1031

Gordon M, Gryfe C I 1981 Hyperthyroidism with painless subacute thyroiditis in the elderly. Journal of the American Medical Association 246: 2354–2355

Gregerman R I, Gaffney G W, Shock N W 1962 Thyroxine turnover in euthyroid man with special reference to changes with age. Journal of Clinical Investigation 41: 2065–2074

Gryfe C I, Ginsberg J, Hazani E, Walfish P G 1978 The prevalence of subclinical hypothyroidism in the aged. XI International Congress on Gerontology, Tokyo 110 (abstr)

Hansen J M, Skovsted L, Lauridsen U B, Kirkegaard C, Siersbaek-Nielsen K 1974 The effect of diphenylhydantoin on thyroid function. Journal of Clinical Endocrinology and Metabolism 39: 785–789

Hodkinson H M, Denham M J 1977 Thyroid function tests in the elderly in the community. Age & Ageing 6: 67–70

Jefferys P M 1972 The prevalence of thyroid disease in patients admitted to a geriatric department. Age & Ageing 1: 33–37

King J O, Zapf P 1972 A review of the value of creatine phosphokinase estimations in clinical medicine. Medical Journal of Australia 1: 699–703

Kritchevsky D 1960 Influences of thyroid hormones and related compounds on cholesterol biosynthesis and degradation: a review. Metabolism 9: 984–994

Larsen P R 1972a Triiodothyronine: review of recent studies of its physiology and pathophysiology in man. Metabolism 21: 1073–1092

Larsen P R 1972b Salicylate-induced increases in free triiodothyronine in human serum: evidence of inhibition of triiodothyronine binding to thyroxine-binding globulin and thyroxine-binding prealbumin. Journal of Clinical Investigation 51: 1125–1134

Larsen P R 1982 Thyroid-pituitary interaction: feedback regulation of thyrotropin secretion by thyroid hormones. New England Journal of Medicine 306: 23–32

McConahey W M 1969 Serum creatine kinase as a test of thyroid function. Annals of Internal Medicine 71: 1022–1023

Melmed S, Geola F L, Reed A W, Pekary A E, Park J, Hershman J M 1982 A comparison of methods for assessing thyroid function in nonthyroidal illness. Journal of Clinical Endocrinology and Metabolism 54: 300–306

Oddie T H, Meade J H, Myhill J, Fisher D A 1966 Dependence of renal clearance of radioiodide on sex, age and thyroidal status. Journal of Clinical Endocrinology and Metabolism 26: 1293–1296

Olsen T, Laurberg P, Weeke J 1978 Low serum triiodothyronine and high serum reverse triiodothyronine in old age: an effect of disease not age. Journal of Clinical Endocrinology and Metabolism 47: 1111–1115

Ormston B J, Cryer R J, Garry R, Besser G M, Hall R 1971 Thyrotrophin-releasing hormone as a thyroid-function test. Lancet 2: 10–14

Perlmutter M, Riggs D S 1949 Thyroid collection of radioactive iodide and serum protein-bound iodine concentration in senescence, in hypothyroidism and in hypopituitarism. Journal of Clinical Endocrinology and Metabolism 9: 430–439

Pittman J A, Brown R W, Register H B 1962 Biological activity of 3,3′,5′-triiodo-DL-thyronine. Endocrinology 70: 79–83

Rainer R G, Lawson M J, Marshall T, Read T R, Beng C G, Davies G T et al 1980 Thyroid, renal, and hepatic function tests following cholecystography with high-dose contrast agents. Digestive Diseases and Sciences 25: 379–383

Rønnov-Jessen V, Kirkegaard C 1973 Hyperthyroidism — a disease of old age? British Medical Journal 1: 41–43

Schimmel M, Utiger R D 1977 Thyroidal and peripheral production of thyroid hormones — review of recent findings and their clinical implications. Annals of Internal Medicine 87: 760–768

Schussler G C 1971 Diazepam competes for thyroxine binding sites. Journal of Pharmacology and Experimental Therapeutics 178: 204–209

Shock N W, Watkin D M, Yiengst M J, Norris A H, Gaffney G W, Gregerman R I, Falzone J A 1963 Age differences in the water content of the body as related to basal oxygen consumption in males. Journal of Gerontology 18: 1–10

Snyder P J, Utiger R D 1972 Response to thyrotropin releasing hormone (TRH) in normal man & thyrotropin response to thyrotropin releasing hormone in normal females over forty. Journal of Clinical Endocrinology and Metabolism 34: 380–385 & 1096–1098

Snyder P J, Utiger R D 1973 Repetitive administration of thyrotropin-releasing hormone results in small elevations of serum thyroid hormones and in marked inhibition of thyrotropin response. Journal of Clinical Investigation 52: 2305–2312

Spaulding S W, Chopra I J, Sherwin R S, Lyall S S 1976 Effect of caloric restriction and dietary compositon on serum T3 and reverse T3 in man. Journal of Clinical Endocrinology and Metabolism 42: 197–200

Stasilli N R, Kroc R L, Meltzer R I 1959 Antigoitrogenic and calorigenic activites of thyroxine analogues in rats. Endocrinology 64: 62–82

Sterling K, Refetoff S, Selenkow H A 1970 T3 thyrotoxicosis: thyrotoxicosis due to elevated serum triiodothyronine levels. Journal of the American Medical Assocation 213: 571–575

Stoffer R P, Hellwig C A, Welch J W, McCusker E N 1961 The thyroid gland after age 50. Geriatrics 16: 435–443

Taurog A, Nakashima T 1978 Dissociation between degree of iodination and iodoamino acid distribution in thyroglobulin. Ednocrinology 103: 633–640

Taylor B B, Thomson J A, Caird F I 1974 Further studies of thyroid function tests in the elderly at home. Age & Ageing 3: 122–126

Thomas F B, Mazzaferri E L, Skillman T G 1970 Apathetic thyrotoxicosis: a distinctive clinical and laboratory entity. Annals of Internal Medicine 72: 679–685

Volpe R 1979 Subacute (de Quervain's) thyroiditis. Clinics in Endocrinology and Metabolism 8: 81–95

Walfish P G, Hazani E, Strawbridge H T G, Miskin M, Rosen I B 1977 Combined ultrasound and needle aspiration cytology in the assessment and management of hypofunctioning thyroid nodule. Annals of Internal Medicine 87: 270–274

38

Diabetes

H. C. Shapiro

CLASSIFICATION

Recent investigations support the premise that diabetes mellitus is a heterogeneous disorder. The National Diabetes Data Group (1979) (NDDG) recommended a revised classification of diabetes mellitus and developed uniformly acceptable criteria for its diagnosis. Previously established criteria used to diagnose diabetes have established blood sugar standards that were too low causing numerous subjects who manifested impairment of glucose tolerance to be inappropriately labelled as diabetic.

Type I (insulin dependent diabetes mellitus), previously referred to as juvenile or brittle diabetes mellitus, presents with the classic picture of insulinopenia. The metabolic derangement is manifest by a dramatic, sudden onset of clinical symptoms. Type II (non-insulin dependent diabetes mellitus), previously referred to as maturity-onset diabetes is the most common form (NDDG, 1979). Approximately 85% of all diabetics, predominantly elderly, fall into this category. These patients are not prone to ketosis and require insulin only in the event that diet and oral hypoglycaemic agents fail to control persistent hyperglycaemia (Reaven, 1983b; Rifkin, 1982).

The revised diagnostic criteria for unequivocally establishing the diagnosis of diabetes mellitus depends upon the presence of any of the following criteria (NDDG, 1979):

1. Overt metabolic decompensation as manifest by polyuria, polydipsia, polyphagia, weight loss, generalised weakness, ketonuria and hyperglycaemia.

2. A fasting plasma glucose concentration exceeding 140 mg/dl, on more than one occasion, in an otherwise asymptomatic patient.

3. A standard oral glucose tolerance test demonstrating a plasma glucose concentration exceeding 200 mg/dl at 2 hours, and at any other time interval, on more than one occasion.

These revised standards for the oral glucose tolerance test following the administration of a 75 g glucose load can be seen in Figure 38.1. The upper limits of normal for the plasma glucose concentration is a fasting level of less than 115 mg/dl, never exceeding 200 mg/dl at any other time

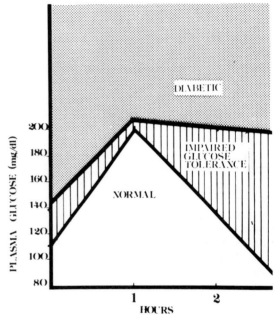

Fig. 38.1 Revised diagnostic criteria proposed by the National Diabetes Data Group for assessing glucose tolerance following a standardised 75 g carbohydrate dose.

period, and falling to less than 140 mg/dl at 2 hours. Post prandial or random blood sugars are not recommended as useful screening procedures (NDDG, 1979).

A considerable number of elderly subjects may demonstrate deviations in glucose disposal following an oral glucose tolerance test (Davidson, 1979; Robert et al, 1982). Abnormalities of plasma glucose concentration may include fasting levels that range between 115 and 140 mg/dl, a 2 hour level approaching 200 mg/dl, or a level exceeding 200 mg/dl for any intermediate period. These subjects were previously labelled as chemical, latent, borderline, subclinical, asymptomatic or stress-induced diabetics. As only a small proportion of these individuals actually develop symptomatic diabetes mellitus, it is unwarranted to classify them as diabetic. A large percentage remain metabolically stable and the glucose

tolerance test reverts to normal in a significant number. It
is impossible to predict with any accuracy which subjects in
this group will develop symptomatic diabetes mellitus. The
revised classification for this group of individuals has now
been amended to a broader unstigmatised category bearing
the descriptive designation of impaired glucose tolerance
(NDDG, 1979; Rifkin, 1982).

INSULIN ACTION

Insulin secretion by the pancreatic beta cells is glucose
dependent. Characteristically, insulin release follows a
biphasic pattern, with the initial release of stored insulin
leading within minutes to a peak plasma concentration,
followed by a larger and more sustained release of newly
synthesised insulin. The plasma half-life of insulin is
approximately 5–6 minutes, with approximately 70% of the
secreted insulin extracted and metabolised by liver and
kidney. The biological effect of insulin is initiated by its
binding to specific, high affinity and low capacity receptors
on the cell membrane surface of its target tissues.
Interaction of insulin with its specific receptor initiates a
series of intracellular events which modulate enzyme
activity. It is also believed that a small portion of the
insulin molecule enters the cell, binding to lysosomal and
golgi membranes.

Numerous target tissues are responsive to insulin action
with a myriad of integrated physiological effects, including
regulation of the synthesis and breakdown of glycogen,
protein, lipid and ketones (Sherwin & Felig, 1978). The
regulation of each of these physiological actions by insulin
is mutually independent, manifesting variable sensitivities
to insulin.

As insulin effectiveness declines progressively with age
(Greenfield et al, 1982; Minaker et al, 1982) an abnormal
glucose tolerance test may reflect impaired utilisation of
glucose by peripheral tissues. Subsequently, the fasting
blood sugar may become elevated due to inadequate
regulation of hepatic glucose production. Finally, impaired
regulation of lipid breakdown may also lead to ketonaemia
and ketoacidosis.

GLUCOSE HOMEOSTASIS

The maintenance of a constant plasma glucose
concentration is essential to provide adequate amounts of
substrate to sustain vital energy dependent functions of
critical organs. Despite prolonged fasting and sustained
periods of starvation, the plasma glucose concentration
remains constant with glucose-dependent organs as the
central nervous system, haematopoetic tissue and renal
medulla, continuing to function normally. These organs
metabolise glucose by a non-insulin dependent process.

In the basal state, a constant level of plasma glucose is
maintained by means of a dynamic balance between glucose
consumption peripherally and hepatic glucose output. In
the absence of food intake, obligatory peripheral glucose
utilisation by glucose dependent organs is satisfied by
hepatic glucose production. Initially, hepatic glucose
output is primarily maintained by the breakdown of stored
glycogen. This source is depleted in 14–24 hours and
hepatic glucose production is then solely derived from
gluconeogenesis.

In the diabetic state, non-insulin dependent tissues
continue to utilise glucose at normal rates. However,
impaired glucose utilisation by insulin-dependent tissues,
such as skeletal muscle, cardiac muscle and adipose tissue
leads to hyperglycaemia. Paradoxically, despite an overall
decrease in glucose disposal, insulin mediated regulation of
hepatic glucose production may also be impaired. The
failure of adequate suppression of hepatic glucose output
further contributes to hyperglycaemia.

Metabolic decompensation in the diabetic patient may
therefore be characterised as a dual physiological
derangement of both peripheral glucose utilisation and
abnormal regulation of hepatic glucose production
(Sherwin & Felig, 1978). The resultant hyperglycaemia
induces a transitory osmotic gradient between plasma and
interstitial-intracellular tissues. Cellular membranes are
freely permeable to water which may enter the vascular
compartment in an attempt to buffer this potential osmotic
gradient. As the tubular maximum for glucose reabsorption
is exceeded by the moderately severe hyperglycaemia,
renal glycosuria induces an osmotic diuresis, further
compounding the degree of dehydration and intracellular
water loss.

HYPEROSMOLAR COMA

The insidious nature of this chronic osmotic-induced
negative water balance may lead to a severe alteration in
mental status which in the extreme case can lead to diabetic
coma. The depth of coma often parallels the degree of
cellular dehydration. Changes in lean body mass that often
accompany advanced age lead to a generalised decrease in
total body water content, increasing the vulnerability of the
elderly patient to hyperosmolar dehydration (Cahill, 1983).

Typically, the patient may have a history of prior glucose
intolerance or mild diabetes, readily controlled by either
diet or oral hypoglycaemic agents. There is often a history
of polyuria, nocturia and progressive mental obtundation
without polydipsia or ketonuria. The syndrome may also be
accompanied by fever due to superimposed infection of
either the lung or urinary tract. The clinical appearance of
the patient reflects moderate to severe dehydration, a
depressed sensorium, and occasionally generalised seizures
refractory to dilantin therapy. The mortality rate

approaches 40% due to the associated high incidence of co-existing diseases.

Predictably, serum chemistries in the hyperosmolar nonketotic dehydrated state reveal a profound hyperglycaemia, ranging from 600 to 1500 mg/dl. In addition, hypernatraemia with levels ranging from 140 to 160 mEq/dl and azotaemia, with the BUN ranging between 60 and 90 mg/dl, may also be observed. The calculated serum osmolarity often exceeding 350 mmol per litre, can be determined by the following formula:-

$$2 \times Na + \left(\frac{BUN}{2.8}\right) + \left(\frac{Blood\ sugar}{18}\right) = mosmoles/l$$

This severe derangement of the metabolic state in association with marked dehydration requires prompt treatment with hypotonic fluids, in the form of half normal saline, and small doses of regular insulin. The rate of fluid infusion should approximate 0.5 litre per hour with close monitoring of vital signs, cardiorespiratory function and the central venous pressure. It is not uncommon for the patient to retain a total of 6–10 litres of fluid replacement in excess of urinary output during the course of the initial 48–72 hours.

A priming dose of 20 units of regular insulin is often administered intravenously. The plasma glucose will initially fall at a rate of approximately 75–100 mg/dl per hour, with treatment directed towards achieving a glucose concentration stabilising at the 250–300 mg/dl level. This nadir serves to prevent the possibility for development of cerebral oedema, which can be manifest by an abrupt onset of hypotension, hypothermia and worsening of mental status in the presence of improving blood chemistries. Following the initial insulin dose, 5–10 units of regular insulin can be administered subcutaneously every 2–4 hours to control the plasma glucose. Characteristically, the patient remains obtunded with full recovery delayed for 4–5 days, despite an improvement in the state of hydration and plasma glucose levels. Antibiotic therapy if mandatory is sepsis is suspected.

The absence of ketoacidosis in this syndrome, is primarily attributable to an intact physiological suppression by hyperglycaemia of growth hormone release in the Type II diabetic. Despite the apparent insulin resistant state, suppression of this potent counter regulatory hormone, enables plasma levels of circulating insulin to remain effective in suppressing peripheral breakdown of triglyceride and thereby inhibiting hepatic ketogenesis. The rate of lipolysis reflected in the plasma concentration on long chain free fatty acids is normal. Ketogenesis, a uniquely hepatic process of fatty acid oxidation and recondensation, is regulated both directly and indirectly by insulin. The anti-lipolytic activity of insulin, the most sensitive parameter of insulin action, regulates precursor availability for ketone production by the liver, despite the decreased insulin effectiveness for regulating peripheral glucose utilisation and hepatic glucose output.

A considerable number of patients admitted with severe hyperosmolar nonketonic coma may subsequently be discharged from the hospital on calorically restricted diets or oral hypoglycaemic agents. A small number may require chronic insulin administration for control of hyperglycaemia.

KETOACIDOSIS

Under severe physiological stress, such as sepsis, bleeding, trauma or shock, the Type II diabetic may also develop ketoacidosis. The clinical presentation is often acute, with rapid metabolic deterioration, presenting with the classic symptoms of polyuria, polydipsia, nausea, vomiting and hyperpnea (Kreisberg, 1978). Elevated plasma concentrations of catecholamines, glucagon, cortisol and growth hormone activate triglyceride lipase stimulating the massive breakdown of triglyceride to free fatty acids. Free fatty acids bind to serum albumin and are transported to the liver where they are selectively oxidised by a process of sequential beta-oxidations to generate large quantities of ketones.

The formation of beta-hydroxy butyrate and acetoacetate, both moderately well ionised organic acids in quantities exceeding the normal physiological capacity for oxidation, contributes to the metabolic acidosis. In the diabetic state, the metabolic clearance rate of plasma ketones is decreased by 40% thereby further contributing to the hyperketonaemia. A low renal threshold for plasma ketones facilitates an osmotic diuresis, with a significant loss of sodium, potassium and other cations. The continued accumulation of ionised organic acids, exceeding the buffering capacity of blood results in a falling arterial pH. Deep, sighing, laboured respirations, described as Kussmaul-type, mediated by chemo-receptors in the brainstem at an arterial pH of 7.2 or less, is an attempt to partially compensate for the metabolic acidosis with a physiologically induced respiratory alkalosis. This type of hyperventilation leads to further lowering of the arterial pCO_2 which is characteristic of a partially compensated metabolic acidosis (Kreisberg, 1978; Sherwin & Felig, 1978).

In comparison to the hyperosmolar state, the degree of dehydration may be relatively mild, reflecting an overall fluid deficit of approximately 2–4 litres. The serum sodium is mildly depressed to 130 mg/dl, reflecting the movement of freely diffusible water from the cellular to the vascular compartment to compensate for the osmotic influence of hyperglycaemia. Fluid administration in the form of either isotonic or hypotonic saline, should be given at the rate of approximately 0.5–1 litre per hour. Insulin, initially administered as a 20 unit intravenous bolus, should be followed by 10 units per hour given either subcutaneously or intramuscularly, for the succeeding 5–6 hours. Hydration and reduction of hyperglycaemia leads to correction of the factitious state of pseudohyponatraemia. During the course of the initial 8 hours, there is a gradual correction in all abnormal parameters including blood sugar, arterial pH and bicarbonate. The blood sugar should be stabilised at about the 250–300 mg/dl range, to prevent the possibility of cerebral oedema. At this point the intravenous fluid should consist of 5% dextrose and 0.45% saline, with regular insulin being given at 4 hour intervals. Intermediate acting insulin preparations can be reordered on the following day. Whenever possible, one should avoid catheterising the urinary bladder to prevent iatrogenic urinary tract infection.

PATHOPHYSIOLOGY

In the basal state, plasma glucose levels are determined by the dynamic equilibrium existing between glucose consumption and hepatic glucose production (Sherwin & Felig, 1978). Seventy per cent of glucose disposal is in insulin independent tissues (central nervous system, renal medulla and bone marrow) (Kolterman et al, 1980). Therefore fasting hyperglycaemia is primarily attributable to defective insulin regulation of hepatic glucose production.

Following the administration of an oral glucose challenge, approximately 60% of the glucose load undergoes hepatic extraction (Felig et al, 1975; Sherwin & Felig, 1978). Skeletal muscle and adipose tissue account for an additional 15%. Non-insulin dependent tissues dispose of the remaining 25%. Thus impairment of 75% of glucose disposal following glucose challenge may be explained by defective insulin action at peripheral sites (DeFronzo & Ferrannini, 1982; Felig et al, 1975). It has been observed that the amount of glucose bypassing hepatic uptake in the diabetic patient challenged with an oral glucose load is twofold higher when compared to non-diabetic subjects (Felig et al, 1978).

Although Type I diabetes has always been associated with insulinopenia, considerable controversy has surrounded the pathogenesis of Type II diabetes. Various studies indicating normal to elevated concentrations of plasma insulin in the presence of hyperglycaemia, have suggested impaired tissue sensitivity to insulin as the primary causal factor (Davidson, 1979).

Studies utilising insulin and glucose clamp techniques have verified a decrease in overall glucose metabolism in diabetic subjects as compared to controls, despite comparable plasma insulin levels (Kalant et al, 1979; DeFronzo et al, 1982 & 1983; Reaven, 1983a). Similarly, radio-isotope dilution techniques have revealed either

normal or slightly elevated hepatic glucose produciton rates in diabetics, despite the presence of hyperglycaemia. (DeFronzo & Ferrannini, 1982). These data suggest that fasting hyperglycaemia in the diabetic may be a consequence of either a relative or absolute defect in the regulation of hepatic glucose production due to insulin insensitivity (DeFronzo et al, 1983).

A variety of disease states may contribute to peripheral insulin resistance by altering insulin action at receptor sites (Kolterman et al, 1983). Counter regulatory hormones e.g. growth hormone, catecholamines, glucagon and cortisol, may influence both receptor number and affinity (Olefsky, 1981). Circulating antibodies to insulin or rarely to insulin receptors may also impair insulin action. In addition, a decreased number of insulin receptors is also seen in association with obesity, cirrhosis and oral contraceptive therapy (Olefsky, 1982). Several studies have been unable to demonstrate a direct correlation between the severity of insulin resistance and the observed decrease in insulin binding (Olefsky & Reaven, 1977; Olefsky, 1981). This supports the view that clinically significant insulin resistance may be attributable to alterations in insulin action at a post-receptor site (Kolterman et al, 1981; Bolinder et al, 1982; Ciaraldi et al, 1982). Studies assessing insulin sensitivity and receptor number in isolated adipocytes have demonstrated that maximal glucose transport can be achieved with only 10% of the total number of receptors occupied by insulin (Olefsky, 1981). This relationship can be best observed by assessing a semilogarithmic insulin dose response curve, plotting maximal insulin effectiveness with insulin concentrations. A rightward shift of the sigmoid curve, with preservation of insulin action at maximal insulin dosage, reflects a decrease in insulin receptors, an impairment of insulin action which can be overcome by increasing the plasma insulin concentration. Failure to achieve maximal insulin action in the presence of increasing insulin concentrations would suggest a pure defect at a post-receptor site. Similarly, a rightward shift of the curve with failure to achieve maximal insulin effect, would suggest a combined defect consisting of a decrese in total number of insulin receptors and a post-receptor defect (Kolterman et al, 1983; Olefsky 1981; 1982).

Obese subjects have a decreased glucose disposal rate in the presence of a decreased total number of insulin receptors. Glucose clamp techniques have demonstrated that the obese population may be heterogeneous, with certain subjects showing an additional defect even at maximal insulin concentrations suggesting insulin insensitivity at a post-receptor site (Ciaraldi, 1981; Olefsky, 1981). Similarly, regulation of hepatic glucose production in obese subjects demonstrates a rightward shift of the insulin dose response curve, implying a primary defect in hepatic insulin receptor number (Olefsky, 1981). Obese subjects with peripheral post-receptor impairment to insulin action, manifest a greater degree of rightward displacement of their hepatic insulin dose response curve, achieving maximal insulin action only at higher plasma insulin concentrations (Olefsky, 1981). The small number of obese subjects who manifest this heterogeneous defect, resemble Type II diabetes regarding tissue insensitivity to insulin at post-receptor sites.

Although obesity may be a factor contributing to the insulin resistance of the Type II diabetic, the degree of impaired sensitivity to insulin seems to be greater than can be accounted for simply on the basis of a pure decrease in total receptor number. Other factors may contribute since insulin resistance is also noted in non-obese Type II diabetics (Table 38.1).

Table 38.1 Presumptive sites of insulin resistance.

	Receptor		Post-receptor Extra-hepatic
Elderly	—	P	—
Impaired glucose tolerance	H	P	—
Obesity	H	P	+ +
Non-insulin dependent diabetes	H	P	+ + +

H – Hepatic P – Peripheral

Despite an apparently normal basal plasma insulin concentration, Type II diabetics demonstrate an impaired capacity to secrete insulin following a glucose challenge. This impairment becomes apparent during fasting hyperglycaemia. The presence of post-receptor insulin resistance predominates in subjects with fasting hyperglycaemia exceeding 200 mg/dl, or basal insulin levels exceeding 30 microunits/ml (Olefsky, 1981). Fasting hypergycaemia has been observed to directly correlate with hepatic glucose production. Type II diabetics, manifest a seemingly paradoxical absolute increase in hepatic glucose production when plasma glucose concentrations exceed 180 mg/dl (DeFronzo & Ferranni, 1982).

Glucose disposal in geriatric subjects may be impaired by as much as 30% when compared to younger controls (DeFronzo, 1979). Glucose clamp techniques in non-diabetic geriatric subjects have demonstrated normal regulation of hepatic glucose production (DeFronzo, 1979; Robert et al, 1982). This supports the general observation that fasting plasma glucose concentrations are generally normal in elderly subjects despite an observed impairment in glucose tolerance.

Maximal rates of glucose transport and oxidation can be dissociated in the experimental animal (Olefsky, 1976). This implies that there are relative degrees of insulin sensitivity regarding glucose transport and oxidation. Insulin directly regulates the permeability of peripheral

tissues to glucose, a primary determinant of glucose disposal. It also regulates the activity of phosphofructokinase, the rate limiting enzyme which regulates anaerobic glycolysis. Lipogenesis, the synthesis of long chain fatty acids from glucose, is also insulin dependent and requires the availability of oxidation–reduction co-factors in the reduced state. The hexose monophosphate shunt pathway, an alternate mechanism of glucose oxidation, is dependent upon oxidation–reduction co-factors in an oxidised state (Randle et al, 1963). In the presence of an altered state of glucose disposal, the preferential oxidation of free fatty acids by peripheral tissues may lead to significantly higher ratios of oxidation–reduction co-factors in the reduced form. Conceivably, clinical situations which exhibit high fatty acid turnover rates, such as diabetes or obesity, may demonstrate similar impairments in insulin sensitivity due to altered rates of glucose oxidation with only moderate changes in glucose transport (Randle et al, 1963).

CLINICAL FEATURES

Although insulin regulates numerous intracellular physiologic functions the clinician is limited in assessing the adequacy of diabetes control to monitoring the degree of hyperglycaemia. A solitary blood sugar determination performed at bimonthly intervals, is often broadly extrapolated as indicative of glucose homeostasis in general. Diabetics predisposed to accelerated atherosclerosis, retinopathy and nephropathy, manifest a twofold increased risk of cardiovascular mortality and a fivefold increase in peripheral vascular disease leading to gangrene. The incidence of blindness and renal failure is respectively 25 and 17 times more common as compared to age and sex matched controls. Individual susceptibility to any of these complications is unpredictable due to the marked genetic heterogeneity of diabetes mellitus. The treatment of any of these disorders in the elderly diabetic patient does not differ significantly from that of the younger diabetic, with the exception that conservative treatment is always preferable.

Caloric restriction has historically been the foremost method of treatment in controlling hyperglycaemia in the Type II diabetic (Reaven, 1983b). It is particularly advocated as the primary mode of therapy in obese patients. The estimated total number of daily calories is dependent upon the ideal body weight in pounds multiplied by a factor of ten. In the non-obese Type II diabetic, the estimated total number of daily calories is determined by multiplying the patient's weight by a factor of fifteen. Calories, in the form of complex carbohydrates with one third of the total fat content in the form of polyunsaturated fats, should be evenly distributed in small frequent meals throughout the day. Regretfully, it is no secret that rigid control of dietary intake in the elderly diabetic is often unsuccessful.

The elderly diabetic is frequently non-compliant, resisting unrealistic demands which interfere with his already well established personal habits determined by years of personal preference, financial considerations and palatability. The astute clinician recognises that the problem is often complex and is reluctant to confront the diabetic patient directly. The physician should strive to develop a mutually acceptable plan of care which is consistent with the patient's established mode of living. Complete acceptance of these dietary recommendations may only be achieved by adapting the nutritional needs of the patient in a flexible and empathetic style. All too often, a conspiracy of silence develops regarding the implementation of rigid dietary control. It is the rare patient, with obsessive-compulsive tendencies, who is willing to accept guidance from enthusiastic dietitians, and faithfully adhere to their recommendations (Jackson, 1980).

The mechanism of improved glucose tolerance following dietary regulation in Type II diabetic with significant post-receptor defects is not clear. Recent studies have suggested that selected oral hypoglycaemic agents may improve glycaemic control by a mechanism independent of their effect on insulin secretion.

In general, patients should be encouraged to maintain their customary programmes of physical exercise (Reaven, 1983b). Although increased physical activity has been associated with improved glucose sensitivity, it would appear somewhat misguided to recommend an active programme of physical activity to a newly diagnosed 65-year old diabetic whose primary activities have always been sedentary. Oral hypoglycaemic agents are recommended in the presence of a fasting blood sugar which exceeds 200 mg/dl, or in the symptomatic patient with polyuria and polydipsia. Initial studies supported the view that oral agents increased the total number of peripheral insulin binding sites, thereby improving glucose disposal rates. Recently, reports have suggested a synergistic effect between oral agents and insulin improving peripheral glucose utilisation at post-receptor sites (DeFronzo et al, 1983; Kolterman et al, 1983; Lockwood et al, 1983; Maloff & Lockwood, 1981). In the elderly diabetic, it is generally safer to select oral agents which have a relatively modest plasma half life and which are primarily metabolised by the liver. Chlorpropamide has a plasma half life of 35 hours and is cleared by renal excretion. It has been associated with a syndrome of profound and sustained hypoglycaemia and occasionally with hyponatraemia. When adminstered in maximal doses, tolbutamide or tolazamide can effectively reduce hyperglycaemia. They have relatively short plasma half lives and are metabolised by hepatic biotransformation. Eventually many elderly diabetics manifest drug failure and require insulin administration to maintain glycaemic control.

Due to the unpredictable absorption of long acting lente and NPH insulin, frequent episodes of unsuspected nocturnal hypoglycamia may occur. Typically the patient is asymptomatic during these episodes of glucopenia. On occasion, subtle symptoms may include morning headaches, lassitude, night sweats, nightmares and early morning fatigue. Due to hypersensitivity to counter regulatory hormones secreted in response to the hypoglycaemia, early morning rebound hyperglycaemia is noted (Somogy, 1959). The counter regulatory hormones induce a sustained increase in hepatic glucose production simultaneous with an enduring inhibition of peripheral glucose utilisation (Rizza et al, 1982). The clinician should resist his initial impulse to further increase the morning dose of long acting insulin to control the unexplained hyperglycaemia. The diagnosis can be established by monitoring glycaemic control during the early morning hours, or by obtaining quantitative, timed urinary samples throughout the day. The patient is observed to have wide fluctuations in glycosuria with alternating ketonuria. Characteristically there is no evidence of weight loss. The patient will often require a split dose of long acting insulin, at reduced dosage to improve regulation of glucose homeostasis.

The best way to monitor glycaemic control in the elderly Type II diabetic is with frequent blood sugar determinations. The absence of glycosuria provides a false sense of security regarding diabetic control due to the decrease in renal function which accompanies the aging process. Haemoglobin A_{lc}, is a useful parameter in monitoring overall glucose homeostasis during the pre-ceeding 6–8 weeks (Bunn, 1981). Increased concentrations of glycosylated haemoglobin have been observed in the elderly consequent to renal insufficiency and impaired glucose disposal. It should not replace the need for frequent monitoring of plasma glucose concentrations. A small number of elderly diabetic patients will accept the principle of home blood glucose monitoring utilising a reflectometer. Treatment with the insulin pump has not been recommended in the management of Type II diabetes. One should strive to achieve a fasting blood sugar ranging between 150 and 200 mg/dl, so as to prevent unanticipated episodes of hypoglycaemia which may lead to either myocardial or cerebral insufficiency.

CONCLUSION

It is well recognised that the incidence of glucose intolerance increases with advancing age. Only a small segment of this aging population is at risk of developing overt diabetes mellitus with its associated complications of premature atherosclerosis, retinopathy, neuropathy or nephropathy. Little justification exists for imposing a rigid, unrealistic life style on elderly patients which generally fails to receive full patient acceptance and compliance. The revised criteria for defining diabetes mellitus requires fasting blood sugars exceeding 140 mg/dl on more than one occasion, or a plasma glucose concentration following a glucose challenge which exceeds 200 mg/dl at the 2 hour interval or at one other time frame.

The majority of Type II diabetics are non-insulin dependent and manifest peripheral insulin resistance. Decreases in either total number of insulin receptors or a post-receptor site defect accounts for the observed impairment in insulin action. Selected oral hypoglycaemic agents appear to act synergistically with insulin to ameliorate the post-receptor defect. Proper management of the elderly diabetic remains a major challenge to the diagnostic talents and clinical judgment of the skilled geriatrician.

REFERENCES

Bloom M E, Mintz D H, Field J B 1969 Insulin-induced posthypoglycemic hypeglycemia as a cause of 'brittle' diabetes: Clinical clues and therapeutic implications. American Journal of Medicine 47: 891–903

Bolinder J, Ostman J, Arner P 1982 Post receptor defects causing insulin resistance in normoinsulinemic non-insulin-dependent diabetes mellitus. Diabetes 31: 911–916

Bunn H F 1981 Evaluation of glycosylated hemoglobin in diabetic patients. Diabetes 30: 613–617

Cahill G F 1983 Hyperglycemic hyperosmolar coma: A syndrome almost unique to the elderly. Journal of the American Geriatrics Society 31: 103–105

Ciaraldi T P, Kolterman O G, Olefsky J M 1981 Mechanism of the post-receptor defect in insulin action in human obesity. Decrease in glucose transport sytem activity. Journal of Clinical Investigation 68: 875–880

Ciaraldi T P, Kolterman O G, Scarlett J A, Kao M, Olefsky J M 1982 Role of glucose transport in the post-receptor defect of noninsulin-dependent diabetes mellitus. Diabetes 31: 1016–1022

Davidson M B 1979 The effect of aging on carbohydrate metabolism: A review of the English literature and a practical approach to the diagnosis of diabetes mellitus in the elderly. Metabolism 28: 688–705

DeFronzo R A 1979 Glucose intolerance and aging. Evidence for tissue insensitivity to insulin. Diabetes 28: 1095–1100

DeFronzo R A, Ferrannini E 1982 The pathogenesis of non-insulin-dependent diabetes. An update. Medicine 61: 125–140

DeFronzo R A, Ferrannini E, Koivisto V 1983 New concepts in the pathogenesis and treatment of noninsulin-dependent diabetes mellitus. American Journal of Medicine 75: 52–81

DeFronzo R A, Simonson D, Ferrannini E 1982 Hepatic and peripheral insulin resistance: A common feature of insulin independent and insulin dependent diabetes. Diabetologia 23: 313–319

DeFronzo R A, Tobin J D, Andres R 1979 Glucose clamp technique: A method for quantifying insulin secretion and resistance. American Journal of Physiology 6: E214–E223

Felig P, Wahren J, Hendler R 1975 Influence of oral glucose ingestion on splanchnic glucose and gluconeogenic substrate metabolism in man. Diabetes 24: 468–475

Felig P, Wahren J, Hendler R 1978 Influence of maturity-onset diabetes on splanchnic glucose balance after oral glucose ingestion. Diabetes 27: 121–126

Greenfield M S, Mondon C E, Rosenthal M, Wright D, Reaven E P 1982 Does insulin removal rate from plasma decline with age? Diabetes 31: 670–673

Jackson R A 1980 The treatment of medical problems in the elderly. Denhan, M.J. editor, University Park Press. 159–208

Kalant N Lebovici T, Rohan I, Ozaki S 1979 Interrelationships of glucose and insulin uptake by muscle of normal and diabetic man. Diabetologia 16: 365–372

Kolterman O G, Gray R S, Griffin J, Burstein P, Insel J, Scarlett J A, Olefsky J M 1981 Receptor and postreceptor defects contribute to the insulin resistance in noninsulin-dependent diabetes mellitus Journal of Clinical Investigation 68: 957–969

Kolterman O G, Insel J, Seakow M, Olefsky J M 1980 Mechanisms of insulin resistance in human obesity. Evidence for receptor and post-receptor defects. Journal of Clinical Investigation 65: 1272–1284

Kolterman O G, Prince M J, Olefsky J M 1983 Insulin resistance in noninsulin-dependent diabetes mellitus: Impact of sulfonylurea agents in vivo and in vitro. American Journal of Medicine 74: 82–101

Kreisberg R A 1978 Diabetic ketoacidosis: New concepts and trends in pathogenesis and treatment. Annals of Internal Medicine 88: 681–695

Lockwood D H, Maloff B L,Nowack J M, McCaleb M L 1983 Extrapancreatic effects of sulfonylureas. Potentiation of insulin action through post-binding mechanisms. American Journal of Medicine 74: 102–108

Maloff B L, Lockwood D H 1981 In vitro effects of a sulfonylurea on insulin action in adipocytes. Potentiation of insulin-stimultated hexose transport. Journal of Clinical Investigation 68: 85–90

Minaker K L, Rowe J W, Tonino R, Pallotta J A 1982 Influence of age on clearance of insulin in man. Diabetes 31: 851–855

National Diabetes Data Group 1979 Classification and diagnosis of diabetes mellitus and other categories of glucose intolerance. Diabetes 28: 1039–1057

Olefsky J M 1976 The effects of spontaneous obesity on insulin binding, glucose transport and glucose oxidation of isolate rat adipocytes. Journal of Clinical Investigation 57: 842–851

Olefsky J M 1981 Insulin resistance and insulin action. An in vitro and in vivo perspective. Diabetes 30: 148–161

Olefsky J M 1982 Insulin resistance in humans. Gastroenterology 83: 1313–1317

Olefsky J M, Reaven G M 1977 Relationships with plasma insulin levels and insulin sensitivity. Diabetes 26: 680–688

Randle P J, Hales C N, Garland R B, Newsholme E A 1963 The glucose-fatty acid cycle: Its role in insulin sensitivity and the metabolic disturbances of diabetes mellitus. Lancet 1: 785–789

Reaven G M 1983a Insulin resistance in noninsulin-dependent diabetes mellitus. Does it exist and can it be measured? American Journal of Medicine 74: 3–17

Reaven G M 1983b Therapeutic approaches to reducing insulin resistance in patients with noninsulin-dependent diabetes mellitus. American Journal of Medicine 74: 109–112

Rifkin H 1982 Recognition and complications of diabetes in the older patient. Journal of the American Geriatrics Society 30 30–35

Rizza R A, Mandarino L J, Gerich J E 1982 Effects of growth hormone on insulin action in man. Diabetes 31: 663–668

Robert J J, Cummins J C, Wolfe R R, Durkot M, Matthews D E, Zhao X H, Bier D M, Young V R 1982 Quantitative aspects of glucose production and metabolism in healthy elderly subjects. Diabetes 31: 203–211

Sherwin R, Felig P 1978 Pathophysiology of diabetes mellitus. Medical Clinics of North American 62: 695–711

Somogy M 1959 Exacerbation of diabetes by excess insulin action. American Journal of Medicine 26: 169–191

39

Osteoporosis

B. E. C. Nordin

INTRODUCTION

Loss of bone is a universal accompaniment of aging in the human species, and probably in the other vertebrates as well. It is associated with a progressive decline in bone strength and rise in fracture rates to a point where in Western societies at least, it represents a significant clinical, social and economic problem among the elderly. The fractures occur because of the small mechanical safety margin in the skeleton; a very small loss of bony tissue appears to increase the fracture risk. This is an indirect consequence of the fact that bone strength is not directly proportional to bone weight, with the result that large animals require relatively heavier skeletons to support them than small animals. The skeleton is simultaneously a mechanical support for the body and a burden that has to be moved around by muscular forces and which needs to be kept as light a possible. In the mouse, the bones only represent about 5% of body weight; in man this has risen to 10%; in the elephant it approaches 30%; in the dinosaur, it must have been even greater; and the whale has of course – very sensibly – taken to the sea. Evolution has ensured that there is no more bone than is required to provide protection against the hazards of ordinary daily life during the reproductive years. The margin of safety is therefore small and any loss of bone increases the fracture risk.

The present chapter will review the significance and pathogenesis of osteoporosis and indicate ways in which it can now be prevented and treated.

DEFINITION

Osteoporosis can only be defined in terms of the amount of bony tissue in an anatomical bone – sometimes called the 'apparent density' of the bone. Thus a bone is osteoporotic when its apparent density falls below the young normal lower limit. This lower limit will of course vary from bone to bone, but in the most commonly used reference site (the second metacarpal of the right hand) the mean cortical area/total area ratio (CA/TA) is about .82 (.70–.94) in men

and .85 (.70–1.0) in women. Male bones are of course generally larger than female bones, but their aparent density is very similar in the two sexes – at least in young adult life. Osteoporosis defined in this way may be of two types. An apparent density which though low is normal for the age and sex of the individual is termed 'simple osteoporosis' and a value which is low even after correction for age and sex is termed 'accelerated osteoporosis'. In simple osteoporosis, no pathogenetic mechanisms need to be sought other than those associated with normal aging, but in accelerated osteoporosis additional factors must also be operating.

A diagrammatic representation of the way in which long bone 'density' falls with age is shown in Figure 39.1, which illustrates how an increasing proportion of the population develop cortical osteoporosis with advancing age. As far as cortical bone is concerned, the entire female population is osteoporotic by the age of 80. Men lose bone proportionately more slowly and about 50% have cortical osteoporosis by age 80.

Trabecular bone behaves somewhat differently (Fig. 39.2). In the iliac crest, the apparent density is about .17–.30 in young normal women. There is a rather rapid loss of trabeculae in middle life in both sexes, but this tends to be self-limiting. In subjects over the age of 60, about 50% of women and a rather smaller proportion of men have simple trabecular osteoporosis.

DIAGNOSIS

There are various ways of diagnosing osteoporosis, but it is usually done by radiography. As already indicated, the most commonly used cortical bone is the second metacarpal of the right hand, and measurement of medullary and total width at the mid-point permits the calculation of the CA/TA ratio (on the assumption that the bone is circular in cross-section) and permits a diagnosis of normal bone, simple osteoporosis or accelerated osteoporosis by reference to published standards (Horsman, 1976).

The diagnosis of trabecular osteoporosis is both more

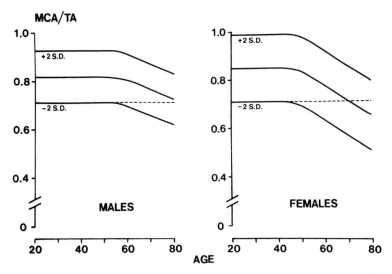

Fig. 39.1 Semi-diagrammatic representation of the fall in metacarpal cortical area/total area ratio in normal men and women with age. Values below the interrupted line represent cortical osteoporosis.

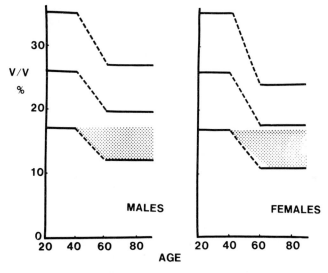

Fig. 39.2 Semi-diagrammatic representation of the change in iliac crest trabecular bone volume with age in men and women. The shaded area denotes the region of simple osteoporosis.

important and more difficult. Until recently, it might have been said that the only sure way was by iliac crest biopsy, although this too is subject to considerable error. Information obtained from iliac crest histology has shown, however, that accelerated trabecular osteoporosis is almost invariably present when the patient has two or more crushed vertebrae which cannot be attributed to myeloma or malignant disease (Horsman et al, 1981). Lesser degrees of osteoporosis are much more difficult to identify, but with the increasing use of computed tomography (CT) scanning (Genant et al, 1982) and of vertebral absorptiometry with gamma-emitting isotopes (Riggs et al,

1982) it is becoming increasingly clear that a vertebral mineral density below about 100 mg/ml should be regarded as osteoporotic; this is a little higher than the fracture threshold value which has been derived from post-mortem studies (Arnold, 1973).

Osteoporosis is in general a systemic disorder; during the course of aging, all the bones are affected to a greater or lesser degree. Localised osteoporosis does of course occur, more particularly in immobolised limbs or after a fracture, but the condition under discussion in this chapter is a generalised disorder of the skeleton characterised by loss of bony tissue.

FRACTURES IN THE ELDERLY

The progressive rise in fracture rates with age which accompanies the loss of bone has been amply documented in many publications (Nordin et al, 1980) and does not need to be recapitulated. The three fractures of particular interest are those of the wrist, vertebrae and femoral neck.

Wrist fractures

The fracture of the distal forearm, involving the radius and the styloid process of the ulna, following a fall on the outstretched hand, is relatively common in children, rare in young adults, but common in post-menopausal women. An interesting feature of this fracture is that it quite often occurs in women within a year or two of the menopause when it seems surprising that sufficient loss of bone could have occurred to cause critical weakening of the distal forearm. The bone status of many of these cases (however it is assessed) falls within the young normal range, although in the patients as a group it is significantly lower than in age-matched controls (Krolner et al, 1982). Perhaps this fracture – in which major trauma is involved – exemplifies the fact that each individual only has a small safety margin and that a small loss of bone in the individual may be critical.

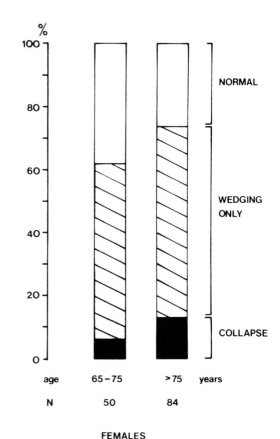

Fig. 39.3 Histograms representing the proportion of elderly women below and over 75 years with normal, wedged and collapsed vertebrae.

Vertebral fractures

This is the syndrome which is regarded as the prototype of 'osteoporosis'. The general impression that patients with crush fractures suffer from severe trabecular osteoporosis is broadly correct, with the emphasis on the trabecular component. However it is important that a distinction be drawn between wedged vertebrae and crushed vertebrae, and that the diagnosis of accelerated spinal osteoporosis should not be made unless there is anterior and posterior compression of at least two vertebrae (malignant disease and myeloma having been excluded). Some degree of vertebral anterior wedging, particularly in the thoracic spine, is common during aging and may affect several vertebrae. Iliac crest biopsy in such cases frequently shows trabecular bone volume that is normal for the age of the subject (Horsman et al, 1981). Only when there are two or more crushed vertebrae can the diagnosis of accelerated osteoporosis be made with confidence – and then only after the exclusion of malignancy and myeloma (see below). This observation is compatible with the fact that some 50% of elderly women may show vertebral wedging but only about 10% have vertebral collapse (Fig. 39.3).

Other radiological signs of osteoporosis may be suggestive without being diagnostic. Vertebral biconcavity is a striking feature of osteoporosis, but is much more likely to be seen in younger cases, possibly because it is associated with young, healthy, turgid intervertebral discs which provide the central axis on which vertebral movement can occur. In the elderly (and the mean age of crush fracture patients is about 62 years), the discs have lost this property and severe osteoporosis with compression of vertebrae may occur without obvious biconcavity.

The bone histology in patients with two or more crushed vertebrae shows a significant reduction in trabecular bone volume. This is associated with a significant increase in percent surface resorption in both sexes and some reduction in forming surface in females (Figs. 39.4–6) (see below).

Femoral neck fractures

Femoral neck fractures are very much more common in women than in men, partly because the actual age-specific rate is higher in females (by a factor of about 2:1), but also because of the increasing proportion of women in the population with advancing age. The fractures may be sub-capital, transcervical, basal or trochanteric, but the great majority are sub-capital or trochanteric in approximately equal proportions. There is a marked seasonal variation in these fractures, most of them occurring in the late winter

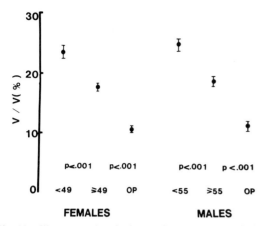

Fig. 39.4 Iliac crest trabecular bone volumes in young, elderly and osteoporotic females and males.

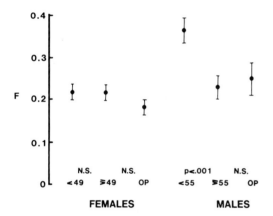

Fig. 39.5 Extent of forming surface in mm^2/mm^3 in iliac crest samples from the same cases Fig. 39.4.

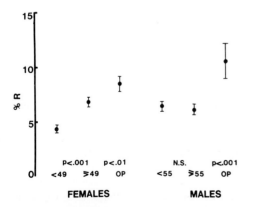

Fig. 39.6 Percentage surface resorption in iliac crest samples from the same cases as Figs. 39.4 & 39.5.

(Evans, 1979) but this cannot be attributed to weather conditions as such because the great majority of the fractures occur in the home and result from a fall at ground level. The incidence of this fracture is increasing (Zetterberg & Andersson, 1982).

Many factors contribute to these fractures, not least of which is the increasing incidence of falls with advancing age due to cerebro-vascular disease, failing eyesight and many other factors (Cook et al, 1982). However the loss of bone with advancing age is undoubtedly an important contributory factor, as evidenced by the fact that the bone status of fracture cases is significantly inferior to that of age-matched controls (Fig. 39.7) (Horsman et al, 1982).

This is true, not only when bone status is judged by the Singh Index (Singh et al, 1970) but also in terms of mid-shaft femoral cortical width (FCW), the thickness of the calcar femorale, the lateral cortical width near the lesser trochanter (FTCW) and the metacarpal cortical area/total area ratio (MCA/TA). However, as shown in Figure 39.7, the significance of these differences is greatest when the measurements are made nearest to the fracture site. A significant difference in forearm density between femoral neck fractures and controls has also been reported by other workers (Elsasser et al, 1980).

However, there are some anomalies Although iliac crest trabecular bone volume is significantly reduced in femoral neck fracture cases (Fig. 39.8) it is not generally as low as it is in the crush fracture syndrome (Compare Figs. 39.4 & 39.8) and the bone-forming surface tends to be increased rather than decreased. Moreover, bone resorption tends to be even higher than it is in the crush fracture cases (compare Figs. 39.6 & 39.8). These features suggest secondary hyperparathyroidism.

Fracture prevalence

From the published data on fracture incidence and the inter-relationships between the fractures, it is possible to construct a diagram representing the prevalence of the three main fractures in the female population in the United Kingdom at the ages of 60 and 80 (Fig. 39.9). By the age of 60, 5% of women have had a wrist fracture, 2.5% a vertebral crush fracture and 0.6% a femoral neck fracture. Some have had two of these fractures and some all three. By the age of 80, 15% have had a wrist fracture, 17.5% a vertebral compression and 6% a femoral neck fracture. After the age of 80, the femoral neck fracture incidence affects at least 1% of the surviving population per annum.

A fracture model

Our interpretation of these data is summarised in Fig 39.10. We suggest that the wrist fracture, which results from major trauma, occurs during the rapid phase of trabecular bone loss illustrated in Figure 39.2. The vertebral fracture, which involves minimal trauma, occurs when trabecular bone volume has reached its lowest level.

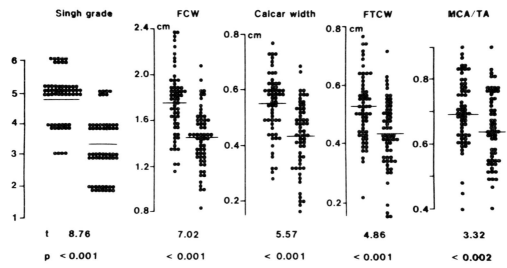

Fig. 39.7 Radiographic bone measurements at five different sites in 63 female femoral neck fracture cases and 63 age matched controls. Note that the 't' value is highest for the Singh grade and lowest for the metacarpal CA/TA ratio. (Horsman et al, 1982).

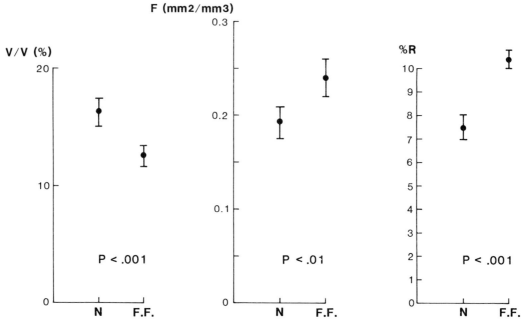

Fig. 39.8 Iliac crest tabecular bone volumes (left) forming surface (centre) and percentage surface resorptoin (right) in 36 normal women over the age of 60 and 133 female femoral neck fracture cases.

The femoral neck fracture on the other hand, results from a weakening of both cortical *and* trabecular bone, and its incidence therefore rises rapidly from the time when cortical bone has lost so much tissue that the combined loss of cortical and trabecular bone produces a critical weakening of the femoral neck. Bone mass and bone strength are of course continuous variables, and the data suggest that the fracture risk is directly related to the bone deficit.

PATHOGENESIS

Osteoporosis is no more attributable to a single cause than is anaemia, but many contributory causes or risk factors can be identified. In the first instance however, it is necessary to consider – as one would with anaemia – whether bone loss in individual cases or groups of cases is due to decreased bone formation, increased bone resorption or a combination of the two.

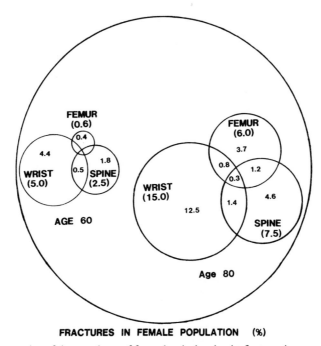

FRACTURES IN FEMALE POPULATION (%)

Fig. 39.9 Diagrammatic representation of the prevalence of femoral, spinal and wrist fractures in women by age 60 and age 80. The outer circle represents the population at risk and the inner circles are drawn to scale. (Supplied by D H Marshall).

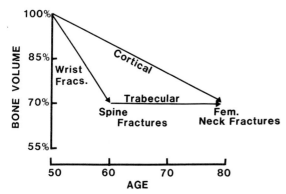

Fig. 39.10 Diagrammatic representation of suggested fracture model.

Examination of iliac crest post-mortem material and biopsies indicates the osteoporosis of aging results from different mechanisms in the two sexes. In women, aging is associated with an increase in fractional surface resorption with no change in the extent of the forming surface (or in the appositional rate (Nordin et al, 1983)), whereas in men a comparable loss of trabecular bone is associated with a decline in the forming surface, but no change in the fractional surface resorption (see Figs. 39.4–6).

There are also differences between the two sexes in respect of accelerated osteoporosis. In females with crush fractures, there is a further increase in surface resorption, but this is associated with some decline in forming surface

(See Figs. 39.5 & 39.6) and a significant reduction in mean seam width, which probably reflects a reduced appositional rate (Nordin et al, 1983). In male crush fracture cases on the other hand, the surface resorption is significantly higher than in age-matched controls, but the forming surface is unchanged — though of course lower than in young normal men (see Figs. 39.5 & 39.6).

Moving one step back in the causal chain, it should be possible to explain these histological changes in hormonal, nutritional and metabolic terms. No definitive explanations can be given but there is a strong presumption that the rise in bone resorption with age in normal women reflects the decline in oestrogen levels at the menopause and it is tempting to speculate that the decline in bone formation with age in normal men reflects declining androgen levels. In this connection it should be remembered that plasma oestrogen levels in the male are higher than in the pre-menopausal female because of the conversion of testosterone to oestradiol (Crilly et al, 1981a). The reduced appositional rate in women with accelerated osteoporosis may be connected with the reduced androgen levels in these cases (Nordin et al, 1981) which is however more significant in patients below the age of 60 than in older osteoporotic cases because of the decline in adrenal androgen levels in the normal population at about the age of 60 (Crilly et al, 1981a). In fact, it might be suggested that this aspect of 'post-menopausal osteoporosis' is not in fact related to the menopause but reflects an early 'adrenopause'. (This would also be compatible with the fact that osteoporotic women below the age of 60 have significantly thinner skin than age-mateched controls whereas this is not true of osteoporotic women over 60.)

The increased bone resorption found in accelerated osteoporosis in both sexes in easier to explain and almost certainly due to malabsorption of calcium (Nordin et al, 1981).

Pursuing the causal chain further back, the next question is the cause of the calcium malabsorption in osteoporosis. Low plasma 1,25 (OH)$_2$D levels have been reported in female osteoporotics by some workers (Gallagher et al, 1979) but not by others (Crilly et al, 1981b). There is no reason to assume however, that this malabsorption of calcium has a single cause. In some cases it may represent a receptor failure in the gastro-intestinal tract, in others a 1,25 (OH)$_2$D deficiency and perhaps in others a 25 OHD deficiency insufficient to cause osteomalacia. In some male cases, there is suggestive evidence that the malabsorption of calcium is in fact due to low plasma 1,25 (OH)$_2$D levels (Francis et al, 1982).

This does not exhaust the risk factors for osteoporosis. Increasing the protein intake raises urinary calcium and causes a negative calcium balance (Hegsted & Linkswiler, 1981); a high sodium intake can do the same (Goulding, 1980); a high alcohol intake can certainly cause osteoporosis (Dalen & Feldreich, 1974) and more recently both tobacco and caffeine consumption have been implicated as risk factors (Daniell, 1976; Heaney & Recker,

1981). Casting the net more widely, there are many other important risk factors such as cortico-steroid therapy, hyperthyroidism and heparin administration. Figure 39.11 represents an attempt to summarise the present state of knowledge.

In femoral neck fractures, vitamin D deficiency may be important. It has already been noted that the bone histology in these cases is suggestive of secondary hyperparathyroidism. This in turn suggests the presence of vitamin D deficiency – either a 25 OHD deficiency from inadequate exposure to sunlight, or a 1,25 (OH)$_2$D deficiency from renal impairment. This sets the scene for the development of osteomalacia.

There are conflicting data on the incidence of osteomalacia in femoral neck fracture cases. Some authors have found an incidence of 20–30% (Jenkins et al, 1973; Aaron et al, 1974; Faccini et al, 1976) but others have not (Hodkinson, 1971; Wicks et al, 1982). However, measurement of plasma 25 OHD in femoral neck fracture cases and controls in Leeds has shown an unequivocal reduction in the fracture cases (Baker et al, 1979) attributable to the fact that many of these cases are housebound before their fracture. Conflicting reports have come from other centresabut a recently completed study in Adelaide has again shown significantly lower plasma 25 OHD levels in fracture cases than controls – again because of the high proportion of housebound cases among the former. It is not yet possible to report the 1,25 (OH)$_2$D

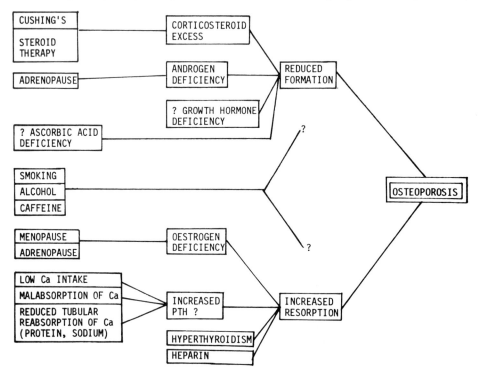

Fig. 39.11 Suggested causal chain in the pathogenesis of osteoporosis. The factors at the top tend to reduce bone formation and those at the bottom tend to increase bone resorption. The way in which smoking, alcohol and caffeine act is quite uncertain.

levels in femoral neck fracture cases, but some degree of renal impairment is common in the elderly, and low values would be expected in at least a proportion of these patients. The seasonal variation in the incidence of osteomalacia among femoral neck fracture cases strengthens the concept that the problem is one of 'nutritional' vitamin D deficiency, but it should be noted that the seasonal incidence of osteomalacia does not coincide with the seasonal incidence of the fractures and the contribution of vitamin D deficiency to the fracture is not necessarily mediated through its bone effect – it might be due to the effect of vitamin D deficiency on muscle function (Baker, 1980).

PREVENTION AND TREATMENT

That postmenopausal loss of bone can be prevented by oestrogen therapy is well documented (Lindsay et al, 1980; Christiansen et al, 1980) and the fact that this tends to reduce fracture rates has also been established by case control studies (Paganini-Hill et al, 1981). However the oestrogen response is dose-related (Genant et al, 1982), and with the increasing use of very low dose oestrogen (because of the risk of side effects) it is likely that oestrogen alone will not provide optimum protection against fractures. It is also apparent, though less well documented, that calcium supplementation can delay post-menopausal bone loss (Recker et al, 1977; Horsman et al, 1977) reflecting the fact that oestrogen deficiency effectively produces an increase in calcium requirement (Heaney et al, 1977). It is possible, though not yet proven, that the combination of low dose oestrogen with a calcium supplement will prove the most satisfactory regime in the future.

However, it would be irresponsible to recommend that all women should take oestrogens, or even supplemental calcium to avoid the fractures which affect 25% of them, and there is therefore a need to identify the subjects most at risk so that preventive measures can be used to the greatest effect. It is likely that it is the faster bone losers who end up with the fractures, and there is a strong presumption that the fast bone losers will prove to be the patients with the lowest oestrogen levels, the highest plasma alkaline phosphatase and the highest urinary hydroxyproline (Horsman et al, 1980). However although calcium and oestrogen clearly have a role to play in the prevention of post-menopausal bone loss, these agents are unlikely to be equally effective in the later years when plasma 25 OHD levels fall and malabsorption of calcium affects an increasing proportion of the population. A strong case can be made therefore for prophylactic use of vitamin D in people over 65, particularly in those who are housebound, and there is a strong presumption in unpublished data from Leeds that this measure would prevent or delay bone loss in this age group.

The treatment of established osteoporosis, generally in women over the age of 60, remains controversial. We will describe our own policy and then review briefly the therapeutic regimens being practised by other workers.

On the clinical scene, the diagnosis 'osteoporosis' generally signifies the crush fracture syndrome. In our opinion, the most important single investigation in these patients is the measurement of calcium absorption, which can be performed very simply with an oral dose of radio-calcium, followed by a single blood sample one hour later (Marshall & Nordin, 1981). If calcium absorption is low, it is our current practice to treat the patient with 0.25 μg daily of 1,25 $(OH)_2D$ (Rocaltrol) combined with a calcium supplement of 0.5–1 g daily. The importance of the calcium supplement lies in the fact that the object of treatment is to reduce bone resorption by suppressing parathyroid activity. We have in the past used vitamin D and its metabolites without calcium in the treatment of osteoporosis with disappointing results (Nordin et al, 1980) and we now believe that this can be explained by the bone-resorbing action of these compounds which we can nullify by the simultaneous administration of calcium. It must be emphasised that the dose of 0.25 μg of 1,25 $(OH)_2D$ cannot safely be exceeed without incurring the risk of hypercalcaemia, but that this dose is safe, even when combined with calcium, if renal function is normal. If calcium absorption is normal, we administer the calcium supplement without the vitamin D metabolite.

The best measure of the success of treatment is a slow fall in the plasma alkaline phosphatase (albeit within the normal range) and a rapid fall in the urinary hydroxyproline. If these values remain high after three months of treatment, it may be necessary to introduce oestrogen therapy if this is not already being done for other reasons – such as dyspareunia. Where oestrogens are not contra-indicated, and the patient is below 65, the recommended dose is 10–15 μg of ethinyloestradiol given for 3 weeks out of 4 or its equivalent in other preparations. Where oestrogens are contra-indicated, or the patient is over 65, a comparable effect on bone resorption can be achieved by the use of norethisterone 5 g daily. If norethisterone is used, and particularly if the patient has had oestrogen in the past, the patient should be warned that she may get some bleeding due to endometrial shedding, in which case the norethisterone should be stopped and not resumed until the bleeding has ceased. If is unlikely to occur again.

Experience to date of this particular policy is very encouraging. Previous data suggested that bone loss and crush fractures could be reduced or prevented by giving a vitamin D metabolite with oestrogen to patients with malabsorption of calcium, or by giving a calcium supplement or oestrogen to patients with normal calcium absorption (Nordin et al, 1980). These treatments also had the most favourable effects on calcium balance (Table 39.1). Reduced fracture rates on calcium and/or oestrogen have also been reported by Riggs et al (1982) who found that the most effective therapy was a combination of these two agents with sodium flouride.

There is a certain logic behind most of the treatments curently in use, and it is possible that all of them have merit; in fact Aloia et al (1982) have recently reported not only a reduced rate of bone loss in osteoporotic patients on calcium supplements but a significant gain of bone in a group of 87 patients given a variety of treatments including calcitonin, fluoride, oestrogens and anabolic steroids. Significant inhibition of bone loss (and a possible gain of bone) has also been reported by Chesnut et al (1979) with calcitonin and with an anabolic agent. However, most current treatments only inhibit bone resorption.

CONCLUSIONS

There are probably as many causes of osteoporosis as there are causes of anaemia. The relatively slow turnover in bone, however, makes it very much harder to assess the response to treatment in osteoporosis than in anaemia. This, and the inaccessibility of bone compared with blood, are the principal reasons why osteology lags so far behind haematology. Nonetheless the causes of osteoporosis are becoming increasingly clear and a defeatist approach to therapy is no longer justified. However, crushed vertebrae do not re-expand and lost bone is only slowly replaced, so the emphasis must clearly be on preventive measures. Enough is now known about bone to make the prevention of osteoporosis possible.

Table 39.1 The effects of various therapies on calcium balance, metacarpal cortical bone loss and vertebral fracture rate in post-menopausal osteoporosis (Nordin et al, 1980).

Therapy	n	Mean Ca Balance (mmol/day ± SE)	n	Mean Loss or cortical area	n	Mean fracture rate (episodes/yr. ± SE)
Hormones + 1-αD	11	0.15 ± 0.40	19	+0.15 ± 0.10	17	0.21 ±0.14
Hormones	13	−0.80 ± 0.52	16	+0.14 ± 0.11	15	0.37 ± 025
Calcium	12	−0.60 ± 0.75	20	−0.06 ± 0.06	17	0
Ca + vitamin D	8	−2.10 ± 1.02	23	−0.22 ± 0.08	20	0.05 ± 0.18
Nil	52	−2.30 ± 0.28	41	+0.26 ± 0.09	32	0.37 ± 0.28
1-αD	15	−2.20 ± 0.49	21	−0.28 ± 0.11	19	0.59 ± 0.31
Vitamin D	21	−2.00 ± 0.40	25	−0.48 ± 0.10	17	0.95 ± 0.30

REFERENCES

Aaron J E, Gallagher J C, Anderson J, Stasiak L Longton E B, Nordin B E C 1974 Frequency of osteomalacia and osteoporosis in fractures of the proximal femur. Lance i: 229–233

Aloia J F, Ross P, Vaswani A, Zanzi I, Cohn S 1982 Rate of bone loss in postmenopausal osteoporotic women. American Journal of Physiology 242: 82–86

Arnold J S 1973 Amount and quality of trabecular bone in osteoporotic vertebral fractures. Clinics and Endocrinology and Metabolism 2: 221–238

Baker M R 1980 The epidemiology and aetiology of femoral neck fracture. Thesis for membership of the Faculty of Community Medicine

Baker M R, McDonnell H, Peacock M, Nordin B E C 1979 Plasma 25 hydroxy vitamin D concentrations in patients with fractures of the femoral neck. British Medical Journal i: 589

Chesnut C H, Ivey J L, Nelp W B, Baylink D J 1979 Assessment of anabolic steroids and calcitonin in the treatment of osteoporosis. In: Barzel U (ed) Osteoporosis II. Grune and Stratton, New York, p 135–150

Christiansen C, Christensen M S, McNair P, Hagen C, Stocklund K E, Transbol I B 1980 Prevention of early postmenopausal bone loss: controlled 2-year study in 315 normal females. European Journal of Clinical Investigation 10: 273–279

Cook P J, Exton-Smith A N, Brocklehurst J C, Lempert-Barber S M 1982 Fractured femurs, falls and bone disorders. Journal of the Royal College of Physicians of London 16: 45–50

Crilly R G, Francis R M, Nordin B E C 1871a Steroid hormones, ageing and bone. Clinics in Endocrinology and Metabolism 10: 115–139

Crilly R G, Horsman A, Peacock M, Nordin B E C 1981b The vitamin D metabolites in the pathogenesis and management of osteoporosis. Current Medical Research and Opinion 7: 337–348

Dalen N, Feldreich A L 1974 Osteopenia in alcoholism. Clinical Orthopaedics and Related Research 99: 201–202

Daniell H W 1976 Osteoporosis of the slender smoker. Archives of Internal Medicine 136: 298–304

Elsasser U, Hesp R, Klenerman L, Wootton R 1980 Deficit of trabecular and cortical bone in elderly women with fracture of the femoral neck. Clincal Science 59: 393–395

Evans J G 1979 Fractured proximal femur in Newcastle Upon Tyne. Age and Ageing 8: 16–24

Faccini J M, Exton-Smith A N, Boyde A 1976 Disorders of bone and fracture of the femoral neck; evaluation of computer image anlaysis in diagnosis. Lancet i: 1089–1092

Francis R, Peacock M, Nordin B E C 1982 Plasma 1,25 (OH)$_2$D levels in male osteoporosis. Journal of Bone and Joint Surgery, In press

Gallagher J C, Riggs B L, Eisman J, Hamstra A, Arnaud S B, DeLuca H F 1979 Intestinal calcium absorption and serum vitamin D metabolites in normal subjects and osteoporotic patients. Journal of Clinical Investigation 64: 729–736

Genant H K, Cann C E, Ettinger R, Gordan G S 1982 Quantitative computed tomography of vertebral spongiosa: a sensitive method for detecting early bone loss after oophorectomy. Annals of Internal Medicine 97: 699–705

Goulding A 1980 Effects of dietary NaCl supplements on parathyroid function, bone turnover and bone composition in rats taking restricted amounts of calcium. Mineral and Electrolyte Metabolism 4: 203–208

Heaney R P Recker R R 1981 Effects of nitrogen, phosphorus and caffeine on calcium balance in women. Journal of Laboratory and Clinical Medicine 99: 46–55

Heaney R P, Recker, R R, Saville P D 1977 Calcium balance and calcium requirements in middle-aged women. American Journal of Clinical Nutrition 30: 1603–1611

Hegsted M, Linkswiler H M 1981 Long-term effects of level of protein intake on calcium metabolism in young adult women. Journal of Nutrition 111: 244–251

Horsman A 1976 Bone Mass. In: Nordin B E C (ed) Calcium Phosphate and Magnesium Metabolism. Clinical Physiology and Diagnostic Procedures: Churchill Livingstone, Edinburgh, p 357–404

Horsman A, Gallagher J C, Simpson M, Nordin B E C 1977 Prospective trial of oestrogen and calcium in postmenopausal women. British Medical Journal 2: 789–792

Horsman A, Marshall D H, Nordin B E C, Crilly R G, Simpson M 1980 The relation between bone loss and calcium balance in women. Clinical Science 59: 137–142

Horsman A, Nordin B E C, Aaron J, Marshall D H 1981 Cortical and trabecular osteoporosis and their relation to fractures in the elderly. In: DeLuca H F, Frost H M, Jee W S S, Johnston C C Jr, Parfitt A M (eds) Osteoporosis: Recent Advances in Pathogenesis and Treatment. University Park Press, Baltimore, p 175–184

Horsman A, Nordin B E C, Simpson M, Speed R 1982 Cortical and trabecular bone status in elderly women with femoral neck fracture. Clinical Orthopaedics 166: 143–151

Jenkins D H R, Roberts J G, Webster D, Williams E O 1973 Osteomalacia in elderly patients with fracture of the femoral neck: a clinico-pathological study. Journal of Bone and Joint Surgery 55-B: 575–580

Krolner B, Tondevold E, Toft B, Berthelson B, Nielsen S P 1982 Bone mass of the axial and appendicular skeleton in women with Colles' fracture: its relatoin to physical activity. Clinical Physiology 2: 147–157

Lindsay R, Hart D M, Forrest C Baird C 1980 Prevention of spinal osteoporosis in oophorectomised women. Lancet ii: 1151–1154

Marshall D H, Nordin B E C 1981 A comparison of radioactive calcium absorption tests with net calcium absorption. Clinical Science 61: 477–481

Nordin B E C, Horsman A, Crilly R G, Marshall D H, Simpson M 1980a Treatment of spinal osteoporosis in postmenopausal women. British Medical Journal 280: 541–454

Nordin B E C, Peacock M, Aaron J, Crilly G, Heyburn P J, Horsman A, Marshall D H 1980b Osteoporosis and osteomalacia. Clinics in Endocrinology and Metabolism 9: 177–205

Nordin B E C, Peacock M, Crilly R G, Francis R M, Speed R, Barkworth S 1981 Summation of risk factors in osteoporosis. In: DeLuca H F, Frost H M, Jee W S S, Johnston C C Jr, Parfitt A M (eds) Osteoporosis: Recent Advances in Pathogenesis and Treatment. University Park Press, Baltimore, p 359–367

Nordin B E C, Aaron J, Makins N, Francis R Sagreiya K 1983 Bone formation and resorption in postmenopausal osteoporosis. In: Dixon A St. J, Russell R G G, Stamp T C B (eds) Osteoporosis — a Multidisciplinary Problem. Royal Society of Medicine London, p 161–171

Paganini-Hill A, Ross R K, Gerkins V R, Henderson B E Arthur M, Mack R M 1981 Menopausal estrogen therapy and hip fractures. Annals of Internal Medicine 95: 28–31

Recker R R, Saville P D, Heaney R P 1977 Effect of estrogens and calcium carbonate on bone loss in post-menopausal women. Annals of Internal Medicine 87: 649–655

Riggs L, Seeman E, Hodgson S F, Taves D R, Fallon W M 1982 Effect of the fluoride/calcium regimen on vertebral fracture occurrence in post-menopausal osteoporosis. New England Journal of Medicine 306: 446–450

Singh M, Nagrath A R, Maini P S 1970 Changes in trabecular pattern of the upper end of the femur as an index of osteoporosis. Journal of Bone and Joint Surgery. 52-A: 457–467

Wicks M, Garrett R, Vernon-Roberts B, Fazzalari N 1982 Absence of metabolic bone disease in the proximal femur in patients with fracture of the femoral neck. The Journal of Bone and Joint Surgery 64-B: 319–322

Zetterberg C, Andersson G B J 1982 Fractures of the proximal end of the femur in Goteborg, Sweden, 1940–1979. Acta Orthopaedica Scandinavica 53: 419–426

40

Osteomalacia

A. N. Exton-Smith

Osteomalacia is a generalised disease of bone characterised by deficient calcification of a normal bone matrix. Histological exmination reveals an increase in the amount of osteoid, that is, non-calcified matrix around the bone trabeculae. It is a disease produced by the lack of vitamin D.

The importance of osteomalacia in old age lies in the fact that it is a very disabling condition which often passes unrecognised, because the skeletal rarefaction is interpreted as due to the much more common osteoporosis. Yet the response to treatment, unlike that of many other conditions in old age, is almost invariably good.

Diagnostic confusion with osteoporosis is understandable:

i) the two conditions can occur together by chance and the problem is to ascertain what proportion of the reduced radiographic density of bone is due to osteomalacia.

ii) there may be common aetiological factors, for example, long continued mild vitamin D deficiency may contribute to osteoporosis through impairment of calcium absorption (Nordin, 1976) and the secondary hyperparathyroidism occurring in osteomalacia may produce new bone remodelling units and thus produce a significant degree of osteoporosis which in older individuals might well be irreversible (Stanbury, 1981).

iii) there is no single non-invasive screening procedure which can be used in surveys of the elderly population to make a diagnosis of osteomalacia (Exton-Smith, 1968).

It is also noteworthy that osteomalacia, often without the usual clinical manifestations, may contribute to the pathogenesis of fractures in old age.

AETIOLOGY

Deficiency of vitamin D may arise from inadequate synthesis in the skin, dietary lack, malabsorption and impaired metabolism.

Sources of vitamin D
There are two forms of vitamin D: cholecalciferol (vitamin D$_3$) and the synthetic ergocalciferol. It reaches the body in two ways, by dietary ingestion and by synthesis in the skin. The main dietary sources are oily fish (sardines, herring, mackerel and tuna) and some dairy products such as eggs. Several foods are fortified with vitamin D, for example, margarine and some beverages taken with milk. Milk itself is a poor source of vitamin D, but in the United States and Canada it is fortified and one US quart contains 10 μg (400 IU) vitamin D. Deficiencies or excess of other substances in the diet may increase the requirements for vitamin D. Phytate (inositol hexaphosphate) which occurs in whole cereal grains interferes with the absorption of calcium by forming insoluble calcium phytate in the intestine. A diet high in phytate and low in calcium and vitamin D is more rachitogenic than one with the same amount of vitamin D but with more calcium and less phytate. A high fibre intake can reduce the availability of calcium (James et al, 1978).

Skin synthesis occurs through the action of ultraviolet radiation (UVR) on 7-dehydrocholesterol which is formed in the liver and stored in the deeper layers of the epidermis. Only solar radiation of a wavelength less than 313 nm is effective in vitamin D skin synthesis. The shortest wavelength of UVR to reach the earth through the atmosphere is about 290 nm so the effective 'window' for vitamin D synthesis is very narrow. The average intensity of UVR declines with distance from the equator and no radiation of less than 313 nm reaches Britain from the end of October to early March; consequently no vitamin D can be formed during this period. Moreover, the intensity of UVR at the earth's surface varies with the time of day. Of the total available radiation in summer the proportion reaching the surface of the earth between 9.30 a.m. and 3.30 p.m. is 68% in Dundee (latitude 56°) and 77% in North Dakota (latitude 47°) (Scotto & Fears, 1977; Frain-Bell, 1979). Cloud cover also reduces the intensity of solar UVR substantially.

In spite of the limited amounts of UVR of wavelengths between 290 and 313 nm reaching the earth's surface in temperate zones and the restricted sunlight exposure of certain sections of the population including the elderly, the main determinant of vitamin D is skin synthesis rather than dietary intake. This has been demonstrated by the experimental work of Haddad & Hahn (1973) who found that over 80% of the circulating 25 hydroxyvitamin D (25 OHD) in six American subjects was present as 25 OHD_3 rather than in the D_2 form in spite of the fortification of milk with vitamin D_2 and consumption of vitamin D_2 supplements in the US.

Variations in vitamin D status

One of the first demonstrations of seasonal variations in vitamin D status in the elderly was that reported by Smith et al (1964) in the United States. They compared a group of elderly women (average age 60.6 years) living in Michigan with a group of similar age living in Puerto Rico. In the Michigan group the level of vitamin D in the blood (as determined by a bio-assay technique measuring antirachitic activity) was significantly lower in those subjects with lower bone density compared with those having normal bones; the level showed marked seasonal variation, being considerably lower in the winter than in the summer months, and it was related to the plasma levels of calcium, phosphate and alkaline phosphatase. By contrast in Puerto Rico, where there is much greater exposure to sunlight, the prevalence of skeletal rarefaction was found to be much lower, the blood levels of vitamin D were much higher and there was no seasonal variation.

Recently, with the development of radio-stereo assay techniques it has been shown that people living in temperate zones have marked seasonal variations in the plasma concentrations of 25 OHD (Stamp & Round, 1974). The mean levels in young healthy white subjects in Britain were 32 nmol/l in early spring and rose to 55 nmol/l in late summer and early autumn; much lower levels with similar seasonal variation were found in the elderly population. Lawson et al (1979) in their studies of elderly people living at home have shown that the summer circulating levels of 25 OHD correlate with the amount of sunlight exposure and are independent of the vitamin D content of the diet, whereas in winter the levels correlate with dietary intake and the degree of sunlight exposure the previous summer. Dattani et al (1984) have examined the effects of increasing age on plasma 25 OHD concentrations. In old people there was a linear decline in the concentration from the age of 65 to 90 years in both sexes; the winter levels were lower than the summer levels and they were lower in women than in men. The summer levels declined faster than the winter levels and by the age of 90 the summer and winter levels were equal. This study clearly shows the effects of limitation of sunlight exposure due to reduction in out-of-doors activity in very old people.

Housebound individuals form the largest group at risk of developing vitamin D deficiency. Not only do they lack sunlight exposure but their dietary intakes are substantially reduced; 48% of housebound women aged 70–79 years had very low dietary intakes of less than 30 IU per day compared with 13% of active women of similar age (Exton-Smith et al, 1972).

Metabolism

Vitamin D itself has no direct action on its target organs, but it is converted in the body to an active hormone in two stages (De Luca, 1974 & 1976; Kodicek, 1974). In the first stage hydroxylation takes place in the liver in the C 25 position of the sterol molecule to form 25 hydroxyvitamin D (25 OHD). This is the main circulating form of the vitamin. In the second stage 25 OHD undergoes further hydroxylation in the renal tubule to form either 1,25 dihydroxycholecalciferol [1,25 $(OH)_2D$] or 24,25 dihydroxycholecalciferol [24, 25 $(OH)_2D$]. The most active of these two metabolities is 1,25 $(OH)_2D$ which is present in minute amounts in the plasma. 24,25 $(OH)_2D$ is synthesised in inverse proportion to the more active form and is usually present in much higher concentrations. It is probable that the production of 1,25 $(OH)_2D$ is regulated by intracellular calcium and/or phosphate levels and is stimulated by low calcium diets, by parathyroid hormone and by low inorganic phosphate levels within the renal cortex.

Actions of vitamin D

The main action of 1,25 $(OH)_2D$ is to promote calcium transport in its target organs. Thus it promotes calcium absorption from the small intestine. When calcium intake is low an adaptation occurs with increased calcium absorption due to enhanced synthesis of 1,25 $(OH)_2D$. In the presence of adequate concentrations of calcium and inorganic phosphate ions in the extracellular fluids surrounding bone and normal concentrations of 1,25 $(OH)_2D$, new bone formation occurs. Similarly the maintenance of skeletal muscle contractility is dependent upon adequate calcium transport. Inadequate concentrations of 1,25 $(OH)_2D$ lead to abnormal bone formation (osteoid) and to muscle weakness (proximal myopathy), features which are characteristic of osteomalacia. Excessive concentrations of 1,25 $(OH)_2D$ promote bone resorption.

Vitamin D deficiency and clinical disorders

The main factors leading to the development of vitamin D deficiency are reduced intake, formation and absorption of vitamin D as well as impaired synthesis of its metabolites in the liver and kidney. In the elderly, several of these factors often operate together to cause osteomalacia, and for example, it should not be assumed that the cause is a dietary deficiency alone.

Simple vitamin D lack

According to Gough and his colleagues (1964) only 3 cases of osteomalacia due to lack of vitamin D had been reported in Britain up to 1962 and consequently it was thought that this was a rare cause. Equally in the United States reported cases of purely dietary origin were extremely rare and indeed Albright & Reifenstein (1948) stated that they 'are cognizant of no single case of osteomalacia in the United States due to a simple vitamin D lack'. Gough et al (1964) described three cases of osteomalacia in old people proved histologically after bone biopsy. One of their cases, a spinster aged 84 years with marked radiological changes of osteomalacia, had an average daily intake of vitamin D of 24 IU. Her diet had been extremely poor for many years and consisted of tea, bread and butter occasionally supplemented by egg and milk puddings. The 'rheumatic' pains associated with osteomalacia were so crippling that she had been unable to leave her room for ten years and no doubt her housebound state contributed to vitamin D deficiency through lack of exposure to sunlight. One of the reasons for the rarity of osteomalacia of dietary origin is that the mature skeleton with its relatively slow turnover rate can withstand short periods of vitamin D deficiency without deleterious effects and vitamin D stores are often more than sufficient to maintain normal mineral homeostasis. Nevertheless, osteomalacia has been reported when the diet contains less than 70 IU of vitamin D per day. The usual dietary history obtained is of avoidance of fatty foods or of being a strict vegetarian. Patients with this form of osteomalacia characteristically respond to small doses of vitamin D.

Sunlight exposure

The importance of sunlight exposure as the main determinant of vitamin D status has already been mentioned. Approximately 8% of the population over the age of 65 years are housebound and the proportion rises steeply in those over the age of 80. Moreover, a high proportion of the very old have disabilities which lead to only limited out-of-doors activity. In the nutritional surveys of the elderly population conducted by the Department of Health and Social Security (DHSS, 1979) the mean plasma alkaline phosphatase activity was significantly higher in the housebound compared with that of subjects who were not housebound. Since there is no skin synthesis of vitamin D in the winter months, even in those who are capable of outside activity, the stores of vitamin D become depleted at this time and the clinical manifestations of osteomalacia often become apparent in the spring.

Malabsorption

Minor and even more severe degrees of malabsorption are not uncommon in old age. Enteropathy resulting from wheat and rye gluten sensitivity and similar to that causing childhood coeliac disease still occurs in patients over the age of 70. In some cases the steatorrhoea is minimal and the bone manifestations can dominate the clinical picture (Moss et al, 1965). The stagnant loop syndrome due to jejunal diverticulosis is a well recognised cause of osteomalacia. Duodenal diverticula are often regarded as innocuous but Clark (1972) discovered two cases of osteomalacia in 15 elderly patients with large primary duodenal diverticula.

Gastrectomy

Osteomalacia (and osteoporosis) can follow gastrectomy and the estimates of its incidence vary from 3–25% according to the diagnostic criteria used. The pathogenesis of the bone disease is virtually unknown but it is usually attributed to defective intake or malabsorption of vitamin D. The development of osteomalacia, however, is not related to the severity of steatorrhoea which in many cases is minimal or absent.

Hepatobiliary disorders

Liver and biliary tract disease can lead to osteomalacia due to impaired absorption of vitamin D and its reduced conversion to 25 OHD. Osteomalacia has often been reported in patients with primary biliary cirrhosis, although osteoporosis is probably the more common form of metabolic bone disease in these individuals. Biliary obstruction, including intrahepatic cholestasis, if unrelieved and sufficiently prolonged, can produce osteomalacia.

Drugs

Dent et al (1970) have drawn attention to the occurrence of osteomalacia in patients receiving anticonvulsant drugs which lead to hepatic microsomal enzyme induction. This form of therapy increases the catabolism of both dietary and endogenously produced vitamin D and directs it towards biologically inactive metabolites. In consequence, body stores of vitamin D and plasma concentrations of 25 OHD are diminished (Hahn et al, 1975). Other drugs commonly used in the elderly and having the potential to stimulate microsomal P 450 enzymatic activity include antidiabetic agents, muscle relaxants, tranquillisers and sedatives.

Renal Impairment

Chronic renal insufficiency produces a characteristic derangement of skeletal metabolism with impaired calcium absorption, secondary hyperparathyroidism and an acquired resistance to the action of vitamin D. The bone disease presents both radiographically and histologically is a mixture of osteomalacia, osteosclerosis, osteoporosis and osteitis fibrosa cystica (Lumb et al, 1971). According to Avioli et al (1968) the reduced ability to synthesise active metabolites becomes apparent when the functional renal mass declines to the extent that the glomerular filtration rate is reduced to 15–25 ml/min. Osteomalacia can occur in renal failure due to both glomerular and tubular disorders and following ureterosigmoidostomy. At present it is uncertain whether impaired metabolism of vitamin D can be attributed to an age-related physiological decline in renal function which is believed to affect all individuals.

PREVALENCE

In the absence of a simple screening test which can be applied to the general elderly population, there are no accurate estimates of the prevalence of osteomalacia in old age. Anderson et al (1966) have drawn attention to osteomalacia occurring in old people in Glasgow. They investigated a group of 100 women aged 68–93 years who had been newly admitted to a geriatric department and who had a possible clinical indication of osteomalacia (Table 40.1).

Table 40.1   Possible indications for the diagnosis of osteomalacia (Anderson et al, 1966).

Vague and generalised pain
Low backache
Muscle weakness and stiffness
Waddling gait
Skeletal deformity
Bone tenderness
Malabsorption states
Long confinement indoors
Malnutrition

In this group 16 cases of osteomalacia were discovered. Subsequently 100 consecutive patients admitted to the female wards were investigated and the incidence of osteomalacia was shown to be 4% of elderly women admitted to this geriatric department. Chalmers (1967), an orthopaedic surgeon in Edinburgh, and his colleagues have described the clinical features of 37 recently recognised cases of osteomalacia. Thirty-four of the patients were women; their ages ranged from 39 to 89 years and the majority were over the age of 70. These investigators consider that osteomalacia is not uncommon in elderly women among whom it is likely to be confused with senile osteoporosis and that there is a need for a thorough screening of all elderly patients presenting with weakness, skeletal pain, pathological fractures or with diminished radiographic density of bone.

CLINICAL FEATURES

In the early stages the disease is often missed altogether because the patient attributes her bodily pains to 'rheumatism'. Owing to the poor localisation of the pain attention may not be directly focused on the bones. At a later stage the pain is nagging, persistent and unremitting and it is the result of strain on tender soft bone rather than fracture of non-tender brittle bone as in osteoporosis. When the pain is very severe breathing becomes difficult and even the weight of the bedclothes pressing upon the ribs becomes unbearable.

Muscle weakness is often a striking feature. It is due to a proximal myopathy affecting chiefly the pelvic and shoulder girdle muscles. The patient may complain of difficulty in climbing stairs or getting up from a chair, difficulty in lifting the feet from the ground when walking and this leads to a typical 'waddling gait' as the patient tilts the pelvis from side to side when attempting to walk. If the shoulder girdle is involved the patient may be unable to brush her hair or lift her arms above her head.

The softening of the bones leads to angulation of the sternum, kyphosis, deformities of the pelvis and bending of the femoral necks. Finally, on account of painful movements and skeletal deformities the patient is forced to her bed.

Osteomalacia and femoral neck fractures

Osteomalacia, often in the absence of the typical clinical features described above, may contribute to the pathogenesis of femoral neck fractures. Aaron et al (1974a) in Leeds have shown that 20–30% of women and about 40% of men with fracture of the femoral neck have histological evidence of osteomalacia. Later they showed (Aaron et al, 1974b) that the proportion with osteomalacia varied with the season of the year. The proportion of cases with decreased calcification fronts or increased osteoid covered surfaces rose from about 15% of the biopsies in the late summer to 40% in the spring. They conclude that the variation in hours of sunshine is responsible for the seasonal change in the incidence of femoral neck fractures.

The significance of vitamin D deficiency as an important factor in fractures of the proximal femur has been confirmed in our studies conducted in London and Manchester (Faccini et al, 1976; Cook et al, 1982). The mean value of trabecular osteoid area in the fracture group was 4% compared with 1% in a control group without fractures, matched for age and sex. Of the fracture patients, 38% had histological evidence of osteomalacia based on the trabecular osteoid area of greater than 2.0% and this proportion was significantly higher than in the control group ($p < 0.01$).

RADIOGRAPHY

The typical findings are of diminished radiographic density of bone, deformities in the softened bone and biconcavity of the vertebral bodies ('codfish vertebrae'). Another characteristic finding is the appearance of Looser's zones or pseudo-fractures. These are bands of decalcification perpendicular or oblique to the surface of bone and on either side of the translucency there may be a denser band of callus which makes the Looser's zone appear more obvious. The common sites are the axillary border of the scapula, the pubic rami, the ribs, the neck of the humerus and the lesser trochanter of the femoral neck. Sometimes the bone changes of secondary hyperparathyroidism, are present, for example, sub-periosteal erosions in the metacarpals or phalanges.

BIOCHEMISTRY

The typical biochemical findings are a low or normal serum calcium, low serum inorganic phosphorus, raised alkaline phosphatase and a diminished urinary calcium excretion. The serum 25 OHD is low and usually less than 10 nmol/l; but there are documented instances of bone disease in association with concentrations of serum 25 OHD of 15–20 nmol/l and others in which concentrations of 5 nmol/l or less show neither clinical, biochemical nor histological evidence of osteomalacia. Patients in whom the serum calcium concentration is within the normal range probably have secondary hyperparathyroidism and this may be demonstrated by the raised levels of serum iPTH. Indeed, according to Stanbury (1981) one of the first consequences of an inadequacy of vitamin D is probably a state of 'normo-calcaemic secondary hyperparathyroidism'.

DIAGNOSIS

In typical cases of osteomalacia diagnosis rests on the history of bone pains and muscular weakness, the radiological findings of Looser's zones, the abnormal biochemical findings including low serum 25 OHD levels and a history of one of the disorders producing osteomalacia. In many cases, however, when osteomalacia is suspected and especially when the presentation is fracture of the femoral neck the diagnosis can only be confirmed by histological examination of an iliac crest bone biopsy specimen.

TREATMENT

Hypocalcaemic nutritional osteomalacia should be treated with small doses of vitamin D, 5–10 μg/day (200–400 IU). A single oral dose of vitamin D may restore the serum 1,25 $(OH)_2D$ from almost undetectable levels to concentrations within the normal range in 24 hours. Continued treatment with the same dosage rapidly produces grossly supranormal concentrations of 1,25 $(OH)_2D$ that are maintained for weeks or months (Stanbury, 1981). Parallel with the increase in serum 1,25 $(OH)_2D$ the serum calcium concentration is restored to normal. This can occur within two weeks but the elevated serum alkaline phosphatase does not fall to normal for several months. There is usually a striking symptomatic improvement with the disappearance of muscle weakness and bone pains.

When malabsorption is an important contributory cause of osteomalacia and when it is due to gluten sensitivity a gluten-free diet should be instituted but the response may be slow over a period of months. If the cause of malabsorption cannot be corrected then the oral dose of vitamin D must be very much greater (0.025–0.125 mg/day). Only when osteomalacia results from a conditioned deficiency of vitamin D due to renal impairment is it necessary to give the 1,25 $(OH)_2D$ metabolite.

REFERENCES

Aaron J E, Gallagher J C, Anderson J, Stasiak L, Longton E B, Nordin B E C, Nicholson M 1974a Frequency of osteomalacia and osteoporosis in fractures of the proximal femur. Lancet i: 229–233

Aaron J E, Gallagher J C, Nordin B E C 1974b Seasonal variation of histological osteomalacia in femoral neck fractures. Lancet ii: 84–85

Albright F, Reifenstein E O 1948 Parathyroid Glands and Metabolic Bone Disease. Bailliére Tindall & Cox, London

Avioli L V, Birge S J, Lee S W, Slatopolsky E 1968 The metabolic fate of vitamin D_3–^3H in chronic renal failure. Journal of Clinical Investigation 47: 2239–2252

Clark A N G 1972 Deficiency states in duodenal diverticular disease. Age & Ageing 1: 14–23

Cook P J, Exton-Smith A N, Brocklehurst J B, Lempert-Barber S M 1982 Fractured femurs, falls and bone disorders. Journal of the Royal College of Physicians of London 16: 45–49

Dattani J, Exton-Smith A N, Stephen J M L 1984 Vitamin D status of the elderly in relation to age and exposure to sunlight. Human Nutrition: Clinical Nutrition 38C: 131–137

De Luca H F 1974 Vitamin D — 1973. American Journal of Medicine 57: 1–12

De Luca M F 1976 Recent advances in our understanding of the vitamin D endocrine system. Journal of Laboratory and Clinical Medicine 87: 7–26

Dent C E, Richens A, Roire D J F, Stamp T C B 1970 Osteomalacia with long-term anticonvulsant therapy in epilepsy. British Medical Journal iv: 69–72

DHSS 1979 Nutrition and Health in Old Age. Report on Health and Social Subjects No. 16. HMSO, London

Exton-Smith A N, 1968 The problem of subclinical malnutrition in the elderly. In: Exton-Smith A N, Scott D L (eds) Vitamins in the Elderly, Wright, Bristol p 12–18

Exton-Smith A N, Stanton B R, Windsor A C M 1972 Nutrition of Housebound Old People. King Edward's Hospital Fund, London

Faccini J M, Exton-Smith A N, Boyde A 1976 Disorders of bone and fracture of the femoral neck. Lancet i: 1089–1092

Frain-Bell W 1979 What is that thing called light? Clinical and Experimental Dermatology 4: 1–33

Gough K R, Lloyd O C, Wills M R 1964 Nutritional osteomalacia. Lancet ii: 1261–1264

Haddad J G, Hahn T J 1973 Natural and synthetic sources of circulatory 25-hydroxyvitamin D in man. Nature 244: 515–517

Hahn T J, Heudin B A, Scharp C R, Boisseau V C, Haddad J G 1975 Serum 25-hydroxycholecalciferol levels and bone mass in children on chronic anticonvulsant therapy. New England Journal of Medicine 292: 550–552

James W P T, Branch W J, Southgate D A T 1978 Calcium binding by dietary fibre. Lancet i: 638–639

Kodicek E 1974 The story of vitamin D: From vitamin to hormone. Lancet i: 325–329

Lawson D E M, Paul A A, Black A E, Cole T J, Mandal A R, Davie M 1979 Relative contributions of diet and sunlight to vitamin D state in the elderly. British Medical Journal ii: 303–305

Lumb G A, Mower E B, Stanbury S W 1971 The apparent vitamin D resistance of chronic renal failure. American Journal of Medicine 50: 421–441

Moss A J, Waterhouse C, Terry R 1965 Glutensensitive enteropathy with osteomalacia but without steatorrhoea. New England Journal of Medicine 272: 825–830

Nordin B E C 1976 Nutritional considerations. In: Nordin B E C (ed) Calcium, Phosphate and Magnesium Metabolism, Churchill Livingstone, Edinburgh

Scotto J, Fears T R 1977 Intensity patterns of solar ultraviolet radition. Environmental Reserach 14: 113–127

Smith R W, Rizek J, Frame B, Mansour J 1964 Determinants of serum antirachitic activity. Special references to involutional osteoporaosis. American Journal of Clinical Nutrition 14: 98–108

Stamp T C B, Round J M 1974 Seasonal changes in human plasma 25-hydroxyvitamin D. Nature 274: 563–565

Stanbury S W 1981 Vitamin D and hyperparathyroidism. Journal of the Royal College of Physicians London 15: 205–217

41

Paget's disease of the bone

R. C. Hamdy

Paget's disease of bone tends to be commoner in old age. It affects about 10% of the population over the age of 85 and only about 0.5% of those aged between 35 and 44 years (Collins, 1956). Both sexes are almost equally affected. Paget's disease of bone has a peculiar geographical distribution. It affects about 4% of the population in the United Kingdom, US, Germany and France, is less common in the rest of Europe, Australia and New Zealand and is rare in Scandinavian countries, Switzerland, Japan, China, the Middle East and Africa. Within the same country variations in the incidence have also been reported. In the UK for instance, in some areas of Lancashire it is as high as 8.3%, whereas in Aberdeen it is as low as 2.3% (Detheridge et al, 1982). The disease also tends to run in families. Several environmental and genetic factors have been thought to play a role in the pathogenesis of the condition, their importance, however, remains controversial.

Virtually any bone can be affected by Paget's disease, the skull and weight bearing bones are, however, more likely to be affected than the rest of the skeleton. The pelvis and sacro-lumbar vertebrae in particular are very frequently affected and whereas the tibia is often affected, the fibula is usually spared. The bones of the upper limbs are much less frequently involved than those of the lower limbs. This distribution, together with several instances where trauma seemed to precede the development of Paget's disease, has led to the assumption that it may have a traumatic aetiology; repeated minimal physical trauma may precipitate a breakdown of the normal mechanism of gradual continuous bone remodelling and lead to the appearance of hyperactive osteoclasts and Paget's disease. The relatively high frequency of skull involvement can be explained by the mechanical stress resulting from mastication, the pull of the muscles of the neck and the continual pulsations of the brain. If however, trauma were responsible for the development of Paget's disease, one would have expected the bones of the hands and feet, as well as the mandible and maxilla to be frequently affected, yet these bones are usually spared. Many other hypotheses regarding the aetiology of Paget's disease have been put forward and rejected. They include neoplastic, vascular, endocrinological and immunological disorders.

Several histological observations suggest that Paget's disease of bone may result from a slow viral infection of the skeleton with a very long latent period. This may explain the relatively low incidence of Paget's disease in those under the age of 40 years and the increasing incidence as age advances. It may also explain the geographical distribution of the condition and its tendency to occur in families. To date however, no virus has been isolated. Final proof of the aetiology of Paget's disease is not an easy task as it is not seen in experimental animals. At present, it seems reasonable to assume a multifactorial aetiology: probably a slow viral infection with trauma acting as a localising factor and heredity a predisposing one.

PATHOLOGY

The basic underlying pathology of Paget's disease is a focal, excessive bone resorption followed by excessive and disorganised new bone formation. The activity of the osteoclasts is usually paralleled by that of the osteoblasts. Waves of bone destruction and new bone formation succeed each other and the bone turnover is greatly increased. The newly formed bone is architecturally abnormal and is in turn rapidly resorbed by the over-active osteoclasts. Paget's disease goes through various phases of activity and may become quiescent. Sometimes, as in the case of osteoporosis circumscripta, the osteoclastic hyperactivity is not paralleled by an excessive osteoblastic activity. This is particularly seen in the skull vault.

Bones affected by Paget's disease are larger than normal. During the active phase the vascularity of the bone and bone marrow is increased. Histologically the cement lines are irregularly deposited and the bone tissue appears primitive, coarse-fibred and disorganised. During the active phase the bone is quite cellular and several osteoblasts and large multinucleated osteoclasts can be seen in close proximity to the bone surface. The osteoclasts exhibit a wide diversity of shape, size, number of nuclei and staining properties, and when examined by electron microscopy, intranuclear inclusion bodies can be seen (Rebel et al, 1976). These are the hallmark of slow viral infections.

Furthermore the presence of deformed, crumbled, convoluted and degenerating nuclei and the release of microfilaments into the cell cytoplasm lend further support to the hypothesis that Paget's disease is due to a slow viral infection. Although the osteoblasts are present in large numbers they appear essentially normal and it is possible that the increased rate of new bone formation is a compensatory homeostatic response to protect the individual from increased concentrations of calcium ions that may result from the excessive bone resorption.

CLINICAL MANIFESTATIONS AND COMPLICATIONS

The clinical presentation of Paget's disease of bone is varied and depends on the affected bone, the state of activity of the lesion and any complications that may have developed. The majority of patients are however, asymptomatic and only about 5% present with signs and symptoms relevant to the disease (Collins, 1956). In most instances more than one bone is affected by the disease.

During the active phase the affected parts feel much warmer than normal and in the legs differences as high as 4°C between normal and affected sides have been reported (Ring et al, 1976). Furthermore, in a few cases if the bone is auscultated a bruit may be heard during the active phase.

Pain

Pain is by far the commonest clinical presentation of Paget's disease of bone. It tends to be worse at night when the limb is warm, is usually not related to exercise and often there is no correlation between the severity of the pain and that of the disease. Several factors may be responsible for pain including increased bone vascularity, stretching of the periosteum by the enlarging bone and microfractures. It is also possible that the hyperaemic bone marrow stimulates the adjacent somatic nerve endings. Pain may also result from direct pressure on sensory nerves by the expanding pagetic bone.

Not infrequently the pain experienced by patients with Paget's disease is due to an associated or complicating arthropathy. By virtue of their age, patients with Paget's

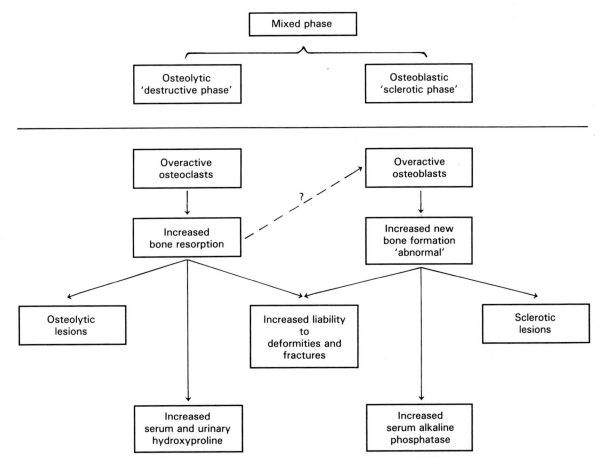

Fig. 41.1 Diagrammatic representation of the pathophysiology of Paget's disease in the mixed phase. (Hamdy, 1981: With the permission of Praeger Publishers)

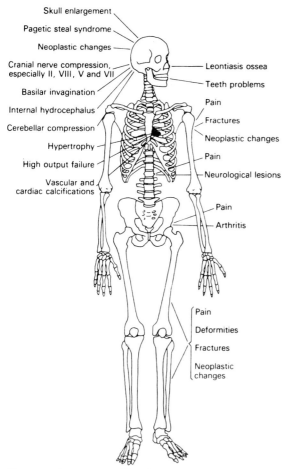

Fig. 41.2 Presentation of Paget's disease at the most frequently affected sites of the skeleton. (Hamdy, 1981: With the permission of Praeger Publishers)

disease of bone are more likely to have osteoarthritic changes than the rest of the population and both pathologies often co-exist. Osteoarthropathies may also complicate Paget's disease of bone because — as a result of the various deformities — non-articular surfaces of the cartilage are brought into contact and articulate with each other. The clinical differentiation of pain secondary to an osteoarthritic process from that secondary to Paget's disease is often difficult. In the former instance it usually tends to be relieved by rest and often responds to mild analgesia, while in the latter the pain is often worse when the patient rests, particularly at night, and does not always respond to mild analgesics. It is however, relieved after two to four weeks of appropriate specific anti-pagetic therapy. This therapy does not affect the course of pain secondary to osteoarthritis.

Deformities

The deformities associated with Paget's disease of bone are characteristic and are the result of bones becoming larger

and mechanically weaker than non-affected bones. When the skull is affected the head becomes larger and as the mandible is usually spared the head tends to become triangular in shape with the base of the triangle along the forehead. The cranium may also appear to have an irregular surface and in severe cases corrugations may be seen and felt.

When the skull base is affected it may become invaginated by the cervical vertebrae, a condition known as platybasia or basilar invagination. Clinically the neck appears disproportionately short and the chin often rests on the chest. When the maxillary bone is affected the face may become asymmetrical and the curvature of the hard palate tends to become shallow and irregular.

When long bones are affected by Paget's disease they also tend to become large and as they are mechanically weaker than normal bone they may become bowed. The direction of bowing is along the line of least resistance. The tibia for instance tends to bow anteriorly because in all other directions it is supported by strong muscle groups, whereas anteriorly it is only covered by skin and subcutaneous tissue. Similarly the femur tends to bow anterolaterally and the humerus laterally.

Fractures

Pathological fractures of long bones are common complications and are often the presenting manifestation of Paget's disease. The fractures are usually situated at right angles to the long axis of the bone and may occur spontaneously. Multiple fractures in the same bone are not uncommon. Fractures are often preceded by pain and the radiological appearance of fissure fractures.

The management of fractures complicating Paget's disease is difficult. If the lesion is active, the excessive vascularity may present serious problems to the operating surgeon. If on the other hand the lesion is quiescent, the bones may be so brittle that the insertion of a prosthesis or pin could be difficult. Furthermore as the bone itself is weak, it may not be able to retain in position any prosthesis which later may become displaced. Finally, although callus formation is good during the active phase, the newly formed bone is often abnormal and mechanically weak. Indeed refractures are not uncommon.

Neurological complications

As the cranial nerves pass through narrow foramina in the skull base they may become compressed by the expanding pagetic bone. The commonest ones to be involved are the second, eight, seventh and branches of the fifth cranial nerves. Patients may therefore present with visual or auditory impairment, facial palsy or atypical trigeminal neuralgia (usually only one or two branches of the trigeminal nerve are affected). Impaired hearing may also result from other complications such as involvement of the middle ear ossicles and infiltration of the inner ear.

Patients with plastybasia may develop signs of cerebellar insufficiency. Furthermore as the aqueduct of Sylvius may become distorted or the foramina of Lushka and Magendie obliterated, internal hydrocephalus may develop. The clinical features include psycho-motor retardation, a spastic gait, urinary incontinence and brain failure. Brain failure may also result from relative brain anoxia as a major part of the cardiac output is monopolised by the enlarged hypervascular skull. Furthermore anastomotic channels shunting blood from the internal to the external carotid circulation have been described (Blotman et al, 1974).

Although the lumbar vertebrae are often affected by Paget's disease, spinal cord lesions and nerve root compression are not frequent complications of the disease. This is probably the result of the gradual remodelling of the vertebrae possibly allowing time for the spinal cord and nerve roots to accommodate themselves to the gradual changes in the space available. Rarely neurological complications are due to interference with the blood supply as a result of the expanding pagetic bone.

The prognosis of neurological complications depends on the speed with which patients are adequately managed. If the condition is diagnosed early and energetically treated, then the prognosis is better than if it is left untreated for sometime.

Neoplastic changes
Just under 1% of patients with Paget's disease develop malignant changes in the affected bones (Poretta et al, 1957). The characteristic presentation is very severe pain of sudden onset, present most of the time and resistant to ordinary analgesics. A vascular swelling is often present. Not infrequently the patient may present with a pathological fracture. The characteristic radiological features of osteogenic sarcomas are often absent. The skull and bones of the upper limbs are more likely to develop malignant changes than the rest of the skeleton. Histologically, osteogenic sarcomas can be classified according to the predominant cells into osteosarcomas, fibrosarcomas, chondrosarcomas, giant cell tumours and reticulosarcomas. Osteosarcomas are the commonest tumours to complicate Paget's disease. They are associated with a poor prognosis, mean survival time ranging from 7 to 12 months. Several factors may be responsible for this poor prognosis and include the higher average age of the patients, the extreme vascularity of Pagetic bone, the increased risk of haematogenous metastatic spread and the often multicentric origin of osteosarcomas complicating Paget's disease. Furthermore about half of the osteogenic sarcomas complicating Paget's disease arise in sites not amenable to radical amputation.

Cardiovascular complications
As a result of the extensive vascularity of pagetic bones and surrounding tissues, the cardiac output is often increased and as the peripheral resistance is frequently reduced, the pulse pressure is usually widened. Patients with Paget's disease appear to be more at risk of developing atherosclerosis, hypertension and ischaemic heart disease than the rest of the population (Acar et al, 1968). The incidence of high output cardiac failure however, has been over-emphasised. This is a rare complication even when the pagetic lesion is extensive and active.

DIAGNOSIS

The clinical diagnosis of Paget's disease of bone is relatively simple if the skull vault or a peripheral bone is affected and the condition is advanced. It is however often difficult to make when the condition affects the pelvis, the vertebrae or even the base of the skull, which are the commonest bones affected by Paget's disease.

Radiological diagnosis
The radiological features of the disease are characteristic, the bones appear larger than normal and are sometimes deformed. The cortical thickness is increased and often irregular, the trabeculae appearing thickened and irregularly deposited. Many areas of bone resorption appearing as osteolytic or radiolucent areas and areas of new bone formation appearing as osteoblastic or radio-opaque deposits can be seen. Sometimes the lesion consists of only excessive bone resorption with no new bone formation as in osteoporosis circumscripta.

When long bones are affected, the lesion tends to start at one end and spreads towards the other end. The initial feature is an area of localised bone resorption. A V-shaped defect is characteristic of Paget's disease. The demarcation line between the area of resorption and the normal bone is clear cut with no intervening sclerosis. The radiolucent V-shaped advancing edge is closely followed by the deposition of new bone and a mixed picture of bone rarefaction and new irregular bone deposition is usually seen (mixed or mosaic pattern). Incomplete transverse fissure fractures of the cortex are sometimes present. They are usually located at right angles to the shaft on the convex aspect of the long bone.

When the skull is affected the bones of the vault are usually greatly thickened and the diploic space is widened. Areas of rarefaction and new bone formation can be seen, the suture lines do not hinder the progress of the lesion and soon cannot be distinguished. When the base of the skull is affected it may become invaginated by the cervical vertebrae (platybasia or basilar invagination). This is diagnosed when the upper end of the odontoid process is above Chamberlain's line (a line joining the posterior lip of the hard palate with the posterior end of the foramen magnum) or 1 cm above McGregor's line (a line joining the posterior lip of the hard palate to the lowermost end of the occipital bone).

When the vertebrae are affected by Paget's disease the body, neural arches and processes are usually involved. Very rarely is the pagetic process limited only to the body of the vertebrae. The affected vertebra is also larger than the other healthy vertebrae.

The main disadvantages of the radiological diagnosis is that it is usually difficult to assess the state of the activity of the lesion and early in the process the X-rays may appear substantially normal.

Biochemical diagnosis

Several biochemical paramaters can be used as indices of bone turnover rate and activity of pagetic lesions. These levels however, reflect the overall picture and not the activity of the individual bones. The two most commonly used parameters are the urinary hydroxyproline excretion and the serum alkaline phosphatase levels.

Urinary hydroxyproline is mainly derived from bone collagen and the 24 hour excretion reflects the degree of collagen degradation and bone resorption and by inference the activity of the osteoclasts. Urinary hydroxyproline is a more sensitive index of bone turnover than serum alkaline phosphatase. Its estimation is not, however, a simple procedure: Firstly it entails the collection of a 24 hour urine sample, which is not always possible particularly in elderly patients. Secondly the urinary hydroxyproline levels may be elevated after a diet rich in collagen has been consumed and it is therefore important to have the patient on a collagen-free diet for about three days before and during the urine collection. Such diets are not appetising. Finally the biochemical estimation of hydroxyproline, although relatively simple, is time consuming.

The bony fraction of the serum alkaline phosphatase reflects the activity of the osteoblasts and bone turnover. As the activity of the osteoblasts usually parallels that of the osteoclasts, the serum alkaline phosphatase can be used as an indirect measure of osteoclastic activity. Immobilisation is usually associated with a significant drop in alkaline phosphatase levels probably as a result of the reduced stimulus to new bone formation. Acute illness — even in the absence of immobilisation — may also cause a similar sharp fall in the serum level (Nagant de Deuxchaisnes & Rombouts-Lindermans, 1974; Woodward, 1959). The serum alkaline phosphatase consists of several isoenzymes and it is relevant to ensure that the elevated value is of bony origin before attributing it to an increased bone turnover rate.

The magnitude of hypocalcaemia following the administration of calcitonin is sometimes used as an index of osteoclastic activity. The acute inhibition of osteoclasts results in an acute reduction in the rate of bone resorption and a reduced shift of calcium ions from bone to blood. As the other compensatory homeostatic mechanisms are not immediately affected, the serum calcium drops. The magnitude of hypocalcaemia is dependent on the activity of the osteoclasts. Although in most patients the maximum drop is 4–6 hours after the administration of calcitonin, several factors may prolong this period (Hamdy et al, 1982).

Skeletal scintimaging

The main advantage of bone scans is that the relative activity of the various bones and their response to therapy can be easily assessed. The higher the degree of bone turnover the more radioactive isotope will be trapped by the affected bone. This will be seen as a hot area on the scan. During the quiescent or sclerotic phases the degree of radiaoctive uptake is less pronounced and may approach that of normal bone. An increased uptake may also be seen in other bone disorders and a conventional X-ray picture is often necessary to differentiate these various pathologies.

Rarely pagetic lesions can be detected radiologically and not visualised on a bone scan. These are mainly sclerotic or quiescent lesions (Shirazi et al, 1974). On the other hand, most lesions observed on scintimaging and not seen radiologically are associated with symptoms and probably represent early lesions in the osteoclastic initial phase.

TREATMENT

As most patients are asymptomatic the decision to treat Paget's disease of bone or not depends on the individual bone affected as well as the potential complications. In many instances Paget's disease is not active, is not likely to be associated with complications and therefore does not require active therapy. It is therefore essential before embarking on a particular line of therapy to assess thoroughly the site, extent, activity and potential complications of the lesion (Hamdy, 1981). Suggested lines of management are shown in Table 41.1.

Calcitonin

Calcitonin specifically inhibits the osteoclasts. At first their activity is reduced (Singer et al, 1976) and later as calcitonin administration is continued the number of osteoclasts is reduced. The rate of bone turnover is decreased and the newly formed bone is architecturally and mechanically better. Following the administration of calcitonin to patients with Paget's disease the urinary hydroxyproline excretion is reduced and this is followed by a reduction in the serum alkaline phosphatase level. Both fall steeply at first and then tend to plateau regardless of the type of calcitonin used. The significance of this plateau is not yet fully understood. If however calcitonin therapy is continued in spite of this levelling of biochemical values, a radiological response may continue to be observed a few months later (Rojanasathit et al, 1974).

Several forms of calcitonin have been synthesised and are commercially available, they include: salmon, porcine,

Table 41.1 Summary of complications and management of Paget's disease. (Hamdy, 1981: With the permission of Praeger Publishers)

Site of lesion	Complications	Management	
		Active phase	*Quiescent phase*
Long bones	Fractures Deformities Arthritis of neighbouring joints Malignancy	(A) No complications: Observe progress. Analgesics if painful. Anti-pagetic drugs indicated if: (i) Risk of fracture substantial: Cortical thickness diminished Transverse pseudo-fractures Marked deformities (ii) Pain not relieved by analgesics (B) Fractures: Anti-pagetic drugs ± surgery (C) Malignancy: Suspected — biopsy Confirmed — radical surgery ± cytotoxic agents	Observe
Skull Base	Cranial nerve compression, especially II, VIII, V and VII Basilar invagination: Involvement of — pyramidal tracts — lower cranial nerves — cerebellum Chronic brain failure: Obsruction of CSF, drainage and hydrocephalus	Anti-pagetic drugs	Regular monitoring: — serum alkaline phosphatase and/or urinary hydroxyproline — fundus examination (papilloedema) — hearing and visual acuity — x-ray skull patient asked to report once symptoms manifest themselves (see text)
Vault	Brain ischaemia and chronic brain failure Malignancy	Observe Anti-pagetic drugs indicated for: Intractable headaches, brain ischaemia, cosmetic reasons.	Observe
Vertebrae Above L2	Paraplegia: Cord compression or ischaemia	Anti-pagetic drugs	As for skull base
Below L2	Cauda equina lesion	As for skull vault	As for skull vault
Ribs clavicles, scapulae, pelvis	Fractures and compression of adjacent structures	Observe Anti-pagetic therapy indicated if: (i) Intractable pain (ii) Compression of neighbouring structures	Observe
Generalized	High output heart failure	Anti-pagetic therapy if: (i) Marked deformities (ii) High output failure	Observe

human and eel calcitonin. Non-human calcitonin is antigenic and antibodies develop in the majority of patients. Only in a minority of instances however do they interfere with the therapeutic action of calcitonin. Salmon calcitonin is less antigenic and more potent than porcine calcitonin.

Calcitonin is remarkably free from side-effects although occasionally some patients may experience nausea and vomiting 1–2 hours after the injection and lasting up to 2–4 hours. Most of these instances are self-limited and disappear after about 4 weeks of continuous therapy. Severe cases may be helped by the administration of calcitonin before retiring to bed or by the concomitant administration of anti-emetic preparations such as metoclopropamide. Facial flushing often follows the administration of human calcitonin. The main drawbacks of calcitonin are the parenteral mode of administration and the cost of the preparation. Most patients or their relatives, however, can be taught how to inject calcitonin and one must weigh the cost of the preparation against the potential complications associated with Paget's disease, such as fractures (and several weeks of hospitalisation), diminished vision, hearing and brain failure (and the need for custodial care).

There is as yet no consensus of opinion regarding the dose, frequency and duration of calcitonin therapy. Various regimes have been suggested. It is however, generally accepted that the longer the duration of therapy the longer lasting is the period of remission. The author usually prescribes 100 units of salmon calcitonin daily for at least 6 months. Alternatively 160 units of porcine calcitonin may be prescribed if the patient does not tolerate the salmon preparation. This period may be increased if the activity is persistent. The dose may also be increased if the risk of complications is serious as in cases of diminished vision and papilloedema resulting from compression of the optic nerve and its blood supply by the expanding pagetic bone.

Diphosphonates

Diphosphonates inhibit bone resorption and mineralisation by binding to the hydroxyapatite crystals and inhibiting their growth and dissolution (Khairi & Johnson, 1977). In addition they have a direct cellular action and interfere with the membrane transport of calcium and the hydrolysis of mucopolysacharides necessary to start mineralisation (Fast et al, 1977). In active cases of Paget's disease diphosphonates rapidly reduce the excessive bone turnover rate and the overactive osteoclasts and osteoblasts are replaced by a more normal bone population. Furthermore, normal haematopoetic cells gradually replace the excessive fibrous tissue seen in the bone marrow. These changes are paralleled by biochemical evidence of regression of the activity of the lesion (Guncaga et al, 1974; Smith et al, 1973).

The main advantage of disphosphonates over calcitonin

is the oral route of administration. Diphosphonate therapy however, is associated with a number of problems particularly in elderly patients. The main side effects are the incidence of bone demineralisation, bone pain and even fractures. These are probably the result of the mineralisation defects and also affect healthy non-pagetic bones. This is particularly serious in elderly patients who have a higher incidence of osteoporosis and osteomalacia. The intestinal absorption of calcium is also reduced (Bonjour et al, 1973). This can be reversed by low doses of 1–25 dihydroxycholecalciferol, but not cholecalciferol or 25 hydroxycholecalciferol, suggesting that diphosphonates may also interfere with the activation of vitamin D. Interestingly, although 1–25 dihydroxycholecalciferol can reverse the defect in intestinal calcium absorption induced by diphosphonates, it cannot reverse the mineralisation defect suggesting that the two mechanisms are probably independent (Russell & Fleisch, 1975). Other side effects occasionally encountered with diphosphonate therapy include abdominal discomfort and diarrhoea.

Several different diphosphonate compounds have been studied. At present only ethane,1-hydroxydiphosphonate (EHDP) is commercially available. The rate of absorption and effects of diphosphonates are dose-related. The presently available evidence suggests that 5 mg/kg per day continued for 6 months is the optimum dosage (Canfield et al, 1977). This dose results in a reduced bone turnover rate and clinical improvement without being associated with an unduly high risk of side effects. After the discontinuation of therapy, various periods of remission have been described.

Diphosphonates may effectively be combined with calcitonin, both agents potentiate each other and the incidence of mineralisation defects is reduced (Hosking, 1982).

Cytotoxic agents

Cytotoxic agents and mithramycin in particular are still sometimes used in the treatment of Paget's disease. They have been largely replaced by less toxic compounds such as calcitonin and diphosphonates. Unlike calcitonin which specifically inhibits osteoclasts, cytotoxic agents inhibit both osteoclasts and osteoblasts. As a result excessive bone formation as well as bone destruction is suppressed. The main advantage of mithramycin is its rapid action. Bone pain is relieved in most patients within a few days, which is followed by an improvement in the biochemical paramaters, and in the appearance of bone scans and a progressive remodelling of bone towards a more normal appearance (Ryan et al, 1972). As mithramycin is also toxic to the liver, kidneys and platelets, careful monitoring is essential. The isocitric dehydrogenase (ICD) serum concentration is a sensitive indicator of hepatic toxicity and it is recommended to check its level before the administration of mithramycin.

The recommended dose of mithramycin is 15 μg/kg body

weight for 10 days administered intravenously in 5% dextrose over a period of 4–6 hours (Russell & Lentle, 1974). Various dosage regimes have been suggested to limit the toxicity of mithramycin including the administration of 25 µg/kg weekly or every 2–3 weeks (Elias & Evans, 1972). Mithramycin has also been successfully used in combination with calcitonin, the effects appearing to be additive and accompanied by minimal toxicity (Hadjipaviou et al, 1976).

CONCLUSIONS

Paget's disease of bone is not an uncommon condition among the elderly population and whereas only a minority of patients complain of pain or deformities, a substantial number of patients may present with complications such as fractures, diminished hearing, diminished vision, cerebellar ataxia and brain failure. Most of these complications have an insidious onset and slow progress and may therefore be erroneously attributed to the aging process. Clinicians now have the means to control the activity of the lesion and attempts should be made to prevent these complications from occurring. Most of these complications are initially reversible. Unfortunately if left untreated for sometime, they may become irreversible and severely impair the patient's physical and mental well-being. The possibility of Paget's disease of bone being responsible for these complications should therefore be considered and if found to be the underlying pathology, should be actively treated.

REFERENCES

Acar J, Delbarre F, Waynberger M 1968 Les complications cardio-vascularies de la maladie osseuse de Paget. Archives des maladies du Coeur et des Vaisseaux 6: 849–868

Blotman F, Suquet P, Labauge R, Simon L 1974 L'hemodetournement carotidien externe par le crane pagetique. In: Hioco D J (ed) La maladie de Paget. Laboratorie Armour-Montagu, Paris

Bonjour J P, Deluca H F, Baxter L, Fleisch H, Treschsel U 1973 Influence of 1, 25 dihydroxycholecalciferol and diphosphonate on calcium metabolism. Experientia 29: 740

Canfield R, Rosner W, Skinner J, McWhorter J, Resnick L, Feldman F, Kammerman S, Ryan K, Kunigonis M, Bhons W 1977 Diphosphonate therapy of Paget's disease of bone. Journal of Clinical Endocrinology and Metabolism 44: 96–106

Collins D H 1956 Paget's disease of bone — incidence and subclinical forms. Lancet ii: 51–57

Dethridge F M, Guyer P B, Barker D J P 1982 European distribution of Paget's disease of bone. British Medical Journal 11: 1005–1008

Elias E, Evans J 1972 Mithramycin in the treatment of Paget's disease of bone. Journal of Bone and Joint Surgery 54: 1730–1736

Fast D, Felix R, Neuman W F, Sallis J, Fleisch H 1977 The effect of diphosphonates on cells in culture. Calcified Tissue Research (Supplement) 22: 449–450

Guncaga Jr, Lauffenberger T H, Lentner C, Dambacher M A, Hass H G, Fleisch H, Olah A J 1974 Diphosphonate treatment of Paget's disease of bone. Hormone and Metabolic Research 6: 62–69

Hadjipavlou A G, Tsoukas G M, Siller T N, Danais S, Greenwood F 1977 Combination drug therapy in treatment of Paget's disease of bone. Journal of Bone and Joint Surgery 59: 1045–1051

Hamdy R C 1981 Paget's disease of bone. Praeger Publishers, Eastbourne

Hamdy R C, Brown I R, Howells D W, Nisbet J A 1982 Vitamin A and Paget's disease. Lancet 2: 1103–1104

Hosking D J 1982 Paget's disease of bone. Update Publications Ltd, London

Khairi M R, Johnston C C 1977 Treatment of Paget's disease of bone with sodium etidronate (EHDP). Clinical Orthopaedics and Related Research 127: 94–105

Nagant de Deuxchaisnes C N, Rombouts-Lindermans C 1974 Exploration biologique de la maladie de Paget. Journal Belge de Rhumatologie et de Médecine Physique — Acta Medica Belgica 29: 243–293

Poretta C A, Dahlin D C, Janes J M 1957 Sarcoma in Paget's disease of bone. Journal of Bone and Joint Surgery 39: 1314–1329

Rebel A, Malkani K, Basle M, Bregeon C 1976 Osteoclasts ultrastructure in Paget's disease. Calcified Tissue Research 20: 187–199

Ring E F, Davies J, Barker J R 1976 Thermographic assessment of calcitonin therapy in Paget's disease In: Kanis J (ed) Bone disease and Calcitonin. Armour Pharmaceutical Co Ltd, Eastbourne, London, p 39–48

Rojanasathit S, Rosenberg E, Haddad J 1974 Paget's bone disease: response to human calcitonin in patients resistant to salmon calcitonin. Lancet ii: 1412–1414

Russell R G, Fleisch H 1975 Pyrophosphate and diphosphonates in skeletal metabolism. Clinical Orthopaedics and Related Research 108: 241–263

Russell A, Lentle B 1974 Mithramycin therapy in Paget's disease. Canadian Medical Association Journal 110: 397–400

Ryan W G, Schwartz T B, Northrop G 1972 Treatment of Paget's disease with mithramycin — further experiences. Seminars in Drug Treatment 2: 57–64

Shirazi P H, Ryan W G, Fordham E W 1974 Bone scanning in evaluation of Paget's disease of bone. CRC Critical Reviews in Clinical Radiology and Nuclear Medicine 5,4: 523–558

Singer F R, Melvin K, Mills B G 1976 Acute effects of calcitonin on osteoclasts in man. Clinical Endocrinology 5: 333–340

Smith R, Russell R G, Bishop M, Woods C, Bishop M 1973 Paget's disease of bone experience with a diphosphonate in treatment. Quarterly Journal of Medicine, New Series 42: 235–256

Woodward H 1959 Long-term studies of the blood chemistry in Paget's disease of bone. Cancer 12: 1226–1237

42

Arthritis

M. F. R. Martin & V. Wright

INTRODUCTION

While rheumatologists have in recent years rightly drawn attention to the fact that arthritis occurs from childhood onwards, few would disagree that older people have more and suffer most from it. Arthritis in old age may present in a setting where there are already multiple aging or degenerate features, and it occurs frequently in conjunction with other diseases.

The importance of an early and accurate diagnosis of arthritis is paramount, for whether symptoms are primary or secondary, joint disease makes a significant contribution to disability in the elderly (Akhtar et al, 1973). This may in turn place a heavy burden on the family and social services, and in cases where disability is so marked that assistance with self-care is required, varying degrees of dependence come to exist, which are very different from those found in the younger age groups.

Recognition of these differences and an increased awareness in old age, particularly in those patients over the age of 75 years, that the disease process is operating in a unique setting, has led to a modified approach in the management and treatment of arthritis in the elderly. The sheer weight of clinical experience imposed by demographic change in the population has made this an urgent consideration (Fox, 1982).

Connective tissue changes with age

The structure of connective tissue changes throughout life (Engel & Larsson, 1969). The individual functional requirements and inheritance determine these alterations. It is recognised that with advancing age the stature diminishes, the back becomes curved, bones brittle, joints stiff and the skin wrinkled, thinned and stiffer (Bourne, 1961; Ridge & Wright, 1966; Goldman & Rochstein, 1975). These commonly observed changes are the result of altered connective tissue structure and function, and help to illustrate its ubiquity, its importance and its possible defects. Defects are commonly related to disease that disturbs the state of dynamic equilibrium.

Articular cartilage

Cartilage is a unique gel reinforced with fibre; it contains a few cells (chondrocytes) and a large proportion of extracellular matrix material (Muir, 1980). The chondrocytes occupy only a small proportion of the tissue volume. They rarely divide but are metabolically active synthesising and catabolising extracellular constituents. The fibrous portion of the matrix comprises proteins of type II collagen and in between are non-fibrous globular molecules called proteoglycans. These proteoglycan molecules consist of a protein core to which are attached several long chain carbohydrate moieties (glycosominoglycans). These attract water, become swollen and hold the collagen bundles in place, thereby giving cartilage its resilience. In addition, a small amount of hyaluronic acid, together with a 'protein link component' present at one end of the proteoglycan molecule, helps to stabilise the aggregates (Hardingham & Muir, 1975).

Much attention has focused on the relations between normal cartilate aging and osteoarthritis (Lawrence et al, 1966). The argument is difficult to assess because the anatomical changes and secondary clinical signs of osteoarthritis become more prevalent with advancing age.

Two patterns of degenerative change are recognised and are found in different areas of load-bearing cartilage surfaces (Byers et al, 1970 & 1977). The first of these disorders becomes more common with age. It comprises increased granularity, softening, splitting and fragmentation (fibrillation) which finally leads to loss of cartilage and subsequent ossification. These changes are not thought to progress and therefore are not considered to be precursors of clinical osteoarthritis. The second pattern of change is much less common; it is not thought of as an age change but may be regarded as part of the degenerative disease process. Well circumscribed zones of granularity progress to complete loss of joint cartilage, and associated with these anatomical lesions osteoarthritis later develops.

Connective tissue

In the studies of aging in the other connective tissues it has been suggested that three fundamental changes occur.

Firstly, variations in water content may considerably interfere with normal connective tissue function. Secondly, there may be a reduced rate of connective tissue synthesis and finally, in the presence of increased degradation, considerable connective tissue loss will occur (Hall et al, 1981).

COMMON ARTHROPATHIES

Osteoarthritis

Osteoarthritis is probably the most important and frequent joint disease affecting the elderly and may account for up to 90% of diagnoses. Osteoarthritis describes the condition which may follow damage to the avascular, aneural hyaline cartilage of synovial joints (Gardner, 1983). Any of man's 190 or so synovial joints may be affected. With increasing age the joints most affected, in decreasing order of frequency, are the knees, acromioclavicular, elbows, first metatarsophalangeal, hips, sternoclavicular and shoulders. Lawrence et al (1966) in a radiological study, concluded that almost all individuals over 65 had minor osteoarthritic changes in joints, but only 15–20% reported clinical symptoms. Most degenerative joint disease involves surrounding tissues, but clearly several other factors must be present before symptoms develop.

Osteoarthritis is not difficult to diagnose and in the elderly the typical features of joint pain, stiffness and deformity are seen. Two categories of disease are recognised. The first group includes those where hyaline cartilage fails with no recognisable hereditary defects, metabolic or endocrine abnormalities and no history of injury, infection or other joint disorders is known. This condition, which is common and yet neglected as a disease entity, is referred to as 'idiopathic' or primary generalised osteoarthritis. This form of the disease is characterised by Heberden's nodes with characteristic X-ray changes in the distal interphalangeal joints. Occasionally, these nodes may be hot and tender, and sometimes the erythrocyte sedimentation rate (ESR) may be raised in these patients. Furthermore, the joint involvement may be more widespread and include small and large joints, degenerative changes being frequently present in the cervical and lumbar spines. In this condition there is a female preponderance and strong genetic factors have been suggested by both family and twin studies (Carter & Fairbank, 1974). A number of careful family studies have demonstrated clear recessive and dominant inheritance patterns.

There is another variant of primary generalised osteoarthritis where Heberden nodes are absent. Interestingly, relatives of these patients have an increased instance of seronegative arthritis, implying that patients with widespread osteoarthritis may have an underlying disease not recognised as an inflammatory arthropathy.

The disease of secondary osteoarthritis occurs where cartilage failure is shown to have been caused by injury, infection, nutrition and metabolic disorders, endocrine dysfunction or other insults. Examples of these include fractures affecting articular surfaces, suppurative and tuberculous arthritis, rickets, gout, acromegaly and late joint changes associated with rheumatoid arthritis. The structure and function of cartilage may also be affected by congenital deformity of the whole joint or skeleton, and these deformities or those associated with metabolic disease may be heritable.

Clinically the commonest sites of joint involvement in osteoarthritis are the knees and hips. The loss of cartilage in the medial compartment of the knee joint frequently leads to the development of a genu varum deformity. Disease of the hips may go completely unnoticed, being accepted by the older person as a normal part of aging. Involvement of any of these major weight-bearing joints may contribute considerably to disability and dependence in a significant proportion of the elderly and this proportion increases with advancing age.

Thus an elderly patient may present to the geriatrician in a non-specific manner with a problem such as immobility, with consequent failure to cope at home; or with urinary incontinence or with falling and all its attendant complications. Patients who present with such features need full clinical assessments, delineation of all problems and finally clear decisions on treatment.

Occasionally osteoarthritis may present as an acute inflammatory condition with a sizeable effusion; care should be taken to distinguish it from other acute arthritic conditions, such as septic arthritis, crystal induced synovitis and rheumatoid arthritis. Aspiration is mandatory if these are suspected. Examination of the joint fluid in osteoarthritis reveals sterile fluid, with a low white cell count (predominantly lymphocytic) and low protein content.

The radiological changes associated with degenerative joint disease consist of narrowing of the joint space, the presence of osteophytes and ossicles, sclerosis of subchondral bone and the development of subchondral bone cysts (Kellgren & Lawrence, 1957). The earliest X-ray changes correspond in most cases to already well established disease, but care must be taken not to overdiagnose, especially in the investigation of falling, for the condition of cervical spondylosis is clinically very common and is often seen radiographically, but it is not always the cause of vertebrobasilar ischaemia.

Rheumatoid arthritis

Though the peak decade of onset of rheumatoid arthritis is the fifth, it is not at all unusual for patients to present first with this condition in their sixties or seventies, and it is common for joint inflammation to persist or to relapse and remit for periods of 30 years and over.

Rheumatoid arthritis is common in the elderly and presents a wide spectrum of disease severity and clinical manifestations (Brown & Sones, 1967). The ravages on the joints accumulate with time, as do the effects on extra-articular tissues, and so may present complex problems in diagnosis and management. Rheumatoid arthritis is much less common than osteoarthritis, but again its recognition, accurate diagnosis and correct treatment are of vital importance.

Rheumatoid arthritis is the commonest diagnosis in elderly patients presenting with an acute arthritis (Gibson & Graham, 1973) and it is generally accepted that an acute onset may be more frequent in the elderly and lead to rapid deformity (Oka & Kytila, 1957). However, overall the disease tends to be milder in old age and is less deforming (Cecil & Kammerer, 1951; Duthie et al, 1964). Extra-articular manifestations, with the exception of anaemia, are less common in the elderly. Female predominance remains but is less marked than in the younger age group (Ehrlich et al, 1970).

As in the young, a peripheral polyarthritis tending towards symmetry over several months is the commonest presentation. The joints most commonly and first involved are the metacarpo-phalangeal, metatarso-phalangeal, proximal interphalangeal and wrists. In contrast elderly patients sometimes present initially with a proximal distribution of joint stiffness and pain involving the shoulders and/or hips; this only becomes distinguishable from polymyalgia rheumatica when clinical and radiological changes of rheumatoid arthritis supervene in peripheral joints.

Occasionally elderly patients may present with systemic complications of rheumatoid disease, for example pleural effusions, pericarditis or an anaemia, and all may occur prior to the development of arthritis. This variable presentation emphasises the importance of repeated assessments in elderly subjects presenting with an undiagnosed rheumatic complaint. Other extra-articular complications of rheumatoid arthritis should also be sought. The presence of nodules and vasculitis suggests a more aggressive form of disease. Frequently tear secretions may be found to be impaired indicating a Sjogren's syndrome. Scleritis, scleral nodules and ulceration may impair vision and any suspicion of these requires urgent ophthalmological assessment. Pulmonary and cardiac involvement is known to occur and should not be overlooked.

In patients with long-standing rheumatoid arthritis iatrogenic complications may supervene, for example steroid induced myopathy occurs with high dosages and osteoporosis develops following prolonged use. Indomethacin may produce fluid retention and anti-inflammatory drugs may occasionally cause anaemia by sudden or intermittent gastric blood loss.

Diagnosis is made in the same way as in the younger age groups and the same criteria are applied. Anaemia and a raised ESR are commonly associated with active disease, and mention should be made of rheumatoid factor titres. The latex and sheep cell agglutination tests are frequently positive in low titres in the elderly and are thus of limited diagnostic value (Lawrence, 1977). Rheumatoid factor titres of 1 in 64 or higher can generally be regarded as diagnostic, but lower levels must always be questioned. Increased specificity utilising other and newer techniques may help to clarify these anomalies.

Synovial fluid aspirated from rheumatoid joints often appears purulent and turbid, but invariably the viscosity is low and the cell count, which is mostly made up of neutrophils, may be in excess of 30 000 mm^{-3}. Early radiographic changes are periarticular osteoporosis with the development of erosions on the articular surfaces. These are best seen in radiographs of the hands and feet and particular attention should be paid to the metacarpal and metatarsal joints and the ulnar styloids (Thould & Simon, 1966) where these lesions are first seen. Osteoporosis is often profound and may be generalised. Later radiographic changes include loss of joint space, bone destruction and rarely ankylosis. Special radiographic views of the cervical spine in flexion and extension should be taken as atlanto-axial subluxation is often present. A gap of more than 3 mm on a standard view between the atlas and the anterior border of the odontoid process is pathological. This is seen in nearly half of rheumatoid patients in hospital, but is rarely symptomatic. However sudden trauma even though it is trivial may produce long tract signs. In the elderly other types of polyarthritis simulating rheumatoid arthritis must be considered and care should be taken to exclude them. They include polyarticular gout, primary generalised osteoarthritis, psoriatic arthritis, calcium pyrophosphate deposition disease, calcific periarthritis at multiple sites and viral arthritis.

Polymyalgia rheumatica

Polymyalgia rheumatica (PMR) is a disease of late middle age and the elderly (Silman & Currey, 1982). In most reported series the mean age of onset is between 65 and 75 years, with few if any cases starting before the age of 50. The onset is more often acute than gradual and symptoms may reach their most severe in less than two weeks. Characteristically they are made up of diffuse, poorly localised muscular pains around the neck and shoulders and also in the lumbar region, buttocks or thighs. The hall mark of PMR is severe morning stiffness, particularly around the shoulders and its absence should leave doubt regarding the diagnosis (Bird et al, 1979).

Local tender areas around the sternoclavicular and acromioclavicular joints, interspinous ligaments and adductor origins are common. The presence of a synovitis often with effusions in other joints can occur, but in view of the age of most patients these features are usually attributable to degenerative arthritis rather than to inflammatory joint disease. Malaise is invariably present, and anorexia, depression, weight loss, night sweats and a low grade fever are all commonly reported.

Polymyalgia rheumatica is one part of a symptom complex that occasionally includes giant cell arteritis. About 30% of patients have apparent temporal artery involvement (Dixon et al, 1966). In patients with giant cell arteritis 50% experience visual disturbances at some time or other, and include 15–20% who may go blind in one or both eyes. Patients may present with severe scalp tenderness and headaches; this sometimes prevents them from washing their hair, wearing spectacles or even produces jaw claudication with eating.

The superficial temporal arteries may be tender and thickened with absent pulsation. Occasionally scalp necrosis in the temporal artery distribution occurs. Vascular bruits are sometimes audible over the orbital or subclavian vessels and abnormal carotid sinus sensitivity may be a useful early sign.

There are no specific diagnostic tests for polymyalgia, although the ESR is invariably raised usually above 50 mm in the first hour, and often may be over 100 mm. Occasionally there have been reports of a normal ESR in the presence of active PMR and biopsy proven temporal arthritis, and this should not be overlooked.

In the early stages of PMR it may be difficult to reach a firm diagnosis. Shoulder girdle symptoms are often associated with cervical spondylosis. The development of muscular and periarthritic pains, constitutional disturbances and a high ESR may suggest such possibilities as systemic lupus erythematosus, polyarteritis nodosa or a prodromal phase of rheumatoid arthritis. Muscle pain may suggest a diagnosis of polymyositis but in contrast this condition produces muscle weakness, muscle enzymes are usually elevated and a muscle biopsy is abnormal.

Crystal Arthropathies

Gout

The intense articular inflammation associated with the presence of intracellular monosodium urate crystals in synovial fluid is often the first and most characteristic manifestation of gout (Arnold & Gröbner, 1977). In the absence of effective anti-hyperuricaemic therapy the clinical syndrome of chronic tophaceous gout may appear, with deposition of urate in the soft tissues, the kidney and the joints with an associated chronic polyarthritis.

The peak incidence of acute gout is in males usually in the fourth or fifth decade and it is rarely seen in women before the menopause. In the elderly the development of gout is often secondary to an underlying disease where there is increased cellular turnover, or it may be associated with drug therapy, the most common being the thiazide diuretics used for the treatment of hypertension and heart failure (De Martini, 1965).

Gouty arthritis is a true intermittent inflammatory condition with distinctive clinical signs and symptoms. Characteristicaly it involves a single joint, although more than one can sometimes be affected simultaneously. The metatarso-phalangeal joint of the grat toe is involved in about 70% of cases, followed in frequency by the ankle or other joints of the foot, knee, fingers, wrists and elbows. Acute gout is also seen in bursae and tendon sheaths. The sensation of discomfort often starts at night, waking the victim and may develop into severe and often excruciating pain. The involved joint becomes red, shiny, swollen and exquisitely tender. Although these characteristic features may not be so marked in larger joints.

Chronic tophaceous gout in relation to articular structures leads to a destructive arthropathy with secondary degenerative changes. These may follow either repeated acute attacks, or less freqently may develop insidiously in a previous unaffected joint. White masses of monosodium urate (tophi) form in periarticular tissues close to the distal interphalangeal joints, causing the skin over these lesions to become thin and shiny, and later these may discharge and ulcerate. In addition tophi are also found in other situations and are particularly common in the external cartilage of the ear, the olecranon and prepatellar bursae and the achilles tendons.

The diagnosis may be from the characteristic history and from the positive identification of crystals in the joint fluid. Crystals of monosodium urate can be observed on ordinary light microscopy, but are detected more readily under a polarising microscope. Morphologically they are seen to be needle shaped, of between 5 and 20 microns in length, and they show a negative birefringence. It is generally necessary to demonstrate a raised uric acid level before the diagnosis can be accepted, but even in the presence of a raised level it does not necessarily mean that a particular symptom is due to gouty arthritis. Failure to appreciate this had led to gout frequently being overdiagnosed.

The differential diagnosis of gout includes other conditions that can give rise to acute inflammatory joint disease, for example rheumatoid arthritis, septic arthritis and other crystal arthropathies, which include calcium pyrophosphate deposition disease.

Pyrophosphate arthropathy (Pseudogout)

Pyrophosphate arthropathy, like gout, results from the deposition of calcium pyrophosphate dihydrate crystals in the joints. These may be visible on X-rays as chondrocalcinosis when it is present within the joint cartilage. Occasionally the condition may be chronic, when it often remains asymptomatic.

This condition is seen more frequently in late middle age and in the elderly. It lacks the male predominance seen in true gout and a positive family history is uncommon. The clinical course is variable, some patients experience only occasional attacks, while others develop a progressive degenerative joint disease without a history of acute attacks. Occasionally a long-standing subacute polyarthritic may develop which mimics rheumatoid arthritis (McCarty, 1976).

The diagnosis may be made from the history. Unlike gout, large joints are affected more commonly than the smaller ones. The most common site is the knee joint and the hips and shoulders are not spared. In most cases the cause of these attacks is unknown, but they may be precipitated by diuretics, surgical operations and blood transfusions. Radiological evidence of chondrocalcinosis should be sought and the diagnosis confirmed by observing crystals within the synovial fluid. Examination under the polarising light microscope shows morphologically that the crystals are short and thick in the shape of a rhomboid, and these show a weakly positive birefringence. Once again the diagnosis must be differentiated from other acute inflammatory arthropathies.

LESS COMMON ARTHROPATHIES

Connective tissue diseases

The connective tissue diseases are a group of disorders of unknown aetiology involving different organs and exhibiting a wide spectrum of clinical manifestations. While they are not common, these conditions occur in the elderly and indeed both scleroderma and vasculitic syndromes are seen most commonly in patients past middle age. However they are generally not considered as diseases of the elderly and are consequently under-diagnosed.

Systemic lupus erythematosus (SLE)

Systemic lupus erythematosus is diagnosed more often in women in the second to fifth decade but it does occur in the elderly. This has often meant delay in making the diagnosis, especially as recent studies have suggested that the clinical expression differs in the older patient (Baker et al, 1979). The onset of clinical features is usually insidious. Constitutional manifestations are common and may dominate the clinical picture. Polyarthritis is a frequent presentation, and patients are often misdiagnosed as having rheumatoid arthritis or a polymyalgic syndrome. Cutaneous manifestations occur less frequently than in younger patients, but pleurisy and to a lesser extent pericarditis are emphasised as prominent clinical features of lupus occurring in the elderly. In contrast, clinically significant renal disease and neuropsychiatric involvement are less frequent.

The most common laboratory abnormality is the anti-nuclear antibody detected by immunofluorescence which is present in 95% of patients. This test is the most sensitive screening test for systemic lupus erythematosus (SLE) but lacks specificity, especially in the elerly. Antibodies to native DNA are present in 60–70% of patients and these antibodies have a much higher degree of specificity for the disease.

Progressive systemic sclerosis (scleroderma)

Progressive systemic sclerosis (PSS) often begins in the elderly (Rodnan, 1963). It is a generalised disorder of connective tissue resulting in diffuse fibrosis of the dermis (scleroderma) and adjacent tissues. Certain internal organs may be involved, notably the intestinal tract, heart, lungs and kidneys. Raynaud's phenomenon is a regular and frequently early symptom and other vascular abnormalities affecting chiefly the micro-circulation constitute a prominent feature of the disease (Maricq & Le Roy, 1979).

A true inflammatory polyarthritic may occur, usually early in the course of the disease, and predominantly involves small joints. Joint limitation and stiffness in advances cases of PSS with skin involvement are related to hardening of the skin and underlying tissues. Joint erosions are only rarely seen radiographically, and bone changes are predominantly confined to the distal phalanges. These usually consist of osteolysis which may occasionally be seen elsewhere. There are no specific laboratory abnormalities, although a variety of serum antibodies are frequently found.

Polymyositis

Polymyositis is a rare inflammatory myopathy of unknown cause. In the presence of a characteristic skin rash the term 'dermatomyositis' is applied (Bohan & Peter, 1975). The onset may be acute or chronic, and in a proportion of cases is associated with an underlying malignancy. Cases have been documented in patients into their eighth decade. The principal clinical features are a symmetrical weakness in the proximal muscles and the anterior neck flexors. The characteristic skin lesion is a purplish, dusky rash on the eye lids (heliotrope), cheeks and light exposed areas with peri-orbital oedema. Arthralgia is common but frank arthritis should alert one to the possibility of an overlap syndrome.

Many patients appear to have overlap syndromes and do not fit into traditional diagnostic categories. Often there is difficulty, in the early stages of the disease, in diagnosis but the subsequent course may resolve the problem as one disease pattern gradually emerges. Less commonly, two or more diseases co-exist and the mixed syndrome persists indefinitely. Commonest amongst these are disorders with features of scleroderma and SLE and/or polymyositis, or of rheumatoid arthritis associated with those of SLE.

Septic arthritis

Infection of a joint with pyogenic bacteria occurs more commonly in the elderly (Willkens et al, 1960). It may present as a complication of infection elsewhere and predisposing factors are frequently encountered, for example underlying diabetes melitus, rheumatoid arthritis, steroid therapy or other debilitating diseases. The symptoms and signs are characteristic, often there is a rapid onset of severe joint pain with swelling, usually monoarticular, with an effusion, tenderness and painful limited movement, and in addition there may be surrounding erythema with peri-articular oedema. In general the patient is systemically ill with an accompanying fever. Joint aspiration is mandatory, the synovial fluid is purulent, with a very high total white cell count, and more than 90% of these are neutrophils. Gram-stain frequently demonstrates organisms and culture is positive in more than 90%. Blood culture may also be positive. The commonest organisms are *staphylococcus aureus* and *streptococcus pyogenes*. Gram negative organisms are less frequently seen and rarely infections with fungi and anaerobic organisms are occasionally encountered (Schmid, 1978).

Malignant disease and arthritis

The incidence of malignant disease increases with age. Arthritis is one of the many ways in which malignant disease may present (Calabro, 1967). The diagnosis is therefore of great importance. Primary malignancy of bone or synovium may occasionally present as a rheumatic problem. Secondary deposits occasionally occur in the synovium, but are much commoner in bone, particularly from primary cancers in the breast, thyroid, kidney, lung and prostate. When they occur near a joint they may simulate arthritis. A clinical condition resembling rheumatoid arthritis occurs principally with carcinoma of the bronchus, prostate and breast. The diagnosis is applicable to cases of arthritis which do not conform to other known patterns of disease. It is important to recognise the underlying disease which, when treated, may help to resolve joint symptoms.

Soft tissue rheumatism

Generalised soft tissue lesions may result from underlying disease, and most of the primary conditions can be diagnosed by careful clinical and laboratory assessment (Dixon, 1979). A large proportion however, occur in the absence of systemic disease. In these circumstances local causes, such as chronic repetitive low grade trauma and excessive and unaccustomed use, may be responsible. These lesions predominate in the middle-aged and elderly.

Painful shoulder

Many of the conditions causing a painful shoulder result from extra capsular soft tissue lesions. Trauma is often slight or unnoticed (Bland et al, 1977). Following hemiplegia it may be associated with mis-handling the paralysed limb.

A tendonitis or even rupture of the supraspinatus close to its insertion on the humeral head may result in a rotator cuff syndrome. Inflammation of the joint capsule may produce pain and immobility of the shoulder or arm, and can predispose to the development of a frozen shoulder.

Shoulder-hand syndrome

Painful disablity of the shoulder may occasionally develop into a secondary reflex sympathetic dystrophy syndrome that involves the hand and fingers. It is characterised by an immobile painful shoulder associated with swelling and pain in the forearm and hand; the skin is cold, shiny and hyperaesthetic and results in a dystrophic-looking hand. In 25% of cases the condition is idiopathic, but usually it is associated with either a previous myocardial infarction or with cervical spondylosis, trauma or hemiplegia. Spontaneous resolution may occur but if the condition persists, permanent restriction of shoulder movement may result.

MANAGEMENT OF ARTHRITIS

It is important to take a complete clinical history and to note details of the main complaint. An enquiry should be made, particularly for underlying skin disease, bowel disorders, urogenital symptoms, inflammatory eye changes, drugs and recent overseas visits. The past medical history may also be appropriate and a careful family history is mandatory. A complete physical examination is essential and must involve every system, including skin and genitalia.

Joint aspiration

The necessity for joint aspiration cannot be over-emphasised. Aspiration may be diagnostic, particularly in cases of crystal deposition disease and in septic arthritis which may be potentially life-threatening if it remains undiagnosed. Therapeutic aspirations of large effusions associated with sepsis and haemarthrosis may produce considerable symptomatic relief. Therapeutic injections of corticosteroids may also be administered to any joint with a persistent localised synovitis with or without effusions. Precautions should include strict asepsis; frequent injections into a single joint should be avoided and the patient should be warned to report if the joint becomes painful and to rest for at least 24 hours, avoiding excessive weight-bearing (Williams & Gumpel, 1980).

General Treatment

Patient education is fundamental to the success of treatment. Educating the patient with regard to the nature of the disease, the general aims of management and the beneficial effects and limitations of currently available therapeutic modalities are all important. In the majority of cases of arthritis, patients should be told that treatment will not cure the disease but that the chances of help are excellent.

Rest is an important part of the management of any acute

arthritis whether present in a single joint or as part of a polyarticular syndrome (Lee et al, 1974). The provision of lightweight plastic splints, particulary for the hands and wrists, may be useful at night or even during daytime. Ill-fitting and uncomfortable footwear may contribute considerably to the general dependence and disability of an elderly arthritic. The provision of suitable custom made footwear may frequently overcome many of these difficulties.

Occupational therapy
There are a wide variety of aids and equipment available to help the arthritic patient lead an independent life and these may be helpful in protecting inflamed joints against stressful use. A careful assessment should be regularly performed by an experienced therapist, who will not only demonstrate simpler ways of doing things than those in current use by the patient, but will also provide the most suitable aids for the individual patient's requirements (Chamberlain, 1981).

Physiotherapy
In order to preserve a normal range of joint motion and maintain muscle strength without excessive joint stress, a programme of heat and graded exercises is important To obtain best results, there measures should be employed regularly, preferably daily. Thus most patients will need to depend on physical therapy at home, performed by themselves or with a family member. Instructions should be provided for methods of application using dry or moist heat. This should be followed by passive or active movements and progressive isometric muscle strengthening exercisees in appropriate instances (Ingberg, 1980). In certain circumstances, part of the programme of physiotherapy and rehabilitation should be in hospital where more intensive treatment can be given.

Social Services
Many elderly arthritics are frequently unfamiliar with state benefits or community services, and referal to a social worker may prove helpful in reducing disability or patient dependence.

Specific treatment
Drugs have an important place in the management of rheumatic disorders (Mowat, 1979; Haslock, 1983). A number of special problems are present in the elderly, particularly with regard to drug metabolism and excretion and a need to monitor drug dose carefully cannot be over-emphasised (Petersen et al, 1979). The mechanisms of action of many of the drugs used are not always fully understood, and in many instances the drug may only relieve symptoms without effecting any fundamental change in the disease being treated.

Simple analgesics that have no anti-inflammatory activity have traditionally been recommended for the treatment of degenerative arthritis, particularly as they avoid the upper gastro-intestinal side effects so common with most non-steroidal anti-inflammatory drugs (NSAID) (Gleeson, 1982). However, clinical signs of mild inflammatory joint disease are commonly found in patients with degenerative osteoarthritis and in the known association of this disease with pyrophosphate deposition. In these cases, and in all patients where there is evidence of an inflammatory process, one of the many NSAIDs should be used.

Aspirin and related drugs have been the corner stone of anti-rheumatic medication for more than a hundred years (Bayles, 1966). Many would continue to advocate their usage as the first drugs in all cases, but this view is now out-dated. The advent of a new range of NSAIDs has allowed us to assess critically each patient's drug needs and to tailor a regime to suit these needs. It is sensible to move in planned stages from the least toxic, and in general least effective, to the most toxic and most effective agents. It is not possible to recommend one drug suitable for all patients. There is probably more variability in the response of an individual patient to any particular drug than there is in the response of a group of patients to different drugs. It is therefore necessary to try more than one drug in turn in an individual patient until the preferred drug for that patient is determined. It is important to ensure that a patient is taking the maximum dose of an NSAID, provided this dose does not result in toxicity, before concluding that it is ineffective (Neumann & Wright, 1983).

Care must be taken in the dyspeptic patient, particularly if an ulcer is present. There is not one NSAID that can be considered safe in all patients with peptic ulcer. Even if it is used as a suppository, there may still be deleterious effects on peptic ulcers because of the systemic effect of these drugs. Phenylbutazone is not now recommended in the elderly (Fowler, 1967), indomethacin is a potent anti-inflammatory drug that suffers from problems of gastro-intestinal toxicity, and central nervous system symptoms occur with high doses. Both these drugs may cause excessive fluid retention that can complicate treatment in the elderly.

The most commonly prescribed group of NSAIDs are the proprionic acids, of which ibuprofen, naproxen and fenbufen have proved of low toxicity in elderly subjects, and these are now preferred as first line drugs in the management of arthritis.

Corticosteroids
Systemic corticosteroids are potent anti-inflammatory drugs which are more effective than NSAIDs, but they have considerably more frequent and serious side-effects which limit their use. In elderly subjects who fail to respond to simple anti-inflammatory agents, the cautious use of corticosteroids may have a dramatic effect on maintaining their mobility and independence (Myles & Daly, 1974).

There are however, some rheumatic conditions in which they are regularly used, their associated toxicity being justified by the serious nature of the underlying disease. Such diseases are polymyalgia rheumatica, temporal arteritis and vasculitis associated with underlying connective tissue disorders. In systemic lupus erythematosus they are of value in the treatment of acute serious manifestations of disease, but their long-term use in patients with mild, non life-threatening symptoms is associated with more problems than benefits, and increasing use is now being made of intermittent corticosteroid therapy. In rheumatoid arthritis, corticosteroids should be used in patients who are failing to benefit from alternative treatment regimes, or where a rapid improvement is essential. It is important to aim for the minimum effective dose.

Specific anti-rheumatic drugs
In general, this group of drugs have a particular place in the treatment of rheumatoid arthritis, although the antimalarial drugs are of value in some patients with systemic lups erythematosus, particularly where skin and joint manifestations predominate.

Sodium aurothiomalate (gold) (Gerber & Paulus, 1975) given intramuscularly and oral penicillamine (Multicentre Trial Group, 1973) are used for the treatment of rheumatoid arthritis. These drugs are slow-acting antirheumatoid agents; they may require 10–14 weeks for their effect to commence and will usually achieve their maximum benefit by 6 months. It is important to remember that they are additional to the other regular therapy that the patient is receiving. Their use is often restricted by toxicity and they are only used in patients whose arthritis is sufficiently severe and progressive to justify these increased risks (Hall, 1980). The major side effects of rashes, thrombocytopenia and proteinuria are usually reversible by stopping the drug. The use of these specific anti-rheumatic drugs should be mainly restricted to patients under regular hospital supervision.

Specific drugs in the treatment of gout
An acute attack of gout may be treated by non-steroidal anti-inflammatory drugs such as indomethacin and azapropazone, which are both effective in reducing the symptoms of acute arthritis. Occasionally in the elderly these drugs may lead to fluid retention and treatment with colchicine may be required. To prevent the frequent disabling attacks or the chronic effects of prolonged hyperuricaemia, the life-long use of the zanthine oxidase inhibitor, allopurinol, can prevent these symptoms from developing. Recently azapropazone, that has both an anti-inflammatory and a weak uricosuric effect, has also been found of value in the long-term management of patients with acute and chronic gout (Dieppe et al, 1981).

Surgical treatment
Surgery has an important part to play in the management of an elderly patient with chronic arthritis (Freeman, 1979). Indications for operation, the type of operation and the timing of any surgical procedure are factors which need careful consideration. The indications for surgery are pain, limitation of movement and progressive deformity.

Low friction arthroplasties of the hip are very successful, especially when combined with good post-operative rehabilitation, which is essential in the elderly. Surgery in the rhematoid patient is more complex since more than one joint may require attention, and arthritis of the hands and feet will limit post-operative rehabilitation after large joint surgery. Minor surgical procedures may therefore have to be undertaken on the hands and feet prior to more extensive arthroplasties. There are a large number of arthroplasties currently being evaluated for the treatment of chronic arthritis, but many of these are still largely experimental and are available only at specialist centres. Hip and knee arthroplasties are now routinely available but shoulder, elbow and ankle arthroplasties are still being developed. Surgery should not be performed for cosmetic reasons alone, the prime aims being pain relief and the restoration of useful function.

REFERENCES

Akhtar A J, Broe G A, Crombie A, McLean W M R, Andrews G R, Caird F I 1973 Disability and dependence in the elderly at home. Age and Ageing 2: 102–111

Arnold W J, Gröbner W 1977 Clinical manifestations of hyperuricaemia. In: Kelly W N (ed) Clinics in Rheumatic Diseases: Crystal Induced Arthropathies, Saunders London

Baker S B, Rovira J R, Campion E W, Mill J A 1979 Late onset systemic lupus erythematosus. American Journal of Medicine 66; 727–732

Bayles T B 1966 Salicylates and rheumatic diseases. Arthritis and Rheumatism 9: 342–347

Benedek T G 1983 Associations of rheumatic diseases and rheumatic symptoms with cancer. In: Wright V (ed) Bone and joint diseases in the elderly. Churchill Livingstone, Edinburgh

Bird H A, Esselinckx W, Dixon A St J, Mowat A G, Wood P H N 1979 An evaluation of criteria for polymyalgia rheumatica. Annals of the Rheumatic Diseases 38: 434–439

Bland J H, Merritt J A, Boushey D R 1977 The painful shoulder. Seminars in Arthritis and Rheumatism 7: 21–47

Bohan A, Peter J B 1975 Polymyositis and dermatomyositis. New England Journal of Medicine 292: 344–347 & 403–407

Bourne G H 1961 Structural aspects of ageing. Pitman, London

Brown J W, Sones D A 1967 The onset of rheumatoid arthritis in the aged. Journal of the American Geriatrics Society 15: 873–881

Byers P D, Contepomi C A, Farkas T A 1970 A post-mortem study of the hip joint including the prevalence of features of the right side. Annals of the Rheumatic Diseases 29: 15–31

Byers P D, Maroudas A, Oztop F, Stockwell R A, Venn M F 1977 Histological and biochemical studies on cartilage from osteoarthrotic femoral heads with special reference to surface characteristics. Connective Tissue Research 5: 41–49

Calabro J J 1967 Cancer and Arthritis. Arthritis and Rheumatism 10: 553–567

Carter C O, Fairbank T J 1974 The genetics of locomotor disorders. Oxford University Press, London

Cecil R L, Kammerer W H 1951 Rheumatoid arthritis in the aged. American Journal of Medicine 10: 439–445

Chamberlain M A 1981 Aids for the Arthritic. Geriatric Medicine 11: 57–60

DeMartini F E 1965 Hyperuricaemia induced by drugs. Arthritis and Rheumatism 8: 823–829

Dieppe P A, Doherty M, Whicher J J, Walters G 1981 The treatment of gout with azapropazone: clinical and experimental studies. European Journal of Rheumatology and Inflammation 4: 392–400

Dixon A St J, Beardwell C, Kay C, Wanka J, Wong Y T 1966 Polymyalgia rheumatica and temporal arteritis. Annals of the Rheumatic Diseases 25: 203–208

Dixon A St J (ed) 1979 Clinics in Rheumatic Diseases, Soft tissue rheumatism. Saunders, London

Duthie J J R, Brown P E, Truelove L H, Baragar F D, Lawrie A J 1964 Course and prognosis in rheumatoid arthritis. Annals of the Rheumatic Diseases 23: 193–202

Ehrlich G E, Katz W A, Cohen S H 1970 Rheumatoid arthritis in the aged. Geriatrics 2: 103–113

Engel A, Larsson T (eds) 1969 Ageing of connective tissue and skeletal tissue. Thule International Symposia Proceedings. Nordiska Bokhaudelns Forlag, Stockholm

Fowler P D 1967 Marrow toxicity of the pyrazoles. Annals of the Rheumatic Diseases 26: 344–345

Fox R A 1982 Arthritis in the elderly. European Journal of Rheumatic Inflammation 5: 285–288

Freeman P A 1979 Joint replacement in the elderly. Age and Ageing 8: 29–32

Gardner D L 1983 The nature and causes of osteoarthritis. British Medical Journal 286: 418–424

Gerber R C, Paulus H E 1975 Gold therapy. In: Pearson C M, Carson Dick W (eds) Clinics in Rheumatic Diseases: Current management of rheumatoid arthritis. Saunders, London

Gleeson M H 1982 Gastro-intestinal complications of NSAIDs. European Journal of Rheumatology 5: 30–34

Gibson T, Grahame R 1973 Acute arthritis in the elderly. Age and Ageing 2: 3–13

Goldman R, Rockstein M (eds) 1975 The physiology and pathology of human ageing. Academic Press, New York

Hall M R P 1980 Rheumatoid arthritis – minimising the side effects of long-term therapy. Geriatric Medicine 10: 81–86

Hall D A, Blackett A D, Zafac A R, Switala S, Airey C M 1981 Changes in skinfold thickness with increasing age. Age and Ageing 10: 19–23

Hardingham T E, Muir H 1975 Structure and stability of proteoglycan aggregates. Annals of the Rheumatic Diseases 34: 26–28

Haslock I, 1983 Arthritis in old age: Drug treatment. In: Wright V (ed) Bone and joint disease in the elderly. Churchill Livingstone, Edinburgh

Ingberg H O 1980 Physical treatment and rehabilitation of arthritis. In: Spittell J A (ed) Clinical Medicine Vol 4, Harper and Row, Hagerstown

Kellgren J H, Lawrence J S 1957 Radiological assessment of osteoarthritis. Annals of the Rheumatic Diseases 16: 494–501

Lawrence J S, Bremner J M Bier F 1966 Osteoarthritis – prevalence in the population and relationship between symptoms and x-ray changes. Annals of the Rheumatic Diseases 25: 1–24

Lawrence J S 1977 Rheumatism in populations. Heinemann, London

Lee P, Kennedy A C, Anderson J, Buchanan W W 1974 Benefits of hospitalization in rheumatoid arthritis. Quarterly Journal of Medicine 43: 205–214

McCarty D J 1976 Calcium pyrophosphate dihydrate crystal deposition disease. Arthritis and Rheumatism 19: 275–285

Maricq H R, LeRoy E C 1980 Disorders of the microcirculation. In: Rodnan G P (ed) Clinics in Rheumatic Diseases: Progressive Systemic Sclerosis. Saunders, London

Mowat A G 1979 Drug treatment of arthritis in the elderly. Age and Ageing 8: 14–25

Muir I H M 1980 The chemistry of the ground substance of joint cartilage. In: Sokoloff L (ed) The joints and synovial fluid, Vol III. Academic Press, New York

Multicentre Trial Group 1973 Controlled trial of D-Penicillamine in severe rheumatoid arthritis. Lancet I: 275–280

Myles A B, Daly J R 1974 Corticosteroid and ACTH Treatment. Arnold, London

Neumann V, Wright V 1983 Non-steroidal anti-inflammatory drugs. Use and abuse. British Journal of Hospital Medicine, In Press

Oka M, Kytila J 1957 Rheumatoid arthritis with onset in old age. Acta Rheumatica Scandinavica 3: 249–258

Peterson D M, Whittington F J, Payne B P 1979 Drugs and the Elderly. Thomas Springfield, Illinois

Ridge M D, Wright V 1966 The ageing of skin; a bioengineering approach. Gerontologia 12: 174–192

Rodnan G P 1963 A review of the recent observations and current theories on the etiology and pathogenesis of progressive systemic sclerosis (diffuse scleroderma). Journal of the Chronic Diseases 16: 929–949

Schmid F R (ed) 1978 Clinics in Rheumatic Diseases, Infective Arthritis. Saunders, London

Silman A J, Currey H L F 1982 Polymyalgia rheumatica in a defined elderly community. Rheumatology and Rehabilitation 21: 235–237

Thould A K, Simon G 1966 Assessment of radiological changes in the hands and feet in rheumatoid arthritis: their correlation with prognosis. Annals of the Rheumatic Diseases 25: 220–228

Williams P, Gumpel M 1980 Aspiration and injection of joints. British Medical Journal 281: 990–992 & 1048–1049

Willkens R F, Healey L A, Decker J L 1960 Acute infectious arthritis in the aged and chronically ill. Archives of Internal Medicine 106: 354–364

43

Renal disease

E. J. Lewis & R. M. Kark

INTRODUCTION

As one ages, the kidneys, in health, appear to perform their varied functions admirably. However, the aging kidney does not function as it had during youth and because of this the elderly patient is vulnerable to many stressful situations which alter the body's internal environment. The kidneys of younger adults have the luxury of a large functional reserve which allows a wide breadth of response to a range of factors which alter the internal environment such as salt, water and potassium. The aging kidney appears to have a narrower response to these factors, so that homeostasis may be more easily threatened in the face of either excessive or diminished intake of an otherwise normal dietary element. The elderly patient is therefore at greater risk when flexibility of homeostatic mechanisms are required. This is frequently noted during intercurrent illnesses where dietary intake may be altered and fluid requirements significantly changed. It is the purpose of this chapter to review these alterations of the aging process.

PHYSIOLOGICAL CHANGES

The potential for homeostatic control related to kidney function changes with age. However, the aging process is also associated with progressive alterations in general metabolic processes which actually decrease basal homeostatic requirements. Much of the latter involves decreased energy requirements which are the result of diminished tissue mass. Thus the mean caloric expenditure of adults decreases progressively from the peak achieved during adolescence. Energy expenditure for an adult male diminishes from 3000 kcal/d at 40 years to 2500 kcal/d at 60 years and 2200 kcal/d above the age of 70 years. Daily caloric expenditure similarly decreases in females from 2200 kcal/d at the age of 30 years to 1600 kcal/d at 70 years. These data must be taken into account when one considers the basal daily caloric and fluid needs of the elderly person (Synder et al, 1976). However, as will be noted below, these needs may change significantly when illness stresses the life of the elderly person.

ANATOMICAL CHANGES AND PATHOPHYSIOLOGY

With aging there is an overall atrophy of the tissues of the musculoskeletal system, which has direct relevance to the evaluation of kidney function in the elderly patient. The muscle energy requirements are decreased with a lessened turnover of creatine phosphate. The decreased catabolism of creatine results in a diminished production of its ultimate metabolic end-product, creatinine. Because of this decreased daily creatinine production, a stabilisation of the concentration of creatinine in the blood occurs despite decreased ability of the kidney to excrete this compound (Fig. 43.1). Rowe et al (1976) and Cockcroft & Gault (1976) have emphasised the danger of misinterpreting the serum creatinine value in the elderly, as it no longer accurately reflects the accepted 'normal' glomerular filtration rate (GFR) of 120 ml/min. The latter 'normal' rate can only be taken seriously in the younger person. With age, the glomerular filtration rate can be expected to decrease. For example a 'normal' serum creatinine level of 1.0 mg in an 80 year-old man may reflect a daily excretion of only 1000

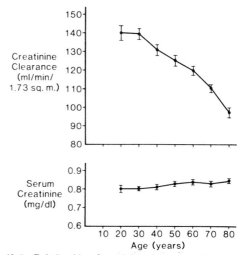

Fig. 43.1 Relationship of creatinine clearance and serum creatinine to age. Despite a large decline in creatinine clearance, serum creatinine remains essentially unchanged owing to a concomitant decrease in muscular mass. (Rowe et al, 1976: With permission of the Journal of Gerontology; Schrier, 1982: With the permission of the publishers)

mg of creatinine and a glomerular filtration rate of 60 ml/min. In this instance, diminished muscle mass is associated with less creatinine production each day. As less creatinine needs to be eliminated, the lower glomerular filtration rate of aging is not reflected in the serum creatinine, which maintains constancy. Thus the serum creatinine by itself does not indicate the progressive loss of glomeruli which attends the aging process and is a poor index of absolute kidney function. For this reason, relatively minor clinical insults may have an apparently dramatic effect on kidney function. The old 'healthy' kidney which has already lost half of its mass will appear to decompensate suddenly with an additional insult, such as decreased renal perfusion resulting from dehydration or cardiac failure. This constriction of response is more evident when new insults impinge on old kidneys, not only in those who have suffered from other disease over the years, such as diabetes, arteriolonephrosclerosis or hypertension, but also in the apparently well but aged person (McLachlan, 1976; Epstein, 1979).

That the kidneys shrink with age has been known for some time (McLachlan, 1978; Griffith et al, 1976; Epstein, 1979). The average renal mass in young adults is about 250 g and decreases to about 200 g in the aged. This shrinkage is associated with various structural changes. For example, many alterations in vascular histology have been described. In the renal arteries, medial hypertrophy and hyalinisation, and intimal proliferation. Basement membrane thickening in both glomeruli and tubules have been noted to be more evident with aging. The interlobar and arcuate arteries were found to have intimal fibrosis, interlobular arteries had fibro-elastic thickening and the pre-glomerular arterioles were involved in irregular hyaline change (McLachlan, 1978; Addis & Oliver, 1931). Shock and his co-workers first demonstrated the progressive functional decline that is associated with these anatomic alterations. Rowe et al (1976) reported a decline in glomerular filtration rate from 140 ml/min 1.73m^2 at age 30, to 90 ml/min 1.73m^2 at age 80. Some acceleration of the rate of decline in creatinine clearance with advancing age was noted. Rowe et al (1976) have emphasised that this decrement in the glomerular filtration rate represents true renal aging and is not secondary to disease. The decline approximates to a loss of 10 ml/min of GFR per decade of life.

The aging, contracting kidney sustains a greater loss of cortical mass as compared to the loss noted in the medulla. The pathophysiology of cortical atrophy was clarified by Hollenberg and his colleagues (1974) who had a unique opportunity to study the intrarenal vasculature in apparently normal adults. These studies were carried out on 207 potential living-related transplant kidney donors aged 17–76 years. Each of these donors required selective renal arteriography to define their renal arterial anatomy before a kidney was removed for transplantation. These subjects had a rigorous clinical and laboratory workup to assure that their kidneys were healthy before they were removed and transplanted. Hence complicating factors such as the effect of hypertension were excluded. Using xenon washout technique in order to determine the distribution of blood flow to the renal cortex, they showed a significant diminution of cortical perfusion with age. Their results indicated a larger reduction in renal cortical blood flow than in anatomic renal mass, suggesting that the change in blood flow was primary to the genesis of renal atrophy. These findings agreed with the morphological observations that have suggested a primary vascular process to be responsible for the development of age-related anatomical changes. While these studies established a progressive decrease in blood flow to the renal cortex with age, presumably due to arteriolar narrowing, the possibility remains that progressive glomerular sclerosis which occurs with aging can also be a primary process contributing to altered cortical perfusion.

From the viewpoint of the renal histologist, glomerular sclerosis must be considered the most dramatic change in the microscopic anatomy of the aging kidney. Moore (1931) showed that the number of functional glomeruli was reduced by one-third to one-half between the ages of 40 to 80. This study demonstrated that nephron dropout proceeds steadily in all men from the third decade onward. Glomerular dropout has been described by several investigators who have studied the age-related incidence of completely sclerotic glomeruli in the kidneys of persons who have died a violent death (Kaplan et al, 1975). The data indicate that one could expect to find acellular global sclerosis of the glomerular tuft in up to 10% of glomeruli in younger adults. In those over 50, the statistical upper limit of acellular global sclerosis is 25%. This tendency to develop global sclerosis must also be considered in the interpretation of renal biopsy material from elderly patients.

What systemic or local changes in the kidney could be responsible for glomerulosclerosis and nephron death? The studies of Addis & Oliver (1931) by nephron dissection and histologic examination, coupled with studies of renal function, convinced them that the renal vascular changes were the primary cause of glomerulosclerosis and renal aging. But there are other views of this. Addis had published extensively (1940) upon the deleterious effects of a high protein diet on kidney function when there is a reduction of renal mass. More contemporary work by Shea et al (1980) and by Brenner et al (1982) in experimental animals suggests that when there is a diminished total number of nephrons, the hydrodynamic effects upon the remaining glomeruli can lead to glomerulosclerosis independent of vascular pathology. Therefore, although there is a tendency for the glomeruli which survive age or an insult to function normally, even super-normally, the hydrodynamic forces within the glomeruli, which cause increased intraglomerular pressure, may lead to chronic damage. In experimental animals, these physiologic changes, and subsequent glomerulosclerosis, can be accelerated by placing the animal on a high protein diet. The stimuli leading to this response has not yet been determined. However, culturally determined dietary habits could conceivably account for progressive glomerulosclerosis in the aging person.

FLUID AND ELECTROLYTE DISORDERS

Changes in renal function in the older patient are accompanied by important alterations in the internal environment. With age the anatomy of distribution of body water and electrolytes also undergoes alterations. As would be expected, the diminished total cell mass is associated with a decreased content of body water (Fig. 43.2). The mean per cent body weight which can be attributed to water at the age of 20 is approximately 60% for males and 50% for females. By the sixth decade this declines to 55% for males and 45% for females (Snyder et al, 1975). The decrease in the total body water is primarily a reflection of decreased water content of the intracellular space (Edelman et al, 1952). Also reflecting on this diminished cell mass is a progressive decrease of the total body potassium with age. On the other hand plasma volume, extracellular fluid volume and total body sodium, as percentages of body weight, appear to vary little over the years (Edelman et al, 1959). Thus the body does dessicate with advancing years and this makes the older person more prone to dehydration and its consequences.

DEHYDRATION AND HYPEROSMOLARITY

It has been a common clinical experience that older patients are prone to develop dehydration and hyperosmolarity

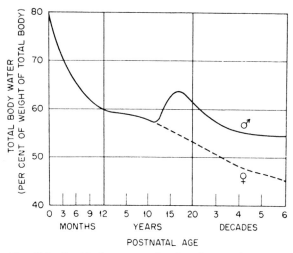

Fig. 43.2 Total body water as a function of postnatal age in males and females. (Edelman et al, 1951: With the permission of the editor, Surgery, Gynecology & Obstetrics)

(Feig & McCready, 1977). This derangement of salt and water balance is often manifested by abnormalities of the sensorium, particularly confusion, but may progress to coma (Minaker & Rowe, 1981). Several factors cause the elderly patient to be vulnerable to the development of dehydration. The ability of the kidney in the adult to maintain normal sodium and water homeostasis differs from that of the older individual who will not respond to salt deprivation in the rapid and precise manner so characteristic of younger persons. When a young adult is placed on a marked sodium restriction, the excretion of sodium in the urine is reduced within 2–3 days to a level no greater than the dietary sodium intake. This is referred to as the attainment of 'sodium balance'. Older people take a longer period of time to attain this metabolic balance. During this time they lose more sodium in their urine. Because of this blunted functional response, the older patient may develop plasma volume depletion before metabolic balance is finally achieved. Hence, in stressful situations when food and water intake may be limited, the older patient is at greater risk of developing plasma volume depletion.

DIURESIS AND DEHYDRATION

In addition to the salt-losing properties of the aging kidney, altered water metabolism has also been described. The ability of the older patient to conserve water is diminished in the face of a deprived intake or negative balance, as is seen in febrile conditions (Rowe et al, 1978). Although there may be no apparent abnormality of the renal handling of water while the elderly patient has free access to oral intake, an impairment in the maximum concentrating ability of the kidney can become clinically obvious during fluid deprivation. Amidst this background of diminished capacity of the aging kidney to respond normally to the deprivation of dietary salt or water, one must recognise common clinical situations which will tend to further place elderly patients at risk of becoming volume depleted. Every effort must be made to identify all the factors and possible causes which can lead to this pathologic condition in the elderly:

1. Negative water balance
   (a) oral water deprivation
   (b) increased water loss
      (1) diminished renal maximum concentrating ability
      (2) lungs–hyperventilation
      (3) skin–fever
      (4) gastro-intestinal tract
2. Osmotic diuresis
      (1) high protein nutrients (tube feedings)
      (2) hyperglycaemic nonketotic coma
3. Pharmacologic agents
      (1) diuretics

Water balance in the elderly may be perturbed not only by diminished intake and increased pulmonary, skin or gastro-intestinal loss, but also by virtue of the imposition of an abnormal dietary osmotic load which can further diminish the renal concentrating ability (Gault et al, 1968). The administration of high protein containing nutrients is often overlooked as a complicating factor in the metabolic management of the aged (Table 43.1). A high protein diet, often taken as tube-feeding, results in the metabolic generation of large amounts of urea, which then imposes an increased osmotic load on the kidney leading to the obligatory loss of sodium and water (Gennari & Kassirer, 1974). In addition to this urea osmotic load, one must be cognisant of the sodium concentration of these tube-feedings, which varies from preparation to preparation. The increased osmotic load which must be excreted by the kidney will cause an obligatory loss of water into the urine irrespective of the patient's state of hydration (Berenyi & Strauss, 1969). Thus the dehydrated patient receiving high protein containing tube-feeding solutions will not be able to conserve fluid appropriately and will continue to sustain a negative fluid balance. High protein nutrients must therefore be administered with caution and an adequate oral water supplement must be assured. Similarly, hyperglycaemic states must be detected and adequately treated in order to avoid the consequences of glucose osmotic diuresis and dehydration (Schwartz & Appelbaum, 1965–1966).

The common use of diuretics for the long-term treatment of congestive heart failure and hypertension imposes still another threat to the elderly patient. This must be recognised in the context of the numerous other factors noted above which are inimical to normal salt and water homeostasis among these patients and tend to predispose the elderly to dehydration and hyperosmolar states.

RENAL DISEASE IN THE ELDERLY

Urinary tract infection

The concurrence of urinary tract infection and dehydration in the elderly is possibly a special problem in the United States and is most commonly seen in seriously ill patients admitted to hospital from nursing homes (Garabaldi et al, 1981; Avorn, 1981).

In this patient population these two nephrologic problems, dehydration and urinary tract infection, are frequently found in association with underlying medical disorders such as dementia and other neurologic diseases, and/or diabetes mellitus. In addition many have septic pressure-point tissue trauma, infections of the lung, as well as neglect of incontinence (Ouslander et al, 1982) and nutrition. Usually, these patients require a high level of skilled nursing care as a result of their multiple medical problems. These patients are likely to be incontinent of urine and faeces and many arrive with long-term indwelling Foley catheters, which predispose them to urinary tract infections.

Urosepsis, with or without septic shock, is a frequent serious complication in this setting, which has a high mortality, even with optimal care (Tunn & Thieme, 1982). It is recognised that many of these patients are infected with resistant gram-negative bacteria when admitted to hospital and therefore require initial treatment with an aminoglycoside in combination with a penicillin or cephalosporin, antibiotic, until the results of culture and sensitivity of the urine and blood are available.

Uncomplicated urinary tract infections

Uncomplicated urinary tract infections present special problems in the elderly, especially in women. In elderly women asymptomatic bacteria without pyuria is more

Table 43.1 The content of commonly used nutrients.

Preparation	kcal/litre*	Protein or amino acid* content/litre	Projected urea production‡ per 1 preparation
Osmolite® (Ross)	1060	35 g	200 mmol
Ensure® (Ross)	1000	35	200
Advance® (Ross) (Undiluted)	540	40	220
Ensure® Plus (Ross)	1500	54	300
Vital® (Ross)	1000	40	220
Vivonex (Norwich-Eaton)	1000	20	110
Vivonex® HN (Norwich-Eaton)	1000	40	220

‡As noted in the text, the osmotic load which must be excreted when high protein nutrients are administered will cause an obligate excretion of water (and possibly sodium) by the kidney. The patient receiving 3000 kcal of a tube feeding containing 35 g protein per 1 must excrete 600 mmol of urea per day. The physiologic effects of a high osmolar load upon the kidney results in a diminished ability to maximally concentrate the urine. In addition, the aged kidney has an intrinsic concentration defect. The patient whose kidneys can concentrate the urine to only 400 mmol/l must excrete 1.5 litres of urine to accommodate this urea load irrespective of that patient's fluid balance. This can lead to hypertonic dehydration.
*Per litre of preparation or one litre of solid preparation diluted in water according to manufacturer's instruction.

common than in men and does not require antibiotics. On the other hand if there is pyuria with significant bacteriuria, antibiotic therapy should be instituted. Many of the elderly have urgency because of age-related loss of control of bladder emptying and are incontinent if a toilet is not within reach. Most elderly women are too embarrassed to volunteer such a history or to seek advice about the common problem of stress-incontinence, even when they have symptoms of urinary tract infection. Thus it is always necessary to question women, particularly those with urinary tract infections, in some detail about dysuria, frequency or urgency.

Urinary tract infection and obstructive uropathy
When the elderly have urinary tract infections, especially elderly men, obstructive uropathy and/or renal infection should always be a consideration. In such elderly patients, symptoms of uropathy may be absent or unusual (Arruda, 1983), and diagnostic radiology and ultrasound studies are of value for assistance after doing routine clinical laboratory studies. The true incidence of renal infections in the elderly with urinary tract infection is not known. Bergan (1982) indicates that approximately half of all adults with urinary tract infection have renal parenchymal infection. This may be greater for the elderly because of the high incidence of obstruction of the urinary conduit in them.

Collecting 'clean-catch' urine for study and culture is usually simple with men. In women urine must be collected by catheterisation and rarely by bladder puncture (Kark & Netter, 1976). We urge initial urinalysis and especially microscopic examination of the sediment for bacteria, leucocytes and white blood cell casts in all patients (Brody et al, 1968; Kark & Netter, 1976). It is also suggested that screening for urinary tract infection be done as a routine on all elderly patients who enter hospital. This is cost effective as it saves time and assists in decisions concerning antibiotic therapy and may also reduce the number of days that patients with urinary tract infection stay in hospital.

Acute Renal Failure
The differential diagnosis of acute renal failure in the elderly encompasses considerations identical to those entertained in younger age groups. However, one must be cognisant of certain special diagnostic considerations among these patients:

I. Pre-renal
  1. dehydration
  2. congestive heart failure
  3. renovascular obstruction
II. Renal
  1. glomerular disease
    (a) glomerulonephritis

  2. tubulointerstitital disease
    (a) ischaemic acute tubular necrosis
    (b) drug-induced
      (1) nephrotoxins: (aminoglycoside antibiotics, CIS-platinum, radio-iodine contrast materials)
      (2) drugs which alter intrarenal perfusion: prostaglandin synthesis inhibitors (nonsteroidal anti-inflammatory drugs)
      (3) acute interstitial nephritis (thiazide diuretics, synthetic penicillin derivatives, radio-iodine contrast materials)
    (c) multiple myeloma
    (d) hypercalcaemic nephropathy
    (e) acute pyelonephritis
III. Post-renal
  1. bilateral ureteral obstruction
  2. bladder outlet obstruction

As noted above, dehydration is a particularly common event in this population. Obviously, severe congestive heart failure and obstructive vascular disease are also significant factors in some elderly patients with acute renal failure. The elderly patient is also at particular risk of being exposed to factors which are associated with acute renal failure. As this population is exposed to a wide variety of therapeutic agents, it is no surprise that drug-associated acute renal failure occurs with some frequency. The use of aminoglycoside antibiotics, a risk factor in all age groups, similarly represents a significant risk in the aged (Whelton & Solez, 1982; Adelman et al, 1982). The inaccuracy of the serum creatinine as an absolute parameter of glomerular filtration rate in the elderly patient is an important consideration when the dosage schedule of an aminoglycoside antibiotic is determined. It is strongly recommended that an appropriate formula or nomogram (see page 374) be applied to determine renal function in the elderly patient in order to avoid a serious overdose.

Non-steroidal anti-inflammatory drugs represent a particular threat in this age group, as they become used with increasing frequency for a wide variety of arthralgic disorders (Appel & Kunis, 1983; Bennett, 1983; Sorahan et al, 1982; Bunning et al, 1982) so common in the elderly (Fig. 43.3). The ability of drugs which inhibit prostaglandin synthetase to cause an abrupt decrease in renal function and acute renal failure is well documented and must be taken into account in the elderly patient. It must be emphasised that in clinical states associated with diminished renal blood flow, such as dehydration, congestive heart failure, cirrhosis and any primary renal disease process, the maintenance of renal function appears to become dependent upon vasodilatory prostaglandins, such as prostacyclin. It is possible, although still unproven, that the aging kidney may also be more dependant upon

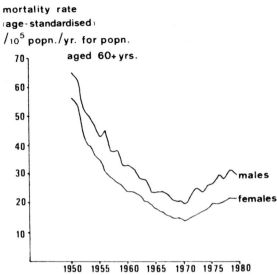

mortality rate
(age-standardised)
$/_{10}^5$ popn./yr. for popn.
aged 60+ yrs.

Fig. 43.3 Annual age standardised rate of mortality from nephritis and nephrosis: England and Wales 1950–79 for population aged greater than sixty years. (Sorahan et al, 1982: With the permission of the authors and editor of the Lancet)

prostaglandins for the maintenance of normal glomerular perfusion and function. Therefore the administration of aspirin, indomethacin or any of the non-steroidal anti-inflammatory agents (NSAIA) to a patient in one of these categories is associated with a rapid decrease in renal function as prostaglandin synthesis becomes inhibited. This adverse effect stands in contrast to the benign appearance of these agents in patients with normal renal haemodynamics who are not prostaglandin dependent. It is not clear whether the high incidence of renal failure in elderly patients taking NSAIA is due to a specific predisposition on their part or simply because so much more of these agents are prescribed in the elderly. However NSAIA must be viewed as a serious threat to renal function in the older patient.

One particular clinical situation which deserves special consideration in the elderly patient with acute renal failure is multiple myeloma (DeFronzo et al, 1975). The appearance of decreased renal function, severe anaemia and proteinuria should alert the clinician to this possibility. Appropriate serum and urine electrophoretic patterns and radiologic diagnostic procedure are required for diagnosis.

Acute renal failure associated with post-renal causes is commonly seen in the elderly population. This may take the form of bladder outlet obstruction, the most common obstructive lesion among elderly men. However, bilateral ureteral obstruction due to pelvic neoplasia, as well as other causes, must be considered.

Overall the elderly do appear to be exposed to more acute insults and risk factors that predispose to the development of acute renal failure. Recently a multivariant analysis of risk factors indicated that age alone did not specifically

appear to be a significant sole risk factor. However hypotension, excessive aminoglycoside exposure, pigmenturia and dehydration were all identified to be very significant risk factors for developing acute renal failure (Rasmussen & Ibels, 1982). Clearly, each of these is seen among the elderly more often than in younger populations. They state that 'an additive interaction between acute insults was demonstrated and the severity of the acute renal failure was related to the number and severity of acute insults'. Often, one or more of these insults is readily preventable.

Determination of renal functional status prior to use of common nephrotoxic agents

As we have noted above, the elderly tend to suffer from the additive effects of different forms of kidney damage. The unplanned addition of a useful but nephrotoxic drug may finally precipitate acute renal failure.

Since the rate at which a drug is eliminated by the kidneys is proportional to the creatinine clearance, it is critical to measure this after the drug history and the environmental history have been ascertained. As it is difficult to collect accurate timed urine specimens from the elderly, the value for creatinine clearance has to be derived from equations, or nomograms. The most popular formula is that of Cockcroft & Gault (1976).

$$\text{G.F.R. (ml/min)} = \text{Creatinine clearance (ml/min)} = \frac{(140 - \text{age in years}) \times (\text{weight in Kg})}{(\text{Serum creatinine ml/dl}) \times 72}$$

The nomogram most commonly used is that developed by Siersbeck-Nielson et al (1971) (Fig. 43.4).*

GLOMERULAR DISEASE IN THE ELDERLY

The spectum of diseases of the glomerulus seen in the elderly essentially reflect those found in younger populations. There are some special circumstances which will be emphasised here.

Acute post-infectious glomerulonephritis

This lesion which are characteristic of older children and adolescents can occur in the elderly. Rare is the case properly diagnosed upon initial contact by the physician. These patients will usually present as acute congestive heart failure or severe hypertension, both clinical patterns attendant on the renal retention of salt and water associated with this lesion. Pulmonary infections are a common complication (Boswell & Eknoyan, 1968; Arieff et al, 1973). It is only after a proper urinalysis is performed and

---

*This nomogram is printed on a pocket size plastic card provided to the medical profession by the manufacturers of gentamicin. It is useful and can be obtained from the manufacturer's representatives.

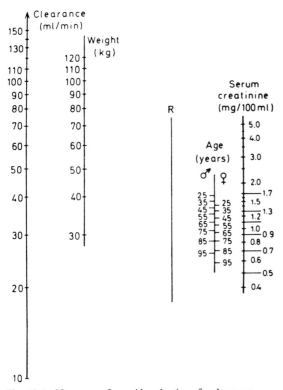

Fig. 43.4 Nomogram for rapid evaluation of endogenous-creatinine clearance from serum creatinine. To accomplish this, take a ruler or marker with a straight edge and with it join 'weight' to 'age'. Keep the straight edge at the crossing point of the line 'R'. Using the point on 'R' as a fulcrum, move the right-hand side of the ruler so the edge is on the appropriate serum creatinine value and read the patient's clearance from the left side of the nomogram. Note that the rate at which a drug is eliminated by the kidneys is commonly proportional to the clearance of creatinine. It is not possible on many occasions to collect a timed urinary sample to measure creatinine clearance. Using the nomogram to estimate the creatinine clearance is adequate in most clinical situations when kidney function is stable or not changing too rapidly. In the presence of shock, severe cardiac failure or oliguria the estimate is too high, as it is in very obese or oedematous patients or in those with generalised muscle wasting. (Siersbaek-Nielsen, et al, 1971: With the permission of the authors and editor of the Lancet).

proteinuria and haematuria with red blood cell casts is found, that the diagnosis is entertained. The clinical, pathologic and serologic alterations usually found in younger patients are also seen in the older population. While it has been stated that older patients while developing this lesion have a decreased tendency to pursue a course to complete resolution, the majority of patients probably have a benign course (Heptinstall, 1983).

Nephrotic syndrome

The glomerular lesions associated with the nephrotic syndrome vary considerably with age. The most common glomerular lesion associated in nephrotic syndrome of childhood is minimal change glomerulopathy (or lipoid nephrosis), however the most common lesion in adults is membranous glomerulonephritis. The distribution of glomerular lesions among older nephrotics is distributed among several diagnostic categories (Fawcett et al, 1971). In our own series of 33 patients with the nephrotic syndrome over the age of 50, 30% had membranous glomerulonephritis, 24% had a proliferative glomerulonephritis, 15% had minimal change glomerulopathy and 25% had amyloid.

Amyloid

The increased incidence of amyloid among older nephrotics clearly distinguishes this group from younger adults and children with this syndrome. Few clinical characteristics distinguish the older nephrotic with amyloid from those with other histologic lesions, although an elevated serum creatinine is found more often among these patients than the other diagnostic groups. An elevated excretion of monoclonal light chains may be noted in the urine, however one does not see an M-spike in the serum. Other organs may be involved with amyloid, however these patients frequently present renal manifestations as their major clinical problem.

Membranous Glomerulonephritis

It is important to recognise that adult patients with membranous glomerulonephritis may harbour an occult solid tumour. Approximately 10% of adults above the age of 50 years have been found to have a neoplastic condition in association with the nephrotic syndrome with membranous glomerulonephritis (Row et al, 1975; Eagen & Lewis, 1977). As these patients present with proteinuria and oedema as the major signs, they require a diagnostic workup for evidence of tumour. The most common tumours seen in this circumstance are of bronchogenic, gastro-intestinal and renal origin.

Proliferative glomerulonephritis

Patients with proliferative glomerulonephritis and the nephrotic syndrome frequently are found to have systemic diseases. Vasculitis, microscopic polyarteritis, Wegener's granulomatosis and Goodpasture's syndrome have all been noted (Moorthy & Zimmerman, 1980). In fact, it appears that rapidly progressive glomerulonephritis associated with anti-glomerular basement membrane antibodies may occur more commonly in the elderly and must be considered in the differential diagnosis of abrupt onset of renal failure.

Focal segmental glomerulosclerosis

This lesion found in about 6% of children and a still larger per cent of younger adults, appears to be an infrequent finding in the elderly nephrotic (Bolton et al, 1978). As noted earlier in this chapter, global sclerosis of glomeruli can be expected to be found in 10–25% of glomeruli in the kidney of the elderly. Hence this must be taken into account when a renal biopsy is interpreted. However segmental sclerosis and hyalinosis, a lesion with a characteristic appearance associated with the nephrotic syndrome, is infrequently seen in this age group.

Minimal change glomerulopathy

This appears to respond normally to high dose steroid therapy. There does not appear to be an increased frequency of non-response to steroids in older patients. Because of the fear of the ill effects of treatment with steroids in elderly nephrotics, particularly their catabolic effects and salt retention, one may elect to wait for a spontaneous remission, if the effects of the proteinuria are not debilitating.

In essence then, the clinical course of the various forms of the nephrotic syndrome in the elderly do not appear to be different from that found in younger adults even though the incidence of the different varieties found seem to be somewhat changed (Moorthy & Zimmerman, 1980).

END STAGE RENAL FAILURE

The elderly patient with chronic renal failure presents certain risks which appear to be greater than that seen in younger populations. While little data is available, the existing wisdom appears to suggest that with transplantation the dangers of adverse affects due to high dose prednisone therapy are excessive among the elderly and that chronic dialysis programmes provide a better alternative to long-term maintenance.

A recent report of overall transplant results according to age of the patient revealed that of 1051 patients over the age of 50 years who had an unrelated donor transplant, 79% survived 1 year and 68% survived 3 years. This patient survival was associated with a graft survival of 52% at 1 year and 42% at 3 years. Among 208 patients receiving related donor transplants, 81% survived 3 years with a graft survival of 68% (Krakauer et al, 1983). These results were not as good as those reported for younger age groups, but not as bad as one might have expected. In any given case, the pros and cons of all modalities of therapy for end stage renal failure must be considered.

Most elderly patients in end stage renal failure are placed on a haemodialysis programme. It has been known for some time that older patients do well in the first two years of haemodialysis provided they do not have a serious generalised disease like diabetes (Lewis et al, 1969). This observation was confirmed in Roberts' study (1976) of over 1000 patients on home haemodialysis. At any age there was about a 74% survival rate at the end of 2 years. Thereafter there was rapid drop-off in those aged 50 years and over, so that 34% were alive at the end of 5 years compared to 55% in those between the ages of 30 and 49, and 64% in those

less than 30 years old. The more recent survey of the European Dialysis and Transplantation Association indicated that the 5 year survival with dialysis for patients 55–64 years old was 40% and for patients over 65 was 27%. After the 2 year experience, older patients survive much more poorly on haemodialysis than do those in younger age groups. Neff et al (1983) reported cumulative survival rates for 58 patients aged 55–74 and compared these to 103 patients aged 35–54 and 42 patients aged 15–34. They showed that there was a rapid drop-off in survival after 2 years and by 6 years only 10% of the older age group was alive as compared to 40% in the middle group and 65% in the youngest group. This is a highly significant difference which most likely represents cardiovascular morbidity (Lindner et al, 1974; Rostand et al, 1979). Nevertheless, although these figures are significantly poorer than those noted in the younger age groups, the opportunity for acceptable rehabilitation clearly exists and should be offered to the elderly.

A final consideration for the treatment of the end stage renal failure patient is that of continuous ambulatory peritoneal dialysis or regular use of the peritoneal dialysis cycling machine. While it is too early to determine comparative data with these treatment modalities, there would appear to be no specific contra-indication in the older age group provided visual and motor skills are intact. The therapeutic approach to a patient in the geriatric age group therefore involves considerations similar to those for younger patients. While the overall outcome is predictably poorer for older patients, haemodialysis, transplantation and ambulatory peritoneal dialysis can all potentially provide effective treatment in a given patient.

SUMMARY AND CONCLUSIONS

Maintaining the health of the older patient represents a challenge to the physician. The disorders of homeostasis serve to emphasise the ways in which the body changes with time. At baseline in the healthy older person, the kidney functions at a level which preserves the internal environment despite the fact that the aging process has caused a diminution in absolute function and a narrowing of the breadth of response that the kidney can make to a given alteration of the internal environment. These changes must be taken into account when the patient becomes ill. Not only may baseline nutritional, electrolyte and fluid requirements change, but the physician must take care to avoid giving either too much or too little of these dietary or parenteral elements to the older patient. It must be remembered that the remarkable flexibility of the younger kidney to retain salt and water in the face of marked deprivation or excrete large quantities of salt and water when intake is high, is partially lost with age. The dangers of volume depletion due to deprivation or volume overload consequent to a high salt and water intake are ever present.

In addition to altered functional capacity, the aging kidney is exposed to a number of therapeutic insults which provide a greater danger to the aging patient than to younger persons. Aminoglycoside antibiotic or digitalis overdose due to an overestimation of functional reserve of the kidney is common. It is emphasised that a normal serum creatinine or 'slightly elevated' serum creatinine does not indicate a normal glomerular filtration rate by the standards of younger patients. Doses of these agents may have to be altered to take into account the normally expected decrease of renal function due to the aging process (10ml/decade after the age of 30) as well as the effects of intercurrent acute and chronic illnesses. The older patient is also more likely to receive therapeutic agents which have potentially serious adverse effects on the kidney. The increased use of non-steroidal anti-inflammatory agents, including aspirin, for various forms of degenerative arthritis, may pose a serious threat to renal function. These agents must be used only when necessary and with great caution, including monitoring of the serum creatinine regularly.

Lastly, the aging kidney is susceptible to all those diseases affecting younger age groups and appropriate diagnostic and the therapeutic procedures are required when a kidney lesion occurs. Elderly patients with end stage renal failure, while having a higher death rate than those who are younger (but not necessarily more youthful), deserve full consideration for end stage renal failure programmes, where the overall results of survival and rehabilitation provide a potential future for these patients.

Acknowledgements

1. Supported in part by donations to the General Nephrology Research Fund (EJ Lewis) and by the John Simon Guggenheim Jr. Memorial Foundation, and the Commonwealth Fund (RM Kark)
2. We wish to thank Helen Follmer, Janet Iapichino and Julia E Kark for their assistance.

The opinions expressed in this chapter are the private ones of the authors and are not to be construed as official pronouncements of the Veterans Administrations.

REFERENCES

Adelman M, Evans E, Schentag J J 1982 Two compartment-comparison of gentamicin and tobramycin in normal volunteers. Antimicrobial Agents and Chemotherapy 22: 800–804

Addis T, Oliver J 1931 The renal lesion in Bright's disease. Paul B Hoeber Inc, New York, p 553

Addis T 1940 The osmotic work of the kidney and the treatment of glomerular nephritis. Transactions of the Association of American Physicians 50: 223–229

Addis T 1984 Glomerular Nephritis. Diagnosis and treatment. MacMillan Company. New York

Appel G B, Kunis C L 1983 Acute tubulo-interstitial nephritis. In: Cotran J H (ed) Tubulo-interstitial nephropathies, Churchill Livingstone, New York p 243

Arruda J A L 1983 Obstructive uropathy. In: Cotran R S, Brenner B M, Stein J H (eds) Tubulo-interstitial nephropathies, Churchill Livingstone, New York p 243

Avorn J 1981 Nursing home infectious — the context. New England Journal of Medicine 305: 759–760

Beaufils H, Alphonse J C, Legrain M 1978 Focal glomerulosclerosis: natural history and treatment. Nephron 21: 75–85

Bennett W M 1983 The adverse renal effects of anti-inflammatory drugs: increasing problems of overrated risk. American Journal of Kidney Diseases 2: 477

Berenyi M R, Straus B 1969 Hyperosmolar states in the chronically ill. Journal of the American Geriatric Society 17: 648–658

Bergan T 1982 The role of broad-spectrum antibiotics and diagnostic problems in urinary tract infections. Archives of Internal Medicine 142: 1993–1999

Bichet D C, Schrier R W 1982 Renal function and diseases in the aged. In: Schrier W R (ed) Clinical Internal Medicine in the Elderly. W. B. Saunders Company, Philadelphia

Bolton W K, Westervelt F B Jr, Sturgill B C 1978 Nephrotic syndrome and focal glomerulosclerosis in aging man. Nephron 20: 307–315

Boswell D C and Eknoyan G 1968 Acute glomerlonephritis in the aged. Geriatrics 23: 73–80

Brenner B M, Meyer T W, Hostetter T H 1982 Dietary protein intake and the progressive nature of kidney disease: the role of hemodynamically mediated glomerular injury in the pathogenesis of progressive sclerosis in aging, renal ablation, and intrinsic renal disease. New England Journal of Medicine 307: 652–659

Brody L H, Webster M C, Kark R M 1968 Identification of urinary sediment with phase-contrast microscopy. Journal of the American Medical Association 206: 1777–1781

Cockcroft D W, Gault M H 1976 Prediction of creatinine clearance from serum creatinine. Nephron 16: 31–41

DeFronzo R A, Humphrey R L, Wright J R, Cooke C R 1975 Acute renal failure in multiple myeloma. Medicine 54: 209–223

Edelman I S, Liebman J 1959 Anatomy of body water and electrolytes. American Journal of Medicine 27: 256–277

Edelman I S, Haley H B, Schloerb P R, Sheldon D B, Friis-Hansen B J, Stoll G, Moore F D 1952 Further observations on total body water: I. Normal values throughout the life span. Surgery, Gynecology and Obstetrics 95: 1–12

Eagen J W, Lewis E J 1977 Glomerulopathies of neoplasia. Kidney International 11: 297–306

Epstein M, Hollenberg N K 1976 Age as a determinant of renal sodium conservation in normal man. Journal of Laboratory and Clinical Medicine 87: 411–417

Epstein M 1979 Effects of aging on the kidney. Federation Proceedings 38: 168–172

Fawcett I W, Hilton P J, Jones N F, Wing K 1971 Nephrotic syndrome in the elderly. British Medical Journal 2: 223–224

Feig P U, McCuroy D K 1977 The hypertonic state. New England Journal of Medicine 297: 1444–1454

Garibaldi R A, Brodine S, Malsuniya S 1981 Infections among patients in nursing homes: policies, prevalence and problems. New England Journal of Medicine 305: 731–735

Gault M H, Dixon M, Doyle M, Cohen W M 1968 Hypernatremia, azotemia, and dehydration due to high protein tube feeding. Annals of Internal Medicine 68: 778–791

Gennari F J, Kassirer J P 1974 Osmotic diuresis. New England Journal of Medicine 291: 714–720

Griffith G J, Robinson K B, Cartwright G O, McLachlan M S F 1976 Loss of renal tissue in the elderly. British Journal of Radiology 49. 111–117

Heptinstall R H 1983 Pathology of the Kidney. 3rd Edition, Little, Brown Company, Boston

Hollenberg N K, Adams D F, Solomon H S, Rasbid A, Abnerus H L, Merrill J P 1974 Senescence and the renal vasculature in normal man. Circulation Research 34: 309–316

Kaplan C, Pasternack B, Shah H, Gallo G 1975 Age-related incidence of sclerotic glomeruli in human kidneys. American Journal of Pathology 80: 227–234

Kark R M, Netter F H 1976 Examination of the Urine, Section III Diagnostic Technique. In: Shafter R K (ed) Netter F H Kidney, Ureter and Bladder. The Ciba Collection of Medical Illustrations, Ciba, Summit, New Jersey p 71

Krakauer H, Grauman J S, McMullan M R, Creede C C 1983 The recent US experience in the treatment of end-stage renal disease by dialysis and transplantation. New England Journal of Medicine 308: 1558–1563

Lewis E J, Foster D M, DeLapuente J, Scurlock C 1969 Survival data for patients undergoing intermittent hemodialysis. Annals of Internal Medicine 70: 311–315

Lindner A, Charra B, Sherrard D J, Scribner B H 1974 Accelerated atherosclerosis in prolonged maintenance hemodialysis. New England Journal of Medicine 290: 697–706

Linton D L, Clark W F, Driedger A A, Turnball D L, Lindsay R M 1980 Acute interstitial nephritis due to drugs — review of the literature with a report of nine cases. Annals of Internal Medicine 93: 735–741

McLachlan M S F, Gaunt A, Fulker M J, Anderson C K 1976 Estimation of glomerular size and number from radiographs of the kidney. British Journal of Radiology 49: 831–835

McLachlan M S F 1978 The aging kidney. Lancet 2: 143–145

Minaker K L, Rowe J W 1981 Behavioural manifestations of renal disease in the elderly. In: Levinson A J, Hall R W (eds) Neuropsychiatric manifestations of physical disease in the elderly, Raven Press, New York p 93

Montoliu J, Darnell A, Torras A, Revert L 1982 Acute and rapidly progressive forms of glomerulonephritis in the elderly. Journal of the American Geriatrics Society 29: 108–116

Moore R A 1931 The total number of glomeruli in normal human kidney. Anatomical Records 48: 153–168

Moorthy A V and Zimmerman S W 1981 Renal disease in the elderly: clinicopathologic analysis of renal disease in 115 elderly patients. Clinical Nephrology 5: 223–229

Neff M S, Eiser A R, Slifkin R F, Baum M, Baez A, Gupta S, Amarga E 1983 Patients surviving ten years of hemodilaysis. American Journal of Medicine 74: 996–1004

Oliver J 1939 Architecture of the Kidney in Chronic Bright's Disease. Paul B. Hoeber Inc, New York

Ouslander J G, Kane R I, Abrass I B 1982 Urinary incontinence in elderly nursing home patients. Journal of the American Medical Association 248: 1191–1198

Roberts J L 1975 Analysis and outcome of 1063 patients trained for home hemodialysis. Kidney International 9: 363–374

Rostand S G, Gretes J C, Kirk A A, Rutsky E A, Andredi T E 1979 Ischemic heart disease in the hemodialysis population. Proceedings of the Clinical Dialysis Transplantation Forum 9: 44–49

Row P G, Cameron J S, Turner D R, Evans D J, White R H R, Ogg C S, Chantler C, Brown C B 1975 Membranous nephropathy: long term follow up and association with neoplasia. Quarterly Journal of Medicine 44: 207–239

Rowe J W 1980 Aging and renal function. In: Eisdorfer C (ed) Annual Review of Gerontology and Geriatrics, Springer, New York, p 161

Rowe J W, Robertson G L 1978 Age-related failure of volume-pressure medicated vasopressin release in man. Kidney International 14: 660

Rowe J W, Andres R, Tobin J D, Norris A H, Shock N W 1976 The effect of age on creatinine clearance in men: a cross sectional and longitudinal study. Journal of Gerontology 31: 155–163

Schrier W R (ed) 1982 Clinical Internal Medicine in the Aged. W B Saunders Company, Philadelphia.

Schwartz T B, Appelbaum R I 1965–66 Nonketotic diabetic coma. In: Yearbook Medical Publishers, Chicago, p 165

Shea S M, Raskov A J, Morrison A B 1980 Ultrastructure of glomerular basement membrane of rats with proteinuria due to subtotal nephrectomy. American Journal of Pathology 100: 513–528

Siersbaek-Nielsen K, Molholm Hansen J, Kampmann J, Kristensen 1971 Nomogram for rapid evaluation of endogenous creatinine clearance. Lancet 2: 1133–1134

Snyder W S, Cook M J, Nasset E S, Karhausen L R, Howells G P, Tipton I H 1975 Report on the Task Group on Reference Man, International Commission on Radiological Protection, No. 23, Pergamon Press, Oxford, p 338

Sorahan T, Kokoszynska R, Adams R G 1982 Trends in mortality from nephritis and nephrosis. Lancet 1: 567–570

Tunn V W, Thieme H 1982 Sepsis associated with urinary tract infection. Archives of Internal Medicine 142: 2035–2038

44

Diseases of the bladder and prostate

P. H. L. Worth

AGE CHANGES IN THE BLADDER

Bladder structure and function alter with age, even in the absence of any local pathology. The changes in function, which are likely to result in incontinence are discussed in the next chapter.

There have been many studies on the prevalence of urinary symptoms in older patients. Stress incontinence in females is found in 57% but in very few men. Pain passing urine may be the presenting urinary complaint in under 5% of patients, but 75% of women and 50% of men will give a past history. Urinary infection is three times as common in women as in men, occurring in 10% of the latter. Under 10% will have a history of frequency on presentation, but this is a symptom that increases with age eventually affecting 70%. Interestingly slightly more women than men get up at least twice at night, although nocturia is present in about 50% of people (Milne et al, 1972).

The incidence of trabeculation and pseudodiverticula is very common in elderly women. Is there an organic basis for obstruction in women or is it due to inco-ordinated detrusor and urethral function? In the male it is easy to incriminate the prostate, but there is no good evidence that a homologous structure exists in women although there are a few protagonists. Careful examination of post-mortem specimens suggested the basis for the changes was probably neuropathic and the inflammatory changes seen at the bladder neck were secondary (Brocklehurst, 1972). Von Brunn's nests are a normal finding in the submucosa of the bladder, but an increased number were found and this was thought to be due to irritation of the bladder epithelium. When glandular ducts get blocked mucus crypts develop. All this gives rise to thickening of the bladder wall and is in no way related to hormonal changes. It is possible that these glandular changes could be precursors of neoplastic change.

Trabeculation as already mentioned is very commonly seen in the aging bladder and is not always associated with detrusor instability or obstruction. In fact it may be due to a decrease in the amount of collagen that gives a false impression of the extent of the trabeculation. In the female the trigonal and urethral epithelium may change to stratified squamous epithelium, which is oestrogen sensitive. In addition the vascularity of the submucosal layer may alter. This is under adrenergic control and may account for the decreased urethral resistance that occurs with age in the female.

URINARY TRACT INFECTION

Urinary infection may present with the symptoms associated with cystitis, but in females it may present with incontinence. The appropriate antibiotics should be given. If the infection is associated with an indwelling catheter it will be very difficult to eradiate and in this situation it is not strictly necessary to treat. However maintaining a good fluid intake and changing the urinary pH — potassium citrate to make it alkaline and vitamin C or mandelamine to make it acid may be helpful. With severe catheter encrustation washouts with hibitane 5% or noxyflex may be necessary. Of course it is important to exclude diabetes in any patient presenting with a urinary infection.

In a man it is important to be certain that the bladder is emptying efficiently and if there is good evidence of obstruction this should be dealt with. In the female stones in the upper tracts must be excluded and it is important to exclude any local gynaecological problem such as prolapse, and to look for oestrogen lack. If it is not possible to eradicate the infection an intravenous pyelogram (IVP) should be carried out, followed by cystoscopy to exclude bladder cancer.

Chronic cystitis, of which interstitial cystitis is an example, gives rise to severe pain and frequency, but is not usually associated with bacterial infection. The bladder mucosa bleeds easily on decompression and there may be characteristic histological appearances. Treatment is difficult, but simple bladder distension may be very effective. Provided that cancer and specific infections such as tuberculosis have been excluded there are two courses of action available. If the bladder can be stretched to a reasonable capacity under general anaesthetic a sensory denervation can be performed, but if the capacity is fixed and small an augmentation cystoplasty using caecum should be considered. This will abolish the pain and give the patient a satisfactory capacity and is preferable to doing a urinary diversion. Age is not a contra-indication to this procedure and good results have been achieved in patients in their seventies (Worth & Turner-Warwick, 1973).

It should be remembered that bowel pathology may present with urinary symptoms because of the proximity of the sigmoid colon to the bladder, especially in the male. Diverticular disease may produce a fistula, but the presence of pneumaturia as a symptom may not be admitted to by the patient who may only have the symptoms of cystitis. Once the diagnosis has been made treatment should be directed at the bowel pathology.

CARCINOMA OF THE BLADDER

The classical presentation of bladder cancer is painless haematuria. If ignored as a symptom or treated inappropriately with antibiotics and allowed to recur, the individual is likely to develop painful frequency and haematuria on account of associated infection. Carcinoma in situ however, may present without any bleeding, but with troublesome frequency and bladder pain and should not be confused with developing obstruction. In women bladder tumours often present with symptoms suggestive of urinary infection. When painless bleeding does occur there is often confusion in the individual's mind as to whether or not the bleeding is gynaecological in origin.

About 30% of bladder cancers occur in the over-seventies and as in other age groups it is twice as common in men as in women. Clinical examination may be very unrewarding. Before carrying out a cystoscopy, which is mandatory in every case, full investigation is necessary. An IVP may give some information about the type of tumour to expect — if high grade and infiltrating a ureter may be obstructed. Cytological screening will be positive in at least 60% at presentation (and in 70% of recurrent lesions).

Tumour staging

At the time of the initial cystoscopy, when a biopsy is taken, it is important to stage the tumour as accurately as possible, because further management will depend on this information as well as the additional help from the pathologists on the histology of the biopsy material (Fig. 44.1). Carcinoma in situ is recognised by red patches on the wall of the bladder without any exophytic lesions. Ta and T1 lesions may be single or multiple papillary lesions. If there is evidence of cancer in the base of the tumour which has breached the lamina propria it is a T1 P1 lesion, otherwise it is a Ta Pa case. A careful bimanual examination should always be done with the patient well relaxed and the bladder empty, but one would not expect to feel any mass with this staging. Once there is evidence of muscle invasion on histology, the tumour is staged T2, but

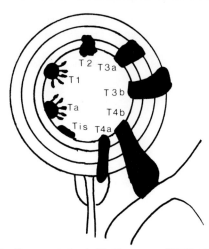

Fig. 44.1 Tumour staging in bladder cancer. TIS Flat in situ tumour; TA Papillary tumour not invading the lamina propria; TI Papillary tumour invading the lamina propria; T2 Tumour invading superficial muscle; T3a Tumour invading deep muscle, but confined to the bladder wall; T3b Tumour extending into perivesical fat and mobile; T4a Tumour involving prostate; T4b Tumour involving adjoining organs and fixed to side wall of pelvis.

it may not always be possible to differentiate this tumour from a T1 endoscopically. Again it is unlikely that any mass will be palpable unless the tumour is very extensive.

T3 tumours are divided into T3a, which are confined to the bladder wall and T3b, which extend beyond the bladder wall. In both a mass will be palpable, but it should be freely mobile.

T4 tumours are also divided into two groups; T4a invade the prostate and T4b invade the adjacent organs and on bimanual examination a fixed mass may be palpable.

Management

Carcinoma in situ is a worrying situation because 50% may become infiltrating within a year. Unfortunately they do not respond to radiotherapy and therefore cystectomy will have to be considered. It may be possible to contain the disease by either systemic cyclophosphamide or intravesical mitomycin and the patient should be followed by cytology.

If the disease is superficial local resection and diathermy at appropriate intervals will usually keep the disease under control. Topical chemotherapy may reduce recurrences, but should only be used for Ta Pa disease. Radiotherapy is reserved for cases resistant to therapy and sometimes cystectomy will have to be undertaken.

Once the disease has invaded the bladder muscle endoscopic control is no longer possible, except for low grade P2 lesions. Cystectomy is not usually considered for people over 70 and so it is likely that the more advanced disease will be treated with radiotherapy and the results can be very encouraging. However, if the disease recurs and causes a lot of local symptoms urinary diversion should be avoided because it does not help local symptoms. In a fit patient and in the under 70s provided there is no evidence of secondaries on chest X-ray or computed tomography (CT) scanning of the abdomen, cystectomy can be considered.

If bleeding is a major problem, Helmstein's distension, when the bladder is distended under epidural anaesthesia at approximately systolic blood pressure for six hours, may be very effective in stopping the bleeding (England et al, 1973). A small dose of radiotherapy may also be very helpful. When metastases are present and surgery is not indicated methotrexate may control the disease and the symptoms for a shortwhile (Hall et al, 1974).

The outlook for bladder cancer depends very much on the staging and histological grading of the disease. T1 tumours have an 80% five year survival, whereas T2 tumours can expect about a 50% five year survival. Once the tumour is deeply invasive as in T3 staging the survival is 25%. However when patients have fixed T4 lesions they are all likely to be dead within a year.

BENIGN AND MALIGNANT PROSTATIC DISEASE

Although there has been an immense amount of work done on the production of testosterone and related compounds in the male, the mechanism of breakdown and distribution of these compounds in the body and in the prostate, no-one has yet produced a satisfactory explanation for the development of benign hypertrophy of the prostate or the development of carcinoma. However it is well known that castrated males do not develop benign hyperplasia.

The major production of testosterone is in the testis, but the adrenal produces a small amount. It is carried in the blood bound to a protein, but it is the unbound hormone that is active. As men get older the serum testosterone (T) levels fall as do also 5a dihydrotestosterone (DHT) which is the primary breakdown compound of testosterone.

Steroid receptor proteins have been demonstrated in the prostatic cells. They are occupied, in the main, by endogenous androgens and the proportion occupied is proportional to the level of circulating androgen. However the number of receptors is in no way related to the pathological condition of the gland. Various changes in hormones have been shown with age and differences can be demonstrated in benign and malignant disease. Testosterone levels are higher in patients with carcinoma than benign hyperplasia, whereas DHT levels are higher in benign hyperplasia than in carcinoma. The ratio of DHT-T is greatest in benign disease and lower in carcinoma than in the normal situation (Chisholm & Habib, 1981). Zinc has been found in the nucleus of prostatic epithelial cells and it has a higher concentration in normal cells than in malignant cells.

PROSTATIC OBSTRUCTION

As men get older the incidence of prostatic obstruction increases but only about 10% of all men will require surgical treatment. However it is likely that 70–75% of all men undergoing prostatectomy are over the age of 65 (Graham, 1977).

The symptoms of obstruction, whether due to benign prostatic enlargement, carcinoma, urethral stricture or bladder neck obstruction are well recognised. If the history is very long it may suggest a bladder neck problem, and if very short and severe it may relate to carcinoma. Difficulty in initiating micturition, poor urinary flow, intermittent flow, terminal dribbling and incomplete emptying are all symptoms of obstruction. Frequency by day, nocturia, urgency and urge incontinence are the symptoms due to the bladder response to the obstruction and relate to detrusor instability. Frequency is a symptom that needs careful investigation and is not per se an indication for operation. As has already been mentioned in the section on urodynamics, one is just as likely to be able to demonstrate obstruction and instability as the cause of the symptoms as instability alone, and if the patient is in the latter group the results of surgery can be disastrous. In the elderly patient it is very likely that other contributory causes for the instability will be present, such as previous stroke, atherosclerosis or Parkinson's disease. However one cannot measure the contribution of an underlying neurological condition or of obstruction. One can however, advise the patient as to likelihood of resolution of symptoms after the relief of obstruction.

Management

The traditional indications for surgical treatment of prostatic obstruction are really very unimpressive. With the availability of urodynamics it should be possible to decide which patient needs surgery, whether his symptoms will resolve quickly or slowly or whether surgery is inadvisable.

The symptoms as have been discussed can be very misleading. The size of the prostate is irrelevant: abnormalities seen on a standard IVP may be late changes which only appear once bladder decompensation has occurred. Ideally one should operate before the changes occur and before a residual urine becomes significant. Bladder trabeculation is not synonomous with obstruction and trying to decide on the endoscopic appearances, whether or not a prostate needs removing is very inaccurate.

Acute retention

Not every patient who develops acute retention requires prostatectomy. There may be a number of precipitating causes such as constipation, enforced bed rest required for the management of some intercurrent illness or following some other surgical procedure. Catheterisation is obviously

DISEASES OF THE BLADDER AND PROSTATE 381

required for the acute stage, but if the individual denies any symptoms of prostatic obstruction prior to the retention he may succeed in re-establishing micturition once the precipitating cause has been dealt with.

If pressure measurements are done in acute retention, the bladder pressure is often quite low, but a urethral pressure profile shows a raised pressure in the mid-prostatic urethra (Caine & Perlberg, 1977). It has also been shown that phenoxybenzamine, an α-blocker, lowers the proximal urethral pressure and may increase the maximum urinary flow rate and decrease the residual urine (Caine et al, 1978) and it has been used to re-establish micturition in acute retention (Boreham et al, 1977). The drug should be used with caution in the elderly because it may cause dizziness and postural hypotension in about 30% of patients.

Chronic retention
Having already suggested that not every patient who develops acute retention requires surgery, it is likely that if he has chronic retention he will need an operation. Very often it is the smaller prostate that causes chronic retention and this may be a manifestation of a long-standing bladder neck problem. One will occasionally meet the patient with tabes dorsalis and therefore a careful neurological assessment is always indicated. Autonomic neuropathies may present in this way and therefore diabetes should be excluded. A patient with chronic retention requires catheterisation if he is significantly uraemic (blood urea in excess of 15 mmol/l) and sometimes it will be necessary to drain the bladder for convenience if he is in a state of overflow incontinence, just for the practical reason of making it easier to manage the patient. In chronic retention it is probably best to decompress the bladder over a 24 hour period to reduce the incidence of bleeding, but it will not effect the diuresis and sodium loss which will occur once the kidneys are allowed to drain more efficiently and effectively. This is something to watch for once the catheter is inserted, because an elderly and infirm patient may have great difficulty in maintaining an adequate fluid intake and if the sodium loss is significant this in itself will cause trouble and it may be necessary to supplement the fluid intake by putting up an intravenous infusion of isotonic saline.

It cannot be stressed too often that it is important to be sure that a patient's symptoms are due to obstruction before he is subjected to prostatectomy. If his symptoms are due solely to detrusor instability without obstruction, the patient will firstly be no better symptomatically without his prostate and secondly he may well be worse when he has not got his bladder neck mechanism and relies solely on his distal urethral mechanism.

Alternatives to surgery have been pursued by various enthusiasts for many years. Although many drugs of various chemical compositions have been prescribed to try to decrease the size of the prostate there is little objective evidence to suggest that there is any improvement even when the patients claim subjective improvement (Claridge, 1975). Injecting the prostate with phenol in acetic acid may cause sufficient reaction to shrink the prostate to allow a patient to pass urine but there is no evidence to suggest that it improves a patient who is not in retention (Angel, 1969).

Prostatectomy
Provided the patient is physically fit and requires treatment one can offer him a safe operation with a low mortality and morbidity (Chilton et al, 1978). In a modern urological department 95% of prostatectomies are done trans-urethrally and the mortality is less than 3%. If the patient is admitted as an emergency the mortality will be trebled and it is the increased incidence of infection and impaired renal function in these cases that is of major importance.

If the patient has had a recent myocardial infarct it is wiser to defer surgery for 3–6 months. If the patient has had a stroke and has made a poor recovery and is operated on within a year the symptomatic results of surgery are likely to be very poor. However it is probably better to have a patient who can empty his bladder completely rather than having a patient in retention who relies entirely on a catheter, because the incidence of infective problems will be much higher in the retained patient and any problem with his catheter is an emergency.

Surgical techniques have changed over the past 15 years mainly because of improved surgical armamentarium. The solid rod lens system designed by Professor H H Hopkins has been a major advance. Fibre lighting means better illumination and with the improved solid state diathermy machines the ease and efficiency of resecting the prostate have made a tremendous difference. All this has meant that the majority of prostatectomies can now be done endoscopically, and it is now very rare to do an open prostatectomy. Most prostates are of a reasonable size but every urologist has a limit to the size of the gland that he is prepared to resect, and not every prostate has to be resected. Firstly the big glands take a long time to resect. This may be unpopular with the anaesthetist and there is the additional problem of the transurethral resection (TUR) syndrome. This relates to the amount of irrigating fluid that flows into the patient during the time of the resection. If the pressure of the irrigating fluid is kept high while the blood pressure is kept low, the influx of fluid into the patient's veins in the prostatic fossa may be of the order of 1–2 litres in a long resection. If an isotonic solution is used (usually 1.5% glycine) haemolysis will not occur but the patient's circulating volume will be increased, cardiac failure may occur and the patient may develop water intoxication which manifests itself as restlessness post-operatively or even unconsciousness. The situation should be recognised and a serum sodium estimation may show it to be quite low (110–130 mmol/l) and occasionally very much lower at 100 mmol/l.

It is essential to eliminate the fluid by promoting a diuresis. If a diuretic is given, an intravenous infusion of saline should be set up so that the serum sodium is not further reduced.

In the post-operative period it is important to maintain satisfactory drainage from the catheter and this can be achieved by using a three way irrigating catheter. Although nowadays a TUR is such a routine procedure it is probably best to manage the patient on a urological ward until the catheter is removed and the patient is voiding satisfactorily. Routine antibiotics are not necessary, but if an urinary infection is present it should be treated with the appropriate antibiotic. If the patient has had an indwelling urethral catheter there is a chance of an infection developing within three days of the catheter being put in. Infection certainly increases the morbidity; secondary haemorrhage is more common and septicaemia is a real risk. It might well be sensible to give the patient an intravenous bolus of a broad spectrum antibiotic at the start of the operation to reduce this risk.

CARCINOMA OF THE PROSTATE

The incidence of carcinoma of the prostate is rising in this country. About 6000 new cases are diagnosed a year, but in addition many cases must go undetected because there are no symptoms. Among men aged 80 years, 80% will have histological evidence of cancer. Screening tests have not helped in making an earlier diagnosis as 80% still present with advanced disease and 33% of carcinomas will present with metastatic disease without urinary symptoms.

If carcinoma of the prostate causes outflow obstruction there are no specific symptoms to distinguish the condition from obstruction caused by benign hyperplasia. Severe symptoms of short duration may suggest it, but haematuria is not a characteristic feature. The diagnosis may be easy to make on rectal examination, but often it is only made as an incidental finding on histology following prostatic surgery. There are no distinctive features on standard urography to suggest the diagnosis, but sclerotic deposits may be visible in the lumbar spine. Renal function may be quite normal; with bony involvement the serum alkaline phosphatase will be raised. With focal disease the acid phosphatase is likely to be normal, but once the disease has spread beyond the confines of the gland both the total and prostatic fraction of the acid phosphatase will be raised. Radio-immuneassay of acid phosphatase is very sensitive and may well be raised with focal disease. In the absence of urinary symptoms a prostatic resection is not indicated but prostatic tissue should be obtained for diagnosis. Franzen aspiration cytology (Franzen et al, 1960) is 82% reliable and can be done as an out-patient procedure. Trucut perineal or transrectal biopsy under antibiotic cover is 95% accurate (Hendry & Williams, 1971). Once the diagnosis has been made a bone scan should be carried out to detect metastatic disease. This examination is 10% more accurate than conventional X-rays. However the two should be compared because Paget's disease and severe osteoarthritis may give false positives.

At the time of prostatic biopsy or resection the tumour should be staged according to the UICC, because further management depends on this (Fig. 44.2). Lymphography for N. staging is not necessary in this age group — if at all,

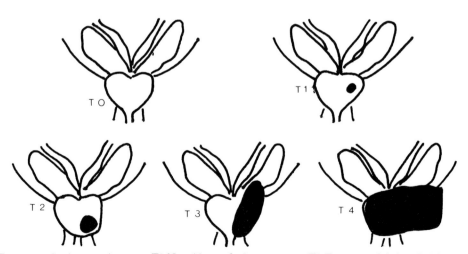

Fig. 44.2 Tumour staging in prostatic cancer. T0 No evidence of primary tumour; T1 Tumour nodule in palpably normal gland; T2 Smooth nodule deforming contour of gland; T3 Tumour extending beyond capsule or into seminal vesicles; T4 Tumour fixed or invading neighbouring structures.

because firstly it is difficult to do and the interpretation is difficult. Once there is lymph node involvement it is likely that there will also be bony involvement and bone scanning is a much easier procedure to carry out and better for the patient.

Management

It has been shown that carcinoma of the prostate is oestrogen sensitive in the majority of cases. Here therefore is a simple way of controlling the disease. However the administration of oestrogen may have a considerable morbidity from increased cardiovascular complications and marked fluid retention. Other problems are nausea and vomiting, gynaecomastia, which can be quite painful, and impotence.

If oestrogens work by suppressing testosterone levels it has been shown that 1 mg of stilboestrol three times a day is quite adequate and so the much bigger doses previously used, 50 mg three times a day, are not necessary and therefore the side effects can be considerably reduced. The Veterans Administration Co-operative Urological Research Group (VACURG, 1967; Byar, 1977), raised this query when much larger doses were being used and the morbidity and mortality from the side effects of the hormones were greater than the mortality from the disease itself. With the smaller dose now used this argument is not so valid, but administering small doses of oestrogen to men over the age of 75 is potentially dangerous.

The question has therefore to be asked whether treatment is justified in the presence of focal disease. With well differentiated disease, which probably represents less than 5% of all cases, no treatment is necessary. However if the histology suggests it is undifferentiated 20% will progress and so early treatment is justified.

Oestrogens and antiandrogens are not now considered for primary treatment for non-metastatic disease. They are reserved for metastatic disease. An alternative is orchidectomy, or more usually subcapsular orchidectomy. This however is not particularly popular even with the older patient. Sometimes it is reserved for patients who have escaped from hormonal control, but Stone et al (1980) have shown that there is no evidence to suggest that orchidectomy in these circumstances is a justifiable procedure.

External beam radiotherapy gives good results and it is probably wise to use this form of treatment in early cases and in localised T3 and T4 disease, giving 48% five year and 30% ten year survival. It is also very useful in treating painful metastases. A recent advance has been the introduction of intraprostatic radioactive iodine implants using rectal ultrasound localisation.

Several chemotherapeutic agents have been identified as being useful in treating escaped cancer. Perhaps the most popular is the combination of oestrogen and nitrogen mustard as estracyt (Chisholm et al, 1977). When widespread bony pain is a major problem hypophysectomy using yttrium introduced trans-sphenoidally gives 71% response (Fitzpatrick et al, 1980).

A major part of a urologist's workload is involved with patients in the geriatric age group. I do not think that this particularly alters one's approach. However, there is no point in being over-enthusiastic in treating advanced bladder cancer in the elderly, but many symptoms can be helped, without resorting to major surgery. With the low mortality associated with prostatectomy one is able to offer a procedure which will make living much more comfortable. Cancer of the prostate is a common condition, but luckily treatment is mainly non-surgical and very successful. We now know a lot about incontinence and there is plenty that can be done to alleviate this symptom and help patients in a practical way. The elderly patient with urinary problems is well worth assessing very carefully and distressing symptoms may be relatively easy to treat.

REFERENCES

Angel J C 1969 Treatment of benign prostatic hypertrophy by phenol injection. British Journal of Urology 41: 735–738

Boreham P F, Braithwaite P, Milewski P, Pearson H 1977 Alpha-adrenergic blockers in prostatism. British Journal of Surgery 64: 756–757

Brocklehurst J C 1972 Bladder outlet obstruction in elderly women. Modern Geriatrics 2: 108–113

Byar D P 1977 VACURG studies on prostatic cancer and its treatment. In: Tannenbaum M (ed) Urologic Pathology: the Prostate. Lea and Febiger, New York, p 241–267

Caine M, Perlberg S 1977 Dynamics of acute retention in prostatic patients and role of adrenergic receptors. Urology 9: 399–403

Caine M, Perlberg S, Meretyk S 1978 A placebo-controlled double-blind study of the effect of phenoxybenzamine in benign prostatic obstruction. British Journal of Urology 50: 551–554

Chilton C P, Morgan R J, England H R, Paris A M I, Blandy J P 1978 A critical evaluation of the results of transurethral resection of the prostate. British Journal of Urology 50: 542–546

Chisholm G D, Habib F K 1981 Prostatic cancer: Experimental and clinical advances. In: Hendry W F (ed) Recent Advances in Urology/Andrology. Churchill Livingstone, Edinburgh, p 211–232

Chisholm G D, O'Donoghue E P N, Kennedy C L 1977 The treatment of oestrogen-escaped carcinoma of the prostate with estramustine phosphate. British Journal of Urology 49: 717–720

Claridge M 1975 Medical treatment of prostatic obstruction. An objective assessment. Investigative Urology 12: 401–404

England H R, Rigby C, Shepheard B G F, Tresidder G C, Blandy J P 1973 Evaluation of Helmstein's distension method for carcinoma of the bladder. British Journal of Urology 45: 593–599

Fitzpatrick J M, Gardiner R A, Williams J P, Riddle P R, O'Donoghue E P N 1980 Pituitary ablation in the relief of pain in advanced prostatic carcinoma. British Journal of Urology 52: 301–304

Franzen S, Giertz O, Zajicek J 1960 Cytological diagnosis of prostatic tumours by transrectal aspiration biopsy: a preliminary report. British Journal of Urology 32: 193–196

Graham A G 1977 Scottish prostates: a 6 year review. British Journal of Urology 49: 679–682

Hall R R, Bloom H J G, Freeman J E, Nawrocki A, Wallace D M 1974 Methotrexate treatment of advanced bladder cancer. British Journal of Urology 46: 431–438

Hendry W F, Williams J P 1971 Transrectal prostatic biopsy. British Medical Journal 4: 595–597

Milne J S, Williamson J, Malle M M, Wallace E T 1972 Urinary symptoms in older people. Modern Geriatrics 2: 198–212

Stone A R, Hargreave T B, Chisholm G D 1980 The diagnosis of oestrogen escape and the role of secondary orchiectomy in prostatic cancer. British Journal of Urology 52: 535–538

Veterans Administration Cooperative Urological Research Group 1967 Treatment and survival of patients with cancer of the prostate. Surgery, Gynecology and Obstetrics 124: 1011–1017

Worth P H L, Turner-Warwick R T 1973 The treatment of interstitial cystitis by cystolysis with observations on cystoplasty. British Journal of Urology 45: 65–71

45

Urinary incontinence

J. Malone-Lee

A patient presenting with urinary incontinence provides the clinician with a fascinating challenge which, if met successfully, will bring extremely rewarding results. It is difficult to overestimate the misery and suffering caused by this common condition and yet the resources available for its control are frequently neglected. Much can be achieved without recourse to sophisticated technology.

AETIOLOGY

Any failure in normal bladder behaviour may result in incontinence and therefore a clear understanding of bladder and urethral function is essential for a successful approach to the problem. The anatomy, pharmacology and physiology of these organs will first be discussed.

The anatomy

The smooth muscle fibres of the detrusor pass over the body of the bladder and are continued into the urethra as longitudinal fibres forming part of the urethral wall. They terminate in the distal urethra in the female and in the veruomontanum of the male. Contraction of these fibres causes a rise in bladder pressure and shortening of the urethra. The muscle fibres of the ureters are continued into the trigone which forms a base-plate at the bladder neck. Fibres continue from the trigone into the urethra and are inserted in a similar manner to the detrusor muscle. When the trigone contracts the bladder neck funnels. There are some smooth muscle fibres which arise in the detrusor and are inserted into the outer surface of the trigone distally. They tend to pull the plates of the trigone apart thus opening the bladder neck, (Brocklehurst, 1978; Hutch, 1972).

At the bladder neck there is a concentration of smooth muscle which is only developed significantly in the male. This is the internal sphincter and its main function is to prevent the retrograde flow of semen during ejaculation (Gosling et al, 1981).

The urethra is a distensible tube which produces a variable resistance to the flow of urine. The degree of resistance is dependent on the urethral elastic tissue, the pressure exerted by intra-mural arteriovenous sinuses, the smooth muscle of the walls, the surface tension of the urethral mucus, the external sphincter and the periurethral striated muscle (Gosling et al, 1981; Creed & Tulloch, 1982).

The external sphincter consists of circularly arranged striated muscle which is slow-twitch in character and capable of sustained continuous contractions. This muscle is quite separate from the periurethral striated muscle which is part of the pelvic sling and fast twitch in character. It should also be noted that the peri-urethral striated muscle aproaches the urethra from behind and does not encircle it. Both these muscles are supplied by somatic efferents from S 2, 3 and 4 which run quite separately from the pudendal nerves, (Brocklehurst, 1978; Hutch, 1972; Gosling et al, 1981; Creed & Tulloch, 1982).

The internal sphincter and the smooth muscle of the urethra and prostate are influenced both by the descending spinal pathways and the sympathetic input via the hypogastric plexus. The smooth muscle and voluntary sphincter mechanisms are also influenced by some neurones originating in the ventro-lateral aspect of the sacral cord. These packets of nerve cells are called 'Onuff Cells', after their discoverer. The Onuff cells are unaffected by the generalised neuronal destruction occurring in motor neurone disease and this may explain why sphincter function is preserved even in the very late stages of this illness. This phenomenon suggests that these sphincter influencing nerves are in some way separated from the central pathways. Both noradrenaline and acetylcholine have been detected in Onuff cells which explains why the external sphincter has been found to be influenced by alpha blockers (Rossier et al, 1980).

The prostate gland provides men with a considerable advantage over women in maintaining continence. It consists of a mixture of glandular tissue and smooth muscle. The latter is known to produce a constant resting tone and to influence the process of micturition (Caine et al, 1975) (Figs. 45.1 & 45.2).

The neuro-pharmacology

The greater bulk of the detrusor muscle is innervated by parasympathetic efferents originating from S 2, 3 and 4.

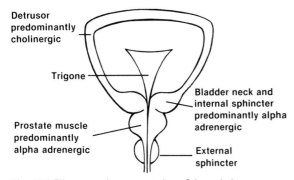

Fig. 45.1 Diagrammatic representation of the male lower urinary tract

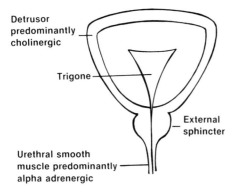

Fig. 45.2 Diagrammatic representation of the female lower urinary tract.

Their influence is excitatory and they are responsible for voiding. Scattered within the detrusor are a limited number of inhibitory beta 2 receptors and excitatory alpha 1 receptors both supplied by adrenergic neurones from the hypogastric plexus. There is evidence to suggest that in certain neurogenic bladders the alpha receptors play a more important role than usual (Fletcher & Bradley, 1978).

The muscle at the bladder neck is richly supplied with excitatory alpha 1 receptors, a number of excitatory cholinergic receptors and a few inhibitory beta 2 receptors (Fletcher & Bradley, 1978).

The smooth muscle of the urethra has a plentiful supply of excitatory alpha 1 receptors. These are also concentrated in the prostatic capsule and adenoma. There are some inhibitory beta 2 receptors in the urethral muscle but their significance is ill-understood, (Caine et al, 1975; Fletcher & Bradley, 1978).

The existence of atropine resistant transmission in both mammalian and human detrusor has been known for many years and accounts for between 30% and 40% of human detrusor activity. It has been suggested that the responsible receptors are purinergic and we do know that quinidine will block their activity (Eaton et al, 1981).

Hindmarsh et al (1977) showed that electrically induced, but not acetylcholine induced, contractions of human bladder muscle were potentiated by very low doses of 5HT and this potentiating effect was not altered by methysergide or morphine. Burnstock (1983) has recently described an inhibitory action of 5HT at the bladder neck.

The effects of prostaglandins F2 alpha and E2 were studied by Khalaf et al (1981) who found that prostaglandin E2 reduced urethral pressure and lowered the threshold for induced detrusor contractions. Prostaglandin F2 alpha in low dose raised urethral pressure but at higher doses also reduced the detrusor threshold.

Owman & Sjostrand (1965) reported fluorescent microscopic studies which demonstrated a rich innervation, with short adrenergic neurones, of the muscular tissue in the prostatic glands in various mammals. Caine et al (1975) reported on in vitro studies of the human prostate, prostatic capsule and bladder neck. The prostatic capsule was found to be very rich in both excitatory alpha and excitatory cholinergic receptors. The prostatic adenoma was moderately supplied with alpha receptors but cholinergic receptors were absent. Beta receptors were absent in the prostatic adenoma and a minimal presence was found in the capsule. When studying the effect of noradrenaline on the prostatic capsule they found that in some cases there was an extreme sensitivity to even very small concentrations of the drug. This would support the view that receptor super-sensitivity may play an important role in some cases of prostatism.

It has been known for a while that the female urethelium is oestrogen sensitive and that it degenerates, as does the vagina, with oestrogen reduction in old age. The result is an atrophic urethra which markedly reduces urethral function. Recently workers have identified large numbers of oestrogen receptors throughout the urethra and these are most concentrated in the distal two thirds. Progesterone receptors have not been detected though there is a sensitivity of the urethra to progesterone, (Wilson et al, 1981; Caine & Ras, 1973).

With the development of immunological methods, the identification of other transmitters in the central and peripheral nervous system has become possible. We now know that neurones innervating the striated sphincter and those innervating the smooth muscle of the detrusor are influenced by the somatostatinergic system (Daa Schrode 1981). There is evidence to suggest that VIP may have an important influence on the prostate (Burnstock, 1984).

The intravenous administration of the opioid antagonist naloxone markedly aggravates the reactivity of the unstable bladder. It has also been demonstrated that the intra-thecal administration of morphine reduces detrusor instability (Murray et al, 1982).

The complexity of the lower urinary tract neuro-anatomy helps to explain the failure of so many pharmacological agents in the treatment of incontinence.

The mechanisms of incontinence

Our understanding of the causes of incontinence has been greatly hampered by the plethora of muddling classifications of bladder pathologies. The subject can be made easier by viewing the pathophysiology as a continuum of varying factors rather than a series of separate diagnostic categories. A failure of one mechanism will influence the significance of pathology in another.

A bladder should store urine in volumes of around 500 ml without leaking. Once emptying becomes appropriate the detrusor needs to develop a sustained co-ordinated contraction that coincides with a similarly sustained relaxation of the sphincters and urethra.

The main neurological control of the bladder and urethra is exerted through the influence of the descending pathways passing from the brain to the sacral cord in the lateral columns. These are frequently, and inaccurately, referred to as the descending inhibitory pathways. They both inhibit and stimulate. In the brain the descending pathways communicate with the frontal lobe centres for micturition on the supero-medial aspect of both frontal lobes; the genu of the corpus callosum; the hypothalamus; the midbrain and the pons. During urine storage these pathways send inhibitory signals to the detrusor. During voiding they emit a series of signals that result in a co-ordinated completed micturition. In the sacral cord there is a reflex arc which if uninhibited will cause unsustained destrusor contractions in response to stimulation through bladder stretch receptors.

As stated earlier, the sphincters are influenced both by central pathways, the hypogastric plexus and the Onuff mechanisms. These all function to ensure an effective resistance to vesicle pressure rises during storage and a sustained adequate relaxation during voiding. It should be noted that the voluntary and involuntary sphincter mechanisms frequently function quite separately and both maintain continence in their own right under different circumstances.

If nerve fibres in the descending pathways carrying inhibitory impulses are damaged the result will be a 'detrusor instability'. The degree of instability will vary according to the extent of the damage. The typical symptoms precipitated will be frequency, nocturia, urgency, urge-incontinence and nocturnal enuresis.

If pathways responsible for voiding are damaged then detrusor activity will become unsustained with the result that voiding will tend to be incomplete. This leads to a chronic residual urine with recurrent infections which will greatly aggravate any existing instability.

Damage to the descending pathways will also affect sphincter function. The finely balanced co-ordination between sphincter relaxation and detrusor activity is lost and the patient has to void against a functional urethral obstruction. This phenomenon is referred to as 'detrusor-sphincter dyssynergia'. It is often very difficult to determine which sphincter mechanism is affected. The symptoms induced by dyssynergia involve hesitancy and a reduction in stream, together with problems incurred by a chronic residual.

A mixed bladder problem is more likely to occur if the lesion is sited where the different pathways co-exist. The spinal cord is an example of such an area. Consequently, patients suffering from multiple sclerosis or any other spinal lesion tend to present with a detrusor instability and a voiding problem secondary to unsustained detrusor activity or dyssynergia. Because of the nature of the causative lesions it is as likely that any of these problems may occur in isolation as in combination.

When assessing patients with an obvious neurological pathology, it is usually simple to identify the cause of the bladder lesion but a number of patients exhibit no neurological symptoms or signs. Under these circumstances, the label 'idiopathic' tends to be used. Caution is required here, as an isolated lesion of the urinary pathways will induce symptoms and signs solely in the lower urinary tract. There is no evidence to support the notion that adults experience symptoms of bladder failure because of neurotic psychological illness.

When a neurological lesion is sited at sacral level or in the peripheral nerves supplying the bladder and urethra then a hypotonic detrusor will result. Hypotonic sphincter failure may co-exist but is seen less frequently. The atonic bladder is most commonly encountered in sacral cord lesions and in diabetes. The typical symptoms are recurrent urinary tract infection, secondary to a chronic high residual, and persistent dribbling incontinence or precipitant incontinence. Women often describe stress incontinence and incontinence precipitated by standing is a strong indicator of hypotonia. Acute retention is a late sequel. It should be noted that, given a mixed pathology, it is quite possible for an instability to co-exist with a hypotonia and for both components to produce symptoms.

The most important sign pointing to any of the voiding problems is the demonstration of an abnormal residual volume by passing a Jacques catheter after micturition.

The sphincter incompetences usually result from physical damage due to childbirth or urethral instrumentation. De-oestrogenisation in later life tends to exacerbate a potentially incompetent urethra. The typical symptom is stress incontinence and an effort should be made to elicit this by examining a patient whilst she is standing, her bladder full and asking her to cough. It must be remembered that coughing and other stresses may induce unstable contractions and these can result in instability masquerading as sphincter incompetence. By the same token both conditions may co-exist.

The stress incontinence resulting from a failure of pelvic floor support will be associated with a urethral dislocation, a cystocele or a cystourethrocele. As the bladder neck drops down posteriorly the urethra may become kinked. The woman will then experience both sphincter incompetence and an intermittent obstruction which demands surgical correction.

The anatomical obstructive lesions of the outflow tract, such as prostatism or other strictures, may lead to incontinence. The term 'over-flow' incontinence is nebulous and rather misleading. I am impressed by the fact that patients with a pure obstruction experience voiding difficulties or complete retention without developing incontinence. Frequency, urgency and urge incontinence are often described by obstructed patients. The usual reason for this is that a detrusor instability tends to develop where a significant obstruction exists and clears with surgical correction. This suggests that the detrusor muscle, when exposed to localised pathology, reacts hyperactively even in the absence of a neurological lesion. A similar response is encountered during urinary infections. If an instability existed before the stricture then surgery will not affect it.

I have described a view of the important pathologies which may lead to incontinence. I would like to emphasise that often a mixed pathology is encountered and this demands careful diagnosis with management aimed at all aspects. A compartmentalised approach may lead to important factors being ignored. It is however essential not to become over-orientated towards the complex pathophysiology. It is quite possible to have a detrusor instability and remain totally continent until non-physiological events precipitate a breakdown. Attention to mobility, manual dexterity, access to lavatories or a transient urinary infection may re-establish continence. A hypotonic bladder may decompensate because of a faecal impaction. A demented patient, with a detrusor instability, who is unable to recognise a lavatory will not be rendered continent by treating the instability. Often these factors are over-emphasised with resultant errors. What is required is a careful conscientious assessment of all the contributory problems.

THE ASSESSMENT OF A PATIENT

The majority of patients presenting with urinary incontinence can be successfully assessed by using an algorithmic approach that does not necessarily demand complex investigations. The method described by Hilton & Stanton (1981) has proved effective in our unit, but with some modifications. The voiding efficiency needs to be measured by a catheterisation. Treating an asymptomatic urinary tract infection is unlikely to alter the symptoms. The possiblity of a mixed lesion needs to be constantly kept in mind.

Care is required in recognising the severity of symptoms. We recently completed a study on the volumes being lost by incontinent patients which demonstrated the very small quantities involved. Ambulant subjects showed a mean 4 hour loss of 10 ml and the incapacitated and highly dependent subjects showed a mean of just 60 ml. Despite these small figures, the incontinence was still having a devastating effect on the lives of the patients. We also noted that many subjects, using incontinence garments, experienced accidents very infrequently but the unpredictability and humiliation associated with these events caused great distress. To those not experiencing the symptoms themselves, the presentation may sometimes appear deceptively trivial.

When a voiding problem is detected, surgery is being considered or initial therapy has failed then a properly interpreted urodynamic study can prove invaluable.

The urodynamic investigation using pure pressure/flow cystometry or video cystometry has been described in a number of texts (Turner-Warwick & Whiteside, 1979; International Continence Society, 1976, 1977 & 1978). The basic principles are easy enough to grasp but accurate interpretation requires considerable practice. There is danger in trying to apportion single diagnostic categories rather than considering the effects of a summation of pathologies.

Two catheters are introduced into the bladder. One is used to fill the bladder with normal saline at a rate of about 60 ml/min. The other is connected to an external transducer mounted at pubic level which records the bladder pressure through the column of water inside the catheter. A representative measure of abdominal pressure is obtained through a rectal catheter, capped with a latex balloon to avoid faecal plugging. This rectal line is also connected to an external transducer mounted at pubic level. The rectal pressure is subtracted from the bladder pressure in order to obtain the intrinsic bladder pressure in cm H_2O. The proper placement of the various catheters and the recording of a balanced representation of abdominal pressure in both lines requires diligence and great care. The bladder is filled to 500 ml or the maximum volume tolerated while the pressures are recorded. At the end of fill the filling catheter is removed leaving both pressure catheters in situ. A stress test is performed standing. The patient is then asked to void while the pressures and voiding flow rate are recorded simultaneously. Once maximum flow rate is achieved the patient is asked to interrupt flow temporarily and then bladder emptying is completed. The interruption of flow, referred to as a 'stop test', gives important information on detrusor-urethral function during inhibition of flow, but only very rarely does it provide information on isometric detrusor function. At the end of micturition the voided volume is recorded and compared with the infused volume Figure 45.3.

The filling study provides information on the stability, compliance and capacity of the bladder. The International Continence Society criteria state that instability is present when uninhibited pressure rises occur during fill to a

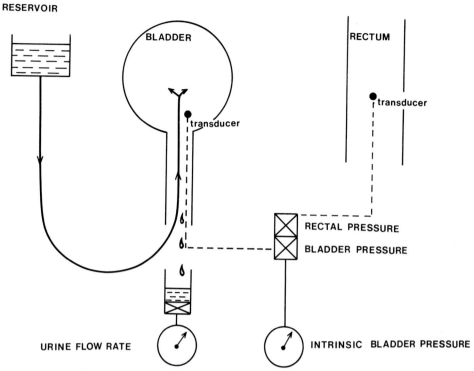

RESERVOIR

BLADDER

transducer

RECTUM

transducer

RECTAL PRESSURE

BLADDER PRESSURE

URINE FLOW RATE

INTRINSIC BLADDER PRESSURE

Fig. 45.3 Diagrammatic representation of a urodynamic study.

pressure of 15 cm water or more. It should be noted however that lower pressure rises, in association with symptoms, in women with reduced urethral resistance, are significant to management. A normal bladder will take in a full capacity without causing a rise in pressure much above 10 cm H_2O and certainly below 15 cm H_2O. A bladder with poor compliance will demonstrate a pressure rise in direct proportion to volume infused. Reduced compliance is classically seen in patients treated with permanent indwelling catheters. The bladder capacity will depend on the presence or absence of instability and the sensory urgency experienced by the patient. I have not found that the volume when the first sensation of fullness is experienced is a useful measure. A totally incompetent urethral sphincter will prevent adequate bladder filling.

One of the most helpful monographs of urodynamics is that written by Griffiths (1980). A significant part of the book is devoted to the voiding study. His method of plotting the detrusor pressure against the voiding flow rate, during micturition, greatly enhances our understanding of the relationship between detrusor and urethra and helps clarify many of the concepts discussed in this chapter. If the voided volume is less than 150 ml the accuracy of the measure of flow rate becomes very doubtful. An effort should always be made to obtain a good representative voiding study.

Figure 45.4 illustrates a graph of the detrusor pressure against the voiding flow rate. If it were possible to establish a constant resistance to flow in the urethra but to increase or decrease the detrusor contractility then the flow rate would change in proportion to the pressure head developed by the contraction. Provided the bladder volume was sufficient to maintain flow then a pressure against flow plot would move up and down the line A–B and the position and gradient of the line would depend on the constant urethral resistance. If it were possible to cause the detrusor to contract to a certain level and then maintain an absolutely constant tone while the resistance of the urethra was increased or decreased then the bladder pressure would vary inversely to the flow rate with changes in urethral resistance. Provided available volume were such as to not limit flow then a pressure against flow plot would move up and down the line C–D and the position and gradient would depend on the constant detrusor tone.

At the beginning of the section on the mechanisms of incontinence I pointed out the importance of a balance between detrusor contractility and urethral relaxation during voiding. It should not be surprising that a pressure/flow plot taken during a normal void should demonstrate a vector made up of the two changing components described above and that this vector should be well balanced. Figure 45.5 illustrates a pressure/flow plot taken from a normal female void. It illustrates beautifully how both the detrusor contractility and urethral resistance are changing in relation to each other throughout micturition.

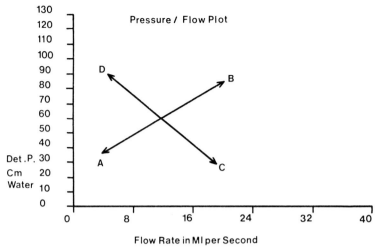

Fig. 45.4 The vectors in a pressure/flow plot.

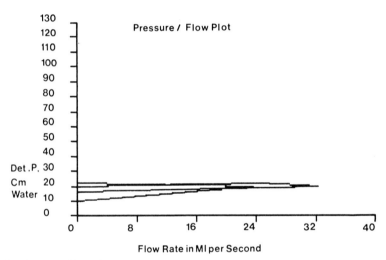

Fig. 45.5 A normal female pressure/flow plot.

It should be noted that the interpretation of this plot must alter at the end of micturition when available volume will influence both components. The plots illustrated here were recorded before the volume factor came into play.

Figure 45.6 illustrates a plot taken from a man with a tight prostatic obstruction. Note how the vector of urethral relaxation is totally absent from this graph and the high pressure void. Figure 45.7 is also taken from an obstructed patient but there is a difference. The direction of the curve shows clear evidence that the urethral resistance is falling during voiding despite the requirement for a high voiding pressure. The former was a rigid obstruction, the latter a destensible obstruction.

Figure 45.8 demonstrates the effect produced when voiding is interrupted at point 'P' by a urethral sphincter contraction without a concomitant fall in detrusor contractility. Figure 45.9 is taken from a young man with

detrusor-sphincter dyssynergia and shows the failure of the sphincters to relax adequately during void. Figure 45.10 demonstrates a relaxing sphincter but lagging behind detrusor contractility.

Figure 45.11 is a typical example of bladder hypotonia. Note the combination of a low voiding pressure and reduced flow rate. Figure 45.12 is taken from a patient with unsustained detrusor activity, the residual volume was 300 ml.

A normal maximum flow rate for a voided volume of 150 ml or more should be at least 15 ml/s. The maximum voiding pressure for a man should be 60 cm H_2O and for a woman 50 cm H_2O. I would accept a residual of 100 ml in an elderly patient but not wish to see it above 50 ml in a younger subject. Normal values are helpful guides but should never be treated as absolutes. A voiding bladder pressure and maximum flow rate provide information on

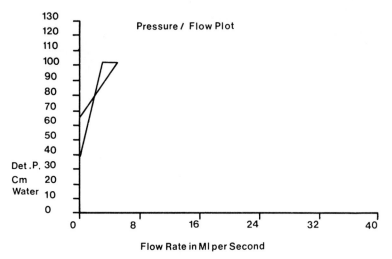

Fig. 45.6 A pressure/flow plot from a tight prostatic obstruction.

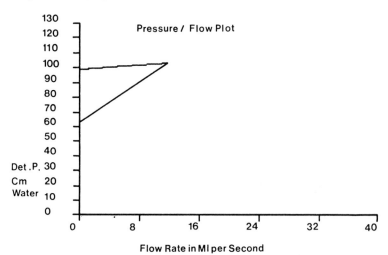

Fig. 45.7 A pressure/flow plot from another obstructed patient.

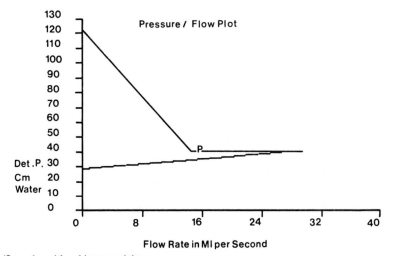

Fig. 45.8 A pressure/flow plot with sphincter activity.

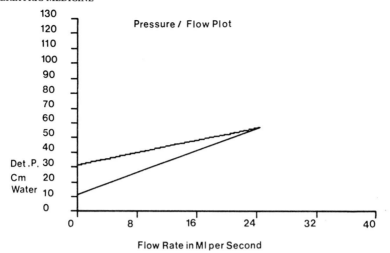

Fig. 45.9 A pressure/flow plot from a patient with dyssynergia.

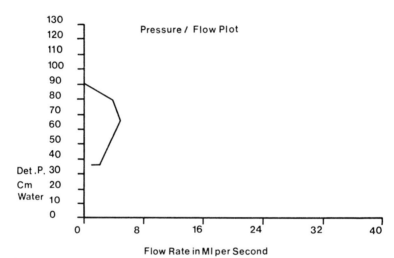

Fig. 45.10 A pressure/flow plot with late sphincter relaxation.

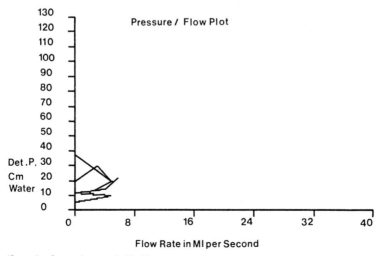

Fig. 45.11 A pressure/flow plot from a hypotonic bladder.

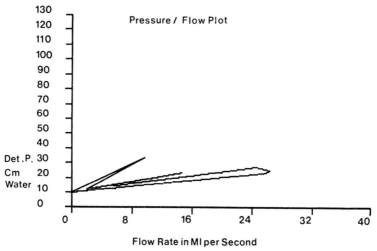

Fig. 45.12 A pressure/flow plot with unsustained detrusor activity.

one brief moment in the whole course of micturition. It is much more important to see how the pressure relates to the flow rate and the pressure/flow plot to the completeness of void. Above all, how does the overall study relate to the symptoms?

The use of video-cystometry adds little   to the information provided by a good voiding cystometrogram and is an expensive investigation. There is little application as far as the elderly are concerned. We tend to use the facility when dealing with the more complex problems. It is certainly helpful to visualise the behaviour of the bladder neck in women with sphincter incompetence prior to surgery.

A cystometrogram may be augmented by the measurement of the urethral pressure profile. This is obtained by pulling a pressure measuring device down the resting urethra at a fixed rate. It will give accurate information on the siting of an obstructive lesion and the competence of a urethra. Unfortunately it does not measure the behaviour of the urethra during voiding. In patients with denervation problems the stimulation of the urethral receptors may give misleading pressure readings because of excessively sensitive reflex arc activity.

THE MANAGEMENT OF INCONTINENCE

The first approach to the problem should be aimed at ensuring that the patient's environment and general condition is conducive to continence. Improving general health, mobility and access to lavatory facilities as well as clearing any faecal impaction or symptomatic urinary tract infection are all important.

It should be noted that any management system may well have to take account of the fact that the pathology is mixed and demands more than one remedy.

The detrusor instabilities

It should be emphasised that by far the most important principle in managing the unstable bladder is the development of a good relationship with the patient involving confidence and compassionate understanding. The bladder retraining regimes are an essential part of any treatment schedule. The aim of these is to increase gradually the interval between micturitions until a normal frequency pattern is established. This requires regular consistent follow-up. It should be remembered that the term 'detrusor instability' is very broad. It presents in many different forms depending on the cause and in the elderly is often complicated by another bladder lesion. When assessing the efficacy of described treatment regimes it is important to consider the type of patients in whom it was found successful. Hypnosis may be effective in treating idiopathic detrusor instability in a young or middle-aged woman but is less likely to succeed in a patient with cerebrovascular disease.

The two anticholinergic drugs most frequently used in the treatment of the unstable bladder are propantheline and emepronium bromide. They are quaternary ammonium compounds which do not readily penetrate biological membranes and therefore have a very low and variable absorption leading to an unpredictable clinical response. Both compounds have marked muscarinic blocking actions with some nicotinic blocking properties. They often produce disturbing systemic side-effects such as paralysis of accommodation, tachycardia, dryness of the mouth, postural hypotension and impotence. Emepronium bromide has also been identified as a cause of oral and oesophageal ulceration (Rich et al, 1977; Leys, 1956).

Flavoxate hydrochloride is a tertiary amine chromone which selectively acts on the muscle receptor producing a muscle relaxant effect without significant anticholinergic action. It is thought to act by influencing one of the steps in the excitation coupling of the smooth muscle of the bladder. This is a papaverine-like action and the toxicity of the drug is of the same order as that of papaverine (Stanton, 1973).

Oxybutinin chloride is a newer antispasmodic agent having a direct papaverine-like effect as its most prominent property. It also inhibits the muscarinic actions of acetylcholine on smooth muscles, but its ability to depress spontaneous activity or spasms of certain smooth muscles is due to a strong direct musculotrophic action. The effectiveness of orally administred oxybutinin is good and the duration of action seems satisfactory for therapeutic use. The side effects can be attributed to its anticholinergic properties and a dry mouth is a very prominent feature (Moisey et al, 1980).

Dicyclomine appears to have a non specific direct relaxant action on smooth muscle though a competitive antagonism of acetylcholine at muscarinic sites is also a feature (Downie et al, 1977).

The publications related to the use of these drugs have been both encouraging and disappointing. Flavoxate has not proved very successful. Dicyclomine has not been used very much and has attracted few publications. Oxybutinin is currently available in the United Kingdom on a named-patient basis only. It has been used extensively in the United States and by all accounts it is a drug very well worth trying and our experience confirms this (Fredericks et al, 1978).

The release of acetylcholine at the neuromuscular junction is dependent on the presence of calcium ions During depolarisation of the muscle cell membrane a slow inward current of calcium ions follows the sodium ion current. The separation of the actin and myosin myofibrils during muscle contraction involves a reaction utilising energy from adenosine triphosphate and requiring the presence of calcium ions. It has been shown that irrespective of how isolated human bladder muscle is activated the contractions can be blocked by inhibiting the inflow of calcium through the cell membrane. Despite these facts, attempts at treating the unstable bladder with calcium ion antagonists have not proved successful. Flunarazine showed initial promise but its action was not sustained. Nifedipine was found to have a very limited action. Terodiline has similar properties to nifedipine but in addition it has an antimuscarinic action which causes it to be more effective than any of the other calcium ion antagonists (Palmer et al, 1981; Gerstenberg et al, 1981).

The influence exerted by prostaglandins on the detrusor has led to their use in treating detrusor instability but responses have been disappointing. Some of their influence could be attributed to an anti-diuretic action mediated through the supression of prostaglandin E2 which thereby enhances the activity of anti-diuretic hormone (Shah et al, 1981).

The tricyclic antidepressant imipramine has anti-cholinergic, alpha agonistic, antihistamine and anti-5HT properties. These multiple actions combine to give imipramine a very effective influence on detrusor instability and it produces good results. Nocturnal enuresis usually responds to a dose of between 10 and 25 mg nocte. Some of the patients with daytime incontinence require an extra dose in the morning though the majority respond to a single nocturnal prescription (Castleden et al, 1981).

Beta receptor agonists, dopamine receptor agonists and membrane stabilising drugs have all been tried in the management of the unstable bladder but the results have not proved impressive.

The voiding problems

Any patient suffering from an anatomical obstruction of the outflow tract requires surgical correction. A person suffering from a physiological voiding problem can be greatly helped by the use of intermittent catheterisation (Lapides, 1976).

The principle behind this technique is to remove the residual volume by means of a catheter using a frequency that prevents infection and maintains continence. In the elderly this rarely requires more than two catheterisations a day. While in hospital, or if performed by a district nurse, the technique must be sterile. If performed at home by the patient or a relative, then a clean non-sterile technique may be used. If done with care the catheterisation is neither painful nor traumatic and can be accomplished very rapidly (Lapides, 1976).

We have used this technique in a number of elderly women and have been successful in re-establishing normal spontaneous voiding. We presume that this coincides with clearing of the infection, associated with a chronic residual and a reduction in the swelling and inflammation of the outflow tract. Clearly, those patients with a mixed pathology may require treatment for a detrusor instability at the same time.

The long-term use of cholinergic therapy to promote voiding has not proved successful in managing the chronic voiding problems.

Sphincter incompetence

It is only the less marked urethral lesions that are likely to respond to pelvic floor exercises. If these are used they can be supported by the use of low dose topical oestrogen therapy. More often a surgical approach is required. It is very difficult to achieve an adequate exercise routine in elderly women.

On occasions it is worth trying an alpha agonist to stimulate the smooth muscle of the urethra so as to increase sphincter tone. Both ephedrine and norephedrine (phenylpropanolamine), have been used for this purpose.

Irreversible incontinence

Inevitably there are some patients whose problems cannot

be corrected. In these circumstances we have to resort to incontinence aids.

The use of penile sheaths in elderly males is throught with problems and very rarely do they prove effective. Latex urinals are even less effective than sheaths. This means that disposable absorbents have to provide the main method of management for both sexes.

Recently there have been a number of advances in the development of absorbents and certainly the newer body-worn disposable pads are proving very effective. It is important to appreciate that different patients have very different requirements and a garment system must be carefully chosen to suit the individual (Malone-Lee et al, 1983).

The permanent indwelling catheter should be a solution of last resort since it will almost invariably produce difficult problems. The aim is to use a small guage silicone catheter with the smallest ballon possible. Drainage should be concealed. Infections should only be treated when sympomatic and bladder washouts reserved for those who recurrently block their catheters. By-passing can often be alleviated by treating a coincident detrusor instability.

REFERENCES

Brocklehurst J C 1978 The genitourinary system. In: Brocklehurst J C (ed) Textbook of Geriatric Medicine and Gerontology, 2nd edn. Churchill Livingstone, Edinburgh, ch 9, p 306

Burnstock G Personal communication 1983

Caine M, Raz S 1973 The effect of progesterone on the adrenergic receptors of the urethra. British Journal of Urology 45: 131–135

Caine M, Raz S, Zeigler M 1975 Adrenergic and cholingergic receptors in the human prostate, prostatic capsule and bladder neck. British Journal of Urology 47: 193–201

Castleden C M, George C F, Renwick A G, Asher M J 1981 Imipramine – a possible alternative to current therapy for urinary incontinence in the elderly. Journal of Urology 125: 318–320

Creed K E, Tulloch A S S 1982 The action of imipramine on the lower urinary tract of the dog. British Journal of Urology 54: 5–10

Daa Schrodoe H 1981 Somatostatin in the regulation of the bladder and the pelvic sphincters. XIth annual meeting International Continence Society, Lund, Skogs Trelleborg

Downie J W, Twiddy A S, Awad S A 1977 Antimuscarinic and non-competitive antagonistic properties of dicyclomine hydrochloride in isolated human and rabbit bladder muscle. Journal of Pharmacology and Experimental Therapeutics 201: 662–668

Eaton A C, Birmingham A T, Bates C P 1981 Evidence for the existence of purinergic transmission in the human bladder and a possible new approach to the treatment of detrusor instability. XIth Annual meeting of the International Continence Society, Lund, Skogs Trelleborg

Fletcher T F, Bradley W E 1978 Neuroanatomy of the bladder. Journal of Urology 119: 153–160

Fredericks C M, Green R L, Anderson A S 1978 Comparative in vitro effects of imipramine, oxybutinin and flavoxate on rabbit detrusor Urology 12: 487–491

Gerstenberg T L, Klanskor P, Ramirez D, Hald T 1981 The effect of terodiline in women with motor urge incontinence. XIth Annual meeting of the International Continence Society, Lund, Skogs Trelleborg

Gosling J A, Dixon J S, Hilary O D, Critchley, Thompson S A 1981 A comparative study of the human external sphincter and periurethral levator ani muscles. British Journal of Urology 53: 35–41

Griffiths D J 1980 Urodynamics Medical Physics Handbooks, Adam Hilger Ltd, Bristol

Hilton P, Stanton S L 1981 Algorithmic method of assessing urinary incontinence in elderly women. British Medical Journal 282: 940

Hindmarsh J R, Idown O A, Yeats W K, Zar M A 1977 Pharmacology of electrically evoked contractions of human bladder. British Journal of Pharmacology 61: 115

Hutch J A 1972 Anatomy and physiology of the bladder, trigone and urethra. Butterworth, London

International Continence Society 1976 First report on storage of urine in the bladder, urinary incontinence and units of measurement. British Journal of Urology 48: 39–42

International Continence Society 1977 Second report on micturition and use of symbols British Journal of Urology 49: 207–210

International Continence Society 1978 Third report on micturition, pressure-flow relationships and residual urine. Scandinavian Journal of Urology and Nephrology 12: 191–193

Khalof I M, Ghoneim M A, Elkiloli M M 1981 The effects of endogenous prostaglandins F2 alpha and E2 and indomethacin on micturition. British Journal of Urology 53: 21–28

Lapides J 1976 Further observations on self catheterisation. Journal of Urology 116: 109–171

Leys D 1956 Value of propantheline bromide in the treatment of enuresis. British Medical Journal i: 549–550

Malone-Lee J G, McCreery M, Exton-Smith A N 1983 A community study of incontinence garments. Department of Health and Social Security Report, Her Majesty's Stationery Office, London

Moisey C U, Stephenson T P, Brendler C P 1980 The urodynamic and subject results of treatment of detrusor instability with oxybutinin chloride. British Journal of Urology 52: 472

Murray K, Howell S, Lewis P 1982 The effect of opioid blockade on idiopathic detrusor instability. XIIth annual meeting of the International Continence Society, Leiden, Netherlands

Owann C, Sjostrand 1965 Short adrenergic neurones and cathecolamine containing cells in vas deferens and accessory male genital glands of different mammals. Zeitschrift Fur Zellforshung 60: 200–320

Palmer J H, Worth P H L, Exton-Smith A N 1981 Flunarizine – a once daily therapy for urinary incontinence. Lancet ii: 279–281

Rich A E S, Castleden C M, George C F, Hall M R P 1977 A second look at emepronium bromide in urinary incontinence. Lancet i: 504–506

Rossier A B, Bushra A, Fam Di Beneditto M, Sarkarati M 1980 Urethro-vesical function during spinal shock. Urological Research 8: 53–65

Shah P J R, Abrams P H, Choa G 1981 Flurbiprofen and the treatment of male detrusor instability. XIth Annual meeting of the International Continence Society, Lund, Skogs Trelleborg

Stanton S L 1973 A comparison of emepronium bromide and flavoxate hydrochloride in the treatment of urinary incontinence. Journal of Urology 110: 529–532

Turner-Warwick R, Whiteside C G (eds) 1979 Clinical Urodynamics, Urologic Clinics of North America, Saunders, Philadelphia 6: 1

Wilson P O, Barker G, Brown A O G, Russel A, Siddle N 1981 Steroid hormone receptors in the female lower urinary tract. XIth Annual meeting of the International Continence Society, Lund, Skogs Trelleborg

46

Gynaecology

E. A. Graber

The number of people over the age of 65 in the United States is now well over 25 000 000 and the majority are women. Contrary to popular myth, they are relatively healthy and most function without help well into their seventies, eighties and beyond.

There is also a popular misconception that older people lose their sexual drive. This is incorrect. According to the National Institute of Aging, many people continue to enjoy sex throughout their life. The women who cannot are usually those who lose their partners because of death or illness, or who themselves have physical or emotional disabilities. Outside of slower response and perhaps less frequent exposure, the enjoyment of orgasm, sensuality of body contact, love and affection is deeply appreciated by most older women. Age is certainly not an indicator of biologic function, and the modern post-menopausal women retains both sexual interest and activity.

It is the function of a gynaecologist to correct any circumstances that interfere with the quality of their patient's lives. We must not assume that older people necessarily will die rather soon and their needs are therefore to be subordinated. The quality of life is paramount, and older women are entitled to the preservation and restoration of genital function should this be desired. This is a most important facet in the maintenance of emotional stability and self worth.

MENOPAUSAL ENDOCRINOLOGY

The menopause is basically identified with a diminuation of ovarian oestrogen and progesterone and a slight decrease in circulating serum testosterone (Korenman, 1982). The lack of menses is due to the fact that there has been an exhaustion of ovarian follicles capable of responding to follicle-stimulating hormone (FSH) and luteinising hormone (LH) stimulation. The term 'menopause' is used when menses are absent for one year. There is a substantial rise in gonadotropins, a marked diminution or absence of progesterone and the level of oestrogen falls precipitously.

Androstenedione levels fall by one third or more and its source now becomes predominantly adrenal rather than ovarian (Longscope et al, 1969). Testosterone secretion from the ovary increases, probably because of excessive gonadotropin stimulation. Testosterone elevation plus the drop in oestrogen may be the explanation of some increase in hirsutism and even defeminisation seen occasionally in older women.

While oestradiol, produced mainly in the functioning ovary, decreases markedly in post-menopausal women, a low level can still be isolated in this group (Judd et al, 1974). Its source has not been determined. Oestrone levels however, are elevated. This results from the peripheral aromatisation of androstenedione in fat, muscle, kidney, brain and adrenal and usually correlates with the patient's weight.

Follicle stimulating hormone and luteinising hormone are elevated because of diminished feedback of ovarian oestrogen and inhibin. There is an increase in the amplitude of pulses of pituitary hormone in the menopause because of increased release of gonadotropin releasing hormone (GNRH) and enhanced responsiveness of the pituitary to GNRH seen with low oestrogen levels.

Symptoms

The results of the above hormonal changes have been variously interpreted. The dominant symptom of the changed hormonal millieu is the hot flush.

A feeling of warmth and perhaps pressure usually starts int he cephalic region and then proceeds to encompass the rest of the torso (Meldrum et al, 1980). It is followed by profuse sweating, predominantly over the upper part of the body. The frequency, intensity and duration varies in different individuals, but there is no doubt that emotional stress is a major factor in accentuating the severity of this symptom. In most instances the patient can tolerate the discomfort, and there is a gradual diminution of hot flushes over a period of 1–2 years. The fact is that this symptom of the menopause is severe enough in only 25% of the menopausal population to cause the patient to seek medical help.

With a flush, there is cutaneous blushing and redness which usually causes more embarrassment than the actual warmth. Patients find this distressing because 'It gives away the menopause'. The onset of redness usually occurs about one minute after the onset of warmth and it persists for 15–30 minutes. Skin warmth measured by finger skin temperature is elevated about 0.2–0.4°F and returns to its baseline in about 30 minutes. There is also tachycardia (80–90 beats per minute) reported in some women.

There is no relationship between the level of sex steroids and the occurence of hot flushes. There is also no correlation with norepinephrine, epinephrin and dopamine levels. There is evidence that LH pulsations and perhaps ACTH pulsation accompanies a flush (National Institutes of Health Consensus Development Conference, 1979; Plotz & Friedlander, 1967).

Anatomical changes

There are certain anatominal changes that should be reviewed before discussing the hormonal therapy for the menopause (Lang & Asonte, 1967). The major change is atrophy of the female hormone dependent organs. The degree of atrophy depends on the individual and is variable depending on the degree and speed of hormonal deprivation. The size and number of cells in these ovarian hormone dependent organs decreases, and nuclear changes consist of a more condensed, tight, compactness of nuclear chromatin. Collagen swells, fuses and tends to become hyalinised. Elastic fibres become fragmented, and lipochrome pigments accumulate within the cells.

Specific changes in the gynaecological organs will be described here and changes in other organs are described elsewhere in this text.

Vulva

Atrophy with diminished prominence of landmarks. Shrinking of the introitus. Loss of subcutaneous fat and thinning of pubic hair.

Vagina

Rugae disappear, depth shortens, and there is diminished calibre and elasticity. Secretions become scant. Bacteriologically, there is a mixed flora with a diminished lactobacillus count. Pap smear shows diminished superficial epithelial cells and an increase in parabasal and basal cells.

Cervix

Decreases in size. The squamocolumnar junction retreats into the cervical canal producing more unsatisfactory colposcopies. Increase in atresia of the canal and decreased secretion of the endocervix is also seen.

Corpus uteri

Becomes much smaller, atrophic with a concomitant increase in fibrosis and calcification. The endometrium becomes atrophic (thinning with single layer of cuboidal cells. Glands diminish in number). The stoma is fibrous and shows areas of hyalinisation.

Ovaries

Decrease in size and atretic follicles gradually disapper. Stromal fibrosis is the major finding.

Fallopian tubes

Marked diminuation in length and diameter. Epithelial atrophy with disappearance of cilia. Increased fibrosis.

Therapy

While the changes in the generative tract are obviously due to ovarian hormone deprivation, other diverse changes ascribed to oestrogen deprivation are controversial.

There are 3 basic changes resulting from oestrogen deprivation that are incontroversial. These are hot flushes; atrophy of the vagina and other gynaecological organs; and acceleration of osteoporosis (Hammond & Dry, 1982). There is no doubt that exogenous hormones will stop the flushes, and local or systemic oestrogens will help to correct atrophic vaginitis, but whether these hormones will correct osteoporosis is open to debate. As mentioned previously, only a relatively small proportion of women will require adjunctive hormone therapy, because there is not a sudden complete deprivation of oestrogen but rather a gradual one. There is still some oestrogen synthesis from the adrenal glands, and from peripheral conversion of androgens.

As far as osteoporosis is concerned, the incidence of fractures of hip, radius, vertebra etc increases in women beyond the age of 50 (Weiss et al, 1980). Those at highest risk are usually thin, light skinned, underweight and sedentary with a relatively poor diet. Food intake is particularly poor in protein, vitamin D, calcium and fluoride. In addition, a high percentage are smokers.

Osteoporosis is due to accelerated bone loss. To maintain bone strength, oestrogen may be used to diminish calcium loss via the urine, but it does nothing to create new bone growth in the bone cortex. The majority of physicians working in this field seem convinced that a high protein diet plus calcium, fluoride, vitamin D, augmented by cessation of smoking and a regular exercise programme will do more for the patient then just the administration of oestrogen. If after a few years oestrogens are terminated, bone loss occurs at an accelerated rate, so that within a short time the bone changes are similar to those who have never taken the drug.

In order for oestrogen to function, there must be a high concentration of oestrogen receptors in the tissue. Oestrogen targets are the brain (hypothalamus), pituitary gland, ovary, uterus, vagina, fallopian tubes, base of the urinary bladder, breasts and the liver. Other organs such as the kidney, pancreas etc have lesser amounts of receptors.

Whether oestrogens are involved with many other symptoms attributed to its diminished levels is open to controversy. The psychological symptoms of depression, anxiety, irritability, headaches, insomnia etc may not be due to hormone deprivation but rather the tension of middle life and normal aging. High blood pressure and atherosclerosis cannot be attributed to oestrogen lack.

This naturally brings up the question 'who do we treat with oestrogens?' The answer, in the opinion of the author, is only those who cannot function adequately without help. Some believe that the menopause is a deficiency disease and should be treated as such by automatic replacement. This thesis was especially popular in the early 1970s and patients paid a price for this. Based on our present knowledge, most physicians who use oestrogens thereapeutically in the menopause advocate their use in terms of the smallest effective dose for the shortest possible time.

One must weight the risk–benefit ratio in the advocacy of hormonal replacement therapy. Endometrial carcinoma has increased in proportion to the increased sale of oestrogen and the popularity of its widespread use (Kaufman et al, 1980; Ziel & Finkle, 1975; Smith et al, 1975; Hulka et al, 1980). Various studies indicate an increase of 2–6 times depending on the dose, duration and predisposing conditions in the patient. The resulting malignancy is not characteristically too aggresive, but there is no doubt that it is there. There is some research that indicates that by using progestins for 10 days during each oestrogen cycle, that the incidence of endometrial malignant changes is diminished. This may or may not be true (Paterson et al, 1980; Whitehead et al, 1981; Mahboubi et al, 1982; McDonald, 1981).

Whether post-menopausal oestrogens increase breast cancer is not settled. Many studies state that there is an increase in the order of 1.5:1, but the findings are not conclusive (Korenman, 1980; Hoover et al, 1976).

If doctors fear the initiation of uterine cancer due to oestrogen therapy they are not alone. A sophisticated public also has significant reservations. The litigious patient will certainly make a case should cancer appear. It is the standard practice of many physicians to do an endometrial biopsy before instituting replacement therapy and repeating it yearly while hormones are continued.

Other side effects such as weight gain, oedema, vaginal spotting and breast tenderness may also cause patient anxiety.

The effects of oestrogen on the liver may cause definite probelms. The bile becomes viscid with a reduction in volume and there is an increase in cholesterol content. Therefore, the incidence of cholecystitis and gall stones increases as does the incidence of gall bladder surgery (Bension & Grundy, 1978). Other side-effects include possible diabetogenic stimulation, increased hypertension and atherosclerosis, increased production of thyroid binding proteins, angiotensinogen and the apoprotcins for high density lipoproteins and very low density lipoproteins, as well as an increase in aldosterone secretion. Oestrogens also inhibit the activity of antithrombin III.

Finally, one should remember that oestrogens are contra-

indicated if there is unexplained vaginal bleeding; liver disease; vascular thrombosis (history or current); any history of or current oestrogen dependent tumour; hypertension or significant arteriosclerosis; gall bladder disease; migraine headaches; epilepsy or other seizures; and endometrial hyperplasia.

If a woman cannot be given oestrogens and is in need of relief for incapacitating correctable symptoms, she can be given Bellergal tablets (combination of phenobarbital and belladona) sedation, reassurance or intramuscular Depo-provera which control the symptoms in the majority of patients.

Hormones should not be used to produce 'Eternal Youth'. They certainly do not prevent aging changes of the skin or degeneration of other organ systems.

A recent analysis of cost vs. benefits of hormone therapy during the menopause found no clear advantage in long-term morbidity or mortality from either taking or not taking oestrogen (Weinstein, 1980). The patient and physician must confer to determine whether oestrogen therapy is appropriate considering the risk vs benefit. If oestrogens are necessary, early termination of therapy is indicated, especially if flushes alone are the indication. Longer therapy may be indicated if they are used for the management of osteoporosis.

GYNAECOLOGICAL SURGERY

In addition to hormone adjustment, elderly women are subject to many local problems associated with their genital and/or urinary tract. The peak incidence of major surgery in women is between the ages of 60 and 69. There are three major gynaecological areas of involvement: urinary tract disease, especially incontinence or bladder descent; pelvic floor and vaginal laceration; and pelvic tumours (benign and malignant).

Basic principles
Before the details of the above are discussed, certain basic principles of surgery in the elderly female must be outlined. There are usually other systemic problems seen in conjunction with the gynaecologic complaints which must be evaluated and taken into account. While age does not accurately reflect the general physical condition of the patient, there is a definite increase in chronic degenerative diseases which in turn increases the complication rate. It is widely accepted that if the patient achieved old age, she has proven that she is a reasonably rugged lady with a strong constitution. Unfortunately this is far from universal. Individualisation, good pre-operative evaluation and careful patient selection are the keys to good results. This saves one from surprises that may well be catastrophic. Generally speaking, older patients take elective surgery well. They do not do well with surgery due to acute

catastrophic events, or if there are major complications during or after elective surgery. Also the outcome may well be influenced by the severity of non-gynaecologic organic disease.

The main areas to be investigated before operation are:

1. The heart and blood vessels (hypertension, coronary heart diseases etc.)
2. Lung disease (emphysema, asthma, chronic bronchitis, chronic obstructive lung disease)
3. Anaemia and blood coagulopathy
4. Malnutrition
5. Gastro-intestinal disease (especially diverticular diesease of colon, mesenteric or retroperitoneal cysts)
6. Renal disease (anatomical anomalies, infection)
7. Chronic neurological dysfunction (central nervous system disease, multiple sclerosis, disc disease)
8. Severe arthritis
9. Diabetes
10. Obesity
11. Neuropsychiatric problems
12. Iatrogenic changes due to drugs.

Evaluation of the elderly patient for surgery is discussed in chapter 4.

Anaesthesia
Anaesthesia management in the elderly is probably one of the most important facets of a successful uncomplicated operation. Unless a physician has a qualified anaesthetist available, the operation should either be postponed until such a person is available or the location of the site of the surgery should be changed. While the ultimate type of anaesthetic chosen should be in the responsibility of the anaesthetist, consultation with the operating surgeon and other physicians involved in the case is very helpful.

The anaesthetist should see the patient before surgery, evaluate her physical condition, and then decide on the optimal anaesthesia. He should anticipate and be prepared for possible complications, and above all should take time to explain the procedure and gain the confidence of his patient. Since the patient will have nothing by mouth after midnight, dehydration becomes a definite factor if the operation is delayed too long thereafter. If the surgery is to take place int he afternoon the patient can be given clear fluids by mouth until 6–8 hours before the operation. Some prefer to give intravenous Ringer's lactate before operation regardless of the time of operation so that the patient has 500–1000 ml of fluid pre-operatively to assure adequate hydration.

There is no safer anaesthesia than local. It can be used with ease and satisfaction in the repair of perineal structures and bladder, rectal or uterine descensus. Further, it can be mixed with vasoconstrictors to diminish blood loss. The anaesthetist can augment their action if necessary with nitrous oxide or any other light

supplemental general anaesthetic, or intravenous Valium or Demerol. This is an excellent anaesthetic for dilatation and curettage (D&C) in the elderly patient with medical complications.

Regional anaesthesia (spinal or epidural) is also safe in the elderly unless there is a definitie contra-indication such as neurological disease, infection at the site of lumbar puncture, low blood volume or bacteraemia. At times, they must be supplemented by intravenous analgesics or light general anaesthesia if the anaesthetic level is not high enough or the patient complains about tugging on her abdominal organs. The usual precautions used for this type of anaesthesia must be followed meticulously.

General anaesthesia is used most frequently for surgery in the elderly. Aspiration of stomach contents is the leading cause of anaesthetic death in this group. Older people are prone to airway obstruction, overdose of anaesthesia, hypoxia, and reflux regurgitation. All patients undergoing major surgery with general anaesthesia should be intubated with a cuffed endotrachial tube. Gastric emptying is delayed by apprehension so that the possibility of aspiration is very real.

VAGINAL OPERATIONS

The basic principles of intra-abdominal gynaecologic surgery are not different than those on any surgical procedure in the abdomen, but a discussion of the basic principles of vaginal surgery is indicated in a chapter concerned with gynaecological surgery in the elderly female. Surgery is usually done to correct prolapse of the pelvic organs or for urologic difficulties (usually stress incontinence). On relatively few occasions, the indication is rectal or urinary incontinence due to the presence of a fistula. While many of the patients are not acutely ill, the fact is that their condition interferes with the quality of life. Repair restores genital integrity and in some cases the ability to again have a satisfying sex life. A vaginal hysterectomy and repair of the endopelvic fascia may be carried out with minimal danger even in women in their seventies. In experienced hands, the operation is relatively short, taking less time than if an abdominal incision must be made and closed. Advantages are less danger of wound hernia and evisceration, less intestinal obstruction, less anaesthesia because the necessary degree of abdominal muscular relaxation is less, breathing is easier post-operatively because there is less splinting because of abdominal pain, less ileus (minimal handling of bowel) and generally greater patient comfort. The important factors regarding feasibility of the vaginal approach are uterine mobility and descensus, no pelvic adhesions from previous operation (free cul-de-sac) and the strength of the uterosacral ligaments.

Two competent assistants for adequate exposure,

adequate illumination and blood on call are also needed. Unless these qualifications are fully carried out, the operation of vaginal hysterectomy or any other vaginal operation should not be undertaken in the elderly. They do not tolerate acute intra-operative catastrophes well. Before surgery one should clean up all infections and ulceration within the vagina, do biopsis on suspicious lesions and check the urinary tract thoroughly.

The question always arises as to whether vaginal relaxation that is relatively asymptomic should be repaired and if so, when. When these patients are seen initially, the pathology may be minimal. If however, on subsequent biannual examination there is progression of the various forms of genital prolapse, this indicates that future progression is almost inevitable. Surgical intervention should be undertaken when the patient is still relatively young and before she gets the degenerative medical problems that may exacerbate as she gets older. The risk–benefit ratio detriorates with advancing years. On the other hand, the repair of a fistula should not be rushed. Clean granulation tissue and eradication of local infection are necessary, or the failure rate is inordinately high.

STRESS INCONTINENCE

One of the more common complaints of the elderly female is urinary stress incontinence. It must be emphasised that cystocele formation or uterine prolapse are not major factors in the production of their annoying symptom. Loss of urinary control occurs in less than 5% of women with cystoceles. With uterine prolapse there usually is no difficulty with urinary control. The above statements are easily explained on the basis of the accepted aetiology of stress incontinence. It results from a loss of the normal angles of the urethrovesical junction and funneling and descent of the base of the bladder. These usually result from pelvic damage at the time of parturition and increases with time and atrophy. If these changes can be demonstrated during examination, the condition can be alleviated by surgery, preferably the Marshall-Marchetti operation which is an abdominal approach. It consists of urethral suspension to the pubic bone to restore the proper urethrovesical angle and elevation of the bladder neck. If the patient refuses surgery or is a poor operative risk, non-operative measures that may be helpful are: the use of oestrogen vaginal cream which helps overcome genital atrophy and increases turgescence of the area; the use of a vaginal pessary to elevate the cystocele and somewhat restore the vesicourethral angle; and the use of perineal exercises to increase levator tone by strengthening the pubococcygeal muscles and elevating the bladder base. While the above suggestions are not as effective as surgery, they are definitely helpful and should be attempted.

The other important causes of incontinence and their management are discussed in chapter 45.

TUMOURS OF THE GYNAECOLOGIC TRACT IN THE ELDERLY FEMALE

Basically tumours in this group are classified as benign and malignant. While the diagnosis and therapy of each tumour is beyond the scope of this chapter, certain basic concepts and conclusions are valid. Tumours that are oestrogen dependent (i.e. uterine fibroids) undergo atrophy. With aging the incidence of malignancy increases. This should be uppermost in the minds of physicians that examine elderly females.

In an office gynaecological examination, careful evaluation of the vulva, vagina, cervix, uterine body, fallopian tubes, ovaries and cul-de-sac should be routine. In addition the rectum should be palpated and the breasts examined in both the upright and prone position.

Benign tumours of the vulva

Papillomas, hidradenoma, mucinous cysts, fibromas, lymphoid hamarteromas and urethral caruncles all can be removed and controlled easily by ablative therapy. Venereal disease may occur, but the incidence is much less than that found in younger women. The most important instrument for diagnosis is a Key biopsy punch. There is no other way of establishing a definitive diagnosis for abnormal dermatological conditions of the vulva. All white lesions should be biopsied as well as red lesions that appear to be inflammatory, ulcerative, or granulomatous disease. Bowen's disease, Paget's disease and in-situ carcinoma of the epithelium all require therapy. It should also be remembered that these lesions are frequently multicentric so multiple biopsies should be performed when indicated. Invasive disease may show ulceration, induration or just a white lesion with only pruritis as the presenting symptom. Vulvar tumours are usually slow growing and this leads to neglect. If diagnosed in the localised stage, the cure rate is very high with surgery. Once it spreads to the lymphatics, the survival rate drops proportionate to the stage of the disease. The important point is 'If in doubt, biopsy'. A second dictum is 'Any lesion that does not heal promptly with what is thought to be appropriate therapy should be biopsied'.

Vaginal tumours

The vagina of elderly females is thin, atrophic and unusually susceptible to trauma. Infection may be present and should be treated in the usual fashion. Atrophic vaginitis, with resulting dyspareunia should respond promptly to intravaginal oestrogens if their use is not contra-indicated. The dose is diminished as healing progresses.

Benign tumours of the vagina consists basically of vaginal cysts, fibromas and leiomyomas. These can be excised if they are symptomatic. Cancer of the vagina is rare and may be primary or metastatic. Vaginal tumour is usually treated by radiation with the five year survival rate about 50%. Early diagnosis by biopsy is the key to success.

Tumours of the cervix

Cervical polyps are perhaps the most common benign tumours of the cervix. Despite the fact that the vast majority are benign, careful pathological examination is mandatory because misdiagnosis or malignant degeneration may occur. Cervical condylomata are occasionally seen. They should be removed by electrodesication, cryosurgery or laser beam.

Cervical carcinoma occurs in the transformation zone and it is now generally accepted that there is usually a gradual progression in most cases through various stages of dysplasia. While mild cases may revert to normal, most will progress through severe dysplasia, carcinoma in situ and finally invasive carcinoma. Earlier stages of cancer are found in the younger population, while invasive cancer occurs on the average of ten years later. There is some debate about cost/benefit ratio of pap smears in older women, because with two negative smears one year apart, it has been suggested that a smear done every three years would be adequate in this age group. This has been questioned by the American College of Obstetrics and Gynecology which recommends that yearly smears should continue to be carried out not only because of screening for cervical carcinoma, but also because it gives the physician the opportunity to do a thorough pelvic and breast examination with its resultant benefits of early diagnosis of other pathology, particularly ovarian, breast and vulvar carcinoma.

Unfortunately early carinoma of the cervix produces no characteristic symptoms with the possible exception of vaginal spotting. Diagnosis by pap smear, colposcopy, endocervical curettage and guided biopsy have made early diagnosis and therapy possible, so that the mortality of cervical cancer has dropped in the past 20 years.

The treatment of dysplasia (moderate to severe) is usually cryotherapy or electrocoagulation. Some use laser therapy. This is done under colposcopic guidance. If carcinoma in situ is found, the treatment in older women should be hysterectomy rather than conisation or local destructive therapy. Invasive carcinoma may be treated by radical surgery and node dissection if the patient is a good risk and is stage 1B or 2A, but all other cases are treated by local irradiation as well as external radiation to the parametria.

Post-menopausal bleeding

One of the most disconcerting symptoms to both patient and physician is the patient with post-menopause vaginal bleeding. If a bleeding lesion can be found, it obviously must be evaluated and treated, but in the majority nothing definitive is seen that accounts for the vaginal bleeding.

A careful history is needed to determine whether the blood came from the rectum, bladder or urethra, or vagina.

The panic of the patient upon seeing blood may interfere with her powers of observation. Careful examination of the rectosigmoid and urinary tract are necessary if there is any doubt as to the site of origin. The important point is that one third of cases in this group of patients have cancer of the vulva, vagina and cervix or uterine fundus. Definitive diagnosis demands endometrial and cervical biopsy and preferably a fractional D&C. Probably the most common cause of post-menopausal bleeding is hormone therapy and since oestrogen may trigger bleeding in early endometrial cancer, again one is obligated to investigate. It is now considered good medical practice to do a yearly endometrial biopsy on all women taking oestrogen in the post-menopause period because of the reported increased incidence of endometrial carcinoma in this group.

Benign lesions that cause bleeding are atrophic vaginitis, endometrial or cervical polyps, urethral caruncles, or bleeding from an atrophic or hyperplastic endometrium. Even with these conditions, the workup should still be complete because the benign condition may be the red herring causing a delay in making an early diagnosis of malignancy.

A disconcerting situation occurs in 10–15% of cases where no reason is found for the bleeding. If no further blood is seen, it is assumed that the condition is healed and is not significant. If further bleeding occurs, it may well mean that an area of pathology has been missed and a second evaluation is attempted. If this too is negative and bleeding persists perhaps the most conservative thing to do is a hysterectomy.

Uterine malignancy

Of uterine cancers diagnosed, 75% occur in women over the age of 50. The predisposed groups of obese, Mulliparous, have a history of menstural dysfunctional bleeding, a history of endogenous or exogenous unopposed oestrogen, hypertension, diabetes, adenomatous endometrial hyperplasia etc. These may not necessarily be present and a patient can still develop cancer.

Routine screening for tumour is rather difficult because it is uncomfortable to the patient. The pap test is grossly inadequate with a definitive diagnosis possible in no more than a minority of cases. Endometrial biopsy with or without suction is 90–95% effective, but the patients frequently do not return for follow up because of the pain or discomfort associated with this procedure. The use of various intrauterine instruments for collection of endometrial cytological material has been controversial. Few cytologists have the expertise to interpret the specimen, especially if the cells are between the normal and outright malignant variety. Some other method of screening will ultimately be found which meets both patient and physician approval.

Fortunately, endometrial cancer usually causes bleeding that alerts the patient at an early stage. The majority of tumours are diagnosed in stage 1. If the tumours are not deep in the myometrium and are well differentiated, the cure rate is 80–90%. The treatment of fundal cancer is total abdominal hysterectomy and bilateral salpingo-oopherectomy in conjunction with radiation. Chemotherapeutic regimens have not been effective.

Ovarian malignancy

The ovary in the post-menopausal woman undergoes marked atrophy about five years after the onset of the menopause. Therefore if pelvic examination reveals what appears to be an ovary with the diameter of that found in a premenopausal woman, this should be looked upon with suspicion and explored.

The diagnosis of ovarian tumours can be made by pelvic examination, ultrasound and computerised axial tomography screening. Unfortunately most ovarian cancers are far advanced at the time of diagnosis because the tumour is silent. Any patient over 40 years of age is in the high risk group. The diagnosis is quite difficult in early cases because the tumour may be small and the index of suspicion low. The malignant tumour usually does not cause symptoms until there is peritoneal spread with involvement of the intestine. The patient's complaints are usually gastro-intestinal, and valuable time is wasted with a GI workup and then perhaps even non-specific treatment for so called indigestion. The diagnosis is finally made when ascites become apparent along with weight loss and cachexia.

The treatment of ovarian malignancy is total abdominal hysterectomy, bilateral salpingo-oophorectomy, omentectomy, appendectomy and prophylactic chemotherapy. If this cannot be completed because of extensive disease, debulking of tumour tissue followed by chemotherapy will at least produce palliation. The important message is that any women in the post-menopause period with an adnexal mass should have an exploratory laparotomy. Any ovarian tumour in this age group should be considered malignant until proven otherwise. There is no place for observation or procrastination.

Breast

In the elderly patient, there is atrophy of the breast parenchymal tissue and an increase in fat deposition. This makes mamographic interpretation much easier and more accurate. In the high-risk patient, a mamogram every 1–3 years will diminish the incidence of advanced cancer with positive axillary nodes. The point to be emphasised is that any older woman with a discrete mass on palpation should have a biopsy unless fluid can be aspirated from a cyst. Biopsy can be carried out under local anaesthesia, after which, if further surgery is deemed necessary after reading of the permanent pathological sections, the surgical procedure should be done within two weeks if possible. There is no increase in treatment failures if this routine is followed.

CONCLUSION

Gynaecologic surgery in older people is usually uneventful if the operation goes well and the patient does not have severe systemic disease. Chronological age is not important. If however the patient has severe systemic disease, elective surgery should be avoided. These cases invite catastrophe. Other means of correcting the pathology such as pessaries or just tolerating the condition and living with it must be accepted. Also in choosing operations, the surgeon's choice must be a procedure that has a maximum chance of success with a minimal chance of severe complications. The mortality increases in surgery for malignancy, co-existing severe degeneration disease, emergency surgery and operative procedures complicated by intra-operative haemorrhage, shock, infection or any undue stress in the cardivascular, neurologic, renal or hepatic systems. These women do not have the resiliency and ability to compensate which can be depended upon in younger women. The older gynaecological patient should be protected, reassured and kept comfortable so that we as physicians make their remaining years secure and happy.

REFERENCES

Bennion L J, Grundy S M 1978 Risk factors for the development of cholelithiasis in man. New England Journal of Medicine 229: 1221–1227

Hammond C, Ory S J 1982 Endocrine problems of menopause. Clinical Obstetrics and Gynecology 25: 19–38

Hoover R, Gray L A, Cole P 1976 Menopausal estrogens and breast cancer. New England Journal of Medicine 295: 401–405

Hulka B S, Fowler W C, Kaufman D E 1980 Estrogens and endometrial cancer. American Journal of Obstetrics and Gynecology 137: 92–101

Hulka B S, Kaufman D G, Fowler W C, Grimson R C, Greenberg G B 1980 Predominance of early endometrial cancer after long term estrogen use. Journal of the American Medical Association 244: 2419–2422

Judd H L, Judd G E, Lucas W E, Yen S S C 1974 Endocrine function of the post-menopausal ovary. Journal of Clinical Endocrinology and Metabolism 39:1020–1024

Korenman S G 1980 Endocrinology of breast cancer. Cancer 46: 874–878

Korenman S H 1982 Menopausal endocrinology and management. Archives of Internal Medicine 142: 1131–1136

Lang W R, Aponte G E 1967 Gross and microscopic anatomy of the aged female reproductive organs. Clinical Obstetrics and Gynecology 10: 454–456

Longcope C, Kato T, Horton R 1969 Conversion of blood androgen to estrogen in normal adult men and women. Journal of Clinical Investigation 48: 2192–2201

McDonald P C 1981 Estrogen plus progestin in post-menopausal women. New England Journal of Medicine 305: 1644–1645

Mahboubi E, Eyler N R, Wynder E 1982 Epidemiology of cancer of the endometrium. Clinical Obstetrics and Gynecology 25: 5–17

Meldrum D R, Tataryn I V, Frumar A M 1980 Gonadotropins, estrogens and adrenal steroids during menopausal hot flush. Journal of Clinical Endocrinology and Metabolism 50: 685–689

National Institutes of Health Consensus Development Conference 1979 Estrogen use and post-menopausal women. Annals of Internal Medicine 9: 921–922

Paterson M E L, Wade-Evands T, Sturedee T U 1980 Endometrial disease after treatment with estrogens and progesterones in the climacteric. British Medical Journal 1:822–824

Plotz E J, Friedlander R L 1967 Endocrinology in women over 65. Clinical Obstetrics and Gynecology 10: 466–480

Smith D C, Prentice R, Thompson D J, Herrman W L 1975 Association of exogenous estrogen and endometrial carcinoma. New England Journal of Medicine 293: 1164–1167

Weinstein M D 1980 Estrogen use in post-menopausal women — costs, risks and benefits. New England Journal of Medicine 303: 308–316

Weiss N S, Ure C R, Ballard H 1980 Decreased risk of fractures of the hip and lower forearm with post-menopausal use of estrogen. New England Journal of Medicine 303: 1195–1198

Whitehead M I, Townsend P T, Pryse-Davies J 1981 Effects of estrogens and prognestin on the biochemistry and morphology of the post-menopausal endometrium. New England Journal of Medicine 305: 1599–1605

Ziel H K, Finkle W D 1975 Increased risk of endometrial carcinoma among users of conjugated estrogen. New England Journal of Medicine 293: 1167–1170

47

Skin disorders

J. Verbov

What can be said about the aging skin? Braverman & Fonferko (1982a) have separated skin changes of sun-exposed skin (actinic damage) from those of chronological aging. They propose (Braverman & Fonferko 1982b) from their studies that the aging process has two major manifestations: elastic fibre abnormalities involving degradation and assembly and vascular wall alterations of widening and atrophy depending on the functional state of the veil cell. Veil cells are flat fibroblast-like cells that surround blood vessels.

Almost all skin diseases may occur in the geriatric patient but leg ulcers, pemphigoid and tumours such as seborrhoeic warts, solar keratoses and skin malignancy occur especially in older individuals. The disorders seen most frequently and accounting for 75% of patients in the over 60 age-group are tumours, eczema, pruritus, leg ulcers and psoriasis. The remaining 25% of patients will have conditions including rosacea, vascular diseases, blistering disorders, infections, drug eruptions and alopecia. I shall confine this chapter to the above conditions and readers wishing to have a more comprehensive discussion of geriatric dermatology are recommended to read elsewhere (Verbov, 1974; Korting, 1980).

Often disease in the older individual is of longer-standing and more florid than it would be in a younger individual because of the tendency of older people not to bother about themselves and to accept disabilities. The patient presenting with a skin problem should be examined in a good light and should undress, at least down to the innermost layer of underclothes. This is essential because skin disease is often more widespread than a patient will admit and examining the skin generally will allow the doctor to see any other blemishes. Unlike younger individuals, older people often have multiple pathology so that both in the letter of referral from the family doctor and in the history from the patient one looks for chronic bronchitis, hypertension, ischaemic heart disease, anaemias, diabetes etc, and notes any drugs the patient is currently receiving. Unfortunately, it is the exception rather than the rule to be given a list of relevant systemic disease or any regular therapy in a referral letter. The elderly housebound patient who rarely sees the light of day

may have osteomalacia from vitamin D_3 lack. Older patients with skin disease should be examined with the possibility in mind that the condition or its poor response to treatment may be due to another pre-existing condition. Thus it is not uncommon to see patients with leg ulcers secondary to oedematous legs where the oedema is the result of untreated undiagnosed right-sided cardiac failure. A leg ulcer may be slow to heal if the patient has an underlying chronic iron deficiency anaemia but once the anaemia is treated healing will be more rapid.

TUMOURS

Benign

Seborrhoeic wart

This is a very common tumour seen most frequently in elderly patients and appearing usually over the trunk and face. Lesions tend to be multiple and of different sizes and colours but it is often a particular one that brings the patient to his family doctor. The warty tumour appears black and brown and looks as though it is stuck onto the skin; often bits of tumour have broken off from the main lesion. Treatment is mainly for cosmetic reasons and curettage or cautery are two simple methods. These warts may become inflamed or irritated by friction and their appearance may then simulate malignant melanoma. If there is any doubt about the nature of the lesions clinically, an excision biopsy must be performed.

Solar keratosis

This common tumour is usually multiple and occurs over exposed areas including the lips. Although most common in elderly patients, younger individuals with a history of prolonged exposure to sunlight are also susceptible. Smaller lesions are often better felt than seen. Clinically, lesions are small, discrete brown or reddish, scaling or horny papules. Long-standing lesions may progress to intra-epidermal carcinoma (Bowen's disease) or squamous carcinoma, so that indurated or prominent keratoses must be treated with suspicion and excised. Simple keratoses over limbs, forehead and cheeks can just be observed,

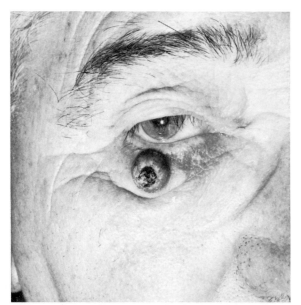

Fig. 47.1 A typical keratoacanthoma showing hemispherical nature with central keratin plug.

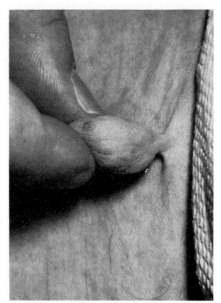

Fig. 47.2 Pedunculated skin tag over thigh.

curetted or treated by twice-daily topical application of a cream containing 5% 5-fluorouracil for about a month. Keratoses over the pinnae are very common and should be treated when seen, either by curettage or excision, because many lesions at this site undergo malignant change without any obvious alteration in their benign appearance.

Keratoacanthoma

This presents as a rapidly growing hemispherical tumour with a central keratin plug (Fig. 47.1) usually over the face but sometimes elsewhere. Growth usually continues for a few months then ceases for some months and this is followed by spontaneous resolution over the next six months or so, usually with a residual scar. Differential diagnosis includes squamous carcinoma in particular, and it is always advisable at least to take a wedge-shaped biopsy from the lesion to confirm its benign nature. My practice is to excise or curette the whole lesion.

Other benign tumours

Skin tag

Small skin tags which are often multiple are commonly found in axillae and groins. Larger ones are also seen frequently (Fig. 47.2). Usually loosely described as 'warts' they are benign connective tissue tumours which can be treated by gentle cautery with or without local anaesthesia. Topical applications are ineffective.

Cutaneous horn

This tumour may arise from a viral or seborrhoeic wart, solar keratosis, squamous-cell carcinoma or occur as such. Treatment is by excision or by curettage.

Arsenical keratosis

This precarcinomatous lesion follows arsenic medication many years previously. Lesions tend to be multiple. Abnormally high retention of arsenic may be an individual metabolic trait and may be an important factor in carcinogenesis (Bettley & O'Shea, 1975).

Post-radiotherapy keratosis

This is still seen in the elderly, occurring years after such treatment for scalp ringworm, acne, hirsuties, chronic eczema and breast or other carcinoma.

Myxoid cyst

This relatively common benign dermal connective tissue tumour usually presents as a small slightly shiny cyst adjacent to a finger posterior nailfold. Glairy fluid often appears at intervals under the fold and nail deformity may be associated. The cyst can be excised but recurrence is common and it is often more sensible to leave the lesion alone. However Sonnex et al (1982) claim success using cryosurgery.

Malignant

Basal cell carcinoma (BCC)

This is the most common malignant skin tumour in the older patient and is a slowly growing tumour which only rarely metastasises. However it does gradually enlarge outwards and over many years may penetrate deeply. it occurs most frequently over the face. It may appear in many clinical forms but the rodent ulcer type is the usual and most well-known. Over a period of years, an enlarging papule ulcerates and the lesion at this stage often scabs repeatedly. The edge of the lesion is raised and pearly and small blood vessels can be seen traversing it. Other forms of BCC include a type that simulates a scar, a type which remains papular and may be markedly pigmented, and a form which clinically simulates eczema or Bowen's disease. Regarding the latter presentation, doctors should be critical in diagnosing eczema or psoriasis where single or few chronic non-irritant patches of reddish scaling skin occur and a skin biopsy may be indicated. Different forms of BCC may occur in the same patient. The recommended treatment of BCC is usually excision but radiotherapy or curettage followed by cautery are other methods.

Bowen's disease

This is a common intra-epidermal carcinoma which will progress to frank squamous carcinoma if untreated. Lesions may be single or multiple and present anywhere as warty lesions or scaling eczema-like patches. Treatment of suspected lesions is by excision usually, but larger patches can be effectively treated by radiotherapy. It is likely that Bowen's disease occurring in covered areas is associated with an increased incidence of internal carcinoma.

Squamous cell carcinoma

This tumour is more rapidly growing than BCC and metastasises readily. It can occur anywhere on the skin or a mucous membrane and often on a site altered by an antecedent lesion such as leukoplakia, varicose ulcer, lupus vulgaris, scar tissue, erythema ab igne or radiotherapy burns. Typical tumours are nodular and hard, show some surrounding induration and commonly ulcerate. They may also be warty. Treatment is by excision.

Melanoma

Clinically, malignant melanoma can be separated into Hutchinson's lentigo (lentigo maligna), superficial spreading melanoma and nodular melanoma. Hutchinson's lentigo is a flat irregularly pigmented macule with its usual site being the face. It appears at middle age or later and is brown to black in colour with an irregular border. After a variable time, sometimes many years, malignancy manifested by nodular thickening develops. Treatment is excision preferably in the pre-malignant stage and prognosis is good. Liquid nitrogen cryotherapy has also been recommended (Dawber & Wilkinson, 1979) for the macular phase and possible also for the nodular phase.

The prognosis of superficial spreading melanoma which is most common on light-exposed areas, and nodular melanomas which can occur anywhere, is closely related to the depth of invasion at the time of treatment but usually requires wide excision with a margin of 3–5 cm, down to but not including deep fascia.

Lymphoma

This may present in various ways. There may be pruritus only, acquired ichthyosis, nondescript slightly irritant erythematous papules or oedematous nodules. Full investigation including biopsy of skin and of a palpable lymph node may be required to confirm the diagnosis. Topical steroids and oral antihistamines are helpful for irritation and superficial X-ray therapy or electron beam therapy, and chemotherapy may be indicated. Mycosis fungoides, which is a lymphoma affecting principally T lymphocytes, typically shows three clinical stages. In the first stage there is a non-specific inflammation which often appears eczematous, then lesions become infiltrated and then frank tumours occur which may ulcerate. Treatment includes the aforementioned but photochemotherapy, a treatment involving use of long-wave ultraviolet light (UVA) in combination with a photosensitising drug 8-methoxypsoralen (P) is another more recent method. An excellent review of mycosis fungoides has appeared recently (Mackie, 1980).

ECZEMA

The term eczema indicates an irritant inflammatory condition of the skin in which papules and vesicles present on an erythematous background. Irritation encourages excoriations and secondary infection and oedema of involved skin may be complicated by exudation. Eczema may be either exogenous and is then termed contact dermatitis, or endogenous (constitutional). Topical steroid applications have an important place in treatment.

Contact dermatitis is seen quite frequently in elderly patients and is diagnosed from the history, distribution of the rash and by patch testing. A patient may have been in contact with an allergen, such as nickel, for many years before developing epidermal sensitivity and this should be borne in mind. Contact dermatitis may also be of primary irritant rather than allergic origin (Fig. 47.3).

Constitutional eczema can be found in a variety of forms but they all have the same pathology. Types including vesicular eczema of palms and soles (pompholyx), discoid eczema, varicose eczema and seborrhoeic dermatitis are all frequently met in the older individual. Seborrhoeic dermatitis favours frictional areas such as groins and axillae and is more common in obese individuals. It is usually complicated by bacterial infection and candidiasis, and a topical steroid-nystatin cream is useful.

Older patients with chronic eczema of various types may become photosensitive in later life presenting with exudative eczema over exposed areas in the warmer weather.

PRURITUS

Dry skin is usual in the elderly and is a common cause of pruritus. It results from a decreased ability of the epidermis

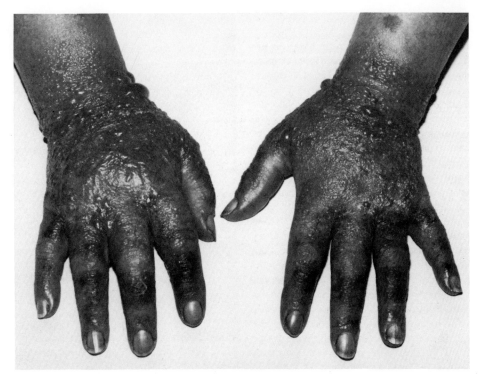

Fig. 47.3 Acute irritant contact dermatitis hands.

to retain water, but environmental factors such as excessive use of soaps which degrease the skin, low humidity in winter and central heating will all promote drying. Treatment is rehydration with lubricants applied to a moistened skin.

Senile pruritus is a diagnosis which should not be made too readily before ensuring that no other causes for pruritus exist; these include many common skin diseases and internal causes such as drugs, iron deficiency, hypothyroidism, hyperthyroidism, psychogenic disorders, reticulosis, internal malignancy, polycythaemia rubra vera, liver disease and chronic renal failure.

Itching in diabetes mellitus is typically confined to pruritus ani and vulvae, and candidiasis is usually present at these sites, but glycosuria must also be an important factor because when it is reduced the itching promptly disappears (Braverman, 1981). It must be admitted that in many patients with widespread pruritus no cause is ever found.

LEG ULCERS

Leg ulcers are a major problem in the elderly patient. In management, the general health of the patient must be assessed and any deficiencies such as dietary, corrected. Most ulcers below the knee are *stasis ulcers,* a consequence of venous incompetence, but skin ischaemia producing pain, superficial ulceration and scars (atrophic blanche) are also often present. *Venous ulcers* vary greatly in size but are usually oval and serpiginous in shape and often multiple. They are usually centred within a hand's breadth of the ankle joint (Leading article, 1982). Venous ulcers may take months to heal and are best treated with weekly medication, namely, impregnated below-knee occlusive bandages covered with an elasticated bandage. Before occlusive treatment is begun infected ulcers should be cleaned twice daily with topical antiseptics such as eusol and any associated cellulitis treated with an oral antibiotic.

Arterial ulcers associated with poor peripheral arterial circulation are less common than the above ulcers and are typically painful. Adequate cleansing of the ulcer, prevention of secondary infection and early referral for surgical opinion may be necessary.

Painless trophic ulcers over the ball of the feet are seen particularly in diabetics and are a real therapeutic problem. Careful paring of the thickened skin and keeping the ulcer clean and buffered from friction are important. In rheumatoid arthritis leg ulcers are common and although most are gravitational, traumatic ulcers, ulceration overlying nodules, arteritic ulcers, and unexplained ulcers also occur. Resolution of ulcers in rheumatoid arthritis is notoriously slow and if in-patient treatment is indicated it is most important to keep the arthritic patient mobile to prevent stiffening of joints.

PSORIASIS

The geriatric patient who presents with psoriasis has usually had the condition for many years and gives a typical history of remissions and exacerbations. Tar or anthralin-containing preparations should be used if possible but for those who cannot tolerate them and for flexures, pustular psoriasis or generalised exfoliative psoriasis, topical steroids are indicated. However the steroid used should be the least potent that is compatible with a reasonable therapeutic response. Thus it is better to have just reasonable control of psoriasis with a weaker steroid than to free the skin of psoriasis but produce widespread skin atrophy and pituitary — adrenal suppression with large amounts of more potent topical steroids. There is also evidence that cosmetically unsightly but harmless ordinary psoriasis can be converted in some individuals to the more serious pustular types by exhibition of corticosteroids whether potent topical ones or systemic ones. Systemic steroids are not normally indicated in psoriasis except for generalised forms or severe unresponsive psoriatic arthropathy. The cytotoxic drug methotrexate, and the vitamin A derivative, etretinate, also have a place in the treatment of the patient with widespread intractable psoriasis. It should be noted that lithium salts tend to worsen psoriasis. Photochemotherapy (psoralen + UVA) is also important in psoriasis therapy.

ROSACEA

A persistent blush appearance over the centre of the forehead, nose and cheeks followed by the appearance of papules and pustules indicates rosacea, a common disease in the older patient (Fig. 47.4). Treatment consists of oxytetracycline 250 mg twice daily for a period of weeks or for as long as six months, and topical 1–3% sulphur cream is helpful. Other oral tetracyclines are also effective. Short courses of oral metronidazole are effective in some cases. Rosacea may be complicated by eye changes including blepharitis and keratitis and these will also improve with the systemic treatment.

VASCULAR CONDITIONS

Chilblains are seen occasionally in the winter in those who lack central heating systems; they result from spasm of small arterioles as a result of cold. Management consists of advice to keep the affected areas warm with appropriate protective clothing.

Erythema ab igne is a common persistent macular erythema and hyperpigmentation occurring in a reticulate pattern in skin areas exposed to continued moderate heat. Histopathology of the small dermal blood vessels suggests that stasis is also important (Shahrad & Marks, 1977). The

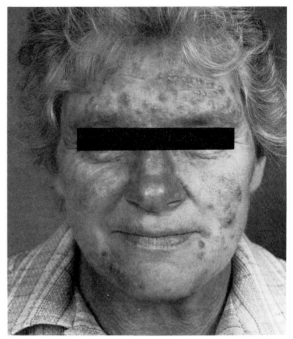

Fig. 47.4 Rosacea showing papules and pustules. This patient also had an inflamed right eye.

legs of women exposed to open fires or electric heaters are the most frequent locations.

Allergic vasculitis presenting as purpura over the lower limbs particularly, but sometimes buttocks and upper limbs, and associated with papules, nodules and blisters, is not rare in the aged (Fig. 47.5). Some lesions may ulcerate leaving areas of necrosis and often leg or upper limb oedema is present. Treatment is bed rest and the prognosis is good generally. However renal involvement (focal nephritis) occurs occasionally and may be progressive. The cause is usually unknown but a preceding streptococcal throat infection or drugs e.g. thiazides, are sometimes incriminated.

Erythema multiforme is a skin reaction usually of unknown cause, but sometimes follows herpes simplex or exhibition of drugs such as barbiturates and sulphonamides. The common form manifests as red round often rather oedematous lesions with a purplish centre which is sometimes vesicular. Limbs are usually mainly affected and ulcers of lips and within the mouth are common.

Clinical scurvy is still seen usually in those living alone and with a poor diet lacking in vitamin C. The patient usually presents with pain, bruises over lower limbs and woody oedema of the legs where haemorrhage has occurred. The swollen leg may simulate a deep vein thrombosis. Perifollicular haemorrhages over the limbs sometimes occur.

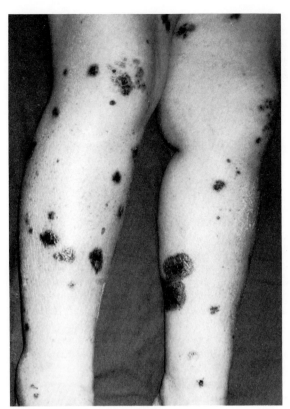

Fig. 47.5 Allergic vasculitis showing purpura and blisters over lower legs.

BLISTERING DISORDERS

Bullous pemphigoid

This uncommon blistering disorder occurs predominantly in the elderly. It is characterised by tense (subepidermal) blisters and erythematous patches. Blisters appear particularly over limbs and abdomen and lesions produce little irritation. The condition is considered an auto-immune disease and is associated with circulating antibody to basement membrane and IgG immunofluoresence can be demonstrated at the basement membrane zone. Treatment is with systemic steroids or adrenocorticotrophic hormone (ACTH) and in some patients methotrexate or azathioprine is also useful. The disease tends to be self-limiting.

Dermatitis herpetiformis (DH)

Although more common in younger adults this uncommon disease is seen in older individuals presenting as a markedly irritant vesicular eruption. Lesions tend to be symmetrical and occur over the scalp, scapular region, elbows, natal cleft, hips and knees. Diagnosis is clinical and confirmed by skin biopsy. In typical DH immunofluorescent studies show granular IgA deposits in the dermal papillae especially in uninvolved skin. Dapsone is effective treatment for the irritant eruption. Many patients with DH

have asymptomatic coeliac disease (diagnosed by jejunal biopsy) and this will respond to a gluten-free diet. Strict adherence to the diet will often enable dapsone therapy to be withdrawn after many months.

Pemphigus vulgaris

Although of unknown cause the presence of circulating antibodies to intercellular epidermal material in pemphigus suggests, like bullous pemphigoid, an immune mechanism. Direct immunofluorescence of lesional skin shows intercellular staining for IgG. The intra-epidermal blisters are widespread, flaccid, easily broken and have a tendency to extend and be complicated by secondary bacterial infection (Fig. 47.6). Lesions often begin in the mouth producing ulceration. The patient is ill through loss of fluid from the lesions and secondary infection and treatment is directed to prevention of both blister formation and secondary infection and combating electrolyte or blood loss by appropriate replacement. High doses of systemic steroids (e.g. 100 mg prednisolone or

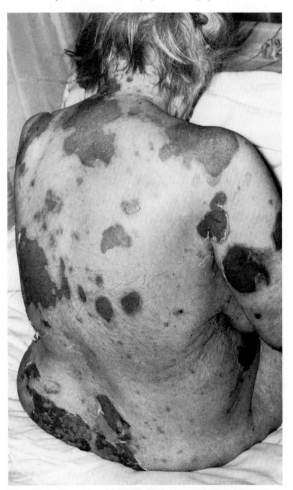

Fig. 47.6 Pemphigus vulgaris. This patient had widespread superficial blistering with affected skin easily separating.

more daily) may be necessary and the dosage is reduced slowly when the blister formation is controlled. Azathioprine or methotrexate also have a place in treatment often reducing the steroid dosage required.

INFECTIONS

Scabies occurs in older people as well as in the young and should not be forgotten in patients with widespread irritant symmetrical eruptions sparing the face, particularly if other members of the household are itching.

Herpes zoster (shingles) is seen regularly and in the elderly post-zoster pain can be very severe. Herpes zoster usually appears for no obvious reason, but an attack may be triggered by radiotherapy, cytotoxic drugs or pressure on nerve roots. A widespread zoster complicating the localised segmental eruption is more common in conditions where immunological resistance is reduced. Analgesics and topical steroid-antibiotic applications are useful in zoster both to treat and prevent secondary infection. Topical use of 5% or 40% idoxuridine in dimethyl sulphoxide is effective in drying up skin blisters rapidly and reducing post-zoster pain but the 40% preparation should be reserved for hospital use. For severe painful attacks of zoster some authorities recommend a three week course of systemic prednisolone commencing with 40–60 mg daily and then reducing the dosage. This therapy reduces both the frequency and severity of post-herpetic neuralgia.

DRUG ERUPTIONS

As a general rule the older the patient the more drugs he is likely to be receiving and the more drugs a patient takes the more likely is a drug eruption to occur. Many types of eruption occur but exanthematic and urticarial rashes are most common. In any unexplained eruption a drug history is most important and purgatives, cough mixtures and all kinds of proprietary preparations should also be considered.

ALOPECIA

With increasing age, as a normal phenomenon, the scalp hair does tend to become less profuse.

Alopecia areata, an auto-immune disease that is genetically determined, can occur at any age including the elderly. Single or multiple well-defined uninflamed areas of hair-fall occur particularly over the scalp. Remnants of broken off hairs (exclamation mark hairs) may be visible at the edge of bald areas. Spontaneous resolution is usual but may take a year or more. In general the more extensive the hair loss the longer it takes to regrow.

Reversible widespread scalp hair thinning may be seen as a toxic effect of cytotoxic drugs and anticoagulants and as a consequence of severe mental or physical stress, the latter including septicaemia or major abdominal surgery.

WHAT CAN BE DONE TO PREVENT OR MODIFY SKIN DISEASE?

Some points have already been mentioned, but early and accurate diagnosis is the prime requisite for correct treatment, and early referral of patients with undiagnosed skin conditions is necessary. Unfortunately in practice this is often difficult because many elderly people with skin disease (or any other disease) delay before consulting their doctor. This may be for various reasons, including their dislike of 'bothering the doctor', failure to appreciate the seriousness of a condition, worry that they may be referred to a hospital or being too occupied with other problems.

Closer liaison between doctors, social service workers and elderly people should allow earlier referral, diagnosis and management of skin diseases. Encouraging the elderly to get out and about and to join friendship clubs and thus meet people of their own age may indirectly hasten an awareness of a skin condition and the desire to do something about it.

Older persons should be advised against excessive exposure to the sun and the young individual should be given similar advice (because he too will become old) particularly if fair-skinned, blond, or redhead. Accepting this advice would help to prevent solar keratoses, squamous carcinomas, melanomas and some basal-cell carcinomas, on sun-exposed areas.

Attention to diet is important because malnutrition or vitamin deficiencies can produce skin disease.

Psychogenic factors are often important in skin disease and appreciation and management of these are necessary. Many systemic diseases may show skin manifestations and as the skin may show the first sign of an underlying disease such signs should not be ignored. Obviously, if possible, the prescribing of too many drugs in any one patient should be avoided. Dangerous drugs and new drugs should be used with care and with full awareness of their toxic effects.

Topical steroids should not be prescribed for direct application to leg ulcers because ulcers may be enlarged in this way and, in addition, bacterial and fungal infection may be encouraged. Application of fluorinated steroids to the face is contra-indicated in rosacea, perioral dermatitis and infections which will all be worsened by such therapy. However, in localised facial lesions of cutaneous lupus erythematosus, application of such steroids is indicated.

CONCLUSION

Nowadays the vast majority of skin conditions can be cured or controlled and the elderly patient must be actively encouraged by both his family and his family doctor to seek treatment of such disease. Although the prime aim of the doctor must be to cure his patient, in some conditions investigation and treatment may be more severe than the disease, and in such patients to provide correct management is far more important than to cure.

REFERENCES

Bettley F R, O'Shea J A 1975 The absorption of arsenic and its relation to carcinoma. British Journal of Dermatology 92: 563–568

Braverman I M 1981 Skin Signs of Systemic Disease 2nd edn, WB Saunders Co, Philadelphia, ch 13, p 655

Braverman I M, Fonferko E 1982a Studies in cutaneous aging: I The elastic fibre network. Journal of Investigative Dermatology 78: 434–443

Braverman I M, Fonferko E 1982b Studies in cutaneous aging: II The microvasculature. Journal of Investigative Dermatology 78: 444–448

Dawber R P R, Wilkinson J D 1979 Melanotic freckle of Hutchinson: Treatment of macular and nodular phases with cryotherapy. British Journal of Dermatology 101: 47–52

Korting G W 1980 Geriatric Dermatology W B Saunders Co, Philadelphia

Leading Article 1982 Diagnosis and treatment of venous ulceration. Lancet 2: 247–248

Mackie R M 1980 Mycosis fungoides. In: Rook A, Savin J (eds) Recent Advances in Dermatology 5. Churchill Livingstone, Edinburgh, p 83–107

Shahrad P, Marks R 1977 The wages of warmth: changes in erythema ab igne. British Journal of Dermatology 97: 179–186

Sonnex T S, Leonard J, Ralfs I, Dawber R P R 1982 Myxoid cysts of the finger: treatment by liquid nitrogen spray cryosurgery. British Journal of Dermatology 107: 21

Verbov J L 1974 Skin Diseases in the Elderly. William Heinemann Medical Books Ltd, London.

48

Pressure sores — prevention and treatment

M. Bliss

INCIDENCE

Pressure necrosis is a serious disorder of the elderly, which, with important exceptions, seldom occurs in young patients. One third of all patients admitted to geriatric wards either have pressure sores or are liable to develop them (Norton et al, 1975), and the same, or greater proportion of patients over the age of 70 years in other hospital departments are similarly at risk. A one day census of a district general hospital in inner London, including medical, surgical, orthopaedic, geriatric and psychiatric beds, showed that 25% of all the patients required special care for the prevention and treatment of pressure sores, 10% of those aged less than 70 years and 40% over this age (Hibbs, 1982). Only about one quarter of these patients had sores, but this is a less significant figure than the number at risk, as it depends on local management and does not indicate the amount of care needed for prevention. About one third of all sores are present on admission and 80% of the remainder develop during the first two weeks of stay (Norton et al, 1975).

AETIOLOGY

Pressure

A pressure sore is caused by the death of an area of tissue which has had its blood supply cut off by pressure or deformation (Reichel, 1958; Scales, 1982) between an internal bony prominence and an outside resistant surface for a critical length of time. Common sites are the sacrum, heels, ischial tuberosities and hips comprising roughly 40, 20, 15 and 10% of all sores respectively (Jordan & Clark, 1977 & 1979; Jordan et al, 1976). Of these sores, 80% are superficial and 20% deep.

A superficial sore is one in which the necrosis has been confined to the skin. It often presents as a blister which breaks down to expose a flat, painful, raw area. Once formed, superficial sores may be exacerbated, or prevented from healing, by friction on rough or wet sheets (Lowthian, 1975).

A deep or gangrenous sore occurs where there has been death of subcutaneous tissue. It appears initially as a blue black patch. The damage in the deep tissue is always greater than that in the skin, so that these sores have overhanging edges, and often deep sinuses, extending for many centimetres.

Experiments in animals have shown that low pressures applied to the tissues for long periods may be even more damaging than high pressures for short periods (Husain, 1953; Kosiak, 1959). However clinical experience suggests that both the pressures and times needed to cause necrosis vary greatly according to the physical condition of the subject.

Susceptible patients

The four principal groups of patients who are liable to develop pressure sores are: 1. patients with spinal cord injury (Reuter & Cooney, 1981); 2. patients with neurological disease e.g. multiple sclerosis (Barbenel et al, 1977), cerebrovascular disease and Parkinson's disease; 3. patients aged over 70 years (Barbenel et al, 1977); and 4. patients who are very ill or dying (Hibbs, 1982; Barton & Barton, 1978). The common factors are probably neurological disease and illness, not age.

Neurological disease

Neurological disease, especially cerebrovascular disease, is very common in the elderly, and almost all patients who develop sores have neurological symptoms. Conversely, alert and normally active elderly patients seldom develop sores, however ill they may be. It is not clear whether neurological disease simply reduces the sensation of pressure pain and mobility (Exton-Smith & Sherwin, 1961), or whether it also affects the responses of the body to intercurrent illness and stress e.g. the vasomotor system (Barton & Barton, 1978; Guttmann, 1976).

Illness

Illness always precedes the appearance of pressure sores (Roaf, 1976). Susceptible patients only develop sores at times of stress, while even patients without neurological disease may develop them if they are sufficiently ill. Common causes of stress which precipitate sores in the elderly are an intercurrent illness, an injury, an anaesthetic, an operation, dehydration, faecal impaction and day sedation. Most elderly patients newly admitted to hospital suffer from at least one of these conditions, thus accounting for the high incidence of sores in the first two weeks of stay. Elderly orthopaedic patients, who have a combination of stress factors, have the highest incidence of all – between 30 and 50% (Barton & Barton, 1978). The incidence in chronically disabled patients at home or in long stay wards is much lower (Barton & Barton, 1978), because of their more stable physical condition; but they are just as liable to develop sores at the onset of illness, which, in these patients, may be indicated only by non-specific symptoms, such as loss of appetite or the development of incontinence.

Incontinence itself does not predispose patients to pressure sores, but the appearance of incontinence, particularly of double incontinence, which often signifies faecal impaction, is an important sign of deterioration in an elderly person's health.

Peripheral vascular disease

Peripheral vascular disease is common in the elderly, and increases their liability to develop sores of the heel. These are commoner in men than in women, and four times commoner in smokers than in non-smokers (Barton & Barton, 1978).

IDENTIFICATION OF PATIENTS AT RISK

The pressure sore score

This is a well known method of assessing an elderly person's state of health and hence his liability to develop pressure sores (Table 48.1) (Norton et al, 1962). It is very effective in identifying newly admitted, acutely ill, susceptible patients, but it is less useful in long stay patients, who cannot be scored daily for years, and in whom deterioration of the score, signifying the onset of illness, is more important than its original level (Bliss et al, 1966).

Pressure marks on the skin

Unfading red blotches or blisters in the pressure areas provide overriding evidence of a patient's susceptibility to sores, but every effort must be made to identify vulnerable subjects before these occur.

Categories of patients at risk

Instead of attempting to identify individuals, it is probably a better policy to regard certain categories of patients as being liable to pressure necrosis until proved otherwise; e.g. all patients with paraplegia or other neurological disease; all patients over the age of 70 years newly admitted to hospital; all elderly patients, in hospital or at home, whose condition is deteriorating; and all very ill or dying patients. These patients should automatically be given antipressure care until they can be shown to be no longer in need of it.

ANTIPRESSURE CARE

Improve the general condition, where practicable, as rapidly as possible

Special effort should be made to prevent and relieve dehydration and faecal impaction, and to avoid non-essential drugs.

Relieve pressure

1. Nurse the patient mainly in bed. The value of bed nursing for preventing and healing sores in paraplegic patients has long been recognised in spinal injury units (Guttmann, 1976; Fallon, 1978), but is only slowly being appreciated in the care of the elderly (Lowthian, 1975; Bliss et al, 1966; Bedford et al, 1961). Contrary to what has often been taught in the past, bed rest is important in the general treatment of patients sufficiently ill to be liable to pressure necrosis and hastens recovery. It also allows the body weight to be distributed over a wide area and antipressure measures to be applied. The patient should be laid as flat as possible, preferably without a back rest.

2. The bed should be made up with a soft, double width drawsheet anchored firmly under the pillow to prevent wrinkling. A fleece next to the skin provides the best relief from friction in the sacral area.

3. Bedwear for both men and women should be of fine material e.g. polyester, which does not cause damaging folds.

4. The whole of the lower third of the bed should be covered with a thick nursing fleece with wide flaps extending up under the drawsheet and at both sides to hold it in place

Table 48.1 The pressure sore score

Physical condition	Mental state	Activity	Mobility	Incontinence
4 Good	4 Alert	4 Ambulant	4 Full	4 Not
3 Fair	3 Confused	3 Walks with help	3 Limited	3 Occasional
2 Poor	2 Apathetic	2 Chairbound	2 Very limited	2 Usually urine
1 Bad	1 Stuporose	1 In bed	1 Immobile	1 Doubly incontinent

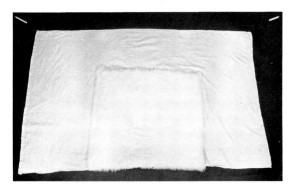

Fig. 48.1 Heel fleece sewn on to a drawsheet to provide proximal and side flaps to anchor it on the bed.

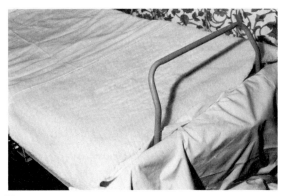

Fig. 48.2 Heel fleece and end-of-bed cradle.

(Figs. 48.1 & 48.2) (Hibbs, 1982). (Heel pads of fleece and other materials are uncomfortable and do not stay in position.)

5. A bedcradle should always be used

6. The bed should be kept as dry as possible if necessary by catheterising the patient.

These simple precautions will prevent about 50% of sacral sores and 90% of heel sores (Hibbs, 1982).

Patients who have gross neurological disease, who are very ill or who have pressure marks on the skin should be given additional anti-pressure care, e.g. regular turning and/or an anti-pressure mattress.

Regular turning

The patient's position is changed at least once every two hours, so that prolonged pressure on any part of the body is prevented. Turning should be carried out where possible, but may be difficult in patients in whom it is most needed, e.g. in those who are heavy or contracted, or in patients with cerebrovascular disease who dislike lying on their sides (Barton & Barton, 1978; Bliss et al, 1966). Elderly patients are often unco-operative or noisy, which discourages nurses from trying to turn them, especially at night. Turning itself increases the danger of hip sores, and in some very ill patients even hourly turning may be insufficient to prevent tissue necrosis, without the help of a special mattress.

Antipressure mattresses

Many types are available but few are suitable for regular use in hospital. The most practical are soft mattresses e.g. pillows, soft foam beds or water beds; and alternating pressure beds.

Pillow beds

Nursing patients on pillows two or three deep, with gaps under bony prominences is an important aid to preventing sores by regular turning (Bailey, 1970), but is difficult with heavy, unco-operative or incontinent patients.

Soft foam mattresses

These are not as effective as might be thought, partly because of the difficulty of finding suitably elastic, waterproof covering materials (Chow et al, 1976). A fitted cover induces shearing stresses by acting like a hammock, while a very loose cover may cause damaging folds. The polyflote mattress (Reswick & Rogers, 1976), a double layer of foam with slits cut in the surface to reduce tension, has been found to be effective only if it is used without a cover. The Vaperm mattress (Scales et al, 1982), made up of sections of foam of different densities, has a vapour permeable cover of Platilon which is elastic but only semi-durable. In general, a soft mattress may be helpful for light patients, but heavy patients tend to concentrate all their weight in the centre which may increase rather than decrease pressure in the dependent areas.

Water mattresses

The deeper the water bed the more effective it is at preventing sores, but the more inconvenient to use. Semiflotation beds, much as the Western Medical (Lowthian, 1975), which has a relatively small mattress, depend for their maximum effect on adjustment of the amount of water for individual patients (seldom attempted in practice). They do not wholly prevent sores, but patients may be turned on them and they are practical and popular.

True flotation beds, such as the Beaufort-Winchester (Andrews, 1981), have a deep bath with a very loose envelope which allows the patient to sink into the water as if he were floating. This distributes the weight evenly over the whole of the undersurface of the body, so that points of high pressure do not occur. These beds completely prevent pressure sores but are difficult to use. Patients cannot easily be lifted in and out of them or positioned on the unstable surface. Bed pans, urinals and catheters all require special management, and dressings and enemas cannot be carried out without removing the patient from the bed. If the undersurface of the mattress becomes contaminated, it can only be cleaned by being emptied and sent away for sterilisation. The beds are cumbersome to install and to dismantle and very heavy, so that once filled, they often remain in a ward occupying a bed space when they are not needed. They are also expensive.

In spite of their disadvantages, water beds have a reputation for being reliable anti-pressure aids. They are useful for nursing light, immobile patients with prolonged terminal illnesses (Hibbs, 1982) but they are not suitable for the routine pressure propylaxis of the majority of ill, elderly patients admitted to hospital.

Alternating pressure beds
These are potentially the most useful anti-pressure aids available (Bliss et al, 1966). The mattresses consist of different patterns of alternating sets of air cells, connected to an electrically operated pump, which causes them to inflate and deflate underneath the patient about every 10 minutes, thus continually altering the supporting points of pressure on the body. Most types can be laid directly on top of an ordinary mattress. For maximum effect, the cells must have sufficient diameter and pressure to lift the body off the bed. Mattresses which do this, e.g. the large celled Ripple bed (Bliss et al, 1967) and the Advanced Pegasus Airwave System (Exton-Smith et al, 1982), have been shown in controlled trials to be able to prevent and heal pressure sores, even in patients who cannot be turned.

Alternating pressure beds are practical and permit all nursing procedures. When they are working properly, they are reasonably comfortable, but unfortunately defective machines are common. No alternating pressure mattress has yet been produced which is sufficiently robust for ward use and hospitals have failed to establish adequate systems for servicing them (Bliss, 1979). A punctured mattress or defective motor does not provide sufficient pressure to lift the body off the bed and pressure sores occur. A mattress which is working properly should feel firm. Doctors and nurses must be taught how to use these beds, to make sure that the pressure settings are correct and that the air tubes are securely fixed and not kinked, and to recognise faulty machines so that they can be replaced immediately.

Emergency anti-pressure care
Two hours of unrelieved pressure in a susceptible patient, e.g. a newly admitted old person with a fractured neck of femur, may be sufficient to cause a gangrenous sore. Hospitals and home nursing services should have anti-pressure kits (Hibbs, 1982), including bedcradles, fleeces and alternating pressure machines, available day and night. Casualty and theatre trolleys, and operating and X-ray tables being used for elderly or paralysed patients should have foam mattresses (Dyson, 1978). Special attention is needed for patients with fractures to prevent sores due to pressure from orthopaedic apparatus (Barton & Barton, 1978).

Time spent out of bed
Unless they are obviously well, newly admitted patients should not be sat out of bed for more than four hours daily, and not at all if their condition is deteriorating. A recent survey has confirmed the growing realisation that helpless patients are more likely to develop sores if they are nursed in a chair than in bed (Barbenel et al, 1977).

Patients who are fit should be sat in comfortable chairs of knee height, so that their feet rest flat on the floor. Fleeces or cushions may be used, but not air rings which prevent the even distribution of pressure (Barton & Barton, 1978). Alternating pressure cushions are not a substitute for rest in bed on an alternating pressure mattress and are seldom necessary for the elderly. As their condition improves patients may be got up for longer periods, but those who are unable to stand unaided should always be laid to rest on their beds for 1–2 hours during the day to provide a radical change in their weight bearing areas.

Removal of anti-pressure aids
When the patient's condition has improved, anti-pressure equipment can usually be removed. Paraplegic or dying patients may need special care indefinitely, but the majority of elderly patients can be safely nursed on an ordinary bed once they are well. Anti-pressure mattresses are a hinderance to patients undergoing rehabilitation.

HEALING SORES

Trunk sores
Unlike sores in some young patients with severe neurological disease, who may have trophic nerve damage affecting healing (Guttmann, 1976), trunk sores in the elderly heal readily once the blood supply is restored by relief of pressure. They may be regarded as accidental wounds in normal tissue which is fully capable of carrying out the processes of repair, provided these are not prevented by continued pressure or over zealous local therapy (Schilling, 1968). The healthy tissue walls off the necrotic area and secretes enzymes which liquify and separate the sloughs in about two weeks. Over the next four weeks the cavity is reduced to about half of its original size by contraction of the surrounding tissue (Barton & Barton, 1978). The remaining defect is then slowly closed by the formation of a scar. The whole process may take from a few weeks to several months depending on the size of the original sore, but the healing time is prolonged or the sore may never heal, if pressure is inadequately relieved.

The principle of pressure relief for the treatment of sores is the same as for prevention. The patient must be nursed mainly in bed with regular turning or an anti-pressure mattress, with minimum pressure on the affected area. A patient with a sacral or ischial sore should not sit in a chair for more than one hour daily, although he may be allowed to walk as soon as he is fit enough.

Heel sores

Heel sores are more difficult to heal than trunk sores, due to poor vascularity and fixation of the surrounding tissue. The sloughs separate more slowly and complete healing may take many months. As in the trunk, speeding healing time depends on improving the circulation. In the heels, two measures are important: 1. local relief of pressure e.g. by use of fleeces, soft slippers etc; and 2. elevation of the legs to a horizontal position.

The arterial blood pressure in the feet is improved by dependency, but venous stasis and fluid retention also occur in ill, elderly patients sitting in chairs, resulting in capillary congestion, anoxia and reduced healing (Barton & Barton, 1978). A horizontal position of the legs appears to offer the best compromise. This is impossible in an upright chair, and the attempt throws great pressure onto the heels, so that patients must be taught to sit on their beds. A pillow should be placed under the calves to relieve pressure on the heels, but the foot of the bed should not be elevated. The patients may be dressed and allowed to walk about and to look after themselves, but must not sit on chairs except for meals. As with most leg ulcers, heel sores improve rapidly with this treatment. Pressure bandages and diuretic therapy do not have the same effect.

Local treatment

This should be minimal for all types of sore (Barton & Barton, 1978). With proper relief of pressure, trunk sore sloughs separate readily, without debrident or enzyme treatment. The artificial removal of the more slowly separating heel slough may accelerate healing, but this is uncertain. Antiseptics, such as Eusol, harm granulation tissue and should not be used (Barton & Barton, 1978; Schilling, 1968). Pressure sores are always heavily infected, but seldom cause a cellulitis, except in immuno-compromised or diabetic patients; these are the only cases where they may need to be swabbed and treated with systemic antibiotics.

Sore cavities should be washed out with normal saline and left empty. They may be dressed with gauze bridged across the opening, but should not be packed with gauze or other material (Barton & Barton, 1978). Packing increases local pressure and prevents discharge and contraction, prolonging healing time and increasing pain.

Superficial sores are probably best left exposed, with a fleece placed next to the skin. Heel sores can also be treated by exposure, but the resolution of very adherent sloughs may be hastened by an emmolient, such as 0.5% cetrimide cream, under an occlusive dressing (Barton & Barton, 1978).

The restoration of the blood supply by relief of pressure stimulates healing to such an extent that additional treatment with ultraviolet light, oxygen etc is unlikely to have any measurable effect. The benefits attributed to these agents are probably due to concommitant increased anti-pressure care (Morgan, 1975; Fernie & Dornan, 1976; Berger, 1957).

Sores in dying patients

With pressure relief, both superficial and deep sores may heal even in dying patients. Thermography shows increased temperature in the surrounding tissues indicating that a healing reaction is taking place (Barton & Barton, 1978). However in some dying patients with very severe sores, the periphery remains cold and lifeless.

Pain relief

The pain of pressure sores is greatly improved by putting the patient to bed with proper relief of pressure, but patients with very severe sores usually also need a powerful analgesic until the acute stage is over. Diamorphine 2.5–5 mg 4-hourly (with an anti-emetic and a laxative) is usually adequate in the elderly. Anti-inflammatory drugs should not be used as they retard healing (Barton & Barton, 1978).

Nutrition

A normal haemoglobin and good nutrition with a high protein diet and vitamins, is important in healing sores, but patients who are not dying usually begin to take an adequate diet naturally as soon as their general health and sores improve with bed rest and relief of pressure.

Plastic surgery

Very large sores can be healed in 2–3 weeks by plastic surgery, provided this is sufficiently radical (Bailey, 1970; Berger, 1957; Constantion, 1981). The sore is excised together with the surface of the underlying bone and skin flaps rotated to cover the defect. Many large sores in young patients can only be healed by these means, but operation is seldom necessary in the elderly and merely exposes the patient to the risk of post-operative complications and further sores. Split skin grafting for heel sores is also seldom necessary, and can cause painful ulceration in the donor areas.

REFERENCES

Andrews J 1981 Prevention and cure of pressure sores. In: Geriatrics for everyday practice. Karger, Basel, New York, p 122–133
Bailey B N 1970 Bedsores. British Journal of Hospital Medicine 3: 223–231
Barbenel J C, Jordan M M, Nicol S M, Clark M 1977 Incidence of pressure sores in the Greater Glasgow Health Board Area. Lancet ii: 548–550
Barton A, Barton M 1978 The management and prevention of pressure sores. Faber and Faber, London, Boston
Bedford P D, Cosin L Z, McCarthy T F, Scott B 1961 The alternating pressure mattress. Gerontologia Clinica 3: 69–82

Berger J C 1957 Surgical treatment of decubitus ulcers. Plastic and Reconstructive Surgery 20: 206–217

Bliss M R 1979 The use of ripple beds in hospitals. Hospital and Health Services Review 74: 190–193

Bliss M R, McLaren R, Exton-Smith A N 1966 Mattresses for preventing pressure sores in geriatric patients. Monthly Bulletin of the Ministry of Health 25: 238–268

Bliss M R, McLaren R, Exton-Smith A N 1967 Preventing pressure sores in hospital: controlled trial of a large celled ripple mattress. British Medical Journal 1: 394–397

Chow W W, Juvinall R C, Cockrell J L 1976 Effects and characteristics of cushion covering membranes. Bedsore Biomechanics. MacMillan Press Ltd, London, Basingstoke p 95–102

Constantion M B 1981 Pressure ulcers: principles and techniques of management. Little Brown, Boston

Dyson R 1978 Bedsores: the injuries hospital staff inflict on patients. Nursing Mirror (15th June): 30–32

Exton-Smith A N, Overstall P W, Wedgwood J, Wallace G 1982 Use of the 'Airwave System' to prevent pressure sores in hospital. Lancet 1: 1288–1290

Exton-Smith A N, Sherwin R W 1961 The prevention of pressure sores — significance of spontaneous bodily movements. Lancet 2: 1124–1126

Fallon B 1978 So you are paralysed. Spinal Injuries Association, London

Fernie G R, Dornan J 1976 The problems of clinic trials with new systems for preventing or healing decubiti. Bedsore Biomechanics. MacMillan Press Ltd, London, Basingstoke p 315–320

Guttmann L 1976 The prevention and treatment of pressure sores. Bedsore Biomechanics. MacMillan Press Ltd, London, Basingstoke p 153–159

Hibbs P 1982 Pressure sores: a system of prevention. Nursing Mirror (4th August): 25–29

Husain T 1953 Experimental study of pressure effects on the tissues. Journal of Pathology and Bacteriology 66: 347–358

Jordan M M, Clark M O 1977, 1979 The incidence of pressure sores in the patient community of the Greater Glasgow Health Board Area on 21st January 1976. Reports of the Bio-engineering Unit, University of Strathclyde and the Greater Glasgow Health Board

Jordan M M, Nicol S M, Melrose A L 1976 The incidence of pressure sores in the patient community of the Borders Health Board Area on 13th October 1976. Report of the Bio-engineering Unit, Univeristy of Strathclyde and the Borders Health Board

Kosiak N 1959 Aetiology and pathology of ischaemic ulcers. Archives of Physical Medicine and Rehabilitation 40: 62–69

Lowthian P T 1975 Pressure sores: practical prophylaxis. Modern Geriatrics 5: 25–30

Morgan J E 1975 Topical therapy for pressure ulcer surgery. Surgery, Gynecology and Obstetrics 141: 945–957

Norton D, McLaren R, Exton-Smith A N 1975 An investigation of geriatric nursing problems in hospital. Churchill Livingstone, Edinburgh

Reichel S M 1958 Shearing force as a factor in decubitus ulcers in paraplegics. 166: 762–763

Reswick J B, Rogers J E 1976 Experience at Rancho Los Amigos Hospital with devices and techniques to prevent pressure sores. Bedsore Biomechanics. MacMillan Press Ltd, London, Basingstoke p 301–310

Reuter J P, Cooney T G 1981 The pressure sore: Pathophysiology and principles of management. Annals of Internal Medicine 94: 661–666

Roaf R 1976 The causation and prevention of bedsores. Bedsore Biomechanics. MacMillan Press Ltd, London, Basingstoke, p 5–9

Scales J 1982 Pressure sore prevention. Care Science and Practice. 1: 9–17

Scales J T, Lowthian P T, Poole A G et al 1982 The Vaperm patient support system: a new general purpose hospital mattress. Lancet ii: 1150–1152

Schilling J A 1968 Wound healing. Physiological review 48: 374–423

Society and the elderly patient

49

Rehabilitation — physical resources

P. H. Millard

A person and his world are changed by illness and afterwards he can be better or worse but never the same. Coming to terms with one's changed state and learning to live with it is the basis of rehabilitation, which is mainly done by verbal and non-verbal communication — a word or smile of encouragement — but sometimes new techniques have to be learnt and thus other professionals are involved.

THE TOTAL APPROACH

The first Aphorism of Hippocrates summarises the need for the total approach to patient care.

'Life is short, the art long; the occasion fleeting; experience fallacious and judgement difficult. The physician must not only be prepared to do what is right himself, but also make the patient, the attendants and the externals co-operate'.

The patient must be visualised in his own world. No-one is independent for everyone interacts with others. The basic system is the informal network of family and friends, who in caring for people in their midst are supported by a formal network of statutory benefits and services.

The informal network

The informal family network — kith and kin — is untrained but has the advantage of familiarity, flexibility, availability and commitment. At times of illness the strength of the family and neighbourhood network is tested — few are found wanting. As stress increases the physiological responses of fight, flight or acceptance come to the fore and few run away. In times of need they turn first to themselves and only if that fails do they turn to the formal network for assistance.

It is untrue to say that the only thing that an aged person requires is the loving care that a daughter would give to her mother, for experience shows that when a mother lives with her daughter, the daughter gradually takes over the role of the mother in running the household, whereas if the unmarried son continues to live with his mother she continues to run the home despite increasing disability. Rehabilitation is about encouraging relative independence not dependence and patients must be encouraged to do those things that they can, and relearn, within the limits imposed by their disability to do some of the things that they at present cannot.

There is a widespread myth, that Western families do not care for the aged but anyone who practises geriatric medicine rapidly comes to realise that this is false. Because elderly people live alone in Western Society it does not imply, either, that they are lonely, or that no-one in their family cares for them or about them. Stearns (1977) pointed out the protective legislation for peasant farmers in France and commented that it may be easier to care for the aged if they live apart from you.

The formal network

The scale and the organisation of the formal network varies from country to country and from town to town for it is dependent upon the economic and social policies of central and local government. In some countries voluntary agencies — usually religious, trade or disease based — play a part. The formal network has the advantage of trained expertise but has the disadvantage that the members of it have been trained to play different roles and thus it tends to be inflexible, to have demarcation disputes, to be not readily available and inappropriate when called (Hemsi, 1982).

Systems of formal care that work in the United Kingdom may not work elsewhere, however, the concepts can gain expression in a different form. Geriatric medicine, for example, arose in the United Kingdom because of the perceived neglect of the elderly in the chronic sick wards run by local authorities and thus, in 1948, the decision was made to place responsibility for the care of those aged people who require long term nursing care on the National Health Service. Out of that decision the whole new specialty of geriatric medicine arose.

Anatomy of social networks

When elderly patients are referred to the now combined Departments of Psychiatry and Geriatric Medicine at St George's Hospital in the suburbs of London, it is surprising how much — not how little — support has been received (much of it unco-ordinated and unplanned). The referral is normally made when someone no longer feels able to cope because the elderly person is falling, confused, immobile or incontinent. To understand the problem, one must take an accurate medical history and this is incomplete if it does not include a full description of the people and services interacting with the aged person. Systematic enquiry should include:

The informal network. Names, addresses, telephone numbers, frequency of contact and contribution — for, or on behalf of the patient — of relatives, neighbours and friends.

The formal network. The frequency of involvement and names of people involved should be specified.

Domiciliary services
  The primary health care team
    General practitioner
    District Nurse
    Health visitor
  Social Services Department — field workers
    Social worker
    Home Help
    Meals on Wheels
Institutional Services
  Hospital based support services.
    Hospital doctors involved
    Outpatient clinics
    Day Hospitals
    Holiday relief/6 weeks in scheme
  Social Services Department — residential and day care
    Luncheon clubs
    Day centres
    Residential homes
    Holiday admissions

Psychology of social networks

The psycho-dynamic factors which exist within social networks need to be handled constructively. All too often doctors erect barriers when what is needed is a sense of partnership. The feelings, opinions and attitudes of the family, the neighbours and the staff are often far more important than minor differences in handicap and mental test scores. Each person holds opinions, some based in prejudice, some in ignorance, some in history, but whatever the reason it is peculiar to that person. The patients' viewpoints also need to be taken note of, for the major factor that decides whether they will rehabilitate to return home is whether they want to. Sometimes the informal network bonds together to oppose the aged person's wish to return home and asks the patient's general practitioner to support the viewpoint that the patient should not be discharged.

Moderate degrees of anxiety can be constructive, but in excess it is destructive. Stresses usually occur because of:

(i) ignorance as to the nature of the illness and its management;
(ii) difficulty in accepting lowered standards of cleanliness etc;
(iii) concern over risk — for example — of falling down stairs and injuring themselves, or setting the house alight (a very rare occurrence), or lying all night on the floor unattended (a not so rare occurrence);
(iv) threat of criticism by others in the informal or formal network;
(v) lack of awareness of the patient's progress in hospital.

Anxiety is reduced if all have the opportunity to express their views. Always be prepared to speak with the relatives when they visit the hospital and put aside a set time each week for them to be able to meet you if they so wish. Do not discuss problems on the telephone, for in that way the nuances of non-verbal communication are lost and one cannot gain a feel for the stress that is involved in coping at home. In difficult cases it is worth arranging a case conference, but only do this if there is a specific reason, for it can be wasteful of time.

The patient's viewpoint

The patient's viewpoint is most important. Most social histories seemingly ignore them and solely record the number and type of services going into the home, the assumption being made, that if something is being done, it must be doing good. However old people often have an entirely different viewpoint. Dependent upon their perception they can feel trapped when there are too many services and they would dearly love to do something for themselves, or they can feel abandoned when they would like more services but are not receiving them.

Presentation of the problem

People consult their doctor if they consider that a symptom that they have warrants attention, but when they decide to consult is dependent upon a host of different factors. Each symptom necessitates a decision — whether or not to seek advice. Symptoms that are commonly seen to be doctor related are swelling of the feet or ankles, breathlessness, pain, bleeding or sudden loss of consciousness. Poor eyesight, bad hearing, inability to chew food and toenails that need cutting are not seen as being doctor related, which is not surprising as three of them — eyesight, teeth and feet — are usually dealt with by other agencies.

Doctors have been trained to deal with the classic presentation of diseases. 'I am sick help me' is the contract between the patient and the doctor. Whatever the age of the patient, the response is to take a history, examine, make a diagnosis, order investigations, commence appropriate treatment and monitor the results. Surveys of the elderly that reveal unmet needs for treatment of eyesight, hearing, teeth or feet reveal a gap in health education of the aged, of their informal caring network and of members of the formal network that have been in contact with them.

Successful aging must be associated with the acceptance of change in one's health status, for deterioration is a natural phenomenon. Some elderly people accept abnormal deterioration as being normal whilst others realise that their symptoms are abnormal but ignore them because of fear. Eventually deterioration in health leads to the classic presentations of disease in old age — falling over, immobility and mental confusion. The inherent strengths and weaknesses of the informal network influence the time of referral. Some refer early, some refer late and some never refer! The call for help when it comes is 'He/she is a problem' — if the doctor responds 'I do not deal with social problems' he demonstrates the poverty of his medical education, for all disease causes social problems. Failure to eat, or an unkempt house precipitate requests for the Social Service Departments whilst falling, immobility and confusion are usually directed to the general practitioner. Inappropriate referrals lead to inappropriate management and thus meals on wheels are given to the elderly person who has myxoedema and home help to those with osteomalacia.

Structure of the home

Before starting on a course of rehabilitation one must be aware of the limitations imposed by the internal structure of the home, for it is pointless to teach a person to be independent in a wheelchair if there are stairs that have to be negotiated. If this is so and wheelchair retraining is the only possible solution, then one should start to arrange rehousing at the beginning — for this may take longer to achieve.

WARD DESIGN

The fundamental knowledge base of consultants in geriatric medicine arises from the attack upon bed rest in the management of illness. At first beds were high and chairs low, but now all the beds are adjustable in height and thus cot sides are rarely necessary, and the chairs are of different heights. Chairs with fixed tables are being phased out and the correct chair is chosen as the one which the patient can most easily get out of. Patients are nursed in bed when they are sick but are out of bed dressed in their own clothes in the stage of rehabilitation. It is preferable for the ward to have lavatories that are in easy reach of all patient areas for this assists the management of incontinence. In one of our most successful units the occupational therapy department and the physiotherapy department are adjacent to the day space, which also has provision for up to eight day patients from home or from other wards in the hospital. In practice this unit works better than those that have separate departments.

MOTIVATION

The basis of rehabilitation is to motivate patients to struggle to overcome their disabilities in a realistic way, making each task just slightly harder than you think they can easily achieve. If they do not want to achieve — perhaps for reasons known only to themselves — they will not. It is essential therefore, to understand what patients want, to discuss with them whether their goals are realistic and then strive to achieve the goal that they want for themselves. Rehabilitation is not about achieving what you or others consider to be right, and success does not come solely when patients are discharged from hospital. Success is solely achieved when they have achieved that which they can accept as being right, taking into account the limitations imposed by their disease, their finances, their housing, the available resources and the inherent strengths and weaknesses of their social network.

Assessment of the degree of disability

An accurate assessment of the degree of disability must be made, and this should be recorded in the notes. There are various scales that can be used for this. We use a three point scale covering 16 parameters which is completed weekly by the team, and displayed graphically in the front of the notes, thus ensuring that problems such as deafness or incontinence are not ignored (Fig. 49.1).

TEAMWORK

Multiple problems either require management by individuals trained to deal with multiple problems or teamwork by people trained to deal with single problems. One of the inherent difficulties in working with aged patients is that hospital-based personnel have been trained to play roles that are more appropriate for single conditions than for multiple pathology. Each one, when faced with a difficult problem, thinks of different solutions, and thus in teamwork there is inherent conflict. Leaderless teams achieve nothing and it is the role of the consultant in geriatric medicine to provide leadership.

Doctors

The biggest falling on the part of the doctors is arrogance when they forget that the other professionals in the team know more about their subject than they do. The houseman/intern is the key medical worker and should be responsible for knowing everything that is happening on the ward. Final responsibility rests with the consultant.

Nurses

The nurses in the ward are key personnel in rehabilitation for they are present at all times, and it is of paramount importance that they should be aware of the goal for each

Fig. 49.1 Disability profile — assessment of the degree of disability in 16 different functions

	Ability	Month 1	Month 2	Month 3
Walking	0 Mobile unaided, including stairs 1 Mobile on flat and aids 2 Independent in wheelchair 3 Chairfast needs aid			
Washing	0 Independent including bathing 1 Needs help for once a week bath 2 Needs help or constant reminder 3 Needs to be washed			
Eating	0 Eats cleanly without help 1 Needs help to cut food 2 Needs help and is messy 3 Needs to be fed			
Dressing	0 Independent 1 Some difficulty e.g. shoes or buttons 2 Needs help with pants or trousers 3 Needs to be dressed			
Sleep	0 Sleeps well 1 Occasional poor sleep 2 Takes regular hypnotic 3 Insomnia			
Urinary Continence	0 No problem (or catheter managed by patient) 1 Needs regular toileting or catheter care 2 Wet at night or infrequently by day 3 Wet day and night			
Faecal Continence	0 No problem 1 Occasionally incontinent 2 Needs bowel care e.g. enema, constipating agent 3 Usually incontinent			
Language or Written Communication	0 Always clear 1 Difficulty in expression but communication adequate 2 Basic communication only e.g. needs food, toilet etc. 3 No communication – able to attract attention			
Sociability	0 Initiates and accepts social contacts 1 Accepts but does not initiate contacts 2 Neither accepts nor initiates social contact 3 Resists attempts at contact			
Memory and Orientation	*Northwick Park Scale* Age Time (to nearest hour) Address to recall at end of test – 43 West Street (This should be repeated by the patient to ensure that it has been heard correctly). Year Name of hospital Recognition of two persons (doctor, nurse) Date of birth Year of First World War Name of present monarch Count backwards (20–1) 0 10–7 1 6–4 2 3–2 3 1–0			

Fig. 49.1 *(Contd)*

	Ability	Month 1	Month 2	Month 3
Mood	0 Normal variation 1 Persistently depressed/euphoric 2 Withdrawn and tearful/euphoric and overactive 3 Mute/maniac excitement			
Behaviour	0 Always co-operative 1 Occasionally verbally aggresive 2 Frequently verbally aggressive 3 Physically aggressive			
Hearing	0 Good with/without aid 1 Poor without aid 2 Poor with aid 3 Completely deaf			
Sight	0 Good with or without glasses 1 Poor without glasses 2 Poor with glasses/partially sighted 3 Completely blind (? registered)			
Teeth	0 Good teeth or good false teeth 1 Own teeth/false teeth need attention 2 Edentulous but masticates well 3 Edentulous, eats only soft food			
Feet	0-1 No problem 2-3 Needs chiropody			

Ability Scale	0	1	2	3
Walking				
Washing				
Eating				
Dressing				
Sleep				
Urinary Continence				
Faecal Continence				
Language				
Sociability				
Memory				
Mood				
Behaviour				
Hearing				
Sight				
Teeth				
Feet				

patient. They must be aware of the achievements of the patient in the physiotherapy department and the occupational therapy department and for this reason I prefer most of the rehabilitation to take place on the wards, for in this way the nursing staff have the opportunity to see what the patient is achieving. The night nursing staff must also be informed of progress. The nursing staff should be encouraged to modify their routines. At first, when sick, patients are nursed in and by their beds, but as independence is regained they should be encouraged to walk to the dining table for their meals, to the day room for group activities and to the lavatory for excretion. Thus maximum use is made of common activities in the ward to encourage independence.

Patients should be dressed in their own clothes and wear their own shoes. Elderly ladies should be encouraged to go to the hairdresser for if they wish to return to the world outside of the hospital it is important that they should look capable of so doing.

Occupational therapy

The occupational therapist assesses the degree of disability and uses her professional expertise to advise on ways and means of improving or maintaining function. She works with the families and the staff to ensure that everyone is aware of the potential and capabilities of the patient. Early referral is essential. In many departments of geriatric medicine all patients are assessed to help ensure that the correct management is instituted from the outset. Assessment is made as to the level of function (eating, dressing, cooking) and reported in terms of the Activities of Daily Living (ADL). An important role is the undertaking of home visits prior to discharge to see what adjustments need to be made. This is not a test that old people can pass or fail; it is an assessment of their needs and of the problems that may beset them when they return. Functions to be taken into account are:

Mobility. Height of chairs, toilet design, floor coverings, tables, stairs, access for walking frames and wheelchairs.

Eating and drinking. This is usually the first area in which the handicapped person can regain independence. Special crockery and cutlery are available.

Toilet management. Crucial for independence and resettlement. Failure in this often breaks the carer's spirit. Toilet seat raises, or a handrail on the wall, or a chemical commode can sometimes *cure* incontinence!

Personal hygiene and dressing. Severe problems are often accounted but perseverance is justified for independence in these functions greatly boosts morale.

Domestic tasks. Guard against the practice of just prescribing every available service on discharge for this is the surest way of making the patient totally dependent upon others. When assessing patients remember that they usually will perform better in their own home, and after a home assessment always ask patients how they thought

they performed and remember that their viewpoint is more important than anyone else's for it is they who have to manage when they go home.

Physiotherapy

Joint working between the physiotherapists and the occupational therapists is essential for their roles are complementary. The task of the physiotherapists ranges from teaching patients to get up off the floor, through building up muscle groups, to helping to reteach the hemiplegic patient to walk.

Socialwork

The social worker enables the person to obtain those services which are appropriate to their needs, and works with them, by counselling, to enable them and others in their caring network to cope.

Other team members

From time to time other disciplines have an important part to play e.g. dietician, speech therapist, hearing aid therapist or chiropodist but the basic team consists of the doctors, nurses, occupational therapists, physiotherapists and the social worker.

Team meetings

A team meeting of all staff on the rehabilitation ward should be held early each morning to plan the day's work. In addition a more formal review should be held weekly in the presence of the consultant.

PHYSICAL RESOURCES

In rehabilitating the aged patient one usually has to make do with the worst facilities available. The unwanted hospitals and wards have been the dowry of many a consultant in geriatric medicine. Marjory Warren (1943) started the revolution in patient management that is gradually changing the practice of medicine throughout the world. Later generations of doctors given responsibility for the development of services for the elderly developed services in individual ways. Prior to Marjory Warren it was unheard of for the chronic sick to be discharged from hospital. Gradually as more and more were rehabilitated out-patients clinics, half-way houses and day hospitals had to be developed. In some hospitals where there had been no physiotherapy or occupational therapy departments the day hospital was developed to provide services for both in and out-patients.

Throughout the history of the development of geriatric medicine the pioneers have had to develop services starting with few resources. The whole language of assessment beds (used to justify beds in the acute hospitals), rehabilitation beds (to justify the need for physiotherapy and occupational therapy) and continuing care beds (perhaps retained solely because it would be thought a folly not to include them) arose because of the need to develop services.

Progressive patient care, wherein the patient was admitted to the assessment ward and if not discharged, was transferred to the rehabilitation ward, and then if not discharged was transferred to long-term care arose solely because that was the way that services had to be run. Some of these words have now been taken on as if they were written down in holy writ. Far from it — no-one really knows what is the correct number of beds to provide for the aged and how these beds should be run. Many people have their opinions and some of these are supported by documents arising from the Geriatric Societies or from Government. It is not the purpose of this short chapter to enter into debate as to the rights or wrongs of the varying viewpoints, for in that I would solely be expressing my own biased views. Suffice it to say that no patients whatever their age, their social class or creed should be admitted for diagnostic purposes to hospitals that lack the basic facilities to undertake modern investigations. If the majority of beds lack these services then progressive patient care must operate. We have now abandoned this practice because we have sufficient resources in active hospitals. If all of the beds are in acute hospitals it may well be that the number of long-term patients is reduced, however, no comparative trials have been carried out.

Mathematics of care
In our part of London the average length of stay in residential homes for the aged is three years and in long-term beds two years. Thus with 360 places in residential homes and 90 places in long-term hospitals, there are only 120 vacancies in homes and 45 vacancies in hospitals each year. There are 90 acute beds to serve a population of 27 500 people aged 65 and over and as the service is referred approximately 1 000 patients a year for admission to its 90 acute beds it can only do this if the average length of stay is 29 days. Of the 1 000 admitted approximately 1 in 5 die, and of the remainder, 1 in 20 can go to a long-term care ward, 1 in 40 can go to a residential home and the remaining 7 out of 10 have to return to the place from which they were admitted — usually their own home, sometimes the home of a relative, or the old people's home where they were previously resident. No more than 10 a year are discharged to private nursing homes for the social class structure of the part of London in which we practise does not make this a viable alternative.

In developing services for the aged patient one is limited by the standard of the accommodation provided and one can only try to do the best one can with the resources available. Geriatric medicine has demonstrated that many of the patients sent for long-term care do not require it. Prevention is said to be better than cure, but despite all of the evidence the aged are still allocated the worst resources.

Aftercare
Rehabilitation has not been successful until the patient has resettled at home. As yet aftercare is only in a primitive early stage in its development. It is my opinion that care, in the first few days after discharge, is best given by ward-based aftercare teams. In the fullness of time I will experiment with this, whilst others will try other methods.

Long-term care
Some people never gain sufficient independence to leave hospital. The major difference between the long-term patient and the patient at home is usually the absence of family.

We, the staff, are thus then surrogate families. The way in which we care reflects our standards, not the patients. Even those who cannot go home can be encouraged to do little things for themselves and rehabilitation should not cease solely because they are not going home. Art therapy, patient committees, music appreciation, drama groups, etc are not solely diversional, they have a therapeutic benefit. The doctor should ensure that such activities take place.

REFERENCES

Hemsi L 1982 Psychogeriatric care in the community. In: Levy R, Post F The Psychiatry of Late Life. Blackwell Scientific Publications, London, ch 9

Stearns P H 1977 Old Age in European Society, the Case of France. Croom Helm, London
Warren M W 1943 Care of the chronic sick. A case for treating chronic sick in blocks in a general hospital. British Medical Journal 2: 822–823

50

Resources for dementia

E. M. D. Grundy & T. Arie

INTRODUCTION

A recent article (Plum, 1979) was entitled 'Dementia — An Approaching Epidemic'. In much of the developed world this epidemic has already arrived and the question of resources is crucial. In Britain and other western countries dementia is now among the biggest problems facing health and social services. As well as looking at resources we shall make some attempt to count the costs of dementia. These extend beyond the simple totting up of expenditure for health and social services, for the burden on the relatives of those with dementia and the contribution which can be expected from the general public are also proper parts of this accounting.

Senile dementia of the Alzheimer type and the less common multi-infarct dementia are both age-related. Kay et al (1970) found that in Newcastle in the late 1960s 22% of the over-80s were moderately or severely demented. The growth in the number of very old people in Britain, America and the rest of the developed world has produced an increase in the number of people with dementia, and there is evidence that the demented are now surviving longer than they did even a few decades ago (Hagnell, 1970; Blessed & Wilson, 1982; Christie, 1982). The number of old people with dementia has thus increased enormously. It is clear that the title 'epidemic' is no exaggeration.

Dementia is a disease which makes great inroads into the individual's capacity to care for herself. This means that enormous resources will be necessary to cope with the scale of problem indicated by demographic trends. These resources will always need to be provided above all by family and friends; but the established health and social services play a fundamental and growing part, as do voluntary organisations, pressure groups and in some cases private profit-making bodies.

Organisation of services in Britain

In Britain statutory resources for dementia are provided by the National Health Service and by Local Authority Social Services Departments. The National Health Service provides both primary health care, based on the general practitioner, and specialist services and is centrally funded.

Local Authority Social Services, like the Health Service, are overseen by the Department of Health and Social Security, but local autonomy is much greater.

THE FAMILY AS A RESOURCE

Where a family exists it usually provides most of the support for the elderly at home. A survey (Abrams, 1978) found that 42% of the over-75s were visited by family and friends more than once a week, while only 6% were visited by social workers and 4% by voluntary workers. Other surveys (Hunt, 1978) have shown the importance of family and friends in providing both friendly visiting and personal care. Isaacs et al (1972) found in their study of patients referred to a geriatric unit in Scotland, that in the very few cases where a son or daughter appeared to be wilfully neglecting the needs of an elderly disabled parent, the reason generally lay in a lifelong poor relationship.

Strain on families

The care of a demented old person can place an enormous strain on the spouse or family providing that care. A number of studies have drawn attention to this and to the impact that 'community care' can have on a family. Grad & Sainsbury (1968) found that families in an area covered by a hospital pursuing a policy of community care were subjected to significantly greater stress than families living in an area served by another hospital which placed more emphasis on in-patient care. Caring for elderly persons so demented that they cannot be safely left alone can be made even more taxing if accompanied by disturbed behaviour. Often care devolves on one 'primary carer' and Isaacs et al (1972) found that great family tension often resulted in these circumstances. Another recent study (Nissel & Bonnerjea, 1982) found that often even husbands and children living in the same household as the disabled old person and the primary carer offered little support.

Supporting the supporters

Given the enormous contribution made by families, it is clear that they often do not receive the help which they need. Moroney (1976) has drawn attention to the tendency of statutory services to provide substitute rather than shared care. The elderly living with relatives are very much less likely than the elderly living alone to receive help from the Social Services (Table 50.1). The priority accorded to those living alone is not surprising, but in the case of old people with dementia this policy may often be

Table 50.1 Elderly people visited by health and social service agencies during a six month period, England 1976, by age and domestic situation (Hunt, 1978).

Visited by	All elderly	Living alone	% visited Living with others	Aged 85+
General Practitioner	33.3	28.4	35.5	49.2
District nurse	7.8	7.6	7.9	19.6
Health visitor	4.4	5.6	3.8	**
Home help	8.9	18.9	4.0	27.3
Meals on wheels	6.0	9.0	4.7	11.5

** not available

inappropriate. Bergmann et al (1978) followed up a small group of demented patients attending a day hospital and found that after a year less than a fifth of those living alone were still in the community, compared with nearly a half of those living with children. It may be that the severely disabled 'solo' dement is beyond adequate support by merely episodic care (which is all that domiciliary services can offer); whilst such support may greatly extend the coping capacity of families.

Apart from providing support at home, services must sometimes of necessity be prepared to provide substitute care. A significant proportion of very old people in Britain and other developed countries have no immediate family. Of women over 65 in England and Wales in 1980, 12% were single (Office of Population, Censuses & Surveys, 1982). Widowhood is the most common marital status of women over 80 in Britain and a recent study (Bowling & Cartwright, 1982) found that 17% of the widowed had no living children. Marital status and family size have an important influence on the probability of an old person living in an institution (Townsend, 1962).

RESOURCES FOR SUPPORT AT HOME

The general practitioner is generally the first person involved; in Britain nearly everyone is registered with a general practitioner. He or she should also be aware of the possibility of dementia whenever consulted by, or on behalf of, an elderly patient and is well placed to detect early cases. Hunt (1978) found that a third of all elderly persons in the community, and a half of those aged over 85, had been visited by a general practitioner in the previous 6 months. The numbers of old people consulting general

practitioners in the surgery ('office') are also high. Demented old persons who live alone are extremely vulnerable and by the nature of their disablity are unlikely themselves to seek assistance. General practitioners must therefore go out of their way to discover such cases and age and sex registers allow identification of the very old at risk. Williamson et al (1964) showed in a survey of the elderly at home that only 13% of those diagnosed as demented by the examining psychiatrist were known to be demented by their family doctor.

Other members of the primary health care team can share the job of ascertainment and surveillance and support.

The health visitor may play a crucial role in follow up of patients discharged from hospital, surveillance of those thought to be precariously supported, and in providing advice to families. Health visitors are now attached to 79% of general practices (Royal College of Physicians, 1983) but Dunnell & Dobbs (1982) recently showed that they still devote only 12% of their time to the elderly. Hunt found that in 1976 only 4.4% of the elderly had been visited by a health visitor in the previous 6 months. Since then the number of health visitor visits to the elderly has actually fallen, despite the increase in the number of very old people.

The district or community nurse is also important in the primary care team. Three quarters of district nursing time is spent with the elderly and one study found that 40% of district nurse patients are mentally ill (Royal College of Physicians, 1983). It seems that district nurses are more often used to ease the burden on carers than are other services; the elderly living with others are slightly more likely to be visited by a district nurse than the elderly living alone. The number of home nurse visits to the elderly has increased in line with the growth of size of the very elderly population, so this important resource is being used.

Apart from the primary care team the GP also has available the resources of local hospitals and their outreach teams. Prominent in the recent development of the latter has been community psychiatric nursing (Carr et al, 1980). It is now official policy that all District Health Authorities employ a psychiatrist with a special responsibility for the elderly and this policy has to date been implemented in nearly half of all health districts (Wattis et al, 1981) and principles for the organisation of such services have been defined (Arie & Jolley, 1982). Where there is no psychogeriatrician the general practitioner must refer to the general psychiatric service. Non-ambulant demented patients are best referred to the geriatric service.

Local authority social work and domiciliary services

The GP trying to arrange support for an old person with dementia will often need to call for help from the Social Services Department. Hospital teams include social workers, but for a patient living at home it is the locally based social services who provide assistance; relatives and friends can also directly seek their help. Goldberg et al (1977) found that 20% of all referrals to a social services area office concerned the 75 and-over age group. Goldberg et al (1978) also showed that assessment, co-ordination and case work by a social worker is less likely to occur in the case of an elderly client than when, for example, a child is referred; more often the social worker decides her chief task is to arrange access to practical services. Of these services it is often the home help that provides the backbone of statutory domiciliary support for the elderly.

Home helps

Today 90% of home help clients are elderly and the home help often does very much more than provide domestic assistance. Home help is undoubtedly the most widely available domiciliary support. In 1979/80 there were 96 elderly households receiving home help per thousand population aged over 65 (DHSS, 1981). Hunt (1978) found that over a quarter of those aged 85 and over were receiving home help at least once a week, but there are big variations between localities; in the Isle of Wight in 1979/80 44 pensioner households per 1000 old people received home help compared with 204 in Doncaster. In some areas a dearth of home help and other domiciliary services may reflect a greater emphasis on residential provision, but a comparison between rates of provision of home help and rates of provision of Part III of the 1948 National Assistance Act suggests planning is generally more haphazard.

The extent to which the home help service can be used to maintain a severely demented person living alone is limited. However home help can provide a useful adjunct to family care and it is unfortunate, if understandable, that it should be a service primarily directed at the elderly living alone. Home helps are under considerable pressure; Moroney has shown that their case loads have grown in recent decades and between 1979/80 and 1980/81 the number of home help whole-time equivalents actually fell by about 1000, despite the increase in the number of very old people.

For the GP, liaison with the home help service is vital. In cases where the elderly dementia sufferer lives alone the home help may be the person in most frequent contact with her.

Meals

The other most widely available local authority domiciliary service is the provision of meals. Differences in rates of provision are even greater than for the home help service. Some authorities deliver meals daily, including weekends, but this is not usual and half of all meals clients receive only one or two meals per week. The DHSS (1979) found that a low Mental Test Score was associated with undernutrition and have recommended that meals on

wheels might be appropriate for mentally confused people alone during the day. Davies (1981) in her survey of meals on wheels clients estimated 2% were 'confused'. For the mildly demented patient a meal delivered regularly may provide a means of orientation in time, an opportunity for surveillance and a source of nourishment. However for the old person with more severe dementia who lives alone, the value of the service is limited as the elderly person must remember to be in at the right time and there is no way of ensuring that the meal is actually eaten. Meals can be very useful in the care of the demented where the sufferer lives with an elderly spouse who perhaps has physical disabilities making shopping difficult, or as a back-up to services provided by other relatives or friends.

Most authorities, as well as delivering meals to the door, also serve meals in luncheon clubs. These clubs are designed for the fit elderly and transport is not provided. The option is of limited use to the demented person living alone, but for the demented patient with a spouse or friend prepared to take her, luncheon clubs can provide some stimulation and company for both, provided that behavioural problems are not severe.

Aids and adaptations

Home help and meals are far from being the only domiciliary service provided by social service departments. Local authorities also employ occupational therapists to visit the homes of elderly people and advise on aids and adaptations, which will often be supplied free or at a subsidised price. For the demented such changes in the physical environment may be disorientating and the ability to learn to use aids limited; but advice on safety may be valuable, for example, substituting electric for gas cookers or fitting safety catches to doors.

Other services

Laundry services are available in some areas, though disposable incontinence pads are more frequently provided. A few local authorities provide other imaginative support for the care of demented old people such as night-sitters. However such extra services are thinly scattered.

Short stay relief care

A few local authorities run special short stay homes but more generally such care is provided in an ordinary home (where, in 1980, 97% of the residents were long stay). Recently a number of authorities have experimented with temporary boarding-out schemes for the elderly. Old people in need of care are temporarily placed with a foster carer who is paid to look after them. This arrangement may be less upsetting for the old person than placement in an institution but careful assessment is essential to make sure that the old person's needs are compatible with the services the carer is prepared to offer. Local authority homes and foster placements are not suitable for the old person with severe physical problems that require nursing care or for those with severe behaviour problems. In these cases relief care may be provided in hospital.

Wherever relief care is provided it is essential that all parties agree beforehand on what is being offered and when the old person is to return home. Moves, particularly into institutions, can be disorientating and disturbing for the old person with dementia, so that extra reassurance from the usual carer and staff of the institution and visits to the home or hospital before admission are helpful.

Day care
Day care, whether day hospital care provided by the NHS or local authority care in day centres is a fairly recent development. The first psychiatric day hospital in Britain was opened in 1946, the first geriatric day hospital followed in the early 1950s and separate provision for mentally ill elderly patients is more recent still.

Psychogeriatric day hospitals seem more likely to offer social care and relief to the primary carer than do geriatric day hospitals. This is reflected in a reduced rate of discharge and longer periods of attendance which, as Greene & Timbury (1979) showed, often only terminate with in-patient admission or death.

Geriatric day hospitals may also cater, albeit unwillingly, for demented patients. Brocklehurst & Tucker (1980) found that 4% of geriatric day hospital patients had a primary diagnosis of dementia and in a further 6% dementia was the secondary or tertiary diagnosis — sometimes demented patients may attend general psychiatric day hospitals.

Old people less seriously affected by dementia and without severe behavioural problems may be best cared for in a local authority day centre. Social services departments provide special day centres for the elderly, day centres for the mentally ill and sometimes day centres which cater for a variety of disabilities. Many authorities have a few day attenders at residential homes. Day centres provide social rather than nursing care, but the distinction between day hospital and day centre is not always clear cut. Hildick-Smith (1977) found that many GPs were unclear about the difference between the two.

There has been a rapid growth in the number of day centre places available and it is one of the few local authority social services which has expanded. In England in 1981 DHSS figures (1982) show that there were 4.1 local authority day centre places for the elderly per thousand populaton aged over 65, just above the 3–4 places per 1000 recommended. Transport is an important part of both day hospital and day centre provision but may not be available for elderly people receiving day care at a residential home.

The value of day care for the demented old person lies chiefly in providing supervision and relieving the prime carer (Brocklehurst & Tucker, 1980). Evaluation of the impact of geriatric day hospital care on patients has shown

a number of benefits with day hospital attenders being less likely than others to enter residential care and less likely to spend time in hospital, however psychogeriatric day hospitals with their greater proportion of demented patients may not have the same effect on admission rates.

RESIDENTIAL AND NURSING HOMES

Under Part III of the 1948 National Assistance Act local authorities are required to 'provide residential care for all persons who by reasons of age, infirmity, or any other circumstance are in need of care and attention not otherwise available to them'. Residential homes for the elderly were not intended to provide nursing care but, as Clarke et al (1979) and others have shown, the residents of Part III accommodation today include large numbers of severely disabled old people. Dementia is the most common of the disabilities likely to lead an old person to enter residential accommodation. Kay et al (1964) found that in Newcastle 26% of the elderly residents of welfare homes had dementia, and old people with dementia were more than three times as likely as other old people to enter institutional care. In the 20 years since this study the growth in the size of the very elderly population, the better provision of services to maintain old people at home and the contraction of mental hospital accommodation has led to greater demands being put on Part III accommodation as a haven for patients with dementia. Studies of residential homes for the elderly in Manchester (Evans et al, 1981) showed that 45% of residents were moderately or severely confused, a similar picture has been found elsewhere (Lowther & McLeod, 1974).

The presence of large numbers of demented old people has put a great strain on the providers of residential care. Degree of dementia and ability to perform the activities of daily living are closely related and the work load imposed by severely demented residents is heavy, as Adolfsson et al (1981) have shown. Often residential homes are short of trained staff and lack the necessary physical resources fully to cope with the increasing numbers of severely disabled old people. Nevertheless, residential care for the elderly is a very expensive and scarce resource; in 1976/77 a quarter of all local authority personal social services expenditure was devoted to it (DHSS, 1980a). The DHSS guideline on the appropriate rate of provision of Part III accommodation is 25 places per 1000 population aged over 65. Rates of provision are substantially below this and it is probably no longer an accurate guide even to what is thought desirable. It would in any case be more realistic to have suggestions on provision related to the population over 75 or 80, as the average age of admission to Part III is now nearly 82 (Grundy & Arie, 1982). Variation in provision by local authorities is considerable; in 1980 the top provider had two and a half times as many places per 1000 elderly as the area with the lowest rate of provision.

For these reasons access to local authority Part III accommodation may be difficult. This may be so particularly for an old person with dementia as the burden of dementia may be felt to be already too great within a particular home. Evans et al (1981) recommended that no more than 30% of the residents at one particular home should be moderately or seriously confused, as higher levels of dementia were considered deleterious for the more lucid residents. Some authorities provide special homes for the elderly mentally infirm, but separate provision has remained controversial.

Private and voluntary homes also provide care for the elderly with dementia. Local authorities are empowered to sponsor residents in private and voluntary homes and in 1976 it was estimated that about a third of people living in institutions were in fact being supported by local authorities (Age Concern, 1981). Some residents are supported financially by central rather than local government through 'board and lodging' allowances from the DHSS. Local authorities are responsible for registering and supervising standards in private homes in their area but this system does not always work dependably and further legislation in this area is currently being formulated.

Nursing homes

For those who need nursing but not medical supervision, a nursing home place may be more appropriate than either Part III accommodation or a place in a long stay hospital ward.

In Britain the NHS has recently decided to introduce, as an experiment which is to be evaluated, three nursing homes. These are intended to cater for geriatric patients who would otherwise be in long stay hospital wards. Apart from these experimental units, the only nursing home provision in Britain is in the private and voluntary sector. This means that access is chiefly for those with private means, although charitable organisations pay for some patients and in other cases the DHSS or local authority may make an allowance to cover some of the cost.

HOSPITAL SERVICES

The hospital has an obvious role in diagnosis and treatment, by advice and support to the primary care team or through short stay admission, as well as in providing longer term or intermittent care.

Old people with dementia make heavy use of hospital in-patient facilities. Kay and his colleagues (1970) found that when followed up two to four years after initial examination, demented old people originally living at home had spent four times as long in hospital (and ten times as long in residential care) as mentally unimpaired old people. Of the total number of admissions to psychiatric units 28%

are of people aged 65 and over, and of these some 30% are demented (DHSS, 1980b).

The importance of open-minded and meticulous assessment of demented old people is obvious. These old people, who often inspire little investigative let alone therapeutic enthusiasm in professional staff, tend to receive only shoddy attention, or even neglect. And yet the results of careful investigation may reveal much that is remediable, or even may result in discarding of the provisional diagnosis of dementia. Even where the patient is frankly demented, there is much that can be done by specific focused management to retrieve and even improve function. Schemata for the investigation and management of such patients are now widely available and the practice of the better units attracts widespread interest and has obvious educational potential (Arie, 1973).

A cardinal feature of services for such old people is that they are likely to have a mixture of mental and physical disabilities. Probably about one third of elderly admissions to geriatric or psychiatric units suffer from mixed disorders of this sort, and co-operation between geriatricians and psychogeriatricians is essential. The Royal College of Psychiatrists and the British Geriatrics Society (1982) have together agreed guidelines for collaboration in this work. The DHSS has recommended joint assessment units in which physicians and psychiatrists co-operate but such units have not been widely established (Wattis et al, 1981). As geriatrics and psychogeriatrics increasingly are established side by side in District General Hospitals (DGH), the need for special joint units should become less. Under the old order, where psychiatry and geriatrics are often practised in single specialty hospitals some distance apart, access to such a joint assessment unit, preferably in the DGH, becomes of great importance, both for bringing the needed resources of the DGH to old people and for acting as a physical focus of collaboration between the geriatric and psychogeriatric service. In Nottingham it has been possible to go a step further and to establish a joint department of Health Care of the Elderly, comprising physicians and psychiatrists and the associated staff and facilities, working together within one teaching department (Arie, 1981).

The organisation of psychogeriatric services has recently been reviewed by Arie & Jolley (1982). Suffice it to say that initial contact with the patient should always be in her own home, preferably in the form of joint consultation by the psychiatrist, the family physician and other relevant staff where necessary. Stay in hospital should be as short as possible, with a planned and active regime instituted without loss of time. Once a problem-orientated diagnosis has been reached, a plan of management is formulated and objectives defined. A wide range of staff will be involved in formulating plans and implementing them and of course the medical component may not necessarily always be paramount. The family and other actual or potential supporters outside the hospital need to be kept involved from the beginning, for the 'hole' left by the demented patient in the community after admission to hospital has a way of closing behind her.

Duration of stay in the assessment ward is not long. Of all patients over 75 leaving mental illness units in 1977, 37% had been there for less than 1 month, and nearly 62% had stays of less than 3 months (DHSS, 1980b). In geriatric wards, the median duration of stay for patients aged 75 and over in 1979 was around 3 weeks (DHSS, 1980c). Since these figures include deaths and discharges from long stay wards, the average length of stay in assessment wards will be even lower.

In Britain long stay care for old people too seriously impaired to be looked after in local authority residential homes is the responsibility of the hospital service. Demented people needing long stay care who are ambulant receive their care in psychiatric units, those who are non-ambulant in geriatric units. Such long stay beds are everywhere in short supply and the recommended provision of 2.5–3.0 beds per 1000 over 65, which is in excess of that available in most localities, has in any case been criticised as too low (Jolley, 1977). Within geriatric services the provision of long stay beds for the demented falls within the overall norm of 10 beds per 1000 over 65 (15 beds in Scotland). Almost everywhere the actual provision is at a far lower level, with a national average of 8.3. The ultimate plan is that longer stay care should be provided in small units close to the localities from which patients come, but for the foreseeable future continuing reliance is certain to be placed on existing single specialty institutions.

THE COSTS OF DEMENTIA

Plum (1979) estimated that the annual cost of caring for the demented in the United States was over 12 billion dollars. In Britain in 1979–80, 10.5 thousand million pounds were spent on health and personal social services (Central Statistical Office, 1981) and Owen (1976) estimated that about 20% of health and social services expenditure was devoted to those aged 75 or more.

It is impossible to judge exactly what proportion of this expenditure is attributable to the care of the demented, but it is known that the demented make heavier use of services, particularly expensive institutional services, than their contemporaries (Kay et al, 1970; Foster et al, 1976). The Office of Health Economics (1979) estimated that in 1976–77 providing resources for those with dementia involved expenditure on health and social services of at least £300 million in England alone.

These estimates of costs are certainly underestimates of spending on dementia and the English figures relate only to health and personal social services expenditure. This means

they do not include, for example, the cost of the extra income support sometimes available to the dementia sufferer or relative. Account must also be taken of the costs borne by families caring for old people with dementia. Caring for an old person with dementia involves extra expenditure on a range of goods and services, such as laundry or domestic help. Opportunity costs are also high; Nissell & Bonnerjea (1982) found a large proportion of female carers had to give up employment. Those who managed to return to a job tended to work shorter hours and earn less money than the average for their occupational group. Rickard (1979) estimated if someone had to give up work to look after an old person at home then this form of care was more expensive than residential care in an old people's home. Opit (1977) suggested that for many elderly sick patients care at home was only cheaper because no account was taken of family support and domiciliary services were often inadequate.

Many of the real costs incurred by the families of old people with dementia cannot be counted. These may include emotional and physical stress, disturbed nights, a severely restricted social life, family problems and a deterioration in health.

FUTURE RESOURCES FOR DEMENTIA

In the next few decades the growth in the number of very elderly people is likely to make the question of resources for the elderly even more crucial. However it is to be hoped that new resources may become available. At the moment there is no specific drug therapy for dementia of the Alzheimer type and the drugs developed for multi-infarct dementia have proved disappointing (Yesavage, 1979). However research activity in this field has increased and with growing understanding of brain chemistry in dementia there now seems more hope of therapeutic advance. Technology and design will certainly prove to be a resource that can be tapped and electronic devices are already available to aid nursing of, for instance, wandering demented patients by keeping them under observation without over-restricting freedom to move around and explore the environment (Langley, 1981). Good practice in the future also depends on the use of education as a resource now.

Education of professional staff

In Britain big strides have been made in establishing the care of the elderly within the curricula of the different health professions. All medical schools now have some teaching in the care of the elderly, though the extent varies greatly. There are now 15 chairs in geriatrics in British universities, and this development has taken place wholly within the last 20 years. Within the field of nursing there has been great emphasis on training in geriatrics, both at the basic level (partly in response to the requirements of the

EEC) and through the activities of the Joint Board of Clinical Nursing Studies which accredits postgraduate courses. The remedial professions have also greatly expanded their training in this field, but in social work and psychology progress has so far been small. There is no doubt that the best resource of all for dementia is proper education for those professionals who are mostly concerned with it — against a background of education too of the public, which in the end votes the cash to provide resources for dementia.

REFERENCES

Abrams M 1978 Beyond three score years and ten. Age Concern, Mitcham, Surrey

Adolfsson R, Gottfries C, Nystrom L, Winblad R 1981 Prevalence of dementia disorders in institutionalized old people. Acta Psychiatrica Scandinavica 63: 225–244

Age Concern Research Unit 1981 Profiles of the elderly: their use of Social Services, Volume 6, Age Concern Publications, Mitcham, Surrey

Arie T 1973 Dementia in the elderly: diagnosis and assessment. British Medical Journal 4: 540–543; Management, ibid. 602–605

Arie T 1981 In: Arie T (ed) Health Care of the Elderly, Croom Helm, London

Arie T, Jolley D 1982 Making services work: Organisation and style of psychogeriatric services. In: Levy R, Post F (eds) Psychiatry of Late Life, Blackwell, London

Bergmann K, Foster E, Justice A, Mathews V 1978 Management of the demented elderly patient in the community. British Journal of Psychiatry 132: 441–449

Blessed G, Wilson I 1982 The contemporary natural history of mental disorder in old age. British Journal of Psychiatry 141: 59–67

Bowling A, Cartwright A 1982 Life after a death. Tavistock, London

Brocklehurst J, Tucker J 1980 Progress in Geriatric Day Care. King Edward's Hospital Fund for London, London

Carr P J, Butterworth C A, Hodges B E 1980 Community Psychiatric Nursing. Churchill Livingstone, Edinburgh

Central Statistical Office 1982 Social Trends 12. HMSO, London

Christie A 1982 Changing patterns in mental illness in the elderly. British Journal of Psychiatry 140: 154–159

Clarke M, Hughes A, Dodd K, Palmer R, Brandon S, Holden A, Pearce D 1979 The elderly in residential care: patterns of disability. Health Trends 11: 17–20

Davies L 1981 Three score years — and then? A study of the nutrition and wellbeing of elderly people at home. William Heineman Medical Books Ltd, London

DHSS 1979 Nutrition and health in old age. Reports on Health and Social subjects no.16, HMSO, London

DHSS 1980a Health and personal social services statistics for England 1978. HMSO, London

DHSS 1980b In-patient statistics from the mental health enquiry for England 1977. HMSO, London

DHSS 1980c Report on hospital in-patient enquiry 1979. HMSO, London

DHSS 1981 Personal social services Local Authority statistics. The home help service during the year ending 31.3.1980. DHSS, London

DHSS 1982 Personal social services Local Authority statistics. Adult training centres for the mentally handicapped and day centres for the mentally ill, the elderly and the younger physically handicapped at 31.3.1981. DHSS, London

Dunnell K, Dobbs J 1982 Nurses working in the community. HMSO, London

Evans G, Hughes B, Wilkin D, Jolley D 1981 The management of mental and physical impairment in non-specialist residential homes for the elderly. University of South Manchester Psychogeriatric Unit Research Section, Manchester

Foster E, Kay D, Bergmann K 1976 The characteristics of old people receiving and needing domiciliary services: the relevance of psychiatric diagnosis. Age and Ageing 5: 245–255

Goldberg E, Warburton W, McGuinness B, Rowlands J 1977 Towards accountability in social work: two year's inake of clients to an area office of a Social Services department. National Institute of Social Work, London

Goldberg E, Warburton W, Lyons L, Willmott R 1978 Towards accountability in social work: long-term social work in an area office. British Journal of Social Work 8: 253–287

Grad J, Sainsbury P 1968 The effects that patients have on their families in a community care and a control psychiatric service: a two year follow up. British Journal of Psychiatry 114: 265–278

Greene J, Timbury C 1979 A geriatric psychiatry day hospital service: a five year review. Age and Ageing 8: 49–53

Grundy E, Arie T 1982 Falling rate of provision of residential care for the elderly. British Medical Journal 284: 799–802

Hagnell O 1970 Disease expectancy and incidence of mental illness among the aged. Acta Psychiatrica Scandinavica 219: 83–89

Hildick-Smith M 1977 A study of day hospitals. Unpublished thesis, University of Cambridge, Cambridge

Hunt A 1978 The elderly at home. HMSO, London

Isaacs B, Livingstone M, Neville Y 1972 Survival of the unfittest. Routledge and Kegan Paul, London

Jolley D 1977 Hospital in-patient provision for patients with dementia. British Medical Journal 1: 1335–1336

Kay D, Beamish P, Roth M 1964 Old age mental disorders in Newcastle-upon-Tyne — 1. British Journal of Psychiatry 110: 146–158

Kay D, Bergmann K, Foster E, McKechnie A, Roth M 1970 Mental illness and hospital usage in the elderly: a random sample followed up. Comprehensive Psychiatry 11: 26–35

Langley G 1981 Alarms or despondency? British Medical Journal 283: 1376–1378

Lowther C, McLeod H 1974 Admissions to a welfare home. Health Bulletin 32: 14–18

Moroney M 1976 The family and the state: considerations for social policy. Longman, London

Nissel M, Bonnerjea L 1982 Family care of the elderly, who pays? Policy Studies Institute, London

Office of Health Economics 1979 Dementia in Old Age. Office of Health Economics, London

Office of Population Censuses and Surveys 1982 Population Trends 28. HMSO, London

Opit L 1977 Domiciliary care for the elderly sick — economy or neglect? British Medical Journal 1: 30–33

Owen D 1976 The costs of ageing. In: In Sickness and in Health, the Politics of Medicine. Quarter Books, London

Plum F 1979 Dementia: an approaching epidemic. Nature 279: 372–373

Rickard J 1979 Economics of health care planning. In: Bennett A (ed) Recent Advances in Community Medicine 1. Churchill Livingstone, London

Royal College of Physicians, College Committee on Geriatrics 1983 Organic Mental Impairment in the Elderly, Implications for Research, Education and the Provision of Services. Journal of the Royal College of Physicians London 15: 141–167

Royal College of Psychiatrists, British Geriatrics Society 1982 Guidelines. In: Levy R, Post F (eds) Psychiatry of Late Life. Blackwell, London

Townsend P 1962 The last refuge, a survey of residential institutions and homes for the aged in England and Wales. Routledge and Kegan Paul, London

Wattis J, Wattis E, Arie T 1981 Psychogeriatrics: a national survey of a new branch of psychiatry. British Medical Journal 282: 1529–1533

Williamson J, Stokoe I H, Gray S, Fisher M, Smith A, McGhee A, Stephenson E 1964 Old people at home: their unreported needs. Lancet i: 1117–1120

Yesavage J 1979 Vasodilators in senile dementias. Archives of General Psychiatry 36: 220–223

51

Death and terminal care

P. H. Millard

The specific function of Medicine is to prevent death by the diagnosis and treatment of disease and it is natural, therefore, for doctors to see death as their failure. The increasing number of aged people throughout the world, is a direct consequence of the postponement of death (mainly in childhood). Death eventually comes to all. Some consider that to be the end, whilst others believe that there is a life after death. This chapter deals with some of the dilemmas inherent in caring for the dying.

THE MANAGEMENT OF DYING PATIENTS

Forecasting death

As Medicine is an inexact science the practice of estimating expected life span should be deprecated. If the patient dies at the forecast time e.g. three months or four months, who is proving whom to be right? It is the decision that imminent death will be the inevitable outcome that is difficult to make, not the management of dying once the decision has been made. In geriatric admission wards, death is a frequent occurrence. In the long-term care wards where the object of the staff is to care for the patients without a discharge objective, death is the eventual outcome for all but the management there is not that of dying but of life until death. The doctor making decisions about the management of the long-term patient must respect the wishes of the staff who care for the patient. If the only thing that he is asked to do is to treat an infection and he refuses, he will be thought by the care staff to be negligent. In the same way, perhaps, as the doctor would look at them if they did not feed the patient. There must be no 'God-like' decisions. In general medical and surgical units the problem is the making of the decision to switch from an active programme of resuscitative treatment, to management of the dying. Many staff feel relieved when they see tube feeding being discontinued in the moribund patient, and respirators being turned off in the intensive care ward in people who are designated as brain dead, for if death is inevitable it is burdensome to prolong life with meaningless treatments. Never forget however, that it is all too easy to give up too early. The task of Medicine is to give

hope for tomorrow – whatever the age of the patient – but if death is seen to be inevitable the majority of general practitioners in the United Kingdom consider that exceptional means should not be used to prolong life. (Keane et al, 1983).

Euthanasia

The proper care of the dying has become mixed up with discussion and debate on euthanasia. In the book 'Beneficient Euthanasia' (Kohl, 1975) the viewpoint is put forward that this is a kindly act. The present medical ethic is not to kill life (that is excepting abortion where human life can be killed up to 24 weeks after conception) and supporters of euthanasia lobby to change the law, so that, in certain circumstances, life after birth can be terminated. In the present state of the law euthanasia without the patient's consent is murder and with the patient's consent is both suicide and murder. (Doherty, 1983). Peope commit suicide because they perceive that their life is no longer worth living. In euthanasia people who wish to die will involve others in their execution. In suicide, despair in the perceived hopelessness of their state reduces patients to kill themselves. Proponents of euthanasia express their own fears of being disabled. Being frightened of the unknown and of their reaction to it they consider that in the perceived future hopelessness of their state they would be better off dead. They see death as the only solution to a difficult problem. The hospice movement has demonstrated that accelerated death is not the answer. The correct response to patients in despair is to give them your time; listen to their problems, show them that they are not alone, that their life is valuable; then build up their confidence and trust in your ability as a doctor to help them to live, whilst dying. If their despair was responded to by a final act of rejection and a swift pain-free death then Medicine itself loses its purpose and this chapter need not be written.

Symptom control

Good terminal care extends far beyond the relief of pain and of other symptoms. It includes supporting the patient during the adjustment to increasing physical disability and through periods of 'anticipatory mourning' for the loss of family and friends and of one's hopes for the future. It also involves supporting the family as they adjust to the fact that their loved one is dying (Linacre Centre, 1982).

Tending

Ensure that the patient is well tended by the nursing staff. Careful attention to state of the sheets and pillows is essential. Lying too long in the same position, especially upon wrinkled sheets, can cause pressure ulceration and thus add to the patient's distress. Small acts show that you care; hold the patient's hand when you talk with him, do not isolate him in a side room – unless such a request is made. Flowers, personal belongings, favourite pictures and cards should be encouraged. There should be no fixed visiting hours, but the visitors should be encouraged to take proper rest themselves. If the patient requests it a favourite pet can be brought in (so long as it does not upset the ward routine). Never pass patients without speaking, always recognise that they are present and occasionally tarry for a while thus giving them the opportunity to talk to you.

Pain control

There is a distinct difference between giving a drug to relieve pain that renders a patient unconscious, and rendering a patient unconscious to relieve pain. Not all deliberate actions that involve risk can be prohibited or legislated against. Death sometimes is a side effect of treatment e.g. when a patient dies on an operating table during an anaesthetic. If the death is due to the use of an empty cylinder of oxygen then the death is caused by negligence and the anaesthetist is culpable in law. If however, death occurs through no-one's fault, as a side effect of the decision to operate, then there is no negligence. Nobody would say that operations should not be performed because occasionally people die. In like manner accelerated death may occur as a side effect of treatment with analgesia, but there is a distinct moral difference between giving drugs to ease pain that may bring about accelerated death and easing the pain by accelerating the death. If the drug is given with the object of accelerating the patient's death, then the position in law is clear – murder has been committed.

In patients with terminal illnesses the correct management of the pain may be surgery, radiotherapy, a root block or a specific treatment. Judgement of the degree of pain and suffering that a patient has is difficult. Doctors have a tendency to underestimate suffering, whilst the carers who are more emotionally involved overestimate it. Reilly & Patten (1981) reported that according to the general practitioner 15% of patients had had severe physical suffering whilst the closest carers considered that 36% had so suffered. Moderate/severe suffering was reported as 54% and 53% respectively.

Pain control with mental alertness is the objective.

Analgesics should not be prescribed on an as required basis, but should be given in small doses regularly. The minimal regular dose that controls the pain is the ideal for which to aim. In moderate to severe pain a useful mixture is:

diamorphine HCl	2.5–40 mg (usually 5–10 mg)
cocaine	10 mg
rectified spirit	2.5 ml
syrup	5 ml
aqua chlor	20 ml

Syrup prochlorperazine 5–10 mg is sometimes added routinely as many patients already have nausea. In severe pain with vomiting use intramuscular diamorphine 5 mg every 4 hours, increasing if necessary to 30 or even 60 mg. In frail elderly people one should commence with no more than 2.5 mg. If necessary it can be potentiated by the use of a phenothiazine such as chlorpromazine 25 mg three times daily.

Nutrition

The mouth should be kept clean and moist. If drinking is difficult a small pipette can be used to put water into the mouth, which helps to assuage thirst. If steroid drugs are being used watch out for monilial infection in the mouth and treat it if it occurs. Ensure that food is attractively presented and suits the patient's taste. Avoid pureed foods, a soft alternative preserves the aesthetic qualities. Small quantities are more tempting than large platefuls.

Infections

Judgement is necessary as to whether a respiratory infection should or should not be treated. There can be no hard and fast rules for each patient has to be treated as an individual. The judgement is solely as to whether the infection forms part of a terminal state and when treatment of it would be seen to prolong the act of dying. The treatment of concomitant infections is indicated if they are not part of the terminal state e.g. parotitis, urinary tract infection.

Sedation

In the aged there is usually quiet acceptance, however if anxiety is a feature then the use of nitrazepam as a night sedative may be helpful, for with its long half-life it sedates the patient by day as well. Chloral hydrate is an effective hypnotic, but its taste is difficult to hide, and in the elderly alcohol can be extremely useful for it has both analgesic and sedative effects. In frank confusion one of the phenothiazines can be helpful but their use should be carefully monitored for they may precipitate hypothermia.

TO TREAT OR NOT TO TREAT

Acceptance is part of normal aging for to age successfully one most come to terms with life and its achievements and disappointments. Elderly patients often accept that their condition is hopeless and part of the art of being a successful geriatrician lies in recognising when and when not to treat. As a good general rule always be energetic the first time you meet the patient, unless of course admission to hospital has been specifically arranged because of terminal illness with a well diagnosed untreatable condition and the reason for hospitalisation was solely because the informal caring network was unable to cope. The first time you meet a patient always ensure that the diagnosis is correct and that in your judgement the investigations and treatment have been properly done. In each case, judgement is necessary as to how far treatment is indicated.

Therapeutic negativism

The fear of precipitating premature death can sometimes adversely influence the decision whether or not to operate. An example of this is when a decision is made not to operate upon an elderly woman with a femoral neck fracture because she might die. However, if she is operated upon successfully there is a good chance that she will leave hospital to return to her home, but if no operation is performed she may never have the opportunity to leave hospital again. If the operation is not carried out she still dies in hospital albeit later.

In all treatment of the elderly there is risk: rehabilitation to discharge may be associated with falling down and fracturing a femur either inside or outside the hospital. Judgement is necessary as to the acceptability of the risk. If the primary act has good intentions but death results, then the primary action is ethical. It must not be forgotten however, that even if the primary act has good intentions, the way that it is carried out may be deemed to be negligent. A negligent act can be either by omission e.g. failing to cross-match blood for the operation from which the patient died from blood loss, or by commission when the correct blood that was cross-matched was given to the wrong patient. Discharging a patient to live at home, who wishes to return home and who falls down the stairs and breaks their neck and dies is different from discharging the patient home because you realised that their stairs were too steep and you hoped that they would fall down them and die!

Therapeutic enthusiasm

Primary decisions that always 'come down on the side' of treatment, may themselves have inherent difficulties; for example whether or not to amputate a gangrenous limb in a patient dying with terminal cancer; whether or not to treat the respiratory infection in a patient dying from Alzheimer's disease; whether or not to tube feed the unconscious patient with a stroke; whether or not to use a respirator in a patient dying with respiratory failure. The views of the patient, the relatives and the carers are important and must be taken into account. The final judgement as to whether further treatment is justified remains medical. Remember too the benefits of obtaining a second opinion from a colleague, for it is preferable to ask advice in life than to be proved wrong after the death. If in doubt, treat. A positive approach to treat has its limitations:

(a) where there is conflict of choice; one dialysis machine and two patients, one old and the other young. Seemingly easy but what if the old person was premorbidly well and the young one has Hodgkin's disease?

(b) where the specialised treatment can be judged on legitimate grounds to be too burdensome e.g. cytotoxic therapy in certain malignancies.

(c) where the treatment is judged to be of such little benefit that it does not justify the use of skill or resources. The decisions to be made are medical and are dependent upon knowledge. Failure to treat the treatable and the patient dies is justifiably considered to be negligence. Omission of treatment, under circumstances where treatment would be considered to be obligatory, makes the doctor just as culpable as if he takes a deliberate action to cause death.

Acceptance of death

The final outcome of life is death, and the time may come when patients are reasonably convinced that life is ending and they consider that their last days would be better spent in composing themselves for death, rather than struggling to prolong life in a profitless way, thus adding to their suffering and that of their friends. Here life is not rejected, but the meaningless attempts to prolong life are. It is easy to be right after death, but, in life, when the decisions have to be made it is not easy. Doctors have been trained to preserve life and reluctance to give up is understandable because:

(a) Misdiagnosis does occur and autopsy sometimes shows that a first class terminal care programme was given to a misdiagnosed treatable condition.

(b) The forecasting of expected life span is notoriously difficult and remissions have been reported in seemingly terminal malignant diseases.

(c) There is always hope that a medical breakthrough will occur (people who pay to have their bodies frozen after death, even take such a hope with them into the grave).

(d) The fear of litigation might affect judgement. Everybody wishes to avoid regret. After the death the doctor might find that his diagnosis was wrong and his treatment inappropriate, or the relatives might consider that their loved one suffered too much.

In making decisions one aproach is to distinguish between Ordinary and Extraordinary means. In this respect Ordinary means are 'all medicines, treatments and operations which offer a reasonable hope of benefit and which can be obtained without excessive expense, pain or other inconvenience' and Extraordinary means are 'all medicines, treatments and operations which cannot be obtained without excessive expense, pain or other hope of benefit'.

The distinction between ordinary and extraordinary means does not in itself make it easy, for as technology continues to advance, what was extraordinary last year may be seen to be ordinary now; rather consider those things that make treatment obligatory. Doctors do sometimes persist in futile treatments but at the time that they made the decision it was difficult to forecast that death was the inevitable outcome. It is the doctor who has to live with the results of his decision.

Decisions to cease treatment

Life does not need to be preserved at all costs but problems may occur when decisions to cease treatment are made. In making the decision, for example, to switch off a respirator, ensure that:

(a) Your intention is not to kill by act or omission – both can be intentional.

(b) The cause of death is the fatal illness which does not support life. Death was not primarily caused by switching off the life support system because the patient already has a fatal illness that did not support life.

(c) The action taken was morally neutral. It in no way compares with injecting a lethal substance, the latter deliberately kills life whilst the former accepts that some diseases do not support life.

The ultimate right of decision to reject further treatment rests with the patient; in the unconscious patient the rights and duties of the family are generally dependent upon the presumed will of the unconscious patient. The duties are usually presumed to be only to use ordinary means to preserve life.

PLACE OF DEATH

Decision about whether or not to treat are easier to make in the patient's own home, rather than in the hospital. In hospitals resuscitation teams are sometimes called to the death bed of a terminally ill patient. An error of judgement that perhaps is to be deprecated, but do not denigrate the nurse who made the decision to call, for it is far better that she called and it was not necessary, than she did not call, and it was! Ward based discussions between doctors and nurses minimise such occurrences, for then everyone should be aware of the expected outcome.

Age alone is not an indication for non-resuscitation. The decision to manage death at home is influenced by the availability of hospital and hospice beds. Only 30% of deaths in the United Kingdom occur at home (Ford & Pincherle, 1978), but those who die in hospital have often been coped with at home for most of their final illness. Parkes (1978) reported that although 60% of deaths occurred in hospital, the amount of time spent at home was three and a half times greater than that spent in hospital.

The decision to manage the patient at home is influenced by the availability of hospital beds. Keane et al (1983) reporting a study of the last illness managed at home by 301 general practitioners stated that in 27 cases the general practitioner's request for admission had been refused. A total of 84% of the deaths occurred in the patient's own home while 8 per cent lived alone. In 35% the family managed alone. The main services used were the district nursing service (56%), the night service (11%), meals on wheels (11%) and the incontinent laundry service (4%). Incontinence was reported as a problem in 23% of the patients managed at home but only 4% had the advantage of the incontinent laundry service, which presupposes that the burden of coping with incontinent laundry at home is carried by the family. Doyle (1980) reported that 29% and 25% of faecally incontinent men and women and 32% of men and 9% of women with urinary incontinence had received no help from the supporting services.

Cartwright et al (1973) reported that 71% of doctors found it easier to arrange the admission of a younger patient who was terminally ill compared with only 28% if the patient was elderly. The aging of the nation will accentuate the problem. Awareness of the impending problems may well have influenced the general practitioners in the study carried out by Keane et al (1983) to want more money to be spent upon the social services rather than on hospital beds (40% agreeing, 30% disagreeing) and on the provision of more hospices to improve the quality of care of the dying (51% agreeing, 17% disagreeing).

The hospice movement

The hospice movement is centuries old, but recently it has gained considerable support. Good hospices teach the proper attributes of care for all patients whether they are dying or not, the principal virtue being to see the person as a whole. Supporters of the movement to expand hospices would claim that only there can the time be given to provide proper care for the dying. The present day hospice movement should however be seen as playing an educative role. The dilemma of education is that if it is successful the behaviour of those who are being taught changes. The care of dying patients in general hospitals is improving and the messages about pain control etc are being passed on. Some hospices are now considering themselves to be pain control centres, but in that role, they conflict with the acute hospitals for the proper control of pain which may necessitate treatment, for example, with radiotherapy, surgery or nerve root blocks. Pain control should properly be the role of hospitals. What then is the role of a hospice?

Its place is in the management of those patients who in the last weeks of their life could be managed at home if they had a strong informal caring network, but in the absence of that network would have to remain in acute hospitals whose resources are best used for others. It would be preferable for their hospital doctor to care for them but in so doing he would deprive others of the resources necessary to treat them. Thus he rejects the patient for the good of others. It would be preferable for hospital doctors not to have to pass on patients when they are terminally ill and in the geriatric medical ward where the pace is slower the need hardly ever arises, for if death is foreseen the unit can cope. It is the perceived imminence of death that differentiates the hospice patient from the continuing care patient because, for both, the outlook is death in hospital. In the hospice the patient goes to live whilst dying and in the long-term care unit they go to live until death.

Attributes in caring for patients

Deaths will continue to occur in hospitals and most will be sudden in onset and unexpected. Important attributes in caring for your patients are:

(a) Do not pass by without acknowledging their presence and try to give them the opportunity to talk with you. Touch them. Linger a while if you can.

(b) Do not be introspective but generate an aura of quiet confidence.

(c) Keep life and death in perspective. Patients can laugh with you and at you on their death bed but do not laugh at them.

(d) Remain a therapeutic optimist. Never remove all hope for today and tomorrow, however one must also be able to accept that at times death is inevitable and further treatment burdensome.

(e) Speak with your staff and with the relatives and give them the time to express their views. Remember that the ultimate responsibility is medical.

(f) After a death express sympathy with the other relatives and take the opportunity to talk with the other patients on the ward, the doctors and the nursing staff thus giving them the chance to express their fears.

Talking to the patient and the relatives

Life is finite. Consultation with a doctor over any symptom is associated with fear that it might herald the inevitable decline to death. If the symptom signifies an illness that, in the present state of our knowledge, cannot be cured then the patient must come to terms and learn to live with it. Lord Horder (1948) stated that dying patients were rarely aware of their true state, whilst Kubler-Ross (1974) found that 'only 1% of our hundreds of terminally ill patients persisted in denial to the very end of their lives compared with 40% of their attendant physicians'. Ward (1974) reported that 46% of 279 patients dying from cancer were thought by the doctor to be aware of their true state, compared with 54% in the opinion of relatives and friends, but the doctor had discussed the probable outcome with only 13%. According to Cartwright and her colleagues (1973), in hospital and in general practice, doctors prefer to tell relatives (58%) rather than the patient (5%).

Keane et al (1983) suggested that the tendency to tell relatives what is not told to the patient would appear to put an unreasonable strain on relationships, and this at a time when frank discussion in the family is best. There may be a legal obligation to tell the truth so that the patient can make important property and business decisions (Ward 1974). Robinson (1973) warns that the 'truth' that we know about another person 'is his truth' and in a sense we have no right to talk about it behind his back. Perhaps we have no right – but most of us do talk with relatives without the patient's express permission. The answer is not simple, and putting theory into practice is not easy. Careful choice of timing and occasion is important and undue pessimism is unwarranted. Many patients with widespread neoplastic disease achieve remarkable remissions with chemotherapy. There is now a trend towards more open discussion. Noyes et al (1977) have reported that between 1971 and 1976, students, recent graduates and faculty staff at the University of Iowa College of Medicine showed a significant increase in the proportion in favour of telling terminal patients their prognosis. However the information is not necessarily retained. Spencer Jones (1981) reported that 90 out of 183 patients with inoperable bronchial carcinoma asked for their diagnosis and 93 deliberately did not. Ten of those told subsequently 'denied' what had been told to them speaking as if their outlook was good. Of the 93 who did not, some explained that they did not want to know, but 42 later showed awareness that they had a fatal illness. Reynolds et al (1981) found that 59 out of 67 patients in a Western Australia oncology clinic wished to be told of their prognosis. In deciding what to tell the patient always give some degree of optimism for although an illness that usually ends in death is present no doctor can forecast exactly when death will occur, and the presence of a terminal illness does not of necessity mean that death is imminent.

Time of death

Forecasts of time of death are notoriously inaccurate. Hope is considered to be life lengthening and despair life shortening. Whether or not this is true is debatable but as the task of medicine is to prevent premature death one cannot but agree with Stoll (1979) that one should always give hope for today and tomorrow.

Throughout life the male is more likely to die than the female, after retirement (Young et al, 1963; Ward, 1976; Casscells et al, 1980), and after bereavement (Rees & Lutkins, 1967; Parkes et al, 1969). The male/female ratio on admission to our department at St George's Hospital in London is 1:2.4 which is equal to the male/female ratio for the population aged 65 and over in the catchment area, but in the continuing care wards the male/female ratio is 1:5, and in my experience the male is more likely to die than the female when he is admitted to hospital or transferred to another ward. In the elderly death is more common in the month after birthdays (Anderson, 1975; Phillips, 1977), on Mondays (MacFarlane & White, 1977) and after admission to residential homes (Smith & Lowther, 1976). There is evidence both for the concept that aged long-term residents die when they are moved and evidence against. Zweig & Csank (1976) reported that death on movement was minimised if patients are given information before transfer and if highly exciting events do not emphasise the relocation. However Roberts et al (1982), reported that there was little mortality when patients were moved in the middle of the night during a riot!

Medicine is an inexact science. We are slowly beginning to understand the complexity of the machine that supports life but as yet we are nowhere near understanding the role of the mind in determining whether a patient lives or dies. Occasionally patients say 'I would be better off dead' but the response they are expecting is 'No you would not'. On a few occasions patients have forecast when they will die. In all of these cases the death occurred at the forecast time without obvious cause.

Bereavement

As caring staff the death of our patients is something that we come to accept. For the relatives it is a deeply personal event. After a death make sure that the relatives are spoken to and that sympathy is expressed to them in their loss.

It is not the purpose of this chapter to deal with bereavement. Remember however that life for the others in the informal caring network must go on. Fight, flight and acceptance are physiological responses to stress. Denial, anger, depression and acceptance are normal responses to any loss. They are not solely factors that occur in association with bereavement, but will occur with any loss. Three books worth reading are those by Ainsworth-Smith & Speck (1982), Kubler-Ross (1974) and Parkes (1975). To overcome bereavement successfully the relatives must come to terms with their grief and take on some of the life roles of the dead person. Discussion can help. Even months after a death relatives sometimes return to the hospital asking questions. Speak to them because it enables them to come to terms with their loss.

REFERENCES

Ainsworth-Smith I, Speck P 1982 Letting Go. Anchor Press, Tiptree

Alderson M 1975 Relationship between month of birth and month of death in the elderly. British Journal of Preventive and Social Medicine 29: 151–156

Bourestom N, Tars S 1974 Alterations in life patterns following nursing home relocation. Gerontologist 14: 506–510

Cartwright A, Hockey L, Anderson J L 1973 Life before death. Routledge and Kegan Paul, London

Casscells W, Hennekens C H, Evans D, Rosener B, De Silva R A, Lown B, Davies J E, Jesse M J 1980 Retirement and coronary mortality. Lancet 1: 1288–1289

Doherty P 1983 Medical ethics. Guild of Catholic Doctors, Bristol

Ford G R, Pincherle G 1978 Arrangements for terminal care in the N.H.S. (especially those for cancer patients). Health Trends 10: 73–76

Gould J (ed) 1971 Your death warrant. Geoffrey Chamberlain, London.

Horder Lord 1948 Signs and symptoms of impending death. Practitioner 161: 73–75

Keane W G, Gould J M, Millard P H 1983 Death in practice. Journal of the Royal College of General Practitioners 33: 347–351

Kohl M 1975 Beneficient Euthanasia. Prometheus Books. New York.

Kubler-Ross E 1970. On Death and Dying. Tavistock. London

Kubler-Ross E 1974 Dying – from the patient's point of view. Triangle Sandoz Journal of Medical Science 13: 25–26

Lieberman M A 1961 Relationship of mortality rates to entrance to a home for the aged. Geriatrics 16: 515–519

Linacre Centre 1982 Euthanasia and clinical practice. Trends, principles and alternatives. The Linacre Centre, London

MacFarlane A, White G 1977 Deaths the weekly cycle. Population Trends. Spring 1977: 7–8

Noyes R, Jochimsen P, Travis T 1977 The changing attitudes of physicians towards prolonging life. Journal of the American Geriatrics Society 25: 470–474

Parkes C M 1975 Bereavement. Penguin, Harmondsworth

Parkes C M 1978 Home or Hospital. Terminal care as seen by surviving spouses. Journal of the Royal College of General Practitioners 28: 19–30

Parkes C M, Benjamin B, Fitzgerald R G 1969 Broken heart: A statistical study of increased mortality among widowers. British Medical Journal 1: 740–743

Rees W D, Lutkins S G 1967 Mortality of bereavement. British Medical Journal 4: 13–16

Reilly P M, Patten M P 1981 Terminal care in the home. Journal of the Royal College of General Practitioners 31: 531–537

Roberts G S, Banerjee D K, Mills G L 1982 The emergency evacuation of a geriatrics hospital in Toxteth. Age and Ageing 11: 244–248

Schulz R, Brenner G 1977 Relocation of the aged – A review and a theoretical analysis. Journal of Gerontology 32: 323–333

Smith R G, Lowther C P 1976 Follow up study of two hundred admissions to a residential home. Age and Ageing 5: 176–180

Spencer Jones J 1981 Telling the right patient. British Medical Journal 283: 291–292

Stoll B A 1979 Is hope a factor in survival? In: Stoll B A Mind and Cancer Prognosis. John Wiley and Sons, Chichester

Ward A W 1974 Telling the patient. Journal of the Royal College of General Practitioners 25: 465–468

Ward A W 1976 Mortality of bereavement. British Medical Journal 1: 700–702

Young M, Benjamin B, Wallis C 1963 The mortality of widowers. Lancet 1: 454–456

Zweig J P, Csank J Z 1976 Mortality fluctuations among chronically ill medical geriatric patients as an indicator of stress before and after relocation. Journal of the American Geriatrics Society 24: 264–269

52

Public policy, health care and aging societies

D. L. Kodner

PUBLIC POLICY AND THE AGING IMPERATIVE

Public policy refers to the philosophies and priorities a government follows in meeting the needs of its citizens (Morris, 1979). Whether public policies are expressed in the form of legislation or programmes, they represent a set of values about governmental responsibility for distinctive problems or groups of people that directly or indirectly determines how a society's political, economic and intellectual resources will be used. The problems important to governments and the nature of their intervention are shared by a number of factors, the most noteworthy being the age composition of the population. It should not be surprising therefore, that the 'greying' of developed nations has emerged as one of the most important public policy imperatives of this century.

The transformation of the United States, United Kingdom and other developed countries into age-heavy societies has firmly established the idea that governments should become involved in the social conditions of the elderly (Binstock & Levin, 1976). It has been suggested that this 'aging explosion' has made policy questions concerning older citizens one of the greatest challenges faced by industrialised societies, save the threat of world war. American health economist Ann Somers (1981) observes that the ever-growing elderly population 'can no more be ignored today than could the baby boom of the post-World War II years.'

By the year 2000, because of low birth rates and increased life expectancy, the fraction of persons age 65 and over in the more urbanised regions of the world will reach 13.2% (United Nations, 1980). In the United States, this proportion is expected to go up to 12%. However the US is far from the world's most 'mature' nation, as the relative number of elderly in the United Kingdom and at least four Western European countries (Austria, East Germany, West Germany and Sweden) has already surpassed the 15% mark (Central Statistical Office, 1976; Saldo 1980). Nowhere will the impact of this swelling elderly population be felt more dramatically than in the health arena.

HEALTH CARE NEEDS OF THE ELDERLY

Health policy for the elderly must account for the unique needs and problems that distinguish older persons from the non-elderly. For the purposes of health policy, an examination of the older population's health status is considered essential for determining the need for health care resources and services. A number of studies reveal that functional ability is more important in planning health care than disease patterns among the elderly (Haber, 1967; Shanas, 1971; Lawton, 1971). This is also the view of the World Health Organization (1959).

The majority of elderly are mobile and in good health. Surveys of people over the age of 65 in Great Britain and the United States show that the great majority view themselves in 'good' or 'fair' health (Somers, 1978). However survival to older ages has produced a predominance of chronic and degenerative disease as both the major diagnosis and principal cause of death (Brody, 1980). A study by Akhtar et al (1973) for instance, shows that the prevalence of disability increases from 12% at the age of 65–69 to over 80% at the age of 85. Increased disability augments emotional, social, economic and environmental handicaps. Because of differences in measurements and methods, it is not entirely clear how many older persons are severely impaired. However Shanas (1971), in a cross-national study of home care needs of the aged, concludes that 'there seems to be a hard-core of bedfast and housebound elderly ranging between 8 and 14% of the total elderly population.'

Before turning to a discussion of the impact of the elderly population on service utilization, it is important to recognize that chronic illness and functional decline mean diminished 'quality of life.' Episodic, curative responses, may meet an acute medical crisis, but do not address issues such as income maintenance, personal social services and housing which are considered essential to overall physical, social and psychological functioning.

Older people naturally require more health care than the general public, especially among the over 75s (the 'old-

old'). The fact that the elderly have more physician visits, greater reliance on drugs, and require more hospital and long-term care services is recognized by the medical profession and amply documented in the literature. Here too, disability appears to be the most significant variable in explaining the interwoven relationship between illness and health care use (Butler & Newacheck, 1981).

The resources devoted to financing these services are greatly out of proportion to the elderly's share of the population. In the United States for example, per capita spending for health care of the elderly in 1977 was almost four times the average direct costs of the under-65 age group (Social Security Administration, 1980). More than two-thirds of these outlays were absorbed by one or another government programme. These expenditures however, belie the United States' total commitment to its older citizens, as funds for related income support and social service programmes are excluded from this figure. This far-reaching investment in programmes for the elderly population is more or less paralleled by other developed countries. At this time of slow economic growth, the need to contain public expenditures is clear. This gives rise to two central policy dilemmas: first and foremost, how can we maintain this existing level of services in the face of rapid increases in the elderly population and diminishing resources for both the old and the young? And second, given the problem of economic scarcity, how should we make the best use of exisiting health services for the elderly? Finding answers to these questions not only urgently demands an examination of the appropriateness, effectiveness and costs of existing models of geriatric health care, but also anticipation of alternate policies and programmes.

CROSS-NATIONAL COMPARISONS OF AGING HEALTH POLICY

Health policy, as in the case of other forms of public policy, not only reflects demographics, but also a society's unique historical, cultural and political environment. Although there are recognisable differences in the policy of industrialised nations, the problems of the elderly and public responses are similar in these countries. Despite differences in national aims and experiences, it is useful to compare and contrast these arrangements and to extrapolate common policy dilemmas and themes. Overall, Binstock & Levin (1976) find that there is a deepening sense of concern in modern societies about their capacity to provide social, economic and health services to the elderly. Kane & Kane (1980) have described old age as 'a land of its own, with a language that will never be fully understood by the younger people who are most often responsible for formulating the policies that affect the elderly'.

The need for adequate income support is often overlooked in discussions of health policy. Inadequate income often portends poor housing and nutrition, as well as a lack of basic necessities of life, the absence of which can be destructive to both physical and mental well-being. For elderly retirees, with little opportunity to replenish savings, this is an especially important issue. The lack of economic security in old age was the first major question of social policy for the elderly faced by developed countries. All industrialised nations now provide some type of public pension system, although there are wide variations in the amount of government spending. Austria, for example, spends 21% of its Gross National Product on retirement benefits as compared to 5% in the US (Saldo, 1980). However, none of these programmes erase lifelong income differentials among older citizens. In some instances, the absence of an adequate income floor deters pensioners from obtaining needed health and social care.

Developed countries also provide health care benefits to their elderly. Needless to say their emphasis, scope and organization varies. While it is beyond the scope of this chapter to describe these different systems in detail, a brief discussion of the more salient characteristics and differences in the specialised arrangements for persons in need of long-term care would be useful.

It is widely recognised that the elderly prefer to remain in their own homes for as long as possible. However, institutional and home care programmes have varying functions and priorities within national health schemes. Kane & Kane (1980) report that the United Kingdom, Sweden, Norway, the Netherlands and Israel have a greater commitment to community-based services than the United States. The range of community programmes supported by these countries is extensive and includes services such as nursing and health-related care and aids, domestic help, sitters, home-delivered meals, assistance with shopping and laundry and day care. Community-based efforts to maintain independence and to postpone institutionalisation is available as in the provision of sheltered or supportive housing. Britain's Warden housing and the Netherlands' 'granny flats' offer two good examples of the importance of supportive living arrangements. Whereas institutional care is considered a last resort in many nations, in the US until recently nursing homes were viewed as almost entirely synonymous with long-term care (Koff, 1982).

Government health care programmes in the United States (Medicare and Medicaid) are oriented to the medical mode, and therefore are far more concerned with covering the elderly's medical bills for hospitalisation, surgery, drugs and follow-up rehabilitation than the need for home-based long-term care services. Even when care is available to chronically impaired older Americans, it is far easier to obtain access to institutions than to home care (General Accounting Office, 1979). Closely related to the availability of home care and other community resources is the system of both evaluating the complex needs of the elderly and controlling inappropriate institutional placement. The countries analysed by Kane & Kane either use geriatric assessment units or national screening programmes to asign individuals to community-based or institutional care. This is in sharp contrast to the US, which has been experimenting with a variety of similar approaches for the last decade, but has not found an acceptable arrangement.

Other significant areas in which the countries reported differ from the US is the recognition of geriatric medicine as a specialty and the degree of the medical profession's dominance in the provision of long-term care. Anderson (1979) identifies Italy, Spain, United Kingdom, Australia and New Zealand as nations which recognise geriatrics as a sub-specialty of general medicine. The US Institute of Medicine (1978) on the other hand, supports integration of geriatrics into appropriate areas of medical education. There is also a major difference in the role physicians play in managing chronically ill patients. In the United Kingdom for example, geriatricians operate out of strong, sophisticated hospital diagnostic units with links to community-based home care programmes and, to a lesser extent, to 'front line' general practitioners. Because of the rapid increase of geriatrics as a medical specialty in the UK, there is a greater tendency to focus attention on the older population's medical needs. In the United States however, there is a general desire to move away from a health care system which is widely perceived as overly 'medicalised' and toward a service framework which incorporates non-physicians as 'case managers'.

Gerontologists in the US are fascinated by the level and range of health and personal social services for the elderly often found in other countries, particularly in the United Kingdom and Europe. While some of the advances in these countries are probably non-transferrable to the American scene, industrialised nations do share a number of common concerns. First, policy planners have long assumed that a wide availability of non-institutional options would help to prevent or forestall institutional placement, thereby minimising national expenditures for long-term care. This assumption is not supported by the studies performed by Kane & Kane in these countries. Not only is there a lack of clear-cut definitions about what community long-term care encompasses in the nations studied, but there is also a paucity of sound research on the costs of these services and whether they truly meet human needs. Second, there is a division of authority between health and social care for older persons which often leads to poor inter-professional communications, fragmented service delivery and wasteful use of resources. Third, there is a question concerning whether the provision of services to the older population is primarily a medical or social problem. And finally, efforts to integrate the care of the physically impaired elderly with mentally ill patients presents a serious dilemma to practitioners. These are some of the major issues which must be addressed in re-thinking health policy for the elderly.

RE-THINKING HEALTH POLICY FOR THE ELDERLY

In all modern societies, as discussed earlier, there is a common concern for rising costs of health care of the elderly and the increase in the numbers of older citizens requiring services. Even in countries like the UK, whose provision of geriatric care is admired throughout the world, there is a surprising degree of anxiety. Bosanquet (1978) for example, fears that the current range, both of services and legislation in the United Kingdom, are inadequate to meet the growing needs of the elderly What is required is a re-evaluation of the way in which health care for the elderly is conceived, arranged and delivered. Surely there is no one simple way to provide needed services to the burgeoning population aged 65 and over while, at the same time, seeking to slow down national health costs. It is not even clear whether these two objectives are entirely compatible. What is apparent is that the problem demands a multi-faceted approach. The following discussion, though far from exhaustive, outlines and addresses a number of issues which are essential to the discussion and formulation of rational and systematic health policies for the elderly.

Income support and employment

The principal aim of a national health policy for older citizens should be to keep this group physically and mentally healthy for as long as possible. Clearly, this will not only require an effective health care system, but perhaps more importantly, an adequate income. It is now recognised that the availability of a reasonably adequate income in old age is a far more important determinant of health status for the elderly than what physicians, hospitals, drugs and long-term care services can do (Somers, 1980). Ball (1981) underscores the importance of an adequate income by noting that older people without enough money to buy food and afford housing cannot possibly lead healthy lives.

Related to the goal of economic self-sufficiency among the elderly is the idea of allowing older people to work as long as possible. The difficulties associated with maintaining upwards of one-fifth of society at a reasonable living standard and in good health without their productive economic participation, is troubling to say the very least. While it appears in the interest of younger workers to see the elderly retire at earlier ages, especially within the context of chronic unemployment, it will be more and more difficult to support such pension policies.

As discussed earlier, most developed countries provide pensions to retirees and supplementary benefits to individuals with little of no income other than the basic benefits. These systems help to maintain many older people at a reasonable standard of living, especially when job-related pensions are included. The one exception is the old-old, who are most vulnerable to poverty and may not be adequately protected by existing social security schemes.

What new policies should be considered in this area? Pensions should be adjusted for inflation with a guaranteed minimum income for the over-75 group. Policies which promote the gradual withdrawal of older workers from the labour force should be evaluated. These could include innovations such as flexible seniority and reduced pay rates. Finally efforts should be directed to protecting the elderly's income. Special attention should be paid to the way in which government taxes its older citizens. Whether the elderly are single and without mortgage commitments or married and own a home, there is a need to carefully examine the effects of taxation on the elderly population and to devise special age-related allowances to offset any negative impacts.

Extension of life vs. quality of life

What should the government's and therefore the health care system's role be, in increasing the length of life and reducing and responding to the human and economic consequences of chronic illness and disability in later life? This is a haunting question which has not received throughtful and practical attention as part of any national policy agenda concerning the elderly population.

Heart disease, cancer and stroke are modern-day plagues, which account for large numbers of deaths among those over the age of 65. The majority of medical research is directed at reducing mortality from these diseases. At the same time, comparatively little funds are spent on chronic disabling conditions such as arthritis and organic brain syndromes. Without such research, we may never understand these diseases well enough so that they might be prevented or detected early enough to be clinically reversed.

The emergence of the hospice movement in the UK and its widespread acceptance in the United States and other countries suggests that modern societies are willing to consider the very complex issues involved in providing services in 'hopeless' cases. Do we want more people to live longer, even if they are physically and mentally impaired to the extent that their life has lost all human meaning and their family and friends suffer much from their care? Can we afford to provide the technical care impaired older people need and, at the same time, assure quality in their living experiences? Do we continue our support of biomedical research into the cause, prevention and treatment of the 'killer' diseases or should we do more in the area of chronic illness?

Obviously, there are no easy answers to these questions. However the unnecessary human and financial costs involved demand serious debate.

Families and family caregiving

In industrialised nations, the family is considered the most important support unit for the older person. Families assist their impaired elderly relatives to maintain indepenent functioning at home by providing domestic help and arranging needed medical care (Kane & Kane, 1980). This reduces reliance upon institutional resources for those in need of long-term care. Informal caregiving to the most impaired is often provided at great emotional and economic costs (Callahan et al, 1979).

Irrespective of the family's importance in caring for their severely disabled relatives, there may be major reductions in the overall amount of support that can be expected of them in the future. This will stem from the pattern of divorce, the re-definition of the woman's traditional caregiving role, increased family mobility and existing housing and working arrangements. Equally as important, there will be many more very elderly living alone with no families or with adult children too old to assume the caregiving role.

It should be self-evident that stable family units, whether they consist of elderly spouses or adult children, reduce demands on the health care system as well as minimise the kind of isolation most frequently related to chronic disability. It therefore follows that an effective health policy for the elderly should include efforts to strengthen the family and encourage their continued role in supporting frail aging people at home. Various economic and legal incentives should be explored, including income and property tax allowances, direct compensation for family-provided personal care services and changes in the divorce law. Another more indirect approach is to find ways to reduce the growing difference between male and female life expectancy. A reduction in excess male mortality from cardiovascular and other diseases would in the long run reverse the family's decline in later years and, therefore, help maintain its natural caregiving capacity.

Prevention and self-care

Some may feel that preventive health measures are inappropriate for elderly persons. This more reflects the attitudes of the medical profession and society-at-large, rather than the actual inability of the elderly to alter their health behaviour and thus their reliance on the health care system.

The old, like the young, have the capacity to greatly influence well-being prior to, at the time of and following illness and disability. Recognising significant symptoms and conditions, understanding diagnoses, asking appropriate questions, following prescribed regimens, modifying habits and carrying out appropriate treatments are some of the variables over which an individual has control. The adoption of more healthful lifestyles (e.g. physical fitness, nutrition, weight loss, stress management) and mastery of self-care skills can reduce morbidity and disability among the older population and improve their daily functioning. Such practices can also enhance feelings of independence, self-confidence and self-worth, and promote a sense of meaning in life. Health promotion, prevention and health maintenance activities may also have an economic value which should not be ignored.

In exploring prevention and self-care for the elderly, a committee of the recent US White House Conference on Aging (1981) recommended that the future American service delivery system be developed within the preventive framework, rather than the more narrow focus of treatment and long-term care. Levin (1976) further concludes that 'barring unforeseen medical breakthroughs or significant changes in patterns of disease, the lay resource may be the only reasonable means of meeting increasing demands of care of chronic illness and the daily requirements of minor illnesses'.

Consideration should be given to widely disseminating information on health promotion, prevention and maintenance skills through simple handbooks as well as formal education, training and counselling programmes for both lay persons and providers. Research should also be undertaken to identify effective prevention and self-care strategies for older persons. These new orientations should assist the elderly and their families in anticipating and coping with the physical and emotional demands of chronic disabling conditions and in making better use of scarce and costly health care resources.

Role of medical profession

In the United Kingdom, as in several other European countries, the evolution of geriatrics as a medical specialty is credited with the emphasis on and development of community supports for the elderly (Somers, 1978). There has also been a tendency to view the problems of the elderly from the physical health perspective as Kane & Kane (1980) point out. This medical orientation has lead to the use of hospitals for both assessment and long-term nursing purposes. Geriatricians are viewed as the prime organisers of the health care system for the older population as well as the leaders of the health care team. In the US on the other hand, the medical profession has lagged behind in development of geriatrics as a field of clinical concentration. While programmes in geriatrics are being established at US medical schools, long-term care and in-home and community-based services have developed separately. Moreover, there is a debate as to whether the medical profession should also serve as the coordinating force to bring together the health and human supports needed by the frail elderly. Dr David Greer (1983) believes that the professionally-trained geriatrician should directly orchestrate the entire spectrum of services. This thesis is strongly supported by Anne Somers (1982), whose recent proposal to reform Medicare (the US government's health insurance programme for the elderly), makes the physician both a 'gatekeeper' to long-term care services as well as the chronically-impaired older person's overall manager. Dr David Rogers (1983) on the other hand, argues that making the physician responsible for non-medical community services represents a serious waste of their technical expertise: It is 'like asking the experienced pilot of a 747 to handle customer services for a major airline'. Weksler et al (1983) further suggest that physicians tend to over-medicalise the health system and that non-medical professionals are usually better prepared to co-ordinate economic, social and community services, which together with the biomedical care of physicians, fulfill the health needs of impaired older patients.

As health care services for the elderly are re-examined, so too must the role of the medical profession in serving the older population. Whether there is a need for geriatrics as a practice speciality or for that matter, for all physicians to become smarter about the needs of their elderly patients, we must question the usefulness of our most highly-priced professional caregivers, that is physicians, in organising the entire service network.

Long-term care

According to the US Department of Health and Human Services (1978), long-term care 'consists of those services designed to provide diagnostic, preventive, therapeutic, rehabilitative, supportive and maintenance services for individuals who have chronic physical and/or mental impairments, in a variety of institutional and non-institutional health care settings, including the home, with the goal of promoting optimum levels of physical, social and emotional functioning'. While this definition is one of several used in the United States, it may differ from definitions adopted in other countries. What is important here is that the variations in definitions reflect the field's 'fuzziness' and lack of a clear and verifiable technology. Probably as a result, there is no all-encompassing solution for the care of the elderly in the countries reviewed by Kane & Kane (1980). Moreover difficulties in measuring the clinical, human and economic consequences of long-term care programmes are inevitable.

Effectiveness and costs

As discussed earlier, the major thrust of most developed countries has been to develop services that would permit the frail elderly to remain at home for as long as possible. This is based on the impression that community support replaces the need for institutional care, maintaining the quality of life and is also less costly. However even in countries which have engaged over the years in systematic national planning, little data exists about the effectiveness and costs of various in-home and community services. In the US where a number of studies have been conducted over the past decade, there is great suspicion about such conclusions. Research fundings summarised by the US Health Care Finance Administration (1981) suggest that while a significant proportion of patients can be effectively treated at lower cost in the community, it is probably less expensive to care for the most disabled in nursing homes.

Moreover, broadened coverage of in-home and community services tends to go to persons who are not at imminent risk of institutional placement and does not appear to improve functional ability. Positive discernable impacts however, are lower mortality rates and increased life satisfaction among community long-term care clients.

While there is recognition that models of geriatric care such as home care, day hospitals and hospices offer society an attractive option to care in an institutional setting, they may only serve to postpone or reduce institutional use and in the long run may actually increase public expenditures. Dunlop (1980) for example, reports that 'at first glance at least, the experience of European countries in reducing the use of nursing homes through the ready availability of home-based services does not appear encouraging'. Moreover there are a number of other important questions. Are community services better delivered in the home on in congregate or out-patient facility? Do these programmes actually improve daily functioning. Are the social needs of bedridden individuals who receive intermittent home care services better addressed in a long-term care institution?

Service co-ordination and integration
Older persons in need of long-term care require a wide range of health and personal social services offered in a variety of settings. Ideally, a long-term care system should provide the most cost-effective care at the right level, time and setting and also ensure maintenance of the individual at the maximum achievable state of well-being or quality of life. Our ability to achieve these desiderata would seem largely to depend on the structures available to co-ordinate and integrate services which are the responsibility of varying government authorities and agencies on the national, regional and local levels.

Resolution of these problems on the community level is most critical, since day-to-day difficulties in targeting, allocating, linking and monitoring services can often result in fragmentation of care as well as costly service duplication and overlap. Inter-professional teams and advisory boards are frequently offered as a solution, but most participants consider these token strategies ineffective. Even in the case of the highly structured Scottish health centre concept and the Norwegian health and welfare centres for example, the co-ordination and integration of services remain a unsolved problem.

In the US two experiments are currently underway which may provide some useful insights. First, the national channeling demonstration project seeks to establish free-standing local entities to manage, co-ordinate and arrange the provision of in-home, community-based and institutional long-term care services. These 'channeling' agencies will identify the population-at-risk, assess needs, determine eligibility, plan and prescribe services, arrange care and monitor its provision. Payment to individual providers and agencies will be based on the channeling

entity's plan of care, irrespective of the source of government reimbursement. The Social/Health Maintenance Organisation (S/HMO), on the other hand, is a prototype health care system for the elderly wherein a single provider assumes total responsibility for a full range of acute in-patient, ambulatory, rehabilitative, extended care, home health and personal support services under a prospectively determined fixed budget (Kodner, 1981: Diamond et al, 1983). In the S/HMO, negotiated per capita premiums from a variety of public financing programmes and individual monthly payments will be pooled to cover the costs of the comprehensive benefit package, with the S/HMO provider sharing financial risk with government payers for costs above the negotiated budget. This arrangement is expected to not only contain the costs of health care for the elderly, but more importantly to correct existing problems of access, inappropriate services and poor co-ordination.

The hospital's function
As discussed, the hospital-based geriatric service is a corner-stone of health care provision for chronically sick patients in the UK. Until recently, hospitals in the United States have avoided this role, in part due to the short-term acute care emphasis of Medicare and their traditional orientation to high-technology, curative medicine. Because there is now recognition that the elderly are rapidly becoming one of the hospital's largest patient groups and therefore key to its social and financial viability, more and more community hospitals have begun to explore ways to diversify their services beyond the acute care institution to emphasise long-term care and continuity of care. According to the American Hospital Association & The Hospital Research and Educational Trust (1980), 'the hospital's unique potential is for providing not only medical care for the elderly during acute episodes of illness, but also for providing care that responds to a much broader range of health and social needs in what may be a more socially acceptable setting for the elderly'. Additionally, Vladeck (1980) argues that the provision of long-term nursing care in hospitals and the acute care institutions's formal link to freestanding nursing homes can vastly improve chronic care services for older persons who require institutionalisation.

There is no question that hospitals currently act as a major focal point for the receipt of medical, health and social services for the elderly population. Consequently, the development of more humane, less technophilic approaches to their in-patient medical treatment is a welcome innovation. However the overriding issue is whether we can afford, in both patient care and economic terms, to have the hospital play a central role in both the provision and co-ordination of long-term care services. Obviously this will depend in large measure, on how the involvement of the medical profession is shaped.

Linking care of physically and mentally impaired

The elderly are at high-risk for physical and mental problems. Mental impairment among the older population is related to a number of factors including organic causes, poor physical health, poverty, bereavement and social isolation. In the case of dementia and other serious mental frailties, there is concern about how to best address the needs of older patients with these illnesses, particularly when they have physical handicaps at the same time.

Some professionals maintain that somatic and mentally ill individuals should be cared for separately. In support of this viewpoint, it is often argued that mentally alert patients are disturbed and frightened by disoriented individuals. Likewise, confused older persons are supposed to feel more comfortable and less inadequate in separate quarters. Furthermore, it is proffered that mentally incapacitated patients require heavier care and, therefore, greater staffing. At the opposite end of the spectrum, there are those who feel that in order to effectively address changes in the mental status of physically impaired persons, care of both somatic and mentally confused individuals should be linked. This may have the added advantage of providing mutually rewarding relationships between mentally alert and mentally incapacitated individuals. Obviously, this problem is extremely complex and demands further experimentation and research both in the in-patient and out-patient sectors.

Quality of care

Brook (1977) has pointed out that the evaluation of health care quality is complicated and that there are no easy approaches. One of the most elusive aspects of long-term care is the meaning and measurement of quality. If long-term care is aimed at achieving optimum physical functioning, emotional well-being and quality of life within certain financial limits, there is a need to define what these terms mean, to agree on concrete indicators and to establish a mechanism to obtain systematic feedback from providers as well as the elderly and their family members.

The task of measuring long-term care quality is complicated by the lack of objective criteria in some areas, and therefore the need to rely on the value judgements of professionals or the opinions of those being cared for. For example, it is easier to evaluate the technical quality of nursing care than the impact of a service on quality of life. Moreover, quality measurement depends on having a universally accepted definition of long-term care, its goals and the elements of a co-ordinated system.

As we begin the task of examining the benefits and costs of existing community and institutional services, there will be a real need to develop objective and meaningful information on all dimensions of quality.

Housing

Long-term care is essentially a problem of housing. The success of community supports depends a great deal on the availability of various sheltered living arrangements. Even in the case of the 'well' elderly, housing is considered essential to healthful and independent living. Despite the importance of housing to the elderly, it is surprising how little policy in this area seems to have taken the special needs of this group into consideration.

In addition to mortgage subsidies which are designed to make housing more affordable, resources are needed to repair the older population's deteriorating housing stock. Assistance could include tax credits, direct improvement grants, low-interest loans and grants for large-scale rehabilitation and redevelopment projects. Funding could also be provided to support the development of local housing repair services.

The most important element of a housing programme for the older population is however the provision of sheltered housing for handicapped individuals. What kind of person should live in such housing? Can we mix individuals of varying degrees of frailty? Should such housing have self-contained services? Are caretakers or wardens required around-the-clock? What special environmental features are absolutely necessary? Is it more cost-effective to build anew or adapt existing buildings? If sheltered housing is to play its proper role, it must be demonstrated that it can act as an effective alternative to institutional care as well as a better way of providing community support. This means that these questions and many others must be carefully examined by experts in both the housing and health care fields.

CHANGES IN THE OVERALL HEALTH SYSTEM

The elderly need the same basic health care services and economic, social and emotional supports as the rest of the population. Therefore as we move towards a more mature society, our new emphasis on geriatric medicine should not diminish the need to make changes in the overall health system. In short, policies for aging people should be formulated within the context of other age groups. This is important for three reasons. First, the well-being of the older generation is grounded in the living conditions of earlier years. For example, Davis & Schoen (1978) forcefully argue that 'many of the untreated acute conditions of childhood and adolescence show up as debilitating and crippling conditions only in middle and old age. The ability of the aged to move about with ease, retain their auditory, visual and mental facilities, and care for themselves is, in part, due to the adequacy of health care in earlier years'. Therefore continuing efforts to reduce health inequalities for the communty as a whole will also benefit the aged. Secondly, such comprehensive strategies can often represent a more effective use of institutional and non-institutional resources and manpower and, finally, one major consequence of special health programmes for older persons may be their broader application to younger people, especially those who are disabled. The focus of geriatrics on caring, rather than curing, can help to rejuvenate medical practice in general. This implies greater attention to social and psychological factors in illness, better doctor-patient communications and more involvement of family members in treatment regimens.

CONCLUSIONS

Maintaining the health of the older population and meeting their needs for both medical and long-term care constitute one of the most important public policy issues confronting the world's developed nations. At a time of steadily rising numbers of elderly citizens (with their very high health costs) and curbs on public spending, there is a serious question whether existing programmes and modes of service delivery can be sustained, no less expanded.

If health policy for the elderly is to be concerned with maximising the level of physical and mental functioning of this age group, a holistic approach must be taken. The underlying social, economic and environmental conditions of the aged must be considred side-by-side with the financing, organisation and delivery of health care services.

This is important for two reasons: First, improved quality of life can prevent or slow down medical and functional decline; and secondly it can buffer disabled older people from many of the side-effects of chronic impairment. In both instances, there is a real saving to society in economic as well as human terms.

The level of resources which will be available in the foreseeable future means that hard public policy choices must be made. These decisions not only require a realistic assessment of the entire range of the elderly's needs and demands for services, but also an understanding of problems and deficiencies in existing programmes and ways in which these resources can be used to obtain the best results. This chapter has provided a sense of the kind of complex issues and questions that must be addressed in re-thinking health policy for the elderly.

The aging imperative must not be seen strictly as a problem; it is also an oportunity. Physicians and other health care professionals are likely to come to understand the link between enhanced living conditions, better nutrition, more adequate incomes and improved access to and quality of medical care among the under 65 age group and the future elderly population. They will also find better ways to use existing services and facilities to benefit their elderly patients and the populace as a whole.

REFERENCES

Akhtar A J, Broe G A, Crombie A, McLean W M R, Andrews G R, Caird F I 1973 Disability and dependence in the elderly at home. Age and Ageing 2: 102–111

American Hospital Association & The Hospital Research and Educational Trust 1980 Office on Aging. American Hospital Association, Chicago

Anderson W F 1979 Achievements in geriatric medicine. In: Recent Advances in Gerontology. Excerpta Medica, Amsterdam

Binstock R H, Levin M A 1976 The political dilemmas of intervention policies. In: Binstock R H, Shanas E (eds) Handbook of Aging and the Social Sciences. Van Nostrand Reinhold Co., New York

Bosanquet N 1978 A Future for Old Age. Maurice Temple Smith, London

Brody S J 1980 The thirty-to-one paradox: health needs and medical solutions. In: National Journal (ed): 17–20 Aging: agenda for the eighties. Government Research Corporation, Washington D C

Brook R H 1977 Quality, can we measure it? New England Journal of Medicine 296: 197

Butler L H, Newacheck P W 1981 Health and social factors relevant to long-term care policy. In: Meltzer J, Farrow F, Richman (eds) Policy options in long-term care.The University of Chicago Press, Chicago

Callahan J J, Diamond L D, Giele J Z, Morris R 1979 Responsibility of families for their severely disabled elders. University Health Policy Consortium Background Paper. Brandeis University,Walham

Central Statistical Office 1976 Social trends, No 7. HMSO, London

Davis K, Schoen C 1978 Health and war on proverty. Brookings Institution, Washington D C p 19

Diamond L M, Gruenberg L, Morris R L 1983 Eldercare for the 1980s: health and social services in one prepaid health maintenance system. The Gerontologist 23: 148–154

Department of Health and Human Services 1978 Long term care: an overview. In: Health, United States. U S Government Printing Office, Washington D C

General Accounting Office 1979 Entering a nursing home: costly implications for medicaid and the elderly. U S Government Printing Office, Washington D C

Greer D S 1983 Hospice: lessons for geriatricians. Journal of the American Geriatrics Society 31: 2

Haber L D 1967 Identifying the disabled: concepts and methods in the measurement of disability. Social Security Bulletin 30: 2: 17–35

Health Care Financing Administration 1981 Long term care: background and future directions. Department of Health and Human Services,Washington D C

Institute of Medicine 1978 Aging and medical education. National Academy of Sciences, Washington D C

Kane R L, Kane R A 1980 Long-term care in six countries: implications for the United States. U S Department of Health and Human Services, National Institutes of Health, Washington D C

Kodner D 1981 Who's a S/HMO? A Look at metropolitan jewish geriatric center and its plans to develop a social health maintenence organisation. Home Health Care Services quartrly 2: 57–68

Koff T H 1982 Long-term care: an approach to serving the frail elderly. Little Brown and Company, Boston

Lawton M P 1971 The functional assessment of elderly people. Journal of the American Geriatrics Society 19: 465–81

Levin S 1976 The layperson as primary health care practitioner. Public Health Reports 91: 3: 207

Morris R 1979 Social Policy of the American Welfare State. Harper and Row, New York

Rogers D E 1983 Where does the geriatrician fit? Journal of the American Geriatrics Society 31: 2: 124

Saldo B J 1980 America's elderly in the 1980s, Vol 35, No 4. Population Reference Bureau, Washington D C

Shanas E 1971 Measuring the home care needs of the elderly in five countries. Journal of Gerontology 26: 37–40

Social Security Administration 1980 Income and resources of the aged. U S Government Printing Office, Washington D C

Somers A R 1978 The high cost of health care of the elderly: diagnosis, prognosis and some suggestions for therapy. Journal of Health Politics, Policy and Law 3: 2: 172

Somers A R 1980 Rethinking health policy for the elderly: a six-point program. Inquiry 17: 1:9

Somers A R 1981 The geriatric imperative: a major challenge to the health professions. In: Somers A R, Fabian D R (eds)

The Geriatric Imperative: an Introduction to Gerontology and Clinical Geriatrics. Appleton-Century-Crofts, New York

Somers A R 1982 Long term care for the elderly and disabled: a new health priority. New England Journal of Medicine 307: 221–226

Vladeck B C 1980 Unloving Care: the Nursing Home Tragedy. Basic Books, New York

Weksler M E, Durmaskin S C, Kodner D L 1983 New goals for education in geriatric medicine. Annals of Internal Medicine 99: 856–857

White House Conference on Aging 1981 Report to the technical committee on health maintenance and health promotion. US Department of Health and Human Services, Washington DC

World Health Organization, Regional Office for Europe 1959 The public health aspects of the aging of the population. World Health Organization, Geneva

53

The geriatric day hospital

J. C. Brocklehurst

Day care as an alternative to institutional care has developed throughout the last 30–40 years in many disparate situations. Psychiatric day hospitals were among the earliest; various other forms of day care now available in Great Britain include those for the elderly (the fit but frail, the physically disabled and the mentally impaired) and for younger people of various types (the mentally handicapped, the physically handicapped and families with problems). The whole range of day care services for adults has been recently reviewed by Carter (1981).

The geriatric day hospital had its root in the practice of elderly patients returning to hospital wards or occupational therapy departments after their discharge. Often this was to make sure they had a meal and were finding their feet back in the community, but sometimes it was for nursing procedures such as the dressing of ulcers. Early day hospitals were adapted from wards and even hospital chapels. The first purpose built day hospital in England was that in Cowley Road, Oxford, opened in 1957. Farndale (1961) reviewed geriatric day hospital development by that time and he described nine day hospitals. He noted that while they were thought to be alternatives to in-patient admission (and at Cowley Road the number of beds was diminished following the opening of the day hospital) it was his impression that day hospitals were serving more as an alternative to clubs and out-patient departments. The emphasis was on occupational therapy and it is interesting that Cowley Road Day Hospital was built in the form of a hollow square to allow confused old people to wander without getting lost.

In the last 20 years there has been a very considerable growth in the number of geriatric day hospitals in Great Britain. There are now over 300 and it is exceptional for a department of geriatric medicine not to include a day hospital among its resources. During that time the purpose and management of geriatric day hospitals has become more uniform but even so there is a fairly wide range both of location and of the nature of provision. There have been three major reviews of the British day hospital movement (Brocklehurst, 1970; Irvine, 1974; Brocklehurst & Tucker, 1980).

Parallel to this development has been the growth of social day centres for old people. These are different from old people's clubs in as much as they provide transport and a midday meal and so are available to much frailer old people than those who generally go to clubs. Most day centres of this type are managed by local authority social service departments although a number of them are in partnership with voluntary organisations. The stimulus to provide the day centre was in part derived from the existance of a day hospital creating a demand for continuing social and recreational facilities for patients no longer needing the therapeutic aspect of the day hospital. While day centres do not overlap in their provision with day hospitals there are a few notable exceptions where the roles have been deliberately combined. Silver (1970) has described a jointly sponsored social club and geriatric day hospital in north London. Picton-Williams (1973) set up a combined purpose-built day unit jointly funded by the social services department and the National Health Service in the geriatric unit of St Thomas's Hospital, London. Some day centres have also taken on the assessment role of the geriatric day hospital notably the day centre of the Newham Social Services Department (Eastman, 1976) where medical, educational, functional and psychological assessment is performed by professionals.

Generally, in Great Britain, the clear distinction between the geriatric day hospital (part of the hospital geriatric service, staffed by physicians, nurses, therapists and social workers) and the social day centre (part of the social services department of the local authority staffed by social caregivers and volunteers) is strongly maintained. In the United States there has also been a considerable development of day care for the elderly over the last fifteen years but here the distinction between the two types of care has been little developed and a whole spectrum of facilities has grown up. The situation was well reviewed by Weissert (1976). He described ten adult day care programmes where the average daily attendance varied from 11 to 52 (with one at 115) and found that despite differences there were sufficient similarities among them to produce two natural groupings. One group did indeed compare with the British geriatric day hospital (although a substantial proportion of attendees were under 65 years old) and the other, a social day centre type, provided social rehabilitation, maintenance and the alleviation of social isolation. However all programmes included general nursing care and social work counselling. More recently psychogeriatric day hospitals have developed in Great Britain as part of specialised departments of psychogeriatrics (or psychiatry of old age).

FUNCTION OF THE DAY HOSPITAL

This may be simply defined as the provision of some hospital facilities without most of the associated hotel facilities – in particular without the need to remain in hospital overnight and at the weekends. This is obviously inappropriate to some forms of hospital care including care of patients confined to bed and those dependent on nurses intermittently or continuously throughout 24 hours. The particular forms of hospital care which the day hospital can provide are assessment and observation, rehabilitation, the maintenance of physical function and the relief of strain among carers of dependent old people. Sometimes these are provided following a period of in-patient care and at other times without the need for admission to hospital at all. The day hospital thus provides an alternative method of management of geriatric patients; it increases the flexibility of the service which the geriatrician can offer and in many although not all, cases it may diminish or remove the need for hospital admission. If it is seen as a substitute for hospital care then it may be cheaper or more expensive depending on the number of days of attendance per week and on other domiciliary facilities that are required (see below).

Patient assessment and observation
Patients may be referred from out-patients or following a domiciliary consultation for assessment of their functional capacity (by an occupational therapist) or for observation of symptoms such as incontinence, falls or episodes of confusion. They may also attend for a period of observation during the initiation of treatment, for instance the drug treatment of Parkinson's disease. These reasons account for about a third of patients attending British day hospitals at the time of the patient's referral.

Rehabilitation and maintenance
Rehabilitation involves physical therapy in an appropriate environment. It is designed to overcome disability and promote independence. It is therefore an important part of the practice of geriatric medicine especially for patients suffering from stroke, Parkinsonism, osteoarthrosis, fracture of the femur and amputation. The day hospital may provide rehabilitation either following a period of in-patient treatment or directly while the patient continues to live at home. This should not simply be a substitute for a short period of attendance at a physical medicine

department – if the latter is appropriate then it should be used. Rather the day hospital provides a continuing process of rehabilitation over several hours and at a slower pace than would be involved in a half hour appointment at a physical medicine department. Patients may attend the day hospital four or five days a week for rehabilitation. Once it becomes clear however, that they are making no further gains towards independence, then rehabilitation ceases to be effective and a decision must be made as to whether the patient should be discharged or should continue to attend on an occasional basis (perhaps one day a week) for 'maintenance' treatment. It is well known that many aged patients having reached an optimal level of functioning following a period of rehabilitation deteriorate once the rehabilitation is withdrawn. For such patients the maintenance provided by the day hospital may well prevent relapse and possible readmission.

Social admissions
Just as short-term intermittent 'holiday' admissions have become a standard part of geriatric practice so attendance at a day hospital for social reasons – and principally to relieve the carer — is also now well recognised. If the day hospital is to be used optimally then patients should only attend for social reasons on the understanding that they would not be able to attend a social day centre. This usually means that they are disabled to the point of needing frequent assistance from nurses. They may be wheelchair-bound or may have problems with continence or confusion. This 'relief of relatives' strain' is another attempt to prevent breakdown and so, long-term institutionalisation. Isaacs et al (1972) showed that many old people were admitted to geriatric units because their relatives collapsed under the strain of trying to cope with them. This type of attendance is particularly relevant to the psychogeriatric day hospital and often allows the spouse of a demented patient to continue giving devoted support for months or years that might otherwise be impossible.

Table 53.1 shows the proportion of patients attending for

Table 53.1 Reasons for attendance at a day hospital (Brocklehurst & Tucker, 1980)

	At time of referral to day hospital (456 patients)		In a random sample of day hospital patients (233 patients)
Rehabilitation	53	73%	43%
Assessment	20		
Maintenance		11%	21%
Social		5%	17%
Medical and nursing observation and treatment		8%	19%

these various purposes both at the time of referral and on a random sample and shows that, overall, maintenance and social reasons account for 38% of attenders. In various areas day hospitals also provide other facilities. For instance in some departments the out-patient clinics are held in the day hospital. In many others in-patient rehabilitation is combined with that of day patients – the day hospital functioning as the rehabilitation unit for the geriatric department. This would seem to be a sensible and economic use of resources.

Two further points should be stressed. First that the principal diagnosis is not a useful indicator of the reason for attendance. For instance a patient with stroke may attend for any of the reasons outlined above. Second, that the day hospital is not always a cheaper alternative to in-patient care.

COST

The average daily cost of a patient attending a day hospital in UK was estimated by Brocklehurst & Tucker (1980) as £13.57, a figure closely relating to an independent study by MacFarlane et al (1979). Of this cost £3.20 was for transport. At that time the average cost of long-term geriatric hospital care was £13.77 per day.

The comparative cost between in-patient and day hospital treatment differs not only on the number of days in the week that the patient must attend the day hospital to avoid in-patient admission, but also the other costs in living outside (for instance, state subsidies of pension, heating allowance, rent allowance and provision of any social services). This again depends on whether the patient would be living alone (in which case all these costs would cease if he were admitted) or whether he is living with his spouse or another person in which case the cost of maintaining the establishment would remain much the same whether the patient was living or not. It is clearly cheaper to maintain a patient at home by once or twice weekly attendance at a day hospital, with the provision of meals on wheels three to four other days a week and a home help once or twice a week, even if other hidden costs have to be added, when compared to long-term hospital care. However, if the alternative is attendance at the day hospital five days a week then institutional care may be cheaper. Most old people of course, would prefer to retain their independence at almost any cost so that this is not a simple financial calculation.

THE MANAGEMENT OF THE DAY HOSPITAL

In most British day hospitals the manager is the consultant geriatrician although in a minority (30%) a consultant does not figure on the staff (Brocklehurst & Tucker, 1980). Nevertheless every patient attending the day hospital is in a consultant's care, and if he does not personally manage the day hospital then he will have delegated that responsibility probably to a clinical assistant or associate specialist. Day to day admission is often in the hands of the head nurse.

There should be a management policy for the day hospital and this will include a method for patient referral, review and discharge, for the organisation of the patient's day, liason with transport, communication with general practice and relatives and the management of drugs.

Perhaps the most important strand running through the whole of this is communication and communication involves meticulous documentation. Patients are referred to the day hospital by the consultant geriatrician and these in turn are either patients in his own care in hospital, those in the care of his colleagues or those in their own homes referred by general practitioners. The referral by the consultant (or his deputy) must be accompanied by a clear indication as to the reason for attendance, the number of times per week, a note of the patient's medication, social and medical problems and particular aspects of therapy or management required.

On his first attendance the patient should be seen by the person in day-to-day medical charge who will summarise his previous case notes or initiate the history and examination. Even before his attendance however, the patient's programme can be arranged if the initial referral provides sufficient information.

Programming meetings should be held weekly and involve representatives of the therapists and the nurses. Careful timetabling is essential if individual needs are to be met and at the same time patients are not to feel that they are hanging around unnecessarily waiting for something to happen.

Patient review

This is generally carried out at case conferences chaired by the consultant geriatrician. It is useful for day hospital patients to be reviewed every second or third week. The review should include information from those concerned about problems of diagnosis and therapy, progress in physiotherapy and speech therapy, the outcome of assessments including social, occupational therapy and possibly home assessment and plans made for the next period of treatment including review of frequency of attendance, the nature of the programme and consideration of discharge. It would seem logical that the patient himself should attend at some stage during this discussion to be appraised of plans and progress and to give his opinion. Curiously, this happens in only a minority of British day hospitals.

Other aspects of communication involve frequent liason with health centres – either with the general practitioner or one of the practice nurses – in relation to changes in therapy, reasons for non-attendance and the exchange of other important information. The general practitioner retains his responsibility to provide medical intervention at any time when the patient requests it outside the hours of attendance at the day hospital.

Another important aspect of communication is with relatives. Interviews with relatives have indicated that many of them have very hazy ideas about the purpose of the day hospital attendance and were anxious to know more so that they too could contribute appropriately to the patient's treatment (Brocklehurst & Tucker, 1980).

The geriatric day hospital marks an important development of the geriatric service in Great Britain with almost every district in the country now having its day hospital. In other parts of the world day hospitals are developing pari passu with the growth of geriatric medicine, but their type and role varies according to different systems of medical and social service.

REFERENCES

Brocklehurst J C 1970 The Geriatric Day Hospital. King Edward's Hospital Fund for London, London
Brocklehurst J C, Tucker J S 1980 Progress in Geriatric Day Care. King Edward's Hospital Fund for London, London
Carter J 1981 Day Services for Adults. National Institute Social Services Library No 40, London, George Allan and Unwin
Eastman M 1976 Whatever happened to casework with the elderly? Age Concern Today 18: 9
Farndale J 1961 The Day Hospital Movement in Great Britain. Pergamon Press Oxford

Irvine R E (ed) 1974 Symposium on day care. Gerontologia Clinica 16: 239
Isaacs B, Livingstone M, Neville Y 1972 Survival of the Unfittest. Routledge & Kegan Paul, London, p 25
MacFarlane J P R, Collings T, Graham K, MacIntosh J C 1979 Day hospitals – modern clinical practice. Age and Ageing 8: 80–86
Silver C P 1970 A jointly sponsored geriatric social club and day hospital. Gerontologia Clinica 12: 235–240
Weissert W G 1976 Two models of geriatric day care: findings from a comparative study. Gerontologist 16: 420

54

Prescribing habits

W. Davison

It is important for the doctor to review his prescribing habits from time to time. Prescribing is not just a straightforward scientific response to a given clinical situation. It is a complex phenomenon with important social and psychological components. The patient's utilisation of the prescription is also complex and perhaps less well understood. Certainly patients cannot be expected to swallow the doctor's pills (or his advice!) in a slavish obedient way.

PRESCRIBING FOR THE ELDERLY

The aim of drug treatment is usually the amelioration of disease to the extent that the elderly person can enjoy his normal way of life. In severely ill patients, with no hope of cure, a comfortable dignified death should be the aim. Mere prolongation of life is rarely warranted. The prescribing of drugs is but part of the total management of the case.

The principles of good prescribing are simple enough:

1. Aim at key problems
2. Use drugs only if likely to do good
3. Use frugal drug schedules
4. Monitor compliance and response.

The implementation of these principles however, is often disturbed by social pressures as well as by casual prescribing habits. Ideally, specific drugs should be used for specific purposes (e.g. vitamin B12 for pernicious anaemia), the dose and duration should be held to a practical minimum and some attempt must be made to assess both patient compliance and response. These simple rules should be followed routinely and probably most doctors would declare that this is their habit. However facts speak otherwise. Prescribing habits are often found wanting (Shaw & Opit 1976; Christopher et al, 1978; Williamson & Chopin, 1980; Tulloch, 1981; Bruce, 1982). The common errors include: prescribing a drug which is not strictly indicated, prescribing more doses each day than is required for satisfactory treatment, continuance of prescriptions long after the indication for the drug

has passed and prescribing unnecessarily hazardous preparations.

Targets for magic bullets

A popular image of modern medical practice is the use of 'magic bullets' (pills) against specific targets and thereby rapidly producing a cure (Dixon, 1978). Some of the treatments we use in geriatrics can be quite magical in their effects, for example, in the treatment of pernicious anaemia, thyrotoxicosis, myxoedema and some infections. More often however, patients do not respond to drugs in this dramatic way. The progress of the disease cannot be halted, palliation is the aim, and even relief from symptoms may be far from complete as, for example, in arthritis, Parkinson's disease, diabetes mellitus, malignant disease and mental disorder. In some major disabling diseases, drugs have a comparatively minor role to play. This is the case in stroke illness, motor neurone disease and multiple sclerosis.

Minimum drug schedules

Each drug prescribed represents a cost both to the patient and to the doctor in time and effort if not in cash. Additionally, even 'full insurance' rarely extends to all drugs especially in ambulatory care. Good medical treatment should represent good value for money whatever system of funding for Health Care is used (see chapter 52). Also each drug consumed produces work for the body's internal economy and many drugs have adverse effects. The doses prescribed must therefore be appropriate to the patient's needs with due regard to his body weight and his ability to metabolise and excrete the drug (see chapter 7). This is especially so with drugs possessing a small therapeutic ratio and it almost always means that smaller doses are required than would be suitable in younger adults. However care must be taken to ensure that the dose given is not so small as to be ineffective. Adherence by the patient to the drug schedule is aided by prescribing fewer medicines and by giving each drug only once or twice in each day rather than three or four times. Adverse drug reactions are of course much less likely when the total exposure to drugs is reduced.

Prescribing 'nothing' and the use of placebos

There are many occasions when pressure is put upon the doctor to prescribe but when he cannot see that any particular drug is indicated. An explanation to the patient of the likely course of events without drug treatment may suffice to allow a period of observation. There is no need for obscurantism. In general the more the patient knows about his illness and its management the better. It is much easier to be frugal in prescribing when the expectations of the patient and his relatives are in accord with those of the doctor. Simply 'doing nothing' or prescribing 'procrastination' (Thomson, 1979) is often the best thing to do while attempting to clarify the diagnosis, while waiting for the results of tests and while giving nature time to heal.

Placebos rather than 'nothing' are sometimes indicated and it is generally observed that some 30% of people are placebo reactors. In these patients many symptoms are relieved by a placebo, especially anxiety, headache, nausea, angina and cough. The pharmacology of the placebo (although a contradiction in terms) includes dose and time-related effects as well as side-effects (drowsiness, giddiness, alteration of bowel habit) but these are never serious. The activity of placebos is influenced by attendants (e.g. the nurse) as well as by the recipient (Kalsbeek, 1972). Placebos are inactive in the unconscious patient.

Placebos should be used sparingly. Doctors and nurses greatly underestimate the frequency and intensity of the placebo reaction and so there is a danger that a good response diverts attention from the need to make a full diagnosis. Placebos cannot be used to prove that the patient's symptoms are not genuine, yet all too often this is attempted. As one resident hospital doctor put it: 'Placebos are used with people you hate, not to make them suffer, but to prove them wrong' (Goodwin et al, 1979).

The medical consultation

As already explained, much of geriatric medicine involves multi-morbidity with chronic incurable illness and the whole picture is perhaps clouded by social malaise (see chapter 2). Major problems include loneliness, fear of being unable to cope and the sheer frustration of suffering a relentlessly increasing handicap together with an inevitable attrition of social activity. At each consultation the doctor must be clear what it is that the patient most requires as an outcome. This is difficult to achieve because the patient's expectations are rarely translated into explicit demands (Stimson, 1976). Nevertheless the attempt must be made. For example, in the patient complaining of backache and pains in the legs, is the main need for reassurance, advice concerning life style or the use of appliances, is it social work help, validation of the sick role or is it actually drug treatment? Sympathetic listening, careful examination and wise counsel can produce a powerful therapeutic effect even when in a strictly scientific sense 'nothing can be done'. However, the physician for the elderly works most effectively in close collaboration with other care practitioners because many of his patients will be greatly helped by them (e.g. the remedial therapist or social worker).

Diagnosis the key to therapeutics

Accurate medical diagnosis is the key to good therapeutics but not uncommonly this also is very difficult to achieve (see chapters 2 & 3). The temptation to prescribe should be resisted until a clear diagnosis indicates a likely target for drug treatment. Difficulties abound because of an inadequate history, the presence of multiple pathology and the altered reaction to disease frequently found in old age. Additionally there may be already polypharmacy and possibly some adverse reactions to the drugs.

Despite the difficulties it is the doctor's job to analyse the problem and give suitable treatment. Simply to prescribe a benzodiazepine for a patient who is anxious, a phenothiazine for the patient who feels giddy on standing up and a 'tonic' for the patient who feels 'run down' is a highly unsatisfactory mode of practice.

THE PRESCRIPTION

In hospital the prescription is an instruction both to the pharmacy and to the nurse attending the patient. It is an integral part of the patient's medical record and there is no transcription. The situation is rather different in family practice and in some hospital clinics where the prescription is not part of the medical record but is solely an instruction to the pharmacist who dispenses and labels the medicine. The transcribed information on the container is available to the patient and attendants (this information is often inadequate and may even be illegible to the patient) (Wandless et al, 1979). When the patient is in a residential home or private nursing home there may be a further transcription to provide a 'drug list' for the attendants. At each stage there is the possibility of introducing error.

There is commonly confusion caused by the different prescriptions of hospital and family practitioners. The patient admitted to hospital still has his own supply of drugs at home and after discharge may revert to these immediately or use them in addition to the drugs provided by the hospital. Alternatively the patient reverts to his old repeat prescription routine as soon as the hospital supply is exhausted (Deacon et al, 1978). Unfortunately this drug regimen may no longer be suited to his needs and may even have caused the recent hospital admission (Williamson & Chopin, 1980).

It cannot be stressed too strongly that the prescribing and consuming of drugs is but one aspect of a complex social interaction between the doctor, patient and society (Stimson, 1976; Smith, 1980) (Table 54.1). In prescribing, the doctor is not just 'treating' the patient before him, but potentially is affecting many of the patient's contacts as well. The writing of the prescription is powerful medical symbolism; the doctor is actually giving something to the

Table 54.1 Latent functions of the prescription (Smith, 1980: Adapted with the permission of Croom Helm Publishers).

Symbolic of	— physician's power to heal
	— sick status of patient
	— overt medical activity
	— patient achievement
	— science versus fate
Exculpatory with respect to	— doctor patient contact
	— failure of patient to cope
	— medical delay (allow natural remission)
	— lack of proper medical explanation
	— termination of consultation

patient. This in turn represents an achievement to the patient who has gained something. The medicine has powers to heal and represents modern science against fate.

The writing of the prescription gives excuses for various social processes and in particular it has a major exculpatory function. It allows patient-doctor contact. Contrariwise, 'other hands' writing of long-term repeat prescriptions may be used to avoid such contact. The patient or relative is kept at bay by the doctor's receptionist and prescription writer. This arrangement may be preferred by the patient or by the doctor. The prescription validates the sick role of the patient in society and helps to explain that the patient cannot cope. The prescription (as mentioned earlier) may be used to 'buy time' to allow a spontaneous recovery or at least a remission of symptoms and of course it is often used by the doctor to terminate the consultation.

Drug use by elderly people

In general practice it has been observed that the number of patients receiving prescriptions rises with age, as does the number of items prescribed for each patient. The increase relates particularly to continued medication (long-term repeat prescriptions) rather than to once only items (Fig. 54.1). The most commonly prescribed long-term repeats are hypnotics, tranquillizers, heart preparations and diuretics. By way of contrast antibiotics, topical preparations and expectorants are mostly prescribed on a one-off or short-term basis.

Some 70–80% of people aged 75 years and over in the UK are on regular prescribed drugs (mostly long-term repeats) and 25–30% also self medicate. Two thirds of regular drug users take 1–3 drugs while one third of them takes 4–6 drugs daily (Law & Chalmers, 1976; Skegg et al, 1977; Williamson, 1978). Over a third of females in this age group are on long-term psychotropic drugs and (perhaps not surprisingly) Williamson & Chopin (1980) found that 13% of all admissions to geriatric wards were suffering from adverse drug reactions (ADR) and in the majority the ADR had contributed to the need for admission. In a retirement community in Dunedin, Florida, USA, Stewart et al (1982) found 6.3% of elderly people to be using

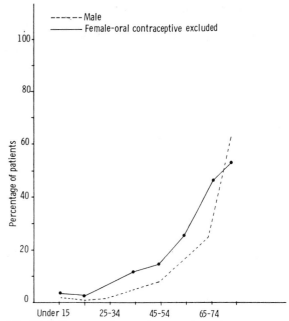

Fig. 54.1 Long-term drug use by age and sex: the percentage of patients in a general practice prescribed any item for 90 days or more (oral contraceptives excluded) (Murdoch, 1980: Adapted with the permission of the Journal of the Royal College of General Practitioners).

hypnotics and 15.6% to be using anxiolytics. Long-term use of these drugs was common and these authors suggested that no real benefit accrued and, in fact, the drugs may have been contributing to the patient's symptoms.

Because long-term treatments are usually on regular repeat prescriptions written by someone other than the doctor medical contact may be scanty. Shaw & Opit (1976) found in one group practice that 30% of those aged 70 years and over who were on long-term drug treatment had made no contact with the doctor for 6 months to 6 years prior to the survey. Much drug use appears to be completely unnecessary or at best of doubtful value. Tulloch (1981) found that almost one third of drugs taken long-term by elderly patients living at home came into this category especially tranquillizers, hypnotics, antidepressants, digoxin, diuretics, antacids and hypotensive agents.

The picture in residential care homes is similar. Bruce (1982) reported over-use especially of drugs acting on the central nervous system and cardiovascular system. By stopping all drugs of doubtful value he was able to reduce the drug expenditure in one home by 50% but at the same time he reduced the profit to his practice. A study of drug use in residential care homes in Scotland showed that 34% of residents were receiving hypnotics and nitrazepam was most often used. Yet with chronic use this drug is known to impair psychomotor performance in elderly people (Murphy et al, 1982). In over a quarter of cases the dose was 10 mg each night. Additionally in 26% of cases phenothiazines and other psychotropic drugs were prescribed irrespective of the psychiatric status (Morgan et al, 1982). Unnecessarily heavy long-term use of hypnotics, sedatives and tranquillizers is reported to occur in the North American Nursing Homes caring for elderly people (US Dept HEW PHS, 1976).

From what has been said it will be clear that a major problem in the care of the elderly is the unnecessarily high incidence of continued (long-term) drug use, especially with psychotropic drugs and drugs for the cardiovascular system. It is also clear that very many patients can benefit from a reduction in the drug burden. Practitioners who have audited their own prescribing usually find that they over-prescribe and are able to become more frugal to their patients' benefit (Tulloch, 1981; Bruce, 1982). In one family practice 36% of elderly patients on long-term treatment were thought to be suffering from unwanted effects of prescribed drugs at the time of the audit (Martys, 1982).

There is evidence to suggest that doctors much more than patients favour drug use as the outcome of a medical consultation. Many patients expecting advice and reassurance are given a prescription instead (Stimson, 1976). Because of the routine nature of the repeats and because of the large numbers involved an increasing proportion of the work is transferred from the doctor to other hands, i.e. non-medically qualified writers. It has been observed that these scripts contain twice the number of errors seen in scripts written by the doctor (Dajda, 1980).

The resolution of these problems depends upon a growing awareness of them and a determination to improve practice organisation. Proper drug use policies are necessary with the meticulous use of clear medical records including a repeat prescription and drug record card (Tomson, 1981; Stuart, 1981; Drury & Sabbagh, 1982). This drug record should be consulted and written up before any prescription is made out. Policies would still allow long-term repeats with infrequent medical review when appropriate (e.g. in many cases with diabetes mellitus, rheumatoid arthritis and hypothyroidism) but would require more frequent medical review in, for example, cases of chronic heart failure or mental depression. Inadequate review of drug use appears to relate more to lack of good practice organisation than to lack of time.

Compliance

Lack of compliance with the prescribed regimen is very common. An American study found lack of adherence or compliance to occur in 40–50% of elderly patients living at home and in most cases it represented under-use of the drug or drugs and it was intentional (Cooper et al, 1982). The non-adherent patients did not believe the drugs to be necessary in the doses prescribed. Patients in this group were more likely to use multiple physicians and multiple pharmacies. A British study found that elderly patients were deviating by more than 10% from the prescription for more the half of all medicines (Wandless et al, 1979) and women complied less well than men. It is impossible for the doctor to guess correctly which patients comply and which do not (Stimson, 1976). Some deliberate assessment is required. This is not always easy (Pearson, 1982) although Wandless et al (1979) found that the use of an interview assessment and an inspection of the prescription records brought to light many cases. Certainly, tablets still in the bottle have not been taken by the patient.

Indirect methods of assessing compliance are most readily available and involve tactful questioning of the patient, pill counts and estimation of fluid preparations remaining in the bottle after a set interval. Direct methods are occasionally needed and include biochemical tests for the drug, its metabolites or a marker, in tissues, body fluids or excreta.

Drugs should be supplied to the patient in suitable containers. The modern child-resistant containers, which have been instrumental in reducing the incidence of accidental overdose of analgesics in children, are increasingly used for all types of pharmaceuticals. Unfortunately many old people find them very difficult to use and even blister packs can be a problem. The old type screw-top bottle suits most elderly people and the addition of flanges or 'wings' to the top makes opening and closing even easier.

Improving compliance

The doctor bears the major responsibility. He must be aware of the likelihood of non-compliance and take preventive action. The advice given to the patient should be brief but specific. He needs to understand what is wrong, what the doctor hopes to achieve and how he expects to do it. The advice should be quite explicit and reinforced by repetition. Clear written instructions are helpful. Regular contact and good rapport with the doctor improves compliance (Sackett & Haynes, 1976; German et al, 1982). Counselling on drug use just prior to discharge from hospital is helpful even in those who have mental impairment and perforce must go home to live alone (MacDonald et al, 1977).

When lack of adherence to the drugs prescribed is detected the need for the drug(s) should be questioned and the drug schedule simplified. The patient's understanding of the illness and treatment should be reassessed and appropriate explanation given. The use of memory aids, written instructions and careful supervision may be required.

It is considered that careful self-audit of prescribing habits using currently available information would provide more effective treatment for elderly patients, a reduced risk of ADR and a reduced demand for hospital care.

REFERENCES

Bruce S A 1982 Regular prescribing in a residential home for elderly women. British Medical Journal 284: 1235–1237

Christopher L J, Ballinger B R, Shepherd A M M, Ramsay A, Crooks G 1978 Drug prescribing patterns in the elderly: a cross-sectional study of in-patients. Age and Ageing 7: 74–82

Cooper J K, Love D W, Raffoul P R 1982 Intentional prescription non-adherence (Non-compliance) by the elderly. Journal of the American Geriatrics Society 30: 329–333

Dajda R 1980 Who prescribes? The illusion of power sharing in the surgery. In: Mapes R (ed) Prescribing Practice and Drug Usage. Croom Helm, London p 147–156

Deacon S P, Hammond L, Thompson B 1978 Drug supply requirement for patients discharged from hospital. British Medical Journal 1: 555

Dixon B 1978 Beyond the Magic Bullet. Allen & Unwin, London

Drury M, Sabbagh K 1982 Four traps for the prescribing doctor. British Medical Journal 284: 634–636

German P S, Klein L E, McPhee S J, Smith C R 1982 Knowledge of and compliance with drug regimens in the elderly. Journal of the American Geriatrics Society 30: 568–571

Goodwin J S, Goodwin J M, Vogel R V 1979 Knowledge and use of placebos by house officers and nurses. Annals of Internal Medicine 91: 106–110

Kalsbeek F 1972 The therapeutic use of placebos. In: Meyler L, Peck H M (ed) Drug-Induced Diseases Vol 4 Excerpta Medica, Amsterdam

Law R, Chalmers C 1976 Medicines and elderly people: a general practice survey. British Medical Journal 1: 565–568

MacDonald E T, Macdonald J B, Phoenix M 1977 Improving drug compliance after hospital discharge. British Medical Journal 2: 618–621

Martys C R 1982 Drug treatment in elderly patients: G P audit. British Medical Journal 285: 1623–1625

Morgan K, Gilleard C J, Reive A 1982 Hypnotic usage in residential homes for the elderly: a prevalence and longitudinal analysis. Age and Ageing 11: 229–234

Murdoch J C 1980 The epidemiology of prescribing in an urban general practice. Journal of the Royal College of General Practitioners 30: 393–602

Murphy P, Hindmarch I, Hyland C M 1982 Aspects of short-term use of two benzodiazepine hypnotics in the elderly. Age and Ageing 11: 222–228

Pearson R 1982 Who is taking their tablets? British Medical Journal 285: 757–758

Sackett D L, Haynes R B 1976 Compliance with therapeutic regimens. John Hopkins University Press, Baltimore

Shaw S M, Opit L J 1976 Need for supervision in the elderly receiving long-term prescribed medication. British Medical Journal 1: 505–507

Skegg D C G, Doll R, Perry J 1977 Use of medicines in general practice. British Medical Journal 1: 1561–1563

Smith M C 1980 The relationship between pharmacy and medicine. In: Mapes R E (ed) Prescribing Practice and Drug Usage. Croom Helm, London ch 10, p 157–200

Stewart R B, May F E, Hale W E, Marks R G 1982 Psychotropic drug use in an ambulatory elderly population. Gerontology 28: 328–335

Stimson G V 1976 Doctor-patient interaction and some problems for prescribing. Journal of the Royal College of General Practitioners 26: 88–96

Stuart D 1981 Practical problems of improving records. British Medical Journal 282: 783–784

Thomson G H 1979 Prescribing procrastination. Journal of the Royal College of General Practitioners 29: 550–552

Tomson P 1981 Medical records: Middle sized group practice. British Medical Journal 282: 1438–1441

Tulloch A J 1981 Repeat prescribing for elderly patients. British Medical Journal 282: 1672–1675

US Dept HEW PHS 1976 Physicians' drug prescribing patterns in skilled nursing facilities: long-term care facility improvements campaign. Monograph No. 2, Washington

Wandless I, Mucklow J C, Smith A, Prudham D 1979 Compliance with prescribed medicines: a study of elderly patients in the community. Journal of the Royal College of General Practitioners 29: 391–396

Williamson J 1978 Prescribing problems in the elderly. Practitioner 200: 749–55

Williamson J, Chopin J M 1980 Adverse reactions to prescribed drugs in the elderly: a multicentre investigation. Age and Ageing 9: 73–80

Index